MEDICAL MICROBIOLOGY

MEDICAL MICROBIOLOGY
THE PRACTICE OF MEDICAL MICROBIOLOGY

TWELFTH EDITION
VOLUME II

ROBERT CRUICKSHANK

C.B.E., M.D., F.R.C.P., F.R.C.P.E., D.P.H., F.R.S.E., Hon.LL.D.(Aberd.)
Professor Emeritus of Bacteriology, University of Edinburgh

J. P. DUGUID

M.D., B.Sc., F.R.C.Path.
Professor of Bacteriology, University of Dundee
Consultant in Bacteriology, Tayside Health Board
Consultant Advisor in Microbiology, Scottish Home and
Health Department

B. P. MARMION

M.D., D.Sc., F.R.C.Path., F.R.C.P.E., F.R.S.E.
Professor of Bacteriology, University of Edinburgh
Chief Bacteriologist, Royal Infirmary, Edinburgh

R. H. A. SWAIN

M.A., M.D., F.R.C.P.E., F.R.C.Path., F.R.S.E.
Reader in Virology, University of Edinburgh
Consultant in Virology, Royal Infirmary, Edinburgh

CHURCHILL LIVINGSTONE
EDINBURGH LONDON AND NEW YORK 1975

CHURCHILL LIVINGSTONE

Medical Division of Longman Group Limited

Distributed in the United States of America by Longman Inc., New York,
and by associated companies, branches and representatives throughout
the world.

© Longman Group Limited 1975

First Edition	1925
Second Edition	1928
Third Edition	1931
Fourth Edition	1934
Fifth Edition	1938
Sixth Edition	1942
Seventh Edition	1945
Reprinted	1946
Eighth Edition	1948
Reprinted	1949
Reprinted	1950
Ninth Edition	1953
Reprinted	1956
Reprinted	1959
Tenth Edition	1960
Reprinted	1962
Eleventh Edition	1965
Revised Reprint	1968
Reprinted	1969
Reprinted	1970
Reprinted	1972
E.L.B.S. Edition first published	1965
Reprinted	1968, 1969, 1970
Twelfth Edition, Vol. 1	1973
Reprinted	1975
E.L.B.S. Edition of Twelfth Edition, Vol. 1	1974
Reprinted	1975
Twelfth Edition, Vol. 11	1975
E.L.B.S. Edition of Twelfth Edition Vol. 11	1975

ISBN 0 443 01111 7 (limp)
       0 443 01203 2 (cased)

Printed in Great Britain

PREFACE

This, the second volume of the 12th Edition of
Cruickshank's Medical Microbiology, is meant for
the professional and technological staffs of
medical, scientific, and veterinary laboratories. It is a
'bench book' containing well tried methods from
previous editions together with many of the most
modern methods of microbiology. Each chapter has
been revised, many have been re-written, and new
chapters on virological techniques have been
added.
Volume II is divided into two parts: Part 1 is
devoted to technical methods, Part 2 to the
identification of microorganisms and the laboratory
diagnosis of specific infections.
Laboratory workers will find that Volume II leans
heavily on the contents of Volume I. Great care
has been taken to avoid unnecessary repetition.
The two volumes are complementary and should
be used together.
Many valuable suggestions and criticisms have
been received by the editors. To their own
colleagues in each of their departments they owe a
great debt of gratitude, and there are also many
microbiologist friends throughout the world to
whom they would express their most sincere
thanks. We are especially indebted to Dr Valerie
Inglis for her care and skill in preparing the index.
Lastly, our particular gratitude goes to our
publishers, who have given so much practical help
both to the authors and the editors.
It is with great regret that we have to inform our
readers of the death of the senior editor, Robert
Cruickshank on 16 August 1974.

April, 1975   The Editors

LIST OF CONTRIBUTORS

and the topics and pathogens in Volume II for which they have
had the sole or shared responsibility

JOYCE D. COGHLAN, B.Sc., Ph.D.[8]

Bacteriology of water etc.; brucella; pasteurella group;
leptospira.

J. G. COLLEE, M.D., M.R.C.Path.[1]

Bacterial cultivation and identification; culture media;
biological standardization; sterilization and disinfection;
clostridia; bacteroides; streptobacillus; donovania.

R. CRUICKSHANK, C.B.E., M.D., F.R.C.P., F.R.C.P.E.,

D.P.H., F.R.S.E., Hon.Ll.D.[1]

Laboratory in diagnosis and control of infection;
streptococcus; pneumococcus; neisseria; bordetella;
haemophilus; corynebacterium; erysipelothrix; listeria;
mycobacterium; vibrio; spirillum.

J. P. DUGUID, M.D., B.Sc., F.R.C.Path.[2]

Safety in Microbiology laboratory; enterobacteria; staining;
sterilization; staphylococcus.

R. R. GILLIES, M.D., F.R.C.P.E., M.R.C.Path., D.P.H.[1]

Actinomyces; nocardia; loefflerella; pseudomonas.

J. C. GOULD, M.D., B.Sc., F.R.C.P.E., F.R.C.Path., F.R.S.E.[9]

Tests for sensitivity to antimicrobial agents.

D. M. GREEN, M.D., F.R.C.Path.[2]

Immunological methods; anthrax.

NANCY J. HAYWARD, B.Sc., Ph.D.[3]

Cultivation of bacteria etc.; culture media; identification
of bacteria.

[1]Department of Bacteriology, University of Edinburgh.
[2]Department of Bacteriology, University of Dundee.
[3]Department of Microbiology, Monash University, Prahran,
Victoria, Australia.
[4]Department of Medical Protozoology, London School of Hygiene
and Tropical Medicine.

W. H. R. LUMSDEN, M.B., D.Sc., F.R.C.P.E., F.R.S.E.[4]

Protozoa.

B. P. MARMION, M.D., D.Sc., F.R.C.Path., F.R.C.P.E., F.R.S.E.[1]

Rickettsiae; mycoplasmas.

W. MARR, F.I.M.L.T.[1]

Culture media; cultivation of bacteria; mycoplasmas; staining.

P. G. SARGEAUNT, A.I.M.L.T., A.I.S.T.[4]

Protozoa.

A. C. SCOTT, M.D., M.R.C.Path.[2]

Sterilization; sensitivity to antimicrobial agents; pseudomonas; loefflerella.

J. D. SLEIGH, M.D., M.R.C.Path.[5]

Salmonella; shigella; escherichia; other enterobacteria.

ISOBEL W. SMITH, B.Sc., Ph.D.[1]

Chlamydia; cell culture; virus isolation; virus serology.

R. H. A. SWAIN, M.A., M.D., F.R.C.P.E., F.R.C.Path., F.R.S.E.[1]

Microscopy; experimental animals; treponema; syphilis serology; borrelia; DNA and RNA viruses.

A. T. WALLACE, M.D., F.R.C.Path., M.R.C.P.E., D.P.H.[6]

Atypical mycobacteria; myco. leprae.

D. M. WEIR, M.D.[1]

Immunological and serological methods in microbial infections.

J. F. WILKINSON, M.A., Ph.D.[7]

Physical and chemical methods.

A. M. M. WILSON, B.M., B.Ch., F.R.C.Path., Dip. Bact.[1]

Pathogenic fungi.

[5] Department of Bacteriology, University of Glasgow.
[6] Bacteriology Laboratory, City Hospital, Edinburgh.
[7] Department of Microbiology, School of Agriculture, University of Edinburgh.
[8] Leptospirosis Reference Laboratory, PHLS, Colindale, London
[9] Central Microbiological Laboratories, Western General Hospital, Edinburgh.

CONTENTS

PART 1 TECHNICAL METHODS

PART 2 IDENTIFICATION OF SPECIFIC MICROBES. LABORATORY DIAGNOSIS OF SPECIFIC INFECTIONS

Volume II: Part 1
Technical Methods

1. Microscopy

The study of the morphology of very small organisms is of such importance that the microbiologist must of necessity be a competent microscopist. It is of paramount importance for him to obtain the best possible performance from his instrument and for this a sound knowledge of the basic optical principles involved and an understanding of the construction of the microscope are essential.

Microscopes designed by different manufacturers differ enormously in their outward appearance, but essentially most consist of three parts—the stand, the body and the train of optical lenses. A typical monocular microscope suitable for microbiology is seen in Fig. 1.1.

The stand comprises a heavy foot, often horse-shoe shaped (1), to give stability and the limb (5) which bears the optical system. The limb is attached to the foot by a hinged joint so that the microscope can be set at a comfortable angle for the observer. The optical system is mounted in the tube which is usually in two parts, (a) an external tube (9) which bears at its lower end a revolving nose-piece (15) in which interchangeable objective lenses of various magnifications are fitted (16 and 17), and (b) an inner draw-tube (13) which carries the eye-piece (12) at its upper end. This whole assembly is held in position by the body (8) which houses two mechanisms, the coarse (7) and fine adjustments (6) whereby the height of the tube can be adjusted in such a way that the objective can be positioned at its optimal working distance (its focal length) from the object (19) to be examined. These focusing mechanisms are operated by milled heads situated on the two sides of the body. The milled head of the fine adjustment is usually graduated in $\frac{1}{50}$ths and one division corresponds to a movement of 0·002 mm of the tube. The stage (18) is a platform which accommodates a glass microscope slide on which the object to be examined (19) is mounted; it is attached to the limb immediately below the level of the objective lens and has an aperture in its centre to permit light to reach the object. The stage may be of the fixed type fitted with two spring clips or of the mechanical type that can be moved in two planes by rack and pinion mechanisms (3). A mechanical stage is of great advantage because it controls small movements of the object accurately and it is really necessary when a large area of the microscopic preparation has to be searched, as in the examination of films of sputum for tubercle bacilli or of blood for malaria parasites. It is possible to obtain attachable mechanical stages for almost all microscopes but the type that is built into the instrument is much more stable and greatly to be preferred.

In some modern microscopes the objective is held in a fixed position and the distance between it and the object is adjusted by the *downward movement of the stage* which is controlled by coarse and fine adjustment screws similar to those used in other models to move the tube. For those accustomed to the standard microscope great care is at first required to avoid the risk of damage to both object and objective.

Beneath the stage is the substage (24) which carries a condenser (20) whose lenses focus light from the illuminating source on the plane of the object. The height of the condenser, and therefore the focus of the light, can be varied at will by a rack and pinion mechanism (2). The horizontal position of the condenser can be adjusted in two planes by centring screws (21). Immediately below the condenser and incorporated in the same mount is the substage iris diaphragm operated by a small lever which protrudes to one side (22). Opening or closing this iris diaphragm controls the amount of light reaching the object. Just below the iris diaphragm is a ring-shaped filter holder (23) designed to carry circular coloured glass filters (e.g. a blue 'daylight' filter) required to reduce excessive red or yellow components in some types of light sources. It is swung in and out of position by a lever which may be situated tiresomely close to that of the iris diaphragm.

3

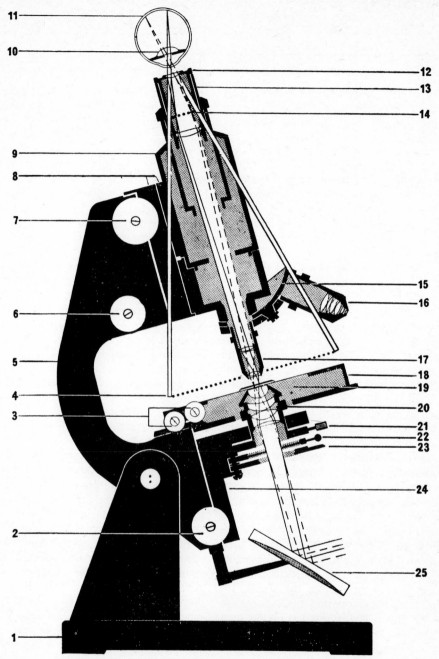

FIG. 1.1

A diagram illustrating the component parts of a monocular microscope and the paths of the optical rays. (1) Foot; (2) Adjusting screw for height of condenser; (3) Controls for mechanical stage; (4) Enlarged virtual image; (5) Limb; (6) Fine adjustment; (7) Coarse adjustment; (8) Body; (9) External tube; (10) Lens of observer's eye; (11) Retina; (12) Eye-piece; (13) Inner draw-tube; (14) Primary image, real and enlarged by objective; (15) Revolving nose-piece; (16) High-power objective; (17) Low-power objective; (18) Stage; (19) Object; (20) Condenser; (21) Centring screw for condenser; (22) Iris diaphragm; (23) Ring filter holder; (24) Substage; (25) Mirror.

The worker must familiarize himself with the relative positions of these two levers. Fitted to the tail piece below the condenser is a hinged mirror (25) that is flat on one side and concave on the other. Many modern microscopes, however, dispense with the mirror and, instead, the whole illuminating source, consisting of a small electric bulb (e.g. 6 volts, 5 amps), is built into the foot of the instrument.

Binocular Microscopes. Where much microscopic work has to be done and for routine examinations we recommend that the microscope should have a binocular body, as, by using both eyes, a considerable amount of eye strain and fatigue is avoided. In the binocular body the rays of light from the objective are divided by a half-silvered surface inclined at an angle of 45 degrees which permits one half of the light to pass vertically, while the remainder is reflected horizontally. Each half of the rays is directed into its appropriate eye-piece by means of prisms (see Fig. 1.2). The eye-piece sockets can be adjusted to the interpupillary distance of the observer, while one of the ocular tubes is adjustable to correct individual differences between the two eyes.

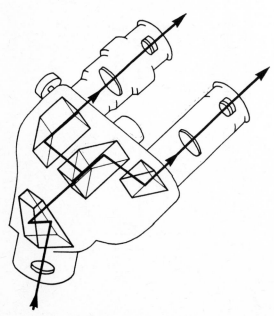

FIG. 1.2
A diagram to illustrate the optical path in the binocular head of a microscope.

Inclined binocular microscopes are very suitable for routine use, as the eye-pieces are inclined towards the observer and it is not necessary to tilt the stand as with the straight binocular or monocular bodies. Consequently the stage is kept horizontal and this is of particular advantage when dealing with wet films or using dark-ground illumination. (Similarly an inclined eye-piece fitting for a monocular tube may be obtained.)

It should be noted that the inclined binocular body may increase the actual magnification by $1\frac{1}{2}$ times. This factor shown as $1\cdot5\times$ is engraved on the body. Lower-power eye-pieces only should be used; $6\times$ is the most convenient, and $8\times$ is the highest practicable for routine use.

Binocular microscopes have interchangeable monocular and binocular bodies, which are removable without disturbing the objectives, so that a monocular body can readily be used for photography, micrometry, etc.

MAGNIFICATION

The purpose of the microscope is to produce an enlarged image of objects too small to be observed with the naked eye; the degree of enlargement is the *magnification* of the instrument. It is perfectly possible to design an optical system which will give enormous magnifications, e.g. hundreds of thousands of times, but after a certain point detail and sharpness begin to be lost. A common example of this is seen when a magnifying glass is used to examine a newspaper photograph; the effect is not to reveal more detail, instead the picture is broken down to a series of black and white dots. Magnification of this type which does not increase the detail observed is known as '*empty magnification*' and is of no value to the microbiologist. As will be seen later there is a fundamental limit to the amount of detail or '*useful magnification*' of any optical system and this is imposed by the wavelength of the light rays used.

The Formation of the Image. It is the lenses composing the objective which initiate the magnifying processes. An objective operates at a distance from the object that is roughly equivalent to its focal length, and admits rays that are transmitted to form a real, inverted, enlarged image (the primary image) in the upper part of the tube. At this point there is interposed another lens—the field lens—whose function is to collect the diverging rays of the primary image (Fig. 1.1 (14)) so that they pass through the eye lens of the eye-piece which magnifies the image still further. The field lens is accommodated in the lower plane of the eye-piece. Rays as they leave the eye-piece to reach the lens of the observer's eye (10) are once more divergent and thus the image seen by the retina (11) is virtual, appearing to be some 10 in. in front of the eyes (see Fig. 1.1 (4)).

The magnification of a microscope is the product of the separate magnifications of the

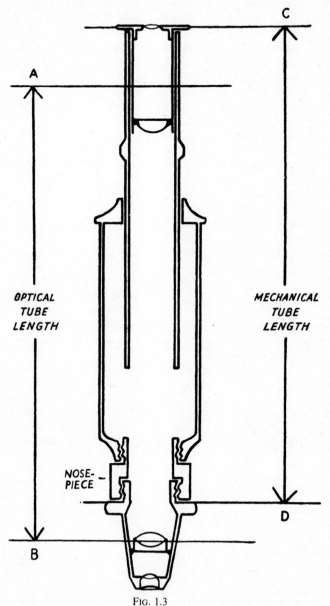

FIG. 1.3

A diagram to illustrate the optical tube of a monocular microscope.

objective and the eye-piece and depends on the following factors:

1. The optical tube length.
2. The focal length of the objective.
3. The magnifying power of the eye-piece.

1. *The optical tube length* is the distance between the posterior principal plane of the lens system of the objective and the plane of the image in the upper part of the draw-tube. This distance is difficult to determine but, for practical purposes, may be taken as equal to the *mechanical tube length* which is the distance between the point where the objective fits into the lower end of the body or the nose-piece and the eye lens of the eye-piece, a measurement easily made with a ruler (see Fig. 1.3). Most modern microscopes have a mechanical tube length of 160 mm, but a few manufacturers employ 170 mm. Objectives are designed to work at a definite tube length and any variation from this distance may seriously impair the quality of the image. This must be borne in mind when buying new objectives, particularly when high-power apochromatic or achromatic lenses are needed.

Many microscopes have an extensile draw-tube that can be used to vary the optical tube length but its use is only required in correcting for coverslip thickness or possibly in calibrating an eye-piece micrometer. The tube length should *not* be used to obtain greater magnification because a serious distortion of the final image results.

2. *The magnification of an objective* is obtained as follows:

Magnification of objective
$$= \frac{\text{size of image}}{\text{size of object}}$$
$$= \frac{\text{distance of image from objective}}{\text{distance of object from objective}}$$
$$= \frac{\text{mechanical tube length}}{\text{focal length of objective}}$$

Examples

(a) 16 mm ($\frac{2}{3}$ in) objective $= \frac{160}{16} = 10$.
(b) 4 mm ($\frac{1}{6}$ in) objective $= \frac{160}{4} = 40$.
(c) 2 mm ($\frac{1}{12}$ in) objective $= \frac{160}{2} = 80$.

The 2 mm objective has, in reality, a shorter focal length than that by which it is designated, and gives a magnification of 95–100 diameters according to the make. Makers now engrave the initial magnification on the objective mount and refer to the objective by its magnification as well as by the numerical aperture thus, the 16 mm ($\frac{2}{3}$ in) objective is designated 10/0·28, the 4 mm ($\frac{1}{6}$ in) is 40/0·65, and the 2 mm ($\frac{1}{12}$ in) is 95–100/1·28 (or 1·3).

3. The *magnification of the eye-piece* is clearly engraved on the mount by the makers.

4. The *total magnification of the microscope* is:

$$\frac{\text{tube length}}{\text{focal length of objective}} \times \text{eye-piece magnification}$$

or

$$\text{objective magnification} \times \text{eye-piece magnification}.$$

NUMERICAL APERTURE

Objectives are rated not only by their focal length but also by their angles of aperture which determine their light gathering powers. A method of expressing the fraction of a wave front admitted to a lens is the use of the measurement of the *Numerical Aperture* (NA). The numerical aperture may be defined simply as the ratio of the diameter of the lens to its focal length.* It is expressed mathematically as follows:

$$NA = n \operatorname{Sin} U$$

where n is the refractive index of the medium between object and objective (air, 1·0; cedarwood immersion oil, approximately 1·5), and 2U the *angle of aperture*, i.e. the angle formed by the two extreme rays of light, which, starting from the centre point of the object, reach the eye of the observer (see Fig. 1.4).

That is,

$$DAC = 2U$$
$$BAC = U$$
$$\operatorname{Sin} U = \frac{EF}{EA}.$$

---

* The numerical aperture has been expressed in this manner to simplify description, but this is true only for objectives of long focal length, where EA is approximately equal to FA (see Fig. 1.4). With short-focus lenses of high numerical aperture this definition is not correct. The length EA is then much greater than the distance of the objective from the slide (FA).

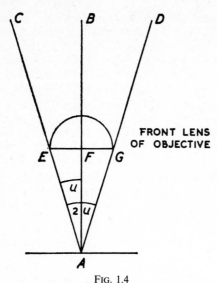

FRONT LENS
OF OBJECTIVE

FIG. 1.4
Diagram to illustrate numerical aperture.

It is thus seen that the numerical aperture, other things being equal, depends on EF, which is half the diameter of the lens. Objectives, therefore, may have equal focal lengths, but different numerical apertures depending on the diameter of the front lens.

The theoretical limit of the angle DAC is 180°, i.e. when the objective is actually on the object—and therefore the theoretical limit of U is 90°. The greatest possible NA of a dry lens cannot exceed 1, since the refractive index of air $(n) = 1$, and Sin 90° = 1. Actually the highest practical NA of a dry lens is 0·95. On the other hand, the introduction of cedar-oil between the objective and object gives n a value of 1·5. The highest theoretical value, therefore, of n Sin U for an oil-immersion objective is 1·5 × Sin 90°—i.e. 1·5. In practice, however, the highest NA of an oil-immersion objective (attained in an apochromat) is 1·4. The ordinary $\frac{1}{12}$-in objective for bacteriological purpose has a NA of 1·28 or 1·3.

RESOLUTION

The limit of useful magnification is set by the resolving power of the microscope, i.e. its ability to reveal closely adjacent structural details as separate and distinct; expressed quantitatively it is its *capacity* to distinguish two neighbouring points as separate entities.

It is this power which determines the amount of structural detail that can be observed microscopically. The minimum resolvable distance between two luminous points (r) is given by the formula

$$r = \frac{0·61 \times \lambda}{\text{NA}}$$

where λ is the wavelength of the light used. In practice, with axial illumination, two points any closer together than about half the wavelength of the light cannot be resolved. Thus, if green light of wavelength $0·55 \times 10^{-4}$ cm and an objective of NA 1·4 are used

$$r = \frac{0·61 \times 0·55 \times 10^{-4} \text{ cm}}{1·4}$$
$$= 0·24 \times 10^{-4} \text{ cm}$$
$$= 240 \text{ nm}$$

Under working conditions the limit of resolution is reached at about 0·00025 mm (250 nm). Thus, using ordinary microscopic methods with an apochromatic objective of NA 1·4, and a high-power compensating eye-piece used at the optimal tube length, the whole optical system and illuminant being carefully centred, stained particles of 250 nm can be seen. It should be realized that when the bodies observed have been coated with a mordant, as in Paschen stain for the vaccinia virus, the stained virus particles may have been rendered larger than the natural ones and are thereby brought within the limits of resolution.

If ultraviolet light is used as the illuminating source greater resolution may be obtained because the wavelength is shorter (about half that of visible light) and thus an effective NA of approximately 2·5 can be obtained. The method, however, requires an optical system composed of quartz lenses because ordinary glass offers too much resistance to the path of the rays; this, with the necessity for photographic recording, makes the apparatus expensive and complicated to use.

In the electron microscope the illumination is provided by a beam of electrons that has an equivalent wavelength as small as 1/100,000th that of ordinary light. The efficiency of the lens systems of the electron microscope, however, does not match that of optical lenses and the resolution of this instrument is therefore only about 250 times better than that of the best light microscope.

DEFINITION

Definition, not to be confused with resolution, is the capacity of an objective to render the outline of the image of the object clear and distinct. It depends on the elimination of optical aberrations inherent in the glass of the lenses.

Spherical aberration is due to the fact that rays passing, for example, through the edge of a lens will seldom be brought to precisely the same focus as those passing nearer the centre (see Fig. 1.5); the result may be serious distortion of the image.

Chromatic aberration occurs because white light as it traverses a lens is diffracted as it would be in a prism to its various component colours, each with its own wavelength (see Fig. 1.6). The rays of different wavelengths are refracted by the lens to varying extents and may not always be recombined in the same focus. Blue rays, for example, are refracted more and come

to a focus nearer to the lens than red rays; the result may be a hazy image fringed with the colours of the spectrum (see Fig. 1.6).

Aberrations are *corrected* by the makers of better quality lenses by combining lenses of different dispersive qualities. Crown glass has a low dispersive power and is used for convex lenses, while flint glass, which has a high dispersive power, is used for concave lenses. In this manner the colours of the spectrum are recombined to form white light and lenses of this type are known as *achromatic lenses*. The best performance from lenses of this type is obtained when monochromatic green light is used.

THE LENSES OF THE MICROSCOPE OBJECTIVES

Microscope objectives are constructed from an intricate assembly of lenses; even the lower powers contain up to four lenses and higher powers eight or more. Essentially the qualities of any objective depend on (1) brightness of image, which, other things being equal, varies

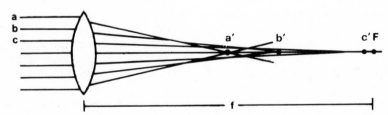

FIG. 1.5

Diagram to illustrate spherical aberration. Light entering a convex lens is brought to a focus at point F, the focal length of the lens being f. Rays a, b and c are refracted to different degrees to reach focus point a′, b′ and c′, which are situated at points apart from each other. The result in an uncorrected lens system would be multiple superimposed images and great blurring.

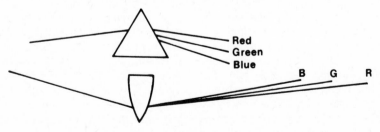

FIG. 1.6

A diagram to illustrate chromatic aberration.

as the *square* of the NA; and (2) the resolution and definition which vary directly as the NA. The depth of focus, while not entirely dependent on the NA, varies in inverse proportion to it. In general, it may be said that in the case of two objectives of equal focal length, the one with the higher NA is to be preferred as the better lens.

In microbiology three objectives are generally adequate for most purposes; a 16 mm or $\frac{2}{3}$ in objective with an NA of at least 0·28, a 4 mm or $\frac{1}{6}$ in with a minimum NA of 0·65, and a 2 mm or $\frac{1}{12}$ in immersion with an NA of 1·28 or greater. Modern achromatic objectives are excellent and are perfectly satisfactory for all routine and much research work. Apochromatic objectives are very expensive and need only be purchased for special purposes, e.g. photomicrography.

Oil-immersion objectives are the types most frequently used in microbiology because their greater magnification and resolution are required in the study of the morphology of objects as small as bacteria. It has been seen that the NA of an objective depends on the angle of the cone of rays that it can admit from the object and that any factor which reduces the rays accepted impairs the quality of the image. In the case of the 2 mm ($\frac{1}{12}$ in) objective such a factor is the air between the front lens of the objective and the coverslip. The 2 mm objective works very close to the object and rays passing from a dense medium (glass of the coverslip) to a less dense medium (air) are refracted obliquely outwards so that many may miss the front lens of the objective altogether. As the brightness of the image depends upon the amount of light entering the objective, and the resolution depends on the effective aperture, this refraction of light diminishes not only the brightness but the clarity of the image. If, however, the space between objective and the object is filled with some transparent fluid with the same refractive index as glass, then the rays of light do not undergo refraction and pass directly into the objective (see Fig. 1.7). The most usual fluid to introduce between the object and the objective is oil of cedar which has a refractive index of 1·515—a figure which is identical with the refractive index of hard crown glass. The refractive indices of other

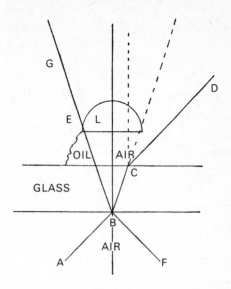

Fig. 1.7
Diagram showing the paths of rays through (1) a dry lens (on right), and (2) an oil immersion lens (on left). Note the refraction of the oblique ray ABCD in passing from the glass slide to air, as compared with the ray FBEG. L is the front lens of the objective.

substances used as immersion or mounting fluids in high magnification microscopy are: dried Canada balsam 1·535, xylol-balsam 1·524, euparal 1·483, glycerol 1·460, water 1·334, and air 1·000. Each of these immersion fluids has its own place in microscopy according to the type of lens being used. The newer designs of objectives are so constructed that the optical train is accommodated in a spring-loaded mount which effectively eliminates the risk to the unwary worker of racking down the objective and damaging the coverslip and slide.

Some objectives are fitted with an adjustable collar that may be turned to move the two back combinations of lenses in order to correct any spherical aberration introduced by the thickness of the coverslip.

Apochromatic objectives represent the highest degree of optical perfection and in consequence are very costly; it is only in critical research work that it is possible to justify the expense of these lenses. In the apochromatic objective, light of at least three different wavelengths (colours) may be united, the aberrations are less, and the NA is usually higher, e.g. a good oil-immersion apochromat may have an NA of approximately 1·4. Apochromats owe this property of almost complete colour correction to the use of the mineral fluorite which endows the objectives with a brilliance and crispness of image not attainable with ordinary lenses, and enables the maximum resolving power to be obtained. Fluorite is so valuable optically because it possesses a high degree of transparency; a low refractive index; and extremely small dispersion. A series of objectives containing a certain amount of fluorite, which are intermediate between apochromatic and achromatic objectives are known as 'semi-apochromatic' or 'fluorite' lenses; some of them have a performance which approximates to that of apochromatic objectives.

Apochromatic objectives must always be used with 'compensating' eye-pieces and a properly centred condenser.

EYE-PIECES

The functions of the eye-piece are (1) the magnification of the real image, (2) the formation of a virtual image of the real image produced by the objective, and (3) to carry measuring scales, markers, cross-hairs, etc. There are many different types of eye-pieces but the most generally useful are simple and comprise two plano-convex lenses with a circular field diaphragm interposed between them according to the system devised originally by Huygens.

Huygenian eye-pieces are constructed with the plane surface of the two lenses facing upwards and the diaphragm is situated between them at the focus of the upper (eye) lens. The lower or field lens collects the rays from as wide a field of view of the image as possible and focuses them at or near the plane of the diaphragm. The upper lens then magnifies this image. The diaphragm limits the field of view to the central and flattest part of the image and reduces glare (Fig. 1.8A). Huygenian eye-pieces are sometimes described as 'negative oculars' because the focus occurs within the eye-piece. In microbiology a 10× Huygenian eye-piece with a monocular tube is most generally useful but a 5× ocular is also useful for locating the object without altering the objective. It is not practical to use this type of eye-piece at a magnification above 12× and even this magni-

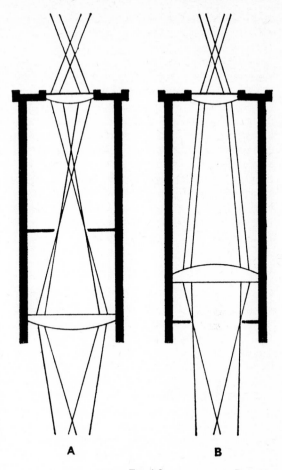

A   **B**

FIG. 1.8
Diagram to illustrate the optical paths in (A) an Huygenian eye-piece, and (B) a Ramsden eye-piece.

fication gives some haziness of outline and distortion. With binocular microscopes, 6× or 8× eye-pieces are perfectly sufficient as, owing to the division of the rays, less light enters each eye-piece. With 10× oculars definition is lost and the field is apt to be too dark when ordinary illuminants are used.

Ramsden or positive eye-pieces are constructed with the convex surface of both lenses facing inwards, the two together forming a single lens unit. In this type of ocular the diaphragm is placed externally *below* the lower lens and in this way has the advantage that any aberration or distortion of the lenses affects equally the image itself and the view of any scale placed on the external diaphragm (Fig.

1.8B). They are therefore admirable for micro-metry and give more accurate results than Huygenian eye-pieces.

Compensating eye-pieces are of the positive type and usually contain a triplet system as the lower lens component. Aberrations are carefully corrected by the makers and they are designed specifically for use with particular objectives. They have an important function in correcting the chromatic difference of magnification inherent in apochromatic lenses. Although designed specifically for use with apochromatic objectives, they can with advantage be used with high power achromats; their use, however, with low power achromats is to be avoided.

CONDENSERS

The function of the condenser is to focus light on the object; it is mounted in the substage with a rack and pinion mechanism for adjusting the focus and should be fitted with centring screws for critical work with highly corrected lenses.

Abbé condensers are the simplest form of 'chromatic' condensers and are often fitted to student microscopes. They are composed of two lenses neither of which is corrected for spherical or chromatic aberration. They are, however, cheap and easily fitted and may be satisfactory for low power work. They should seldom be used in microbiology because they give a poor image at higher magnifications. The light rays are not brought to an accurate focus and only a poor image of the light source can be obtained. Thus, there is flooding of the image with stray light and considerable glare results. In designing apochromatic and semi-apochromatic objectives it is assumed that the light reaching the lenses is corrected and it is essential that a condenser of similar optical quality is used with them.

Aplanatic condensers contain a third or middle lens which corrects for spherical aberration but not for colour. Such condensers give reasonable results especially when used with monochromatic light.

Achromatic condensers, which approach objectives in their complexity, give the best results because they place most of the light where it is needed, i.e. in the plane of the object, and very little escapes to produce glare.

The NA of a condenser should ideally be equal to that of the objective. A good achromatic condenser has an NA of 1·37 and supplies a solid cone of light to the limit of its aperture. This is adequate to fill the aperture of the highest power objective and is sufficient to meet the needs of all the commonly used objectives. The NA of such a condenser can be adjusted to that of lower power objectives by the use of its iris diaphragm mounted below the lowest lens component. It must be remembered that the highest NA of any dry lens is 1·0 and that for critical high-power work it is necessary to introduce immersion oil (refractive index = 1·50) between the top lens of the condenser and the lower surface of the microscope slide.

Centration of the Condenser

If the condenser mount of the microscope possesses centring screws, the centration of the condenser with respect to the objectives must be checked from time to time as follows. After the microscope and the illuminant have been set up as described (see page 14) close the condenser iris diaphragm to its limit. Rack down the condenser until the image of the condenser iris appears in the field. If it is not concentric, adjust the centring screws until it is so. It will be of advantage to open up the condenser iris until its aperture is almost that of the field for the final centration. Then open the iris diaphragm fully and rack up the condenser to its normal position.

For more detailed accounts of the microscope and its uses see Barer (1959) and Wredden (1947).

Brief Specification of a Microscope
Suitable for Routine Bacteriological Work

Microscope, with coarse and fine adjustments, fitted with a removable inclined binocular body. Built-in mechanical stage with verniers, quadruple nose-piece, rackwork substage with centring screws.

Objectives
> Achromatic 10× (16-mm)
> 40× (4-mm)

Fluorite $45\times$ (3·5-mm) oil-imm. (magnification and focal length may vary slightly according to make)

Achromatic $95\times$ (2-mm or $\frac{1}{12}$-in) oil-imm.

Paired eye-pieces

$6\times$ and $8\times$

Condenser

Aplanatic or achromatic

Note

(*a*) Some makers supply a $10\times$ objective specially computed to work with compensating eye-pieces. As it is an advantage to use this type of eye-piece with the other three objectives, it is recommended that this objective and compensating eye-pieces should be specified when ordering.

(*b*) If micrometry or photographic work is to be done, an interchangeable monocular tube is required.

(*c*) For dark-ground illumination, a special concentric condenser is necessary, and also a funnel stop for the $\frac{1}{12}$-in objective.

(*d*) When more than one condenser is used it is advisable to have a substage in which the condensers can easily be changed.

MICROSCOPE LAMPS

The clarity and sharpness of the microscope image depends not only on the excellence of the optical system but also on the illuminant employed. For a monocular instrument with an Abbé condenser, and particularly for lower powers, a 40- or 60-watt opal bulb in a simple lamp housing is sufficient, but for a modern instrument with an inclined binocular body, well corrected oil-immersion objectives and an aplanatic or achromatic condenser, this type of illuminant is far from satisfactory. Unless the bulb is much over-run there is not sufficient light to see small details, and the advantages of modern optical systems can be nullified by poor illumination. If the opal bulb lamp is used it is of advantage to over-run the bulb, e.g. a 200-volt bulb on a 240-volt mains supply. The life of the bulb is shortened, but that is not a serious matter compared with the illumination obtained. The opal bulb should be in a well ventilated housing with a hood over the aperture to prevent direct light from reaching the eyes and should preferably be fitted with an iris diaphragm. The latter is very useful for centring the light in the microscope field and helps to diminish glare. The amount of light required for a good visual image depends on many factors: the intensity of the bulb, the magnification used (for example, less light is required for a 16-mm objective than a 2-mm), the amount of light in the room (less light is required if the microscope is at the back of the room than on the bench at the window), and the time of day (much more illumination is required if there is sunshine than on a dull day or in the evening). With microscopical work, therefore, the amount of illumination required is always changing and a variable resistance of 250 ohms to carry 0·75 or 1 amp fitted with a switch is strongly recommended. This is most desirable if an over-run bulb is used, and an absolute necessity if a high-intensity projection type of bulb is employed. The resistance is placed in series with the opal bulb and in series with the primary winding of the transformer if a low-voltage projection bulb is used.

The full resistance should always be used when the lamp is switched on so that the bulb warms up comparatively slowly, and then the resistance is moved until optimum illumination is reached. With a change of objective it is easy to adjust the intensity of light required, and this method of control is of great value when much microscopic work is done and where the objectives are changed frequently as in histological work.

High-intensity Lamps

With binocular microscopes the amount of light reaching each tube is only about one-third of that of a monocular instrument as light is absorbed by the glass prisms. In consequence a more intense source of light must be used. In order that the whole of the field shall be evenly illuminated, a corrected lamp condenser lens is necessary and this must be capable of being focused. An iris diaphragm in front of this condenser is essential, and provision for a filter holder, preferably of the sliding type, should be made.

High-intensity lamps of this type are produced by several makers and a model specially suitable for high-power microscopy has been described (McCartney, 1951). This lamp uses a large 'solid source' filament bulb of 12-volt 250-watt capacity, but it is actually run at 6 volts and the intensity is controlled by a sliding resistance in the primary of the transformer. The lamp is not only suitable for ordinary microscopy but is useful for dark-ground illumination and phase-contrast microscopy. Its high intensity ensures ample illumination even with dense filters. It is particularly useful for photomicrography.

It may be desirable sometimes to have a more intense beam of light than is possible with a 6-volt transformer, as when filters are required, with dark-ground illumination, or when high-power photomicrography is undertaken. In these cases a 9-volt transformer to take 18 amps and tapped at 6 volts should be used. The 6-volt tapping is employed for ordinary work and the higher voltage output only for special purposes.

Other sources of light may be used for special types of work, such as a mercury vapour lamp for fluorescence microscopy, or even a high-intensity DC arc-lamp as in cinephotomicrography.

Light Filters

A blue daylight filter such as is supplied by most manufacturers should be fitted in the substage ring underneath the microscope condenser when artificial light is used. Filters, however, are not specially required in bacteriological work except for the methods used in fluorescent microscopy. Where much microscopic work has to be carried out, particularly with unstained objects as in dark-ground illumination or phase-contrast microscopy, the use of a pale-green filter, Wratten No. 66 (supplied by Kodak Ltd.) can be recommended. This filter cuts out glare, sharpens detail and is very restful to the eyes. After a short time in use, the green colour is not noticed. It can also be recommended when searching for malaria parasites or tubercle bacilli. In the latter case the organisms appear darker and are more easily recognized when only scanty bacilli are present.

ILLUMINATION OF THE OBJECT

It is common practice in microbiology to use a high-intensity lamp with a binocular microscope and it is important for the worker to obtain the full advantage of this apparatus. It must be remembered that high-intensity lamps have their own optical axis which must be aligned with the optical axis of the microscope. It is recommended that the *Köhler method* of illumination is used because it has the great advantage of providing a variable, uniformly illuminated field of view even with an irregular light source. The essential features of Köhler illumination are (1) the condenser lens of the lamp focuses an enlarged image of the light source (the filament) on the iris diaphragm of the substage condenser; (2) the image of the iris diaphragm in front of the lamp condenser is focused on the object plane by means of the substage condenser.

Method of using a high-intensity lamp:

1. Rack up fully the substage condenser of the microscope.

2. Check that lamp filament has been centred correctly with respect to the lamp condenser lens.

3. Place the lamp so that its distance from the mirror is 8–10 in.

4. Switch on the lamp, open its iris fully and decrease the resistance so that there is a bright beam of light shining on the plane side of the mirror. Adjust the lamp by altering its vertical tilt and by moving the base so that the beam of light is in the centre of the mirror.

It is important to ensure that (*a*) before switching on the lamp the full resistance is in and then for the illumination to be increased or decreased as desired, and (*b*) before switching off the lamp the bulb is dimmed to the full amount. If these precautions are taken, the life of the bulb will be much prolonged.

5. Close the substage iris diaphragm and focus the lamp condenser so that a sharp image of the filament is obtained on the closed diaphragm. A small hand mirror, placed in a suitable place on the bench, facilitates this manoeuvre.

6. Open the substage iris diaphragm and move the lamp backwards or forwards until the size of the image of the filament is large enough to fill the lowest lens of the microscope condenser.

7. Pull back the resistance until the light is

much dimmed, place a stained specimen with good contrast on the stage and focus it with the objective to be used.

8. Close the lamp iris and adjust the mirror so that the image of this iris is in the centre of the field.

9. Open the lamp iris until its image just fills the field.

10. Remove the eye-piece and inspect the back lens of the objective. An image of the filament should be seen to be symmetrically placed and large enough to fill the back lens of the objective.

To obtain the maximum definition, the lamp iris should be closed and focused in the field for each objective. These adjustments, with practice, should only take a few seconds; they are possible with the 16 mm, 4 mm and 3·5 mm oil-immersion objectives but not with the 2 mm oil-immersion objective.

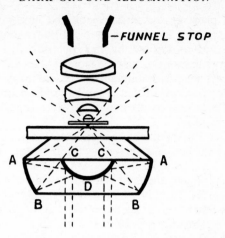

FIG. 1.9

Diagram showing the paths of rays through the condenser and a $\frac{1}{12}$-in oil-immersion lens fitted with a funnel stop. AB and CDC are reflecting surfaces. The surface at CC is opaque. (After E. Leitz.)

DARK-GROUND ILLUMINATION

This method renders visible delicate organisms, such as the spirochaete of syphilis, which cannot be seen in unstained preparations with an ordinary microscope.

By means of a special condenser the specimen is illuminated by oblique light only. The rays do not enter the tube of the microscope, and, in consequence, do not reach the eye of the observer unless they are 'scattered' by objects (e.g. bacteria) of different refractive index from the medium in which they are suspended. As a result, the organisms appear brightly illuminated on a dark background.

There are three requisites for adapting a microscope for dark-ground illumination:

1. A 'dark-ground' condenser.

2. A suitable illuminant of sufficient intensity.

3. A device which reduces the numerical aperture of the objective to less than 1·0.

The Condenser. A special condenser must be employed and may be of the paraboloid or of the concentric spherical reflecting type. The latter is recommended. The function of the special condenser is to focus the light on the object, the paths of the rays being such that no direct light passes into the front of the lens. Figure 1.9 shows the paths of rays through the concentric reflecting condenser. The condenser should be furnished with a centring device, and it must be emphasized here that success with dark-ground illumination depends on the accurate centring of the condenser. There must be immersion oil between the slide and condenser.

The Illuminant. A lamp of sufficiently powerful intensity should be employed.

Alternating current is now almost universal, and high-intensity low-voltage lamps worked through a transformer and having a condensing lens are satisfactory for this purpose. Complete lamps are obtainable from several makers.

The Funnel Stop. When the objectives employed for dark-ground illumination have a numerical aperture of more than 1·0 (as in the case of ordinary oil-immersion lenses), a special stop to reduce the NA to less than 1·0 must be employed. This consists of a small funnel-shaped piece of metal or vulcanite which fits into the objective behind the back lens. It is advisable to procure the stop from the maker of the lens employed. The stop is easily inserted and removed, and the objective can at once be converted for ordinary use.

Alternatively an *objective adaptor*, with a small iris diaphragm, may be used. The front part of the oil-immersion objective is removed and screwed to the adaptor, which then takes the place of the objective on the nose-piece. The numerical aperture of the objective may be reduced as desired by manipulating the iris diaphragm in the adaptor. Some makers incorporate an iris diaphragm in the mount of the objective itself so that it can be used for bright or dark-ground illumination without further alteration.

Certain manufacturers have introduced for dark-ground illumination with bicentric condensers, special oil-immersion fluorite objectives, which are used without a funnel stop. These are 2 mm NA 1·15, and 3·5 mm NA 0·95. The latter lens can be recommended for routine dark-ground observation at low magnification.

The Preparation. The preparation should be as thin as possible in order to secure a satisfactory dark background, and so that the moving objects shall, as far as possible, be in one plane. A preparation which is too thick greatly diminishes the contrast in the dark field, and in order to obtain satisfactory contrast the objective has to be stopped down considerably, thus diminishing its resolving power. The preparation should not be too dense, otherwise there is an excessive number of particles which 'scatter' the light. This causes lack of contrast even to a greater degree than a thick preparation. Some manufacturers supply special cells for dark-ground work so that when the coverslip is placed over the cell the preparation has a definite and uniform thickness.

The thickness of the slide employed is important. The slides should be 1·0–1·1 mm thick, and when a suitable supply has been obtained they should be used only for dark-ground work. They should be thoroughly clean and free from grease. The object to be examined must be at the focus of the condenser, the focal length of which is about 1·2 mm. If, therefore, too thick a slide is used, the focus of the condenser will be below the specimen and poor illumination will result; if the slide is too thin, the distance between the condenser and slide is such that a large amount of oil must be employed to make contact.

Method of Using Dark-Ground Illumination with the Oil-Immersion Objective

The microscope with special condenser, and with the NA of the objective reduced by a funnel stop or iris diaphragm adaptor, is placed in front of the illuminant. It is advisable to have the microscope in the upright position and not inclined, to avoid running of the oil. The condensing lens of the lamp is adjusted so that a slightly converging beam of light is obtained. With the plane side of the mirror, direct the light into the dark-ground condenser. Using the low-power (⅔-in or 16 mm) objective, focus the surface of the condenser so that the engraved concentric rings on the surface come into view. These rings show the centre of the condenser, and if the condenser is out of centre adjust the centring screws so that the rings become concentric with the edge of the field.

Should the condenser have no engraved rings the centring may be accomplished as follows.

A slide preparation is placed on the stage, and oil contact between it and the condenser established. The preparation is focused with the ⅔-in objective, and, if the mirror is properly adjusted, a bright ring of light is noticed in the field. Focus the condenser cautiously up or down so that the ring of light contracts to the smallest bright spot obtainable. If this spot of light is not in the centre of the field, alter the centring screws of the condenser accordingly.

The accurate centring of the condenser is of the utmost importance and the time spent in this manipulation will be amply rewarded by the brilliant illumination obtained. The preparation to be examined must be covered with a No. 1 coverslip, and it is advisable to ring round the coverslip with petroleum jelly to prevent evaporation. Place a large drop of immersion oil upon the under surface of the slide and also on the upper lens of the condenser, and a similar drop on the coverslip. Place the slide on the microscope stage, taking care that the upper surface of the condenser is well below the slide. Rack up the condenser until oil-contact is made between the whole surface of the upper lens of the condenser and the slide; then bring the oil-immersion lens into position so that it touches the oil on the coverslip. Now carefully focus the specimen. A slight adjustment of the condenser, up or down, may be necessary, and some manipulation of the mirror may also be required. After a little practice an evenly illuminated field with an intensely dark background and brilliantly lit objects may be obtained with a minimum of trouble.

Where much dark-ground work has to be done, it is recommended that a microscope be reserved solely for this work and kept ready with the illuminant in position, so that it is always available for immediate use. It is convenient to have the lamp and microscope fixed to a board for this purpose. The microscope, when not in use, should be covered to exclude dust.

After use, the condenser and objective should be carefully wiped free from oil.

Dark-Ground Illumination with Low- and Medium-Power Lenses

Dark-ground illumination is easily obtained with a low-power lens whose NA does not exceed 0·3, e.g. the $\frac{2}{3}$-in objective, by placing a central patch or stop below the condenser. Most manufacturers supply a set of stops which fit into the ring below the iris diaphragm. Alternatively, a circle of glass with a central patch of black gummed-paper about 10–12 mm in diameter may be used. The ordinary source of illumination is quite sufficient. Such dark-ground illumination may be used for observing slide-agglutination and for cells, casts, etc., in urinary deposits. With the higher power dry lenses, however, it is not so easy to secure satisfactory dark-ground illumination unless special condensers are used. Some microscope manufacturers make dry dark-ground condensers to work with $\frac{1}{6}$-in objectives up to numerical apertures of 0·65, but these are expensive and usually require a high-intensity lamp to work satisfactorily. The results, however, are very beautiful.

Where the NA of the objective does not exceed 0·65, dark-ground illumination can be secured with an 'achromatic' or 'aplanatic' condenser (not an Abbé condenser), an expanding iris or suitably large central stop being used. As such condensers are suitable for ordinary microscopy it is possible to change over from direct transmitted light to dark-ground illumination, without removing the condenser, by merely inserting the stop. A high-intensity illuminant is, however, necessary, and

immersion oil is placed between the condenser and slide. An intermediate objective adaptor with iris diaphragm is often of value in reducing the NA of the $\frac{1}{6}$-in objective sufficiently to obtain a uniform dark field.

PRACTICAL INSTRUCTIONS FOR THE USE OF A MICROSCOPE

When an observer has to examine a specimen for a long time, as when scanning a film for tubercle bacilli or malaria parasites, he must adopt a comfortable position with the height of his chair adjusted so that the oculars of the microscope are level with his eyes. Many workers who wear spectacles are able to dispense with them when using a microscope. If, however, the visual defect is that of astigmatism spectacles will often need to be worn, and if this is so workers must take care to avoid contact between the eye-piece and the spectacle lenses or they may scratch each other. If a monocular microscope is used the worker should keep both eyes open if possible, in order to reduce strain. It is wise to ease the burden on the eye by changing from one eye to the other from time to time. Both forearms should rest on the table, and if there is no mechanical stage the slide is moved with the left hand while the right hand controls the fine adjustment. Before beginning to examine a specimen the microscope is checked to ensure that:

1. the objectives are clean and free from immersion oil;
2. the eye-pieces are free from dust;
3. the plane side of the mirror is in position;
4. the substage condenser is racked up until its top surface is 1–2 mm below the object slide.

For microbiological work it is recommended that artificial light should always be used. A 60-watt opal bulb or a high-intensity lamp is employed according to the type of microscope used. It is not advisable to place the microscope at a window because daylight, and especially bright sunlight, entering the eyes renders vision less acute. A suitable arrangement is to use the microscope on a table at one side of a room so that the observer's back is to the window.

When examining an object, using a simple 40- or 60-watt opal bulb lamp, the manipulations of the microscope should be carried out in the following order:

1. Set up the microscope, place the object on the stage, and adjust the plane side of the mirror to the illuminant so that the light is reflected into the condenser.

2. Focus the specimen with the low-power objective, using the coarse adjustment.

3. Manipulate the mirror until the image of the illuminant is seen in the centre of the field; if the lamp has an iris diaphragm this should be closed and the mirror adjusted until the aperture of the iris is concentric with the edge of the field. Rack the condenser up or down until the edge of the iris is sharply focused.

It is essential, particularly when examining tissues, to use the low power first, in order to locate organisms and observe the tissue changes. A suitable field having been obtained, the slide must be kept in place by means of the right-hand clip if a mechanical stage is not used.

4. Rack up the objective a short distance and place a drop of cedar-wood immersion oil on the portion of the specimen immediately below the objective.

5. Raise the condenser so that its upper surface is practically level with the stage. (This is not necessary if the lamp iris has been focused as in (3).)

6. Make sure that the iris diaphragm of the substage condenser is widely open.

7. Rotate the nose-piece until the oil-immersion lens is in position.

8. With the eye at the level of the stage and using the coarse adjustment lower the objective until it makes contact with the oil; at this moment the drop of oil 'lights up'. Next, the objective is gently lowered a little further towards the slide but great care must be exercised not to carry this movement too far or too harshly. The working distance of oil-immersion lenses is extremely short and there is a great risk that with pressure, the tiny front lens of the objective may be displaced and its performance ruined. Some modern objectives, but not all, have a special guarding device to prevent this, or are set in a spring-loaded mount.

9. Apply the eye to the microscope and observe if the field is well illuminated; if not, adjust the mirror until maximum illumination is secured.

10. Next, slowly and carefully *focus up* with the coarse adjustment until the object is brought into view and then use the fine adjustment to secure a sharp focus.

In using a binocular microscope the same directions should be observed, but, in addition, the eye-pieces should be adjusted to the correct interpupillary distance of the observer when the specimen is focused with the low-power objective (see direction No. 2).

Care of the Microscope

The microscope is an instrument of precision, and care must be taken to preserve its accuracy. The instrument should be kept at a uniform temperature and not exposed to sunlight or any source of heat. When not in use it must be protected from dust under a transparent plastic cover or in its box. Failing these, it should be covered with a clean cloth. The microscope should be cleaned at intervals, and its working surfaces very lightly smeared with soft paraffin. With binocular microscopes dust may collect on the surfaces of the prisms. This may be removed by passing a soft camel-hair brush down the eye-piece tubes after removing the eye-pieces. On no account must the prism case be opened and the prisms removed, as this will completely alter the optical alignment and necessitate the return of the instrument to the maker before it can be used again.

If the microscope has to be moved, it should be lifted by the upright limb and not held by the body-tube.

The oil-immersion objective must be cleaned each day after use by wiping the front lens with a well-washed silk or cotton handkerchief. Alternatively, a fine tissue paper known as 'lens paper' may be used (books of which are supplied by most manufacturers), and this is very suitable for the purpose. Oil remaining on the lens-front dries and becomes sticky; later it hardens and is then difficult to remove. Canada balsam accidentally present on the lens from a mounted microscopic specimen may also dry hard in the same way. When cleaning the objective *do not use alcohol*, as the cement that unites the component lenses may be soluble in alcohol, and, in consequence, the lens systems may become disorganized and the objective spoiled. Benzol or xylol must be used to remove dried oil, and if the oil is hard, repeated applications on a soft cloth are necessary.

Dry objectives, e.g. $\frac{2}{3}$-in and $\frac{1}{6}$-in, are cleaned with a piece of well-washed silk or fine cotton, or lens paper. If any oil or Canada balsam is accidentally present on the front lens it must be removed with a soft cloth moistened in benzol or xylol and the lens quickly dried with a soft cloth. On no account should the component parts of an objective be unscrewed.

Eye-pieces from time to time may be contaminated with dust and fuzzy specks are seen in the field of view. The trouble is easily located because the specks move when the eye-piece is rotated in its mount. If the dust is situated on the upper lens the specks will move if the eye-piece is raised a little with one hand while the upper lens is unscrewed with the other. If the dirt is on the bottom lens the specks will move when the lower component is rotated. When the position of the dirt has been located, remove it by blowing a jet of dry air on it with bellows or a large rubber teat. Alternatively, use a soft camel-hair brush. If the brush is held for a few seconds against a hot electric bulb it acquires an electric charge and will then attract dust particles easily. If these methods fail then use a silk cloth or lens paper moistened with *distilled* water. Never rub the surface of a lens with a dry cloth because any hard particles on its surface may scratch the glass.

Common Difficulties in Microscopy

A number of troubles may be encountered by those beginning microscopy and the following hints are given to help overcome them:

1. *Inability to obtain a sharp image with the oil-immersion objective:*

(*a*) Check that there is no dirt or dried oil adherent to the front lens of the objective. If there is clean it off.

(*b*) Check that the microscope slide carrying the object has not been put in upside down.

(*c*) Check that the immersion oil being used it not so viscous that the slide adheres firmly to the objective and travels upwards with movements of the coarse adjustment.

(*d*) Check whether the specimen slide and coverslip has a film of dried immersion oil and dirt left on it by a previous viewer.

(*e*) Some high-power objectives have so short a working distance that a thick coverslip or a thick layer of Canada balsam beneath the coverslip may prevent the objective approaching near enough to bring the object within its focal length.

If none of these steps improves matters, exchange the objective with one from another microscope; if a sharp image is obtained with the new objective the faulty one should be returned to the makers.

2. *A dark shadow passes into the field* with loss of definition of the image. This is usually caused by the movement of an air bubble in the immersion oil. The trouble may be cured by raising the objective so that the contact between the oil and the objective is broken and then refocusing. If this fails, clean objective and coverslip with a little xylol and begin again.

3. *Poor illumination or the field of view in semi-darkness:*

(*a*) Check that the flat and NOT the concave surface of the mirror is being used and adjust the mirror so that the light beam fills the field of view.

(*b*) Check that the condenser has been racked up to its full height. Occasionally it slips downwards in its mounting ring and must be pressed up as far as possible before it can be racked up close to the microscope slide.

(*c*) Check that the substage iris diaphragm is fully open.

Examination of Living Unstained Organisms

In the case of bacteria, 'hanging-drop' preparations are frequently used for this purpose, and a glass slide having a circular concavity in the centre is employed.

There should be no difficulty in observing a satisfactory specimen if the following procedure is adopted:

1. By means of a match dipped in petroleum jelly, a ring or square (according to the shape

and size of the coverslip) is outlined round the concavity.

2. With a wire loop place a drop of fluid containing the organisms on a coverslip laid on the bench.

For this purpose a fluid culture is used or the condensation fluid of a slope culture. A further alternative is to emulsify a small amount of culture from the surface of a solid medium in a drop of broth or normal saline, taking care that the emulsion is not too dense.

3. Invert the slide over the coverslip, allowing the glass to adhere to the jelly, and quickly turn round the slide so that the coverslip is uppermost. The drop should then be 'hanging' from the coverslip in the centre of the concavity.

4. Place the slide on the microscope, rack down the condenser slightly and partially close the iris diaphragm. (Excessive illumination renders the organisms invisible.)

5. With the low-power objective, focus the edge of the drop so that it appears across the centre of the field.

6. Turn the high-power ($\frac{1}{6}$-in or 4-mm) lens into position and focus the edge of the drop. Obtain the best illumination by lowering or raising the condenser, and secure sharp definition by reducing the aperture of the iris diaphragm.

Instead of employing a hanging-drop preparation, a film of the fluid between an ordinary slide and coverslip may be used, but in this case the edge of the coverslip should be sealed with vaseline or nail varnish to prevent evaporation of the fluid.

Motility of organisms can be detected in this way, and their shape, approximate size and general structure can be observed. *It is advisable to use the high-power dry lens* and not the oil-immersion objective. Owing to the viscosity of the oil, the coverslip is apt to move during focusing, and currents are thus caused in the fluid, which produce an appearance of motility in the organisms.

It is essential to distinguish between true motility, where the organism changes its position in the field, and Brownian movement, which is an oscillatory movement possessed by all small bodies (whether living or not) suspended in fluid.

A warm stage is very convenient when examining fresh unstained preparations for amoebae and other protozoa. There are several types of warm stages available, some of which consist of a thin, flat metal box filled with hot water, or through which warm water can circulate, and having an aperture in the centre by which the light passes to the preparation. Improved forms are electrically heated and have an automatic temperature control. The warm stage keeps the preparation at body temperature, and enables the movements of organisms to be studied, because these movements may cease if the material is kept for any length of time at room temperature.

A simple warm stage may easily be improvised from a sheet of thin copper (18-gauge) shaped like the letter T, with the long arm 5–6 in in length. The top of the T is the size of a microscope slide (3 in × 1 in) and in the centre is an aperture $\frac{1}{2}$ in in diameter. The copper T is placed on the microscope stage with the long arm projecting forward, and the aperture over the condenser. The preparation is placed on the copper strip and secured by the stage clips. The projecting part of the T is warmed by means of a small Bunsen flame or spirit lamp. Care must be taken that the preparation is not overheated.

MICROMETRY

In bacteriological work the unit of measurement is 0·001 mm, designated a micrometre or μm. The measurement of microscopic objects is accomplished by means of the stage micrometer in conjunction with a micrometer eye-piece. The stage micrometer consists of a 3 × 1 in slide on which is a millimetre scale graduated in hundredths of a millimetre. This scale may be engraved, but is usually made by a photographic process. The micrometer eye-piece consists of a special eye-piece in which a graduated scale, mounted on the diaphragm of a positive type eye-piece, can be focused by means of the movable eye-lens.

When measurements are to be made, the micrometer eye-piece is inserted into the draw-tube, the tube length is accurately noted, and the rulings on the stage micrometer focused by the appropriate objective according to the size of the object to be measured. The number of divisions on the eye-piece scale corresponding to a definite number of divisions of the millimetre stage scale is determined. The stage micrometer is removed, and the object to be measured is next focused. The number of divisions of the eye-piece scale which just cover the object are noted.

The millimetre value of each division of the eye-piece scale depends on the objective used and the tube length employed, and is usually determined each time a measurement is taken. Sometimes it is advisable to increase or diminish the draw-tube length or to move the adjustable collar of the objective so that the stage and eye-piece scales coincide or bear a geometric relation to each other—e.g. 1 division of the former to 10 of the latter.

Example: Using a $\frac{1}{12}$-in objective and a $6\times$ micrometer eye-piece at 165 mm tube length, it was found that 100 divisions on the eye-piece scale exactly covered 11 divisions of the stage micrometer. Each division of the stage micrometer is $\frac{1}{100}$ mm.

$$100 \text{ eye-piece divisions} = 11 \text{ stage divisions}$$
$$= 0.11 \text{ mm}$$
$$1 \text{ eye-piece division} = 0.0011 \text{ mm}$$

1 eye-piece division, therefore, with the given objective, eye-piece and tube length $= 1.1 \ \mu m$.

The stage micrometer was removed and a stained slide of blood showing malaria crescents was substituted. The diameter of a red blood corpuscle covered 7 divisions of the eye-piece scale, i.e. $7.7 \ \mu m$. A polymorph leucocyte covered 11 divisions, while the length of a malaria crescent was equal to 10 divisions, showing the sizes of these objects to be 12.1 and $11 \ \mu m$ respectively.

If the draw-tube is so adjusted that 1 division of the stage micrometer equals 10 of the eye-piece scale, then each division of the latter corresponds to $1 \ \mu m$.

The Screw Micrometer Eye-piece employs a vertical fine hair line which is made to traverse a fixed scale situated on the eye-piece diaphragm. The eye-piece is of the Ramsden, or compensating, type and is fitted with an accurate screw contained in a drum which is divided into a hundred parts, each of which represents a displacement of 0.01 mm of the hair line. The fixed scale is not intended for direct measurement but is constructed so that with each complete revolution of the drum the hair line traverses one division. Calibration is made by comparison with a stage micrometer (Needham, 1958) in the way described for the eye-piece micrometer. The screw micrometer eye-piece is more precise and accurate than the eye-piece micrometer and measurements to one-hundredths of the fixed scale divisions are possible.

Photographic Method of Micrometry. An accurate method is to photograph a film of the organisms or cells under a high magnification. Without disturbing the microscope or camera, the slide is removed from the microscope stage and the stage micrometer substituted. A photograph of the stage micrometer is then taken at exactly the same magnification. By means of a pair of fine dividers the length of the organism on the print is taken, and its exact measurement found by applying this distance to the micrometer print.

Electron-microscopical Method of Micrometry. Optical methods of micrometry have, to a large extent, been replaced by electron-microscopical techniques. A suitable suspension of the organism to be measured is made and to it is added a suspension of latex particles of known diameter (e.g. 250 or 88 nm). Measurements of the organism and the reference particles on the electron micrograph give a highly accurate estimate of size. It must, however, be remembered that during examination in the electron microscope an organism may be distorted by drying or heat. Most of these difficulties, however, can be overcome by careful fixation.

PHASE CONTRAST MICROSCOPY

One of the difficulties of examining microscopically living, unstained biological specimens is that they are immersed in a fluid of almost the same refractive index as themselves. In order to see them distinctly it is necessary either (*a*) to close considerably the iris diaphragm, thereby reducing the numerical aperture, or (*b*) to use dark-ground illumination. The latter procedure is satisfactory with very small or slender objects such as spirochaetes, but its use in bacteriology is limited.

By means of phase contrast microscopy, it is possible to examine living cells with the full aperture of the objective. In consequence internal details are effectively brought out.

Phase contrast microscopy can be used with any type of microscope, either monocular or binocular.

It is necessary to have:

1. A special condenser which usually incorporates a rotating metal disk carrying a series of annular diaphragms. These are disks of glass rendered opaque but with a narrow ring of clear glass. Each objective requires a different size of annulus according to its numerical aperture; thus, for the 16-mm objective the ring is narrow and about $4\frac{1}{2}$ mm in diameter, whereas for the 2-mm objective it is wider and about 18 mm in diameter. The size of the annulus is such that the condenser forms an image of it in the back focal plane of the objective.

2. Special phase objectives. These are ordinary objectives at the back of which, i.e. in its back focal plane, is inserted a phase plate consisting of a disk of glass having a circular trough etched in it and of such a depth that the light after passing through it has a phase difference of a quarter of a wave-length compared with the rest of the plate (see Fig. 1.10).

The objective is focused on the specimen. The appropriate annulus for the objective is rotated into position under the condenser. The condenser is then focused so that the image of the annulus is superimposed on the phase plate at the back of the objective. A special telescope (supplied with the outfit) is inserted in place of the eye-piece and through it the back focal plane of the objective is observed. The annulus and phase ring should coincide. If they are not exactly coincident the centring screws under the condenser are adjusted to achieve this. The eye-piece is now re-inserted and the specimen examined.

All powers of the microscope can be used, provided that each objective has its own phase plate fitted, and there is an appropriate annulus for it below the condenser.

The *optical principle* briefly is as follows. If a diffraction grating is examined under the microscope, diffraction spectra are formed in the back focal plane of the objective. The

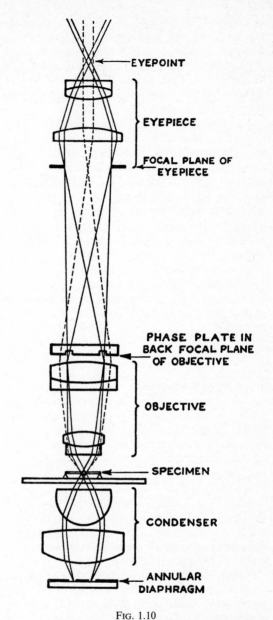

FIG. 1.10
Diagram illustrating the paths of light rays in phase contrast microscopy.
Reproduced by permission of American Optical Company.

detail observed in the image is due to interference between the direct and diffracted beams. Unstained objects such as bacteria or cells may be considered as similar to a diffraction grating; that is, the detail consists of alternative strips of material with slightly different refractive indices, through which light acquires small phase differences, and these form the image. With ordinary illumination, however, such slight differences are almost completely obscured by the intensity of the direct light beam, and hardly any detail can be observed at all.

As will be seen from Fig. 1.10, the direct light from the annular diaphragm passes only through the trough in the phase plate. The diffracted beam having a slightly different path goes through the thicker glass of the phase plate outside the trough and in consequence is retarded one-quarter of a wavelength with respect to the direct beam. When these two beams (direct and diffracted) unite they are not in phase, and these phase differences are apparent as appreciable changes in intensity. The details of the object stand out sharply and distinctly on a grey background, and being observed at full aperture, there is maximum resolution.

As there is a great difference in intensity between the direct beam and the diffracted beam, the trough of the phase plate through which the direct beam passes is covered with a light-absorbing material, usually a thin deposit of silver or other metal, so that the intensity of the direct beam is much reduced and approaches that of the diffracted beam. In consequence of this, and as the illumination is much restricted by the narrow annular diaphragm, a high-intensity lamp must be used.

Phase contrast microscopy is most valuable in general biology, but has less application in bacteriological work. It is useful, however, in examining the growth and subdivision of bacteria, flagellar movement, intestinal and other protozoa, such as amoebae, *Trichomonas*, etc., living blood cells and the cytopathic effect of viruses on tissues and cell cultures.

The interference microscope permits the measurement as well as the observation of the various phase changes produced by transparent objects. The illumination system splits the light reaching the object into two beams; one passes through the object while the other acts as a comparison beam. Both beams may, in fact, pass through the object, but the image in one is out of focus with respect to that in the other. When the two beams are recombined they are

allowed to interfere and the image of the object is defined by interference contrast in the field.

The Baker-Smith and Dyson interference microscopes both employ a built-in rotating polariser and a rotating analyser graduated in degrees. A quarter wave retardation plate of mica is placed below the analyser. The optical systems used are complex and for further information the reader should consult a monograph by Hale (1958).

Phase differences in the object up to 1/300 wavelength can be measured by the interference microscope and from them, with the aid of a mathematical formula, the refractive index of living cells can be calculated. By immersing cells in media of different refractive indices the concentration of dried substances in them can be estimated. Thus, interference microscopy can be used to determine the dry mass of living cells or their nuclei and as a quantitative cytochemical method (Davies *et al.*, 1954).

FLUORESCENCE MICROSCOPY

When certain materials as, for example, uranium ores, uranium glass, oil or fat droplets, solutions of aesculin and various dyes, are exposed to ultra-violet (UV) light, they alter the wavelength of the invisible light and so become luminous and are said to fluoresce. If tissues, cells or bacteria are stained with a fluorescent dye and are examined under the microscope with ultra-violet light instead of ordinary visible light, they become luminous and are seen as bright objects against a dark background. Moreover, these fluorescent dyes have a selective action for the various microorganisms and cells and for their constituents which thus become readily recognized and identified. Dyes specially suited for fluorescent staining are auramine O, acridine orange R, berberine sulphate, primulin, thioflavin S, trypaflavine, thiazo-yellow G, and morin.

Immunofluorescence

Certain other fluorescent dyes can be used to label serum antibodies. They are coupled to gamma globulins (or to any chosen protein) by chemically reactive groups and render the resulting conjugates fluorescent. Two dyes are used, fluorescein isothiocyanate which has a brilliant apple-green colour, and lissamine rhodamine B (RB200) which has an orange colour. Labelled antisera have an important application in immunological work and the techniques of immunofluorescence are described in Chapter 11 and by Nairn (1969).

Many manufacturers supply complete units for fluorescent microscopy but it is possible to adapt the ordinary microscope for this work.

The most satisfactory light source is a high pressure mercury vapour lamp and is preferred to the tungsten or carbon arc lamps formerly used because it emits a very powerful beam of ultra-violet light at a steady intensity. The wavelength range required is 290–325 nm for fluorescein and 310–350 nm for rhodamine; these two dyes have emission peaks at 525 nm and 595 nm respectively. The HB200 (Osram)* lamp is recommended for this purpose and has a wavelength range of 280–600 nm with peaks at 365 and 435 nm. The lamp requires a special starter unit to provide a high tension initial impulse to start the mercury arc, followed by a continuous flow of low tension current to maintain the lamp. The average life of an HB200 lamp is 200 h and it is wise to keep a record of the burning time. The lamp should be enclosed in a protective housing because there is a small risk of explosion that increases when the lamp is used beyond its stated life. Within the housing an aluminium-coated reflecting mirror is needed and adequate centring devices are required.

The collector lens of the lamp should be made of ultra-violet transmitting crown glass or, better still, of 'fused quartz' (quartz glass) because it is more heat-resistant than ordinary glass. Quartz condensers, and lenses in the optical path are, however, quite unnecessary and in any case they are extremely expensive. Thus, the absence of quartz condensers and lenses should on no account discourage the worker from undertaking fluorescence microscopy; the one essential is a satisfactory light source.

Condensers. Two types of substage condenser may be used. For fluorochrome stained preparations a bright ground, three lens, aplanatic condenser is satisfactory, but for immune fluorescence a dark ground condenser gives better results, especially with the higher powered dry or oil-immersion objectives.

Objectives. Achromats are preferred to apochromats because the glass of their lenses has less tendency to fluoresce.

Filter systems. (a) Primary filters. Light of wavelength 480 nm is required and satisfactory filters, which must be sited close to the lamp, are available from Kodak Wratten 18B, Chance Pilkington OX7, in Great Britain, U.G.1 of Schott & Genossen in West Germany, and Corning 5840 in the U.S.A. (b) Secondary filters are situated in the eye-pieces and have the dual purpose of cutting off any UV rays which might damage the cornea of the observer's eye while at the same time giving a satisfactory colour contrast. A Kodak Wratten 2B filter is satisfactory, but a variety of green-yellow filters may be used.

Immersion oil. Special non-fluorescent immersion oil is essential and that supplied by E. Leitz & Co. is recommended.

ELECTRON MICROSCOPY

With improvement in design and the evolution of new preparatory techniques, the modern electron microscope has become indispensable in microbiological research. The greatly increased resolving power of the instrument enables details of the fine structure and of the nature of the component parts of bacteria, viruses, cells and tissues to be visualized in a way that is impossible with the light microscope.

Although the electron microscope is complex, costly and technically difficult to maintain, the principles of its construction are closely paralleled by those of the optical microscope and easily understood. The resolution of the light microscope depends on the wavelength of the light used and the numerical aperture of the lens. When electrons move they behave somewhat like light waves and have properties of refraction, diffraction and interference. The wavelength of electrons is inversely proportional to their velocity and the particular wave-

---

* Manufactured by the 'Osram' Company and marketed in the U.K. under the name of 'MERON'.

length used in an electron microscope is 0·005 nm, i.e. about 100 000 times shorter than that of ordinary light, and thus high resolution and great magnifications are possible. Theoretically, if conditions were identical in the optical and electron microscopes, resolution down to 0·0025 nm would be possible. However, the NA of an electron microscope lens is very small (the diameter of the aperture is only a few microns) and does not approach the width of that of an optical microscope objective. In practice, the best resolution that can be obtained is 0·3–0·5 nm. Thus the resolution of the electron microscope is approximately a hundred times better than that of the light microscope.

The electron microscope (see Fig. 1.11) consists of a column or 'stack' (4) at the top of which is mounted the source of illumination, the 'electron gun' (6) which emits electrons from a hot tungsten-wire filament (7). Beneath this filament a cathode shield (8) is placed. A high voltage (5) which can be varied from 50 to 100 kV is applied to the anode. The life of the tungsten-wire filament is limited and it usually requires to be replaced after some 15 h viewing. A pencil beam of electrons (9) moving at high velocity is projected through the hole in the anode and onwards down the stack. The high accelerating voltage used must be stabilized with an accuracy better than 1 in 100 000 in order to ensure uniform velocity of the electrons. Because the electron beam would be scattered by any atoms with which it might collide, the air in the stack is completely evacuated and a vacuum of the order of 10^{-6} mmHg is maintained (3).

As in the light microscope, focusing and magnification are achieved by a series of 'lenses' which, in fact, are accurately controlled electromagnetic fields. There is a condenser lens system (10 and 11) which bends the rays of electrons so that a parallel beam is directed onto the object (12) placed below it. The electrons are scattered to a degree that is proportional to the thickness and density of the various parts of the specimen. An objective lens (14) gathers the scattered electrons through a very small aperture (13) and brings them to a focus where a real primary image (2) is formed and is magnified about a hundred times. Two projector lenses (16), which have the function of the eye-piece of the light microscope, magnify a part of the primary image a further 300–500 times. The focal length of electromagnetic lenses can be changed by varying the current flowing through the lens and thus a continuously variable magnification is obtained and controlled at the turn of a dial.

The final image (18) is observed on a fluorescent screen (19) situated at the lower end of the stack and is viewed through a glass window. The screen can be withdrawn by a lever to allow the electrons to impinge on a photographic plate (1) or film held in a camera (20) placed immediately below. Owing to the high resolving powers of the electron microscope it is possible to take negatives at any magnification from 2000 to 100 000 and these may be enlarged photographically up to ten times. Thus, a useful magnification of up to 1 000 000 diameters can be obtained.

The specimen to be examined is placed in a special holder and then introduced into the stack between the condenser and objective lenses through an air lock. Finally, when the vacuum has been restored, it is lowered into position by a lever and its examination can be made. A $10\times$ binocular microscope (17) is used to facilitate accurate focusing before taking photographs.

The controls of the electron microscope are accommodated in panels on its desk. They include dials for variation of the magnification, a mechanical stage to move the specimen, switches and meters to control and check the voltage used, vacuum gauges, and controls for electron optical alignment. The electronic circuits for stabilizing and controlling the high voltage and lens currents form a separate unit, as also do the rotary and diffusion pumps.

THE PREPARATION OF MATERIALS FOR ELECTRON MICROSCOPY

The electron beam, with an accelerating voltage of 50–100 kV, has a very poor penetrating power and for this reason only small objects or very thin sections of tissues can be examined in the electron microscope. The specimens must be mounted on films no thicker than 20 nm and of high transparency to electrons. Such films are naturally very fragile and have to be

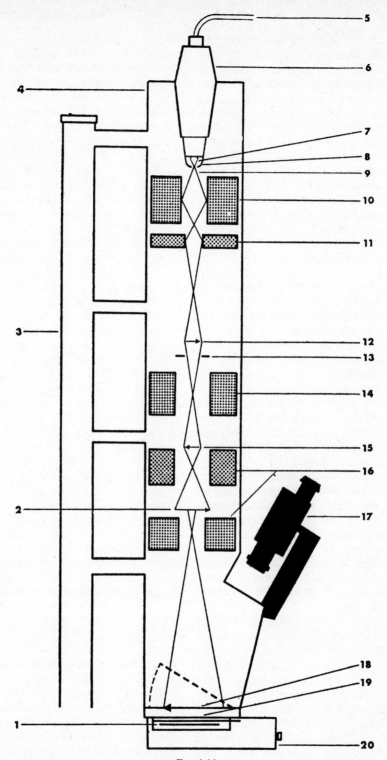

FIG. 1.11

A diagram to show the optical system and component parts of an electron microscope. (1) Photographic plate; (2) Primary image; (3) Connections from stack to
vacuum pumps; (4) Stack; (5) 100000-volt supply; (6) Electron gun; (7) Hot
tungsten-wire filament; (8) Cathode shield; (9) Electron beam; (10) First condenser
lens; (11) Second condenser lens; (12) Object; (13) Objective aperture; (14) Objective
lens; (15) Intermediate image; (16) First and second projector lenses; (17) Focusing
binoculars; (18) Final image; (19) Fluorescent screen; ;20) Camera.

mounted on small copper supporting disks that are perforated with many apertures regularly arranged to form a 40000 per in² mesh. Suitable grids for the AEI and other electron microscopes can be obtained from Smethurst Highlight Ltd., Bolton, Lancs.

They are made with a shiny surface on one side and a matt surface on the other for maximum adhesion of the film. Handling grids of this type requires very fine pointed forceps and is easier if the grids are bent very slightly. Traces of fluid may adhere to the points of the forceps as the grids are being manipulated through various solutions rendering the grids adherent, with the risk of damage to or loss of the specimen. This difficulty can be avoided if it is made a rule always to take a strip of filter paper and blot away traces of fluid from between the points of the forceps before transferring the grid to any dry surface.

Preparation of Support Films

Collodion Cast on Water

The following are required:

1. A 2 per cent solution of nitrocellulose in amyl acetate ('Collodion').
2. A brass ring $\frac{1}{4}$ in deep and about 3 in in diameter which is covered on one side by a disk of fine copper gauze (200 in mesh).
3. A 4-in Petri dish or a shallow glass bowl of similar diameter standing on the lid of a 6-in Petri dish.

PROCEDURE:

1. Place the ring, gauze side uppermost, in the small Petri dish and pour in clean distilled water until it is covered and the water just reaches the brim of the dish.
2. Pick up electron microscope grids with fine forceps, moisten them carefully and place them in even rows, shiny surface down, on to the copper gauze.
3. The surface of the water is now cleaned by allowing two drops of the collodion to fall on it from a dropping pipette. A solid film is formed within a few seconds entrapping any dust particles on the surface and is then swept away with a glass rod.
4. A second film is now formed in the same way.

5. With minimum disturbance pipette the water out of the Petri dish into the surrounding trough. The collodion membrane sinks gently on to the grids on the copper gauze.
6. The gauze on its ring is now lifted from the dish and set to dry over calcium chloride in a desiccator.
7. When the grids are required for use they are freed by cutting the membrane at their edges with a fine needle, and then transferred to a holding clip.

Formvar Cast on Glass

The following are required:

1. A 0·125 per cent solution of polyvinyl formal (Formvar) in chloroform.
2. Microscope slides and short length of glass rod cleaned with a detergent and polished with a clean cloth.
3. The materials required for collodion films.

PROCEDURE:

1. Place a drop of the Formvar solution on a microscope slide and spread it to cover the whole surface with the glass rod. Allow a few seconds for the chloroform to evaporate. Ideally the film should have a pale straw colour.
2. Breathe heavily on the film.
3. Float off the Formvar membrane by lowering the slide at a shallow angle into the water in a Petri dish in which grids have been placed on copper gauze.
4. Proceed as in making collodion films.

Formvar films are much stronger than collodion films and resist the heat of the electron beam much better. They suffer, however, from the disadvantage that they may have a coarser grained surface than collodion and thus are not desirable if the specimen to be viewed is comprised of small particles or macromolecules.

Evaporated Carbon Films are prepared by the method of Bradley (1961). They can be obtained by evaporating carbon on to the surface of a glass slide and floated off as for Formvar. They have a thickness of only 5 nm. They have the finest grain of any film so far described. They are, however, fragile and some workers prefer to evaporate a layer of carbon 2–5 nm thick on to a grid previously covered with a collodion membrane.

Preparation of Suspensions of Microorganisms for Electron Microscopy

Suitable cultures containing large numbers of bacteria or virus particles must be obtained. In the case of viruses an infectivity or haemagglutinating titre of 10^7 or greater is desirable. The original cultures are centrifuged to deposit the microorganisms into a pellet which is then resuspended in a small volume of sterile culture medium. Extracts of virus infected cells or tissues may require several cycles of differential centrifugation.

Fixation

Bacteria and the larger viruses require some form of fixation though this may be omitted with some of the smaller viruses. Usually the suspension or the centrifuged pellet is added directly to the fixing solution. If sections are to be cut the pellet may be embedded in 2·0 per cent molten agar (Difco, Noble agar).

The following three fixatives are of general usefulness:

Kellenberger's Method for the Fixation of Microorganisms (Kellenberger, Ryter and Séchaud, 1958)

Prepare the following:

1. Michaelis veronal-acetate buffer:

Sodium barbitone . . .	2·94 g
Sodium acetate (hydrated) .	1·94 g
Sodium chloride . . .	3·40 g
Distilled water to make .	100 ml

2. Kellenberger buffer:

Veronal-acetate buffer . .	5·0 ml
Distilled water . . .	13·0 ml
0·1 N HCl	7·0 ml
$M/1$ CaCl$_2$ . . .	0·25 ml

   Adjust to pH = 6·0 with the 0·1 N HCl or buffer. Prepare freshly on the day of use.

3. Kellenberger fixative:

Osmium tetroxide . . .	0·1 g
Kellenberger buffer . .	10·0 ml

   The pH does not change.

4. Tryptone medium:

Bacto-Tryptone (Difco) . .	1·0 g
Sodium chloride . . .	0·5 g
Distilled water to make .	100 ml

5. Sterile agar solution:

Agar (Noble) . . .	2·0 g
Distilled water to make .	100 ml

Sterilize in the autoclave in 5 or 10 ml amounts.

6. Kellenberger washing solution:

Uranyl acetate . . .	0·5 g
Kellenberger buffer to make .	100 ml

   This solution keeps for several weeks at 4°C.

PROCEDURE

1. Mix 30 ml of a suitable suspension of microorganisms with 3·0 ml of Kellenberger fixative. Centrifuge 5 min at 1800 g.

2. Decant the supernatant and resuspend the deposit in 1·0 ml of Kellenberger fixative to which has been added 0·1 ml of tryptone medium.

3. Stand overnight (about 16 h) at room temperature.

4. Add 8·0 ml Kellenberger buffer and centrifuge 5 min at 1800 g.

5. Decant the supernatant and resuspend the pellet in distilled water for direct electron microscopy.

6. If ultra-thin sections are to be cut proceed as follows:

   (*a*) add about 0·03 ml of molten agar at 45°C to the suspension and mix carefully;

   (*b*) pour a drop of the molten agar suspension on to a clean microscope slide and allow it to set firm;

   (*c*) cut the solid drop of agar into 1-mm cubes with a razor blade;

   (*d*) place the cubes into the uranyl acetate washing solution for 2 h at room temperature.

   The cubes are now ready for dehydration and embedding.

For the techniques of embedding and the preparation and staining of ultra-thin sections, the reader is referred to Glauert (1965) and to Pease (1965).

Palade's Fixative (Palade 1952)

1.

Osmium tetroxide . . .	1·0 g
Distilled water . . .	50 ml

   Store in a clean dark glass bottle away from the light. It keeps for several months at 4°C.

2.

Sodium barbitone . . .	2·89 g
Sodium acetate (hydrated) .	1·9 g
Distilled water . . .	100 ml

3. Prepare the fixative as follows:
   Mix together—

2 per cent osmium tetroxide	.	12·5 ml
Veronal-acetate buffer	.	5·0 ml
0·1 N HCl	. approx.	5·0 ml
Distilled water	.	2·5 ml

   Adjust to pH 7·3–7·4 using 0·1 N HCl. The fixative can be stored for a few days at 4°C. It is used mainly for fixing protozoa, cells and tissues.

Glutaraldehyde Fixation

1. Stock solution 25 per cent of glutaraldehyde (L. Light, Colnbrook)
2. Phosphate buffer pH 7·4
   Fixative:

Glutaraldehyde	.	5 ml
0·1 M phosphate buffer	.	20 ml

   If sections are to be stained with lead salts, substitute 0·067 M sodium cacodylate for the phosphate buffered saline in order to avoid the precipitation of lead. Adjust to pH 7·4.

Glutaraldehyde is an excellent fixative and much superior to formaldehyde.

Mounting. The fixed bacteria are spun down in the centrifuge and resuspended into a suitable volume in distilled water. A light or phase contrast microscope is used to ensure that the suspension is neither too dense not too dilute. A drop of the suspension is now placed on the surface of a supporting film on a grid. This can be done with a *very finely drawn* Pasteur pipette or a platinum loop. Experience is required to judge the size of drop used but it must not be so large that fluid spills and flows off the grid to adhere to its under side. After 2–3 min the organisms have settled on to the film and the fluid is removed by touching the drop with a fine strip of filter paper. The grid is now dried for a few hours over calcium chloride in a desiccator and is ready for examination.

Contrast Enhancement

Microorganisms fixed in this manner are seen in outline under the electron microscope but if their components and the minute details of their structure is to be seen some form of contrast enhancement is required (Valentine, 1961). This is usually achieved by the use of 'shadow casting' or by negative or positive staining techniques.

Shadow casting or metal shadowing consists of a technique whereby an atomic vapour of electron dense material is directed at an angle and deposited over the specimen. Heavy metals such as gold, platinum, palladium or their alloys are evaporated under a high vacuum in a special plant designed for the purpose (Bradley, 1961). The effect is that the side of the object farthest from the source of the heavy metal vapour is protected from the impinging atoms; these areas are more electron transparent than the overlaid areas and in electron micrographs look like shadows. The method is of particular value in the examination of bacteria bearing flagella, fimbriae and also in visualizing the filaments of spirochaetes.

Negative Staining. When virus particles or other small objects are added to a neutral solution of potassium phosphotungstate and the mixture is transferred to electron microscope grids the particles appear under the electron microscope as surrounded by an electron-dense background. Furthermore, any surface contours and depressions attract the tungstate so that details of the external characters of the object are revealed (Horne and Wildy, 1963). The method has been particularly successful in the study of the fine structure of animal viruses and bacteriophages but has many applications in microbiology.

Phosphotungstate Staining. The method is that of Brenner and Horne (1959). Specimens for examination are suspended in a volatile buffer such as 1 per cent ammonium acetate and then are added to an equal volume of 2·0 per cent phosphotungstic acid adjusted to pH 7·0 by the use of N/1 KOH. The mixture is placed on electron microscope grids in the way described or sprayed on them with a 'Vaponefrin' spray (Horne and Naginton, 1959). Sometimes the phosphotungstate fails to spread and forms dense masses in which the particles are completely buried. This may be corrected by the addition of a trace of serum albumin to reduce the surface tension or by reducing the concentration of phosphotungstate. If, on the other hand, the phosphotungstate spreads too widely and forms only a thin film the trouble can sometimes be overcome by increasing the tungstate concentration and/or diluting the virus preparation a little.

Uranyl acetate in a 1 per cent solution can be used in a similar way. It does not produce so great a contrast as phosphotungstate but is valuable for the very smallest particles and macromolecules. The deposited uranyl acetate has an even texture and is less 'grainy' than phosphotungstate.

Positive Staining has its main application in microbiology in the enhancement of the contrast in ultra-thin sections of bacteria, protozoa and other cells. Solutions of heavy metal compounds such as phosphotungstic acid, phosphomolybic acid, uranyl acetate, barium hydroxide, lead acetate and lead tartrate are all used.

Much information is obtained from the study of ultra-thin sections and the techniques involved include embedding in epoxy resins, the use of the ultra microtome and special staining methods. For the details of these techniques the reader is referred to Glauert and Phillips (1965) and Pease (1965).

REFERENCES

BARER, R. (1959) *Lecture Notes on the Use of the Microscope.* 2nd edn. Oxford: Blackwell.

BRADLEY, D. E. (1961) The preparation of specimen support films. In *Techniques for Electron Microscopy.* Chap. 3. Edited by D. Kay. Oxford: Blackwell.

BRENNER, S. & HORNE, R. W. (1959) A negative staining method for high resolution electron microscopy of viruses. *Biochemical and Biophysical Acta,* **34,** 103.

DAVIES, H. G., WILKINS, M. F. H., CHAYEN, J. & LA COUR, L. F. (1954) The use of the interference microscope to determine dry mass in living cells and as a quantitative cytochemical method. *Quarterly Journal of Microscope Science,* **95,** 271.

GLAUERT, A. M. (1965) The fixation, embedding, and staining of biological specimens. In *Techniques for Electron Microscopy.* Edited by D. Kay. 2nd edn. Oxford: Blackwell.

GLAUERT, A. M. & PHILLIPS, R. (1965) The preparation of thin sections. *Ibid.,* Chap. 9.

HALE, A. J. (1958) *The Interference Microscope.* Edinburgh: Livingstone.

HORNE, R. W. & NAGINTON, J. (1959) Electron microscope studies of the development of and structure of poliomyelitis virus. *Journal of Molecular Biology,* **1,** 333.

HORNE, R. W. & WILDY, P. (1963) Virus structure revealed by negative staining. *Advances in Virus Research,* **10,** 101.

KELLENBERGER, E., RYTER, A. & SÉCHAUD, J. (1958) Electron microscope study of DNA containing plasms. *Journal of Biophysical and Biochemical Cytology,* **4,** 671.

MCCARTNEY, J. E. (1951) An improved microscope lamp. *Journal of Clinical Pathology,* **4,** 234.

NAIRN, R. C. (1969) *Fluorescent Protein Tracing.* 3rd edn. Edinburgh: Livingstone.

PALADE, G. E. (1952) A study of fixation for electron microscopy. *Journal of Experimental Medicine,* **95,** 285.

PEASE, D. C. (1965) *Histological Techniques for Electron Microscopy.* 2nd edn. New York & London: Academic Press.

VALENTINE, R. C. (1961) Contrast enhancement in the electron microscopy of viruses. *Advances in Virus Research,* **8,** 287.

WREDDEN, J. H. (1947) *The Microscope.* London: Churchill.

2. Staining Methods

As bacteria consist of clear protoplasmic matter, differing but slightly in refractive index from the medium in which they are growing, it is difficult with the ordinary microscope, except when special methods of illumination are used, to see them in the unstained condition. Staining, therefore, is of primary importance for the recognition of bacteria.

The use and general principles of bacterial staining have been discussed in Vol. I, Chap. 2.

METHODS OF MAKING FILM OR SMEAR PREPARATIONS

Before describing the various staining processes, details of the methods employed in making films must be considered.

Film preparations are made either on coverslips or on the 3×1 in glass slides, usually the latter. It is essential that the coverslips or slides should be perfectly clean and free from grease, otherwise films will be uneven.

Cleaning Slides and Coverslips

Slides. A satisfactory method for ordinary use is to wipe the slide with a clean dry cotton cloth and then, holding its end with forceps, roast it free from grease by passing it 6–12 times through a blue Bunsen flame. The heating should be as strong as is possible without cracking the slide. Cracking is rendered less likely by allowing the slide to cool somewhat before laying down, or by laying it on a warmed metal rack. Another method of cleaning is to moisten the finger with water, rub it on the surface of some fine sand soap, and then smear the surface of the slide. After removing the soapy film with a clean cloth the surface is clean and free from grease. For special purposes, slides are cleaned by immersion in concentrated sulphuric acid saturated with potassium dichromate for several days at room temperature. If the slide is perfectly clean a drop of water can be spread over its surface in a thin even film; otherwise the water collects into small drops and a film cannot be made.

After the films have been made and examined the slides should be discarded. *They should not be cleaned and used again, since it is difficult to ensure that all organisms are removed.*

Coverslips. These should be $\frac{3}{4}$ or $\frac{7}{8}$ in^2 and of No. 1 thickness, i.e. 0·1 mm thick. (Thicker coverslips—No. 2—may prevent the oil-immersion objective from coming near enough for the specimen to be focused.) They are cleaned by the dichromate-sulphuric acid solution as described for slides; they are then well washed, first in tap water and later in distilled water, and stored in a stoppered jar in 50 per cent alcohol. Before use they are dried with a soft clean cloth, such as an old handkerchief. For routine use, the coverslips may be sufficiently clean as supplied by the maker and require only to be wiped free from grit and dust with a clean dry cloth. The newer plastic coverslips should not be used when staining as they melt or buckle during the process. They should be used only for unstained 'wet' preparations.

Making Films

In the case of fluid material, e.g. broth cultures, urine, sputum, pus, etc., one loopful (or more) is taken up with the inoculating wire and spread thinly on the slide. A little experience will soon determine the amount required, and in spreading the films it will be found that there are both thick and thin portions, which is not disadvantageous. The slide is then held in the palm of the hand high over a Bunsen flame and dried. The film is fixed by passing the *dried* slide, film downwards, three times slowly through the flame, or by heating through the glass slide. In the latter method the slide is held, film upwards, in the top of the Bunsen flame for a few seconds so that the slide becomes hot. Care must be taken not to char the film, and when the slide is just too hot to be borne on the back of the hand, fixation is complete.

In making films on coverslips and staining them, Cornet's forceps are used to hold the slip in a horizontal position, the forceps resting on the bench.

With solid material, such as cultures on agar, etc., it is necessary to place a loopful of clean water on the slide. The loop is then sterilized and a minute quantity of material, obtained by just touching the growth, is transferred to the drop, thoroughly emulsified, and the mixture is spread evenly on the slide. The resulting film is fixed and dried as above. *Beginners are apt to take more material than necessary from the culture and thus make too thick a film.*

STAINING OF FILMS

The stains are poured directly or filtered on to the slide. When staining is completed, the dye is washed off with water, and the slide is allowed to dry in the vertical position or is placed between two sheets of white fluffless blotting paper or filter paper. The drying of the film is completed over the Bunsen flame. Such stained films may be mounted in Canada balsam under a coverslip, or may be examined unmounted with the oil-immersion lens, a small drop of cedar-wood oil being placed directly on the film. If it is desired to mount the preparation later, the oil can be removed with xylene or benzene.

STAINING OF TISSUE SECTIONS

The sections being embedded in paraffin, it is necessary to remove the paraffin so that a watery stain may penetrate. The paraffin is first removed with xylol (xylene) or benzol (benzene), the xylol or benzol is then removed with alcohol (95 per cent ethanol), and the alcohol is replaced with water. The staining is then done. After staining, the section must be dehydrated with absolute alcohol, cleared in xylol and mounted in Canada balsam under a coverslip. The Canada balsam (which is a resin) is dissolved in xylol in order to render it suitable in consistency.

Alcohol (Ethanol) Solutions. The reagents most commonly employed in preparation of sections are 'absolute alcohol', which is 100 per cent ethanol, and '95 per cent alcohol', which is a 95 per cent solution of ethanol in water by volume (i.e. 95 ml absolute alcohol plus water to give 100 ml solution).

Industrial methylated spirit (not mineralized) may be used for making up stains, decolouriz-ing stained preparations, dehydrating tissues and treating sections. The type known as 'Toilet spirit, acetone free (66 OP)' is quite satisfactory for use instead of 95 per cent alcohol. Similarly, industrial methylated spirit, absolute (74 OP), can be used instead of absolute alcohol. Not only are these industrial spirits much cheaper than rectified spirit (90 per cent alcohol) and absolute alcohol, but permits for obtaining them duty-free are more readily granted by the customs authorities.

Technique. The slide bearing the paraffin section is placed in a jar of xylol for some minutes to remove the paraffin. The section is then treated with a few drops of absolute alcohol (ethanol), when it immediately becomes opaque. A few drops of 50 per cent alcohol are poured on, and the slide is finally washed gently in water. If the tissue has been fixed in any mercuric chloride preparation, such as Zenker's fluid, the section should be treated with Gram's iodine solution for a few minutes, then with 95 per cent alcohol and finally with water. The sections are now ready to be stained by the appropriate method. After staining and washing with water, the slide is wiped all round the section with a clean cloth to remove excess of water. The bulk of the water in the section may be removed by pressing between fluffless blotting paper. The section is treated *immediately* with a few drops of 95 per cent alcohol and then with absolute alcohol. The slide is again wiped all round the section, a few more drops of absolute alcohol are poured on and the slide is then immersed in xylol. When cleared, the slide is removed, and excess of xylol round the section is wiped away, a drop of Canada balsam is applied and the section mounted under a No. 1 coverslip. It is essential that the section should not be allowed to dry at any period of the process, and that dehydration with absolute alcohol should be complete in order that the section may be thoroughly cleared.

When the bacteria are readily decolourized with alcohol, aniline-xylol (aniline, 2 parts; xylol, 1 part) should be used for dehydration. After washing, when the slide has been wiped round the section, the preparation is blotted and then treated with the aniline-xylol mixture, which clears as well as dehydrates. The aniline-xylol is then replaced with xylol. This can be done conveniently by holding the slide almost vertically and dropping xylol from a drop bottle on to the slide just above the section. The xylol flows over the section and quickly removes the aniline. The preparation is mounted immediately in Canada balsam.

DPX Mounting Medium

A mounting medium that replaces Canada balsam has been devised by Kirkpatrick and Lendrum (1939, 1941). It consists of polystyrene (a synthetic resin) dissolved in xylol, with a plasticizer—dibutyl phthalate—to ensure flexibility. There is, however, much shrinkage and the mounting fluid should be applied generously. The mountant termed DPX is made up as follows:

Mix dibutyl phthalate (BDH) . 5 ml
with pure xylol. . . . 35 ml
and dissolve 'Distrene 80'. . 10 g

DPX medium is water-clear, inert and does not become acid or cause fading of stained preparations. It is used in the same way as Canada balsam.

If polystyrene of a low molecular weight (about 3000) is used, much less xylol is required and no plasticiser need be added. Moreover, there is practically no shrinkage, which is a great advantage over DPX.

SIMPLE STAINS

These show not only the presence of organisms but also the nature of the cellular content in exudates.

METHYLENE BLUE

Of the many preparations of this dye, Löffler's methylene blue is generally the most useful:

Saturated solution of methylene
blue in alcohol . . . . 300 ml
KOH, 0·01 per cent in water . . 1000 ml

Films. Stain for 3 min, then wash with water. This preparation does not readily over-stain.

Sections. Stain for 5 min or longer. The application of the alcohol during dehydration is sufficient for differentiation. Aniline-xylol can also be used for dehydration and clearing.

Polychrome Methylene Blue

This is made by allowing Löffler's methylene blue to 'ripen' slowly. The stain is kept in bottles, which are half filled and shaken at intervals to aerate thoroughly the contents. The slow oxidation of the methylene blue forms a violet compound that gives the stain its polychrome properties. The ripening takes 12 months or more to complete, or it may be ripened quickly by the addition of 1·0 per cent potassium carbonate (K_2CO_3) to the stain. The preparation is used in a manner similar to Löffler's methylene blue. It is also employed in McFadyean's reaction (Chap. 33).

Borax Methylene Blue (Masson)

This gives similar staining results to polychrome methylene blue:

Methylene blue . . . . 20 g
Borax . . . . . 50 g
Water . . . . . 1000 ml

Warm the water to 60°C, stir in the solids, and allow to cool slowly. This staining solution improves with age.

DILUTE CARBOL FUCHSIN

Made by diluting Ziehl-Neelsen's stain (see below) with 10–15 times its volume of water. Stain for 10–25 s and wash well with water. Over-staining must be avoided, as this is an intense stain, and prolonged application colours the cell protoplasm in addition to nuclei and bacteria.

NEGATIVE STAINING

'Negative staining' is exemplified by Burri's India ink method, which was formerly used for the spirochaete of syphilis. A small quantity of India ink is mixed on a slide with the culture or other material containing bacteria, and then by means of another slide or loop a thin film is made; this is allowed to dry before being examined. The bacteria or spirochaetes are seen as clear transparent objects on a dark-brown background. (See below, also India ink methods for capsules.)

FLEMING'S NIGROSIN METHOD

A 10 per cent solution of nigrosin (G. T. Gurr) is made in warm distilled water (solution is effected in about an hour) and filtered. Formalin 0·5 per cent (i.e. formaldehyde 0·19 per cent) is added as a preservative. A small drop of the dye is placed on a slide, bacteria are mixed with it and a smear is made with a loop or another slide. A number of preparations can be made on the same slide. Dry and examine.

Nigrosin gives an absolutely homogeneous background, and this is the simplest method of making a preliminary examination of a culture to show shape, size and arrangement of bacteria. Most bacteria stand out as clear objects on a dark field, but some bacilli, such as those of the coliform and haemophilic groups, show in their central portion a slightly dark patch somewhat resembling a nucleus.

GRAM'S STAINING METHOD

This is the most important staining method in bacteriology, and must be employed for the diagnostic identification of various organisms. The principle of the method has been dealt with in Vol. I, Chapter 2.

Certain bacteria when treated with one of the basic para-rosaniline dyes such as methyl violet, crystal violet or gentian violet (which is a mixture of the two preceding dyes), and then with iodine, 'fix' the stain so that subsequent treatment with a decolourizing agent—e.g. alcohol or acetone—does not remove the colour. Other organisms, however, are decolourized by this process. If a mixture of various organisms are thus stained and subjected to the decolourizing agent, it is found that some species retain the dye, and these are termed 'Gram-positive', whereas others are completely decolourized and are termed 'Gram-negative'. In order to render the decolourized organisms visible, and to distinguish them from those retaining the colour, a contrast or counterstain is then applied. This counterstain is usually red, in order that the Gram-negative organisms may easily be differentiated from the Gram-positive organisms, which retain the original violet stain.

If Gram's method is properly carried out, Gram-positive organisms and fibrin are stained dark violet in colour. Gram-negative organisms, the nuclei and protoplasm of pus cells and tissue cells are stained pink with the counterstain. To obviate errors from overdecolourizing, a control film of a known Gram-positive organism (e.g. a pure culture of *Staphylococcus aureus*) may be made at one side of the film to be examined. For the recognition of Gram-negative organisms such as gonococci or meningococci in pus, this control must retain the violet stain while the nuclei of the pus cells are stained only with the counterstain.

In the original method of Gram (1884), the smear was stained with aniline-gentian violet, treated with Lugol's iodine (iodine 1 g, KI 2 g, water 300 ml), decolourized with absolute alcohol, and counterstained with Bismarck brown. Later modifications, however, have given better results.

KOPELOFF AND BEERMAN'S (1922) MODIFICATION
(Decolourization with acetone)

This method, which is a modification of Burke's (1922) method, is recommended for general use.

Solutions Required

1. Methyl violet stain
   Solution A
   Methyl violet 6B . . . 10 g
   Distilled water . . . 1000 ml
   Solution B
   Sodium bicarbonate (NaHCO$_3$) 50 g
   Distilled water . . . 1000 ml

Shortly before use, mix 30 volumes of solution A with 8 volumes of solution B. (The mixture is apt to precipitate within a few days and so cannot be kept. Methyl violet solution *without* the addition of bicarbonate acts almost as well in Gram staining and has the advantage of keeping indefinitely. For critical work, however, a freshly made mixture of stain with bicarbonate is to be preferred.)

2. Iodine solution
   Iodine . . . . . 20 g
   Normal solution of sodium hydroxide (i.e. 1N NaOH, or 4 per cent NaOH) . . . 100 ml
   Distilled water . . . 900 ml

Dissolve the iodine in the NaOH solution and, when it is dissolved, add the distilled water.

3. Basic fuchsin stain

Basic fuchsin	. .	0·5 or 1·0 g
Distilled water	. .	1000 ml

Procedure for Staining Films

1. Make a smear on a slide according to the instructions given on p. 31. Dry thoroughly in cool air or in warm air *far above* a Bunsen flame. Then, fix by flaming in the usual way (p. 31).

2. Cover the whole slide with methyl violet stain and allow this to remain on the slide for about 5 min.

3. Tip off the methyl violet stain, hold the slide at a steep slope and wash off the residual stain with an *excess* of iodine solution; begin by pouring the iodine on the upper end of the slide and rapidly work downwards. (It is important to use enough iodine solution to wash away all the crystalline deposit that forms when the stain and the iodine mix.)

4. Cover the whole slide with fresh iodine solution and leave it thus for about 2 min.

5. Decolourize with acetone (100 per cent). First tip off the iodine and hold the slide at a steep slope. Then pour acetone over the slide from its upper end, so as to cover its whole surface. Decolourization is very rapid, and is usually complete in 2–3 s. After this period of contact the acetone must *at once* be removed by washing thoroughly with water under a running tap. To avoid delay, the tap should be running before the acetone is applied to the slide.

(Kopeloff and Beerman recommended that the acetone should be added to the slide drop by drop until no colour is seen in the washings; they noted that decolourization generally requires less than 10 s and that the time should be reduced to a minimum. We have found that, with thin smears, successful results are obtained more consistently if the acetone is flooded over the slide and then washed off with water after only 2 seconds' contact.)

6. Cover the whole slide with basic fuchsin stain and allow this to remain for about 30 s.

7. Wash thoroughly (for about 5 s) in water from the tap, blot and dry in air.

Normally a Gram-stained film is examined under oil-immersion without mounting under a coverslip. The oil can be removed with xylol or benzol if it is desired to preserve the film.

Procedure for staining sections

1. Remove paraffin with xylol or benzol.

2. Treat the section with absolute alcohol (ethanol) and wash in tap water.

3. Cover the slide with methyl violet stain and allow to act for 5 min.

4. Wash off stain with an excess of iodine solution, cover with more iodine and allow to act for 2 min.

5. Decolourize with acetone (see above). The visible violet staining should be removed from the section and this may take one or two seconds longer than is necessary in the decolourization of films.

6. Wash slide in water from tap.

7. Counterstain with basic fuchsin for 30 s.

8. Wipe carefully around the section to remove as much water as possible, dehydrate quickly in absolute alcohol, clear in xylol or benzol and mount in Canada balsam or DPX.

Use of acetone-alcohol as decolourizer

Kopeloff and Beerman's method is sometimes modified by the substitution of acetone-alcohol in the place of pure acetone as decolourizer. Acetone-alcohol is a mixture of 1 volume of acetone with 1 volume of 95 per cent ethyl alcohol (ethanol). It acts rather more slowly than pure acetone and decolourization may be prolonged to 10 s or more, and can be more carefully adjusted in duration. It is not, however, considered to be quite as satisfactory as pure acetone in producing specific differential decolourization.

BURKE'S (1922) MODIFICATION OF GRAM'S METHOD
(Decolourization with acetone)

1. Make smear, dry in air, and fix by flaming.

2. Cover the slide with 1 per cent aqueous methyl violet (or crystal violet). Then add 5 drops of a 5 per cent solution of sodium bicarbonate to the dye on the slide, mix, and allow to act for 3 min.

3. Tip off the stain and flush the slide freely

with iodine solution (iodine 10 g, potassium iodide 20 g, and distilled water 1000 ml). Cover slide with fresh iodine solution and allow to act for 1–2 min.

4. Wash in water from tap, blot off all free water, but do not allow smear to dry. (Alternatively, blot the iodine from the slide.)

5. Decolourize with acetone (100 per cent) or acetone-ether (1 volume of ether and 2 volumes of acetone). Cover the slide with the decolourizer, stand for a few seconds, drain off, cover with fresh decolourizer for 1–2 s and drain off. Decolourization usually requires a total duration of contact of less than 10 s.

6. At once blot slide and allow to dry in air.

7. Counterstain for 10 s or longer with a 2 per cent aqueous solution of safranine (or neutral red).

8. Wash off counterstain by flushing with water for a few seconds, blot and allow to dry in air.

JENSEN'S MODIFICATION OF GRAM'S METHOD
(Decolourization with alcohol)

This modification can be recommended for routine bacteriological work. It has been used especially in examination of exudates for gonococci and meningococci.

Solutions Required

1. Methyl violet stain
   Methyl violet 6B (or crystal
   violet) .   .   .   .   . 5 g
   Distilled water   .   .   . 1000 ml
The solution should be made up in bulk and filtered. It keeps indefinitely, and does not precipitate, but should be filtered again before use.

2. Iodine solution*
   Iodine .   .   .   .   . 10 g
   Potassium iodide   .   . 20 g
   Distilled water   .   .   . 1000 ml
Dissolve 20 g potassium iodide in 250 ml

water, and then add 10 g iodine; when dissolved make up to 1000 ml with water.

3. Counterstain—neutral red solution
   Neutral red .   .   .   . 1 g
   1 per cent acetic acid   .   . 2 ml
   Distilled water   .   .   . 1000 ml

Procedure for Films

These are made, dried and fixed in the usual way.

1. Cover the slide with methyl violet solution and allow to act for about 30 s.

2. Pour off stain and, holding the slide at an angle downwards, pour on the iodine solution so that it washes away the methyl violet. Cover the slide with fresh iodine and allow to act for about 30 s.

3. Wash off the iodine with absolute alcohol (ethanol) and treat with fresh alcohol, tilting the slide from side to side until colour ceases to come out of the preparation. This is easily seen by holding the slide against a white background.

4. Wash with water.

5. Apply the counterstain for 1–2 min.

6. Wash with water and dry between blotting paper.

This method is very simple and gives excellent results with freedom from deposit. Safranine, 0·5 per cent in distilled water, may be substituted for neutral red as counterstain. Basic fuchsin, 0·05 per cent, may be used for up to 30 s, but dilute carbol fuchsin should not be used because it tends to stain Gram-negative bacteria so intensely that they may appear Gram-positive.

For the gonococcus and meningococcus in films, *Sandiford's counterstain* is useful, particularly when the organisms are scanty.

Malachite green   .   .   . 0·05 g
Pyronine .   .   .   . 0·15 g
Distilled water   .   .   to 100 ml
(The stain keeps for about a month only.)

---

* Iodine solution does not keep well and it is convenient, especially where stains are distributed from a central source, to have potassium iodide and iodine mixed ready for solution when required. Potassium iodide tends to be hygroscopic and must be dried, otherwise the mixture becomes sticky and lumpy. Place the potassium iodide in a thin layer in a Petri dish overnight in a desiccator over calcium chloride. Mix two parts of potassium iodide by weight with one part of iodine in a mortar. Weigh out at once amounts of 7·5 g and place them in 1-oz screw-capped bottles and screw down the caps. This is sufficient for 250 ml of solution. The mixture keeps indefinitely and easily 'pours' from the bottle. For use, place the contents of one bottle into an empty 10-oz screw-capped bottle. Add about 50 ml distilled water and agitate until the iodine is dissolved. Make up to 250 ml with distilled water.

Apply the counterstain for 2 min, flood off with water (but do not wash) and blot. Cells and nuclei stain bluish green. Gram-positive organisms are purple-black and gonococci red. It should be noted that not all samples of pyronine are satisfactory for this stain, so that with each new purchase of pyronine the made-up stain should be tested on a film known to contain gonococci or meningococci.

WEIGERT'S MODIFICATION OF GRAM'S METHOD
(Decolourization with aniline-xylol)

Solutions Required

1. Carbol gentian violet
   Saturated alcoholic solution of
   gentian violet . . . 1 part
   5 per cent solution of phenol in
   distilled water . . . 10 parts
   (This mixture should be made up each day, as it tends to precipitate.)
2. Gram's (Lugol's) iodine
   Iodine . . . . . 1 g
   Potassium iodide . . 2 g
   Distilled water . . 300 ml
3. Aniline-xylol
   Aniline . . . . 2 parts
   Xylol . . . . . 1 part
4. Carmalum solution
   Carminic acid . . . 1 g
   Potassium alum . . 10 g
   Distilled water . . 200 ml
   Dissolve with gentle heat; filter and add 1 ml formalin as preservative.

Procedure for Sections

Weigert's modification is specially recommended for the staining of sections.
1. Remove the paraffin with xylol or benzol, treat with alcohol, wash with water and counterstain with carmalum for 10 min.
2. Stain with carbol gentian violet for 2–3 min.
3. Pour off stain, replace with Gram's iodine solution and allow to act for 1 min.
4. Dry thoroughly by blotting.
5. Decolourize with aniline-xylol, using several changes until the stain ceases to be removed.

Now examine at this stage under the low power of the microscope; the nuclei of the pus cells should be of a pale-violet colour; if the nuclei are deeply stained, then decolourization is incomplete.
6. Wash with several changes of xylol and dry.
7. Mount on Canada balsam or DPX.

PRESTON AND MORRELL'S (1962) MODIFICATION OF GRAM'S METHOD
(Decolourization with iodine-acetone)

This method is recommended as giving reliable results without the need for taking great care in adjusting the duration of decolourization.

Solutions Required

1. Ammonium oxalate-crystal violet
   Crystal violet . . . 20 g
   Methylated spirit (64 OP) . 200 ml
   Ammonium oxalate, 1 per cent
   in water . . . . 800 ml
2. Iodine solution
   Iodine . . . . . 10 g
   Potassium iodide . . 20 g
   Distilled water . . 1000 ml
3. Liquor iodi fortis (BP)
   Iodine . . . . . 10 g
   Potassium iodide . . 6 g
   Methylated spirit (74 OP) . 90 ml
   Distilled water . . 10 ml
4. Iodine-acetone
   Liquor iodi fortis . . 35 ml
   Acetone . . . . 965 ml
5. Dilute carbol fuchsin
   Ziehl-Neelsen's (strong) carbol
   fuchsin . . . . 50 ml
   Distilled water . . 950 ml

Procedure for Films

1. Cover slide with ammonium oxalate-crystal violet and allow to act for about 30 s.
2. Pour off and wash freely with iodine solution. Cover with fresh iodine solution and allow to act for about 30 s.
3. Pour off iodine solution and wash freely with iodine-acetone. Cover with fresh iodine-acetone and allow to act for about 30 s.

4. Wash thoroughly with water.

5. Counterstain with dilute carbol fuchsin for about 30 s.

6. Wash with water, blot and dry.

It is essential that the whole slide is flooded with each reagent in turn, and that the previous reagent is thoroughly removed at each step.

STAINING OF TUBERCLE AND OTHER ACID-FAST BACILLI
ZIEHL-NEELSEN METHOD

This method is a modification of Ehrlich's (1882) original method for the differential staining of acid-fast bacilli with aniline-gentian violet followed by strong nitric acid. It incorporates improvements suggested, successively, by Ziehl and Neelsen, and is described in a footnote in a paper by Johne (1885).

The ordinary aniline dye solutions do not readily penetrate the substance of the tubercle bacillus and are therefore unsuitable for staining it. However, by the use of a powerful staining solution that contains phenol, and the application of heat, the dye can be made to penetrate the bacillus. Once stained, the tubercle bacillus will withstand the action of powerful decolourizing agents for a considerable time and thus still retains the stain when everything else in the microscopic preparation has been decolourized.

The stain used consists of basic fuchsin, with phenol added. The dye is basic and its combination with a mineral acid produces a compound that is yellowish brown in colour and is readily dissolved out of all structures except acid-fast bacteria. Any strong acid can be used as a decolourizing agent, but 20 per cent sulphuric acid (by volume) is usually employed. Acid-alcohol may also be used.

In order to show structures and cells, including non-acid-fast bacteria, that have been decolourized, and to form a contrast with the red-stained bacilli, the preparation is counterstained with methylene blue or malachite green.

Solutions Required

1. Ziehl-Neelsen's (strong) carbol fuchsin
   Basic fuchsin . . . 10 g
   Absolute alcohol (ethanol) . 100 ml

Solution of phenol (5 per cent in water) . . . . 1000 ml
Dissolve the dye in the alcohol and add to the phenol solution.

An alternative and quicker preparation is as follows:
   Basic fuchsin (powder) . . 5 g
   Phenol (crystalline) . . 25 g
   Alcohol (95 per cent or absolute) . . . . . 50 ml
   Distilled water . . . 500 ml

Dissolve the fuchsin in the phenol by placing them in a one-litre flask over a boiling water-bath for about 5 min, shaking the contents from time to time. When there is complete solution add the alcohol and mix thoroughly. Then add the distilled water. Filter the mixture before use.

2. Sulphuric acid, 20 per cent solution

Place 800 ml water in a large flask. Add 200 ml concentrated sulphuric acid (about 98 per cent; about 1·835 g per ml). The acid should be poured slowly down the side of the flask into the water, about 50 ml at a time. The mixture will become hot. Mix gently; add remainder of acid in same manner.

Note. The acid must be added to the water. It is *dangerous* to add the water to the acid. Great care must be taken to avoid spilling the acid on skin or clothing, or elsewhere. Especial care must be taken to avoid splashing or spurting into the eye. In event of such an accident occurring the eye should at once be washed with an excess of clean water and medical advice sought.

3. Alcohol 95 per cent
   Ethanol 95 ml plus water to 100 ml
4. Counterstain
   Löffler's methylene blue (p. 33)

Procedure for Films

These are made, dried and fixed by flaming in the usual manner.

1. Cover the slide with filtered carbol fuchsin and heat until steam rises. Allow the preparation to stain for 5 min, heat being applied at intervals to keep the stain hot. The stain must not be allowed to evaporate and dry on the slide; if necessary, pour on more carbol fuchsin to keep the whole slide covered with liquid.

(*Note*. The slide may be heated with a torch prepared by twisting a *small* piece of cotton wool on to the tip of an inoculating wire and soaking it in methylated spirit before lighting. When steam rises from the slide, remove and extinguish the torch. After about 1 min recharge the torch with spirit, relight it, and again heat the slide until the steam rises. Continue in this way for 5 min.)

2. Wash with water.

3. Cover the slide with 20 per cent sulphuric acid. The red colour of the preparation is changed to yellowish brown. After about a minute in the acid, wash the slide with water, and pour on more acid. Repeat this process several times. The object of the washing is to remove the compound of acid with stain and allow fresh acid to gain access to the preparation. The decolourization is finished when, after washing, the film is only very faintly pink.

Decolourization generally requires contact with sulphuric acid for a total time of at least 10 min.

4. Wash the slide well in water.

5. Treat with 95 per cent alcohol for 2 min. This step is optional, and may be omitted; see below.

6. Wash with water.

7. Counterstain with Löffler's methylene blue or dilute malachite green for 15–20 s.

8. Wash, blot, dry and mount.

Acid-fast bacilli stain bright red, while the tissue cells and other organisms are stained blue or green according to the counterstain used. If tissue cells appear red, the preparation has not been adequately decolourized with sulphuric acid.

Note. The practice of using staining jars in the Ziehl-Neelsen method is to be condemned, as with a positive sputum, stained tubercle bacilli may become detached and float about in the staining fluid or decolourizing agent. After a number of strongly positive films have been passed through the staining jars the number of free stained tubercle bacilli may be considerable. Negative material may, during the staining process, pick up these bacilli and so appear positive when examined microscopically. These false positives can give rise to serious errors of diagnosis. Each slide, therefore, should be stained individually by pouring on the stain from a bottle, the washing done with a stream of tap water and the subsequent decolourizing and staining fluids added to the film from bottles. When drying with blotting paper, a fresh clean piece of paper is used for each slide and then discarded. The practice of using a number of large sheets for drying a succession of slides is also condemned as tubercle bacilli from a positive film may adhere to the blotting paper and subsequently be transferred to a negative film.

Use of alcohol for secondary decolourization. After primary decolourization with sulphuric acid, the film may be treated with 95 per cent alcohol as a secondary decolourizer (step 5, above). The basis of this practice is the fact that tubercle bacilli are alcohol-fast as well as acid-fast. One advantage of using alcohol is that decolourization is completed more quickly and the margins and underside of the slide are more completely cleaned and freed from deposits of stain.

Another advantage of using alcohol when the staining is being done for identification of tubercle bacilli, is that certain other acid-fast bacilli, which may be encountered in pathological specimens and may otherwise be confused with tubercle bacilli, are decolourized by alcohol. Thus, specimens of urine often contain the smegma bacillus, an acid-fast bacillus that is a harmless commensal inhabitant in the region of the urethral orifice. Some, though not all strains of smegma bacillus are decolourized with alcohol and the use of alcohol thus lessens, though it does not entirely remove the likelihood of confusion arising in the diagnosis of urinary tract tuberculosis.

Acid-alcohol as decolourizer. Instead of employing 20 per cent sulphuric acid as a decolourizing agent, 3 per cent hydrochloric acid in 95 per cent alcohol (industrial methylated spirit) may be used (i.e. concentrated HCl, 3 ml, and 95 per cent alcohol, 97 ml). The necessity for subsequent treatment with alcohol, as in the original method, is obviated. Acid-alcohol is a more expensive reagent than sulphuric acid, but it is much less corrosive and more convenient to make up and employ, while its use definitely excludes organisms that are acid-fast but not alcohol-fast.

Malachite green as counterstain. Malachite

green is also recommended as a counterstain in the Ziehl-Neelsen method. A stock solution of 1 per cent in distilled water is made, and for use a small quantity is diluted with distilled water in a drop-bottle so that 15–20 seconds' application of the weak stain gives the background a pale green tint. Deep counterstaining must be avoided. The pale green background is pleasant for the eyes, and is required for the method in which a deep blue-green filter is used for the easy recognition of tubercle bacilli.

Procedure for Sections

Sections are treated with xylol to remove paraffin, then with alcohol, and finally are washed in water.

1. Stain with Ziehl-Neelsen's stain as described for films, but heat gently, otherwise the section may become detached from the slide.

2. Wash with water.

3. Decolourize with 20 per cent sulphuric acid or acid-alcohol as for films. The process takes longer owing to the thickness of the section, and care must be exercised in washing to retain the section on the slide.

4. Wash well with water.

5. Counterstain with methylene blue or malachite green for $\frac{1}{2}$–1 min.

6. Wash with water.

7. Wipe the slide dry all round the section, blot with filter paper or fluffless blotting paper, and treat with a few drops of absolute alcohol. Pour on more absolute alcohol, wipe the slide again and clear in xylol.

8. Mount in Canada balsam or DPX.

Modifications of the Ziehl-Neelsen Method

1. Leprosy bacilli are also acid-fast, but usually to a less degree than the tubercle bacillus. They are stained in films or sections in the same way as the tubercle bacillus, except that 5 per cent sulphuric acid is used for decolourization.

2. Sections of tissues containing 'clubs' caused by *Actinomyces*, *Mycobacterium* and *Nocardia* can be treated with 1 per cent H_2SO_4 to demonstrate the acid-fastness of the clubs.

3. Cultures of some *Nocardia spp.* are acid-fast when decolourized with 0·5 per cent H_2SO_4.

4. Most spores are acid-fast; for methods see p. 41.

5. *Brucella differential stain:* a useful differential stain for the demonstration of *Br. abortus* in infected material. Dilute (1 in 10) carbol-fuchsin is allowed to act, without heating, for 15 min. The slide is then decolourized with 0·5 per cent acetic acid solution for 15 s, washed thoroughly and counterstained with Löffler's methylene-blue for 1 min. This method may also be used for demonstrating chlamydia in tissue sections.

STAINING WITH FLUOROCHROME DYES

AURAMINE O. This dye can be substituted for carbol fuchsin in the Ziehl-Neelsen method with the effect that the tubercle bacilli fluoresce and become much easier to detect.

Staining solution

Auramine 'O' . . .	0·3 g
Phenol . . .	3·0 g
Distilled water . .	97·0 ml

Dissolve the phenol in water with gentle heat. Add the auramine gradually and shake vigorously until dissolved. Filter and store in a dark stoppered bottle.

Decolourizing solution. 75 per cent industrial alcohol containing 0·5 per cent NaCl and 0·5 per cent HCl.

Potassium Permanganate Solution. 1 in 1000. Stain a thin smear of sputum with auramine solution for 15 min. Rinse under the tap and decolourize for 5 min with the acid-alcohol. Wash well in tap water, apply permanganate solution for 30 s, wash well in tap water and allow to dry. (Do not use blotting paper to dry.)

The film is examined dry with a $\frac{1}{6}$-in (4 mm) objective, or preferably with an 8-mm objective and a high-power eye-piece. The tubercle bacilli are seen as yellow luminous organisms in a dark field. A darkened room is an advantage. When fluorescent bacilli have been detected with the low power objective their morphology is checked by observation under the oil immersion objective.

This method has the advantage that large areas of a film of sputum can be scanned in a short space of time.

STAINING OF DIPHTHERIA BACILLUS AND VOLUTIN-CONTAINING ORGANISMS

The diphtheria bacillus gives its characteristic volutin-staining reactions best in a young culture (18–24 h) on a blood or serum medium.

ALBERT-LAYBOURN METHOD

Laybourn's (1924) modification, in which malachite green is substituted for methyl green, is given here instead of the original method of Albert. It is recommended for routine use.

Toluidine blue . . . . 1·5 g
Malachite green . . . . 2·0 g
Glacial acetic acid . . . 10 ml
Alcohol (95 per cent ethanol) . . 20 ml
Distilled water . . . . 1000 ml

Dissolve the dyes in the alcohol and add to the water and acetic acid. Allow to stand for one day and then filter.

Albert's Iodine

Iodine . . . . . 6 g
Potassium iodide . . . . 9 g
Distilled water . . . . 900 ml

Note. The iodine solution used in Jensen's modification of Gram's method works equally well.

Procedure

1. Make film, dry in air, and fix by heat.
2. Cover slide with Albert's stain and allow to act for 3–5 min.
3. Wash in water and blot dry.
4. Cover slide with Albert's iodine and allow to act for 1 min.
5. Wash and blot dry.

By this method the granules stain bluish black, the protoplasm green and other organisms mostly light green.

NEISSER'S METHOD (Modified)

The following modification of Neisser's method gives better results than the original:

Neisser's Methylene Blue Stain

Methylene blue . . . . 1 g
Ethyl alcohol (95 per cent) . . 50 ml
Glacial acetic acid . . . 50 ml
Distilled water . . . . 1000 ml

Procedure

1. Stain with Neisser's methylene blue for 3 min.
2. Wash off with dilute iodine solution (iodine solution of Kopeloff and Beerman's modification of Gram's method, diluted 1 in 10 with water) and leave some of this solution on the slide for 1 min.
3. Wash in water.
4. Counterstain with neutral red solution for 3 min, using the same solution as that employed in Jensen's modification of Gram's method (p. 36).
5. Wash in water and dry.

By this method the bacilli exhibit deep blue granules and the remainder of the organism assumes a pink colour.

STAINING OF SPORES

If spore-bearing organisms are stained with ordinary dyes, or by Gram's stain, the body of the bacillus is deeply coloured, whereas the spore is unstained and appears as a clear area in the organism. This is the way in which spores are most commonly observed. If desired, however, it is possible by vigorous staining procedures to introduce dye into the substance of the spore. When thus stained, the spore tends to retain the dye after treatment with decolourizing agents, and in this respect behaves similarly to the tubercle bacillus.

ACID-FAST STAIN FOR SPORES

Films, which must be thin, are made, dried and fixed in the usual manner with the minimum amount of heating.

1. Stain with Ziehl-Neelsen's carbol fuchsin for 3–5 min, heating the preparation until steam rises.
2. Wash in water.
3. Treat with $\frac{1}{4}$ or $\frac{1}{2}$ per cent sulphuric acid for one to several minutes, the period being determined by trial for each culture. *Alterna-*

tively, excellent results are obtained by de-colourizing in a 2 per cent solution of nitric acid in absolute ethyl alcohol; the slide is dipped once rapidly in the solution and immediately washed in water.

4. Wash with water.

5. Counterstain with 1 per cent aqueous methylene blue for 3 min.

6. Wash in water, blot and dry.

The spores are stained bright red and the protoplasm of the bacilli blue.

It should be noted that the spores of some bacteria are decolourized more readily than those of others and that lipid inclusion granules may stain dark red, appearing like small spherical spores.

MALACHITE GREEN STAIN FOR SPORES
(Method of Schaeffer and Fulton, modified by Ashby (1938))

Films are dried and fixed with minimal flaming.

1. Place the slide over a beaker of boiling water, resting it on the rim with the bacterial film uppermost.

2. When, within several seconds, large droplets have condensed on the underside of the slide, flood it with a 5 per cent aqueous solution of malachite green and leave to act for 1 min while the water continues to boil.

3. Wash in cold water.

4. Treat with 0·5 per cent safranine or 0·05 per cent basic fuchsin for 30 s.

5. Wash and dry.

This method colours the spores green and the vegetative bacilli red. Lipid granules are unstained.

STAINING OF CAPSULES

Capsules. The capsules of bacteria present in animal tissues, blood, serous fluids and pus are often clearly stained when these materials are treated by one of the common stains such as basic fuchsin, polychrome methylene blue, Leishman's stain and Gram's stain (which colours them with the red counterstain). Special capsule stains may be of little advantage in such cases. On the other hand, when artificial cultures of bacteria are being examined, the capsules normally are not coloured by ordinary staining methods and special methods must be employed for their demonstration, e.g. 'negative' or 'relief' staining.

The best method for staining capsules on bacteria from cultures in either liquid or solid media is the wet-film India ink method. Dry-film negative staining methods using India ink, nigrosin or eosin are somewhat less reliable since occasionally shrinkage spaces give the appearance of capsules around bacteria that are non-capsulate and occasionally, especially in thick films, capsules may be shrunken or obscured to the point that they are rendered invisible. Dry film methods in which *positive* staining of capsules is attempted are the least reliable and are not recommended. The advantages and disadvantages of all these different methods are discussed by Duguid (1951).

Loose slime. Many capsulate and some non-capsulate bacteria secrete extracellularly a viscid material, generally polysaccharide in composition. This may be seen in preparations made by some of the methods used for staining of capsules. The wet-film India ink method and the dry-film eosin method (see below) are recommended for this purpose. The slime appears as irregular masses of amorphous material lying between the bacteria and outside the capsules of capsulate ones.

DEMONSTRATION OF CAPSULES IN WET INDIA INK FILMS

If a permanent preparation is required for demonstration of bacterial capsules, it is necessary that a dry-film method should be employed, as described below; otherwise capsules are best observed in very thin wet films of India ink. This is the simplest, most informative and most generally applicable method of demonstrating capsules. The capsules do not become shrunken, since they are not dried or fixed, and they are clearly apparent even when very narrow.

A microscope slide is carefully wiped free from grit particles. A loopful of India ink is placed on it. A small portion of solid bacterial culture is emulsified in the drop of ink, or else a loopful of liquid culture is mixed with the ink. A clean coverslip is placed on the ink drop; it is pressed down firmly through a sheet of blotting paper so that the ink film becomes very thin and thus pale in colour. The film should be so thin that the bacterial cell with its capsule is 'gripped' between the slide and coverslip, neither being overlaid by ink nor being capable of moving about.

Some practice is required in making satisfactory films. A *large* loopful of ink should be used and a *very small* speck of solid culture material. The latter is rubbed on the slide just beside the drop of ink before mixing it into the ink.

On microscopical examination with the oil-immersion objective the highly refractile outline of the bacterium is seen. Between this refractile surface-membrane and the dark background of ink particles there is a clear space which represents the capsule; the capsular zone may be from a fraction of a micrometre to several micrometres in width. Non-capsulated bacteria do not show this clear zone; the ink particles directly abut the refractile cell wall and, in consequence, these bacteria are not easily seen. When solid bacterial culture is newly mixed with the ink, any *loose slime* in it can be seen as irregular strands and masses, lighter than the ink, which gradually disperse from the bacteria and dissolve in the ink. Loose slime is generally invisible if the preparations are made from cultures in a liquid medium.

Note. Sometimes a bottle of India ink becomes contaminated with a capsulated saprophytic bacterium. To avoid error from this cause, a film of the ink alone should be examined microscopically and proved to be free from capsulated bacteria.

Use of phase-contrast microscope. It is recommended that wet India ink films should be examined with a phase-contrast microscope. Since the bodies of the bacteria are not stained in such films their outlines are only faintly visible under the ordinary microscope. With the phase-contrast microscope the bodies of the bacteria appear dark and are seen in clear contrast to the bright capsular zones surrounding them.

DEMONSTRATION OF CAPSULES IN DRY INDIA INK FILMS
(Method of Butt, Bonynge and Joyce (1936))

1. Place a loopful of 6 per cent glucose in water at one end of a slide. Add a small amount of bacterial culture to this and mix to form an even suspension. Add a loopful of India ink to the drop, and mix.

2. Spread the mixture over the slide in a thin film with the edge of a second glass slide. Dry thoroughly by waving in the air.

3. Fix the film by pouring over it some undiluted Leishman stain or methyl alcohol. Drain off excess at once and dry thoroughly by warming over a flame.

4. Drop on methyl violet solution as used in Gram's stain, and stain for one or two minutes. Wash in water. Blot and dry over a flame.

5. Examine directly with the oil-immersion objective.

DEMONSTRATION OF CAPSULES BY RELIEF STAINING WITH EOSIN
(Method of Howie and Kirkpatrick (1934))

Staining solution

10 per cent water-soluble eosin, 'yellowish' or 'bluish', or erythrosin in distilled water . . . . 4 parts
Serum (human, rabbit, sheep or ox, heated at 56°C for thirty minutes) . 1 part
Crystal of thymol

Allow the mixture to stand at room temperature for several days. Centrifuge and store the supernatant fluid at room temperature; it will keep for several months.

On a slide with a 1-mm diameter wire loop, mix one drop of exudate (or fluid culture, or a suspension in *broth* from an agar slope culture) with one drop of the eosin solution and leave for about 1 min. Spread a film with the edge of another slide as in making a blood film. Allow to dry without heating and examine with the oil-immersion objective.

Capsulated organisms stained by this method show a practically homogeneous red background with an unstained or lightly stained capsular area and bacterial bodies stained red of about the same intensity as the background. The capsules are thus seen by 'relief staining'. If free slime is present in the culture, it is often seen as a light granular or fibrous deposit distributed throughout the red background between the bacilli.

DEMONSTRATION OF FLAGELLA

Because of their extreme thinness, flagella are best demonstrated with the electron microscope; metal-shadowed films or films made with phosphotungstic acid (PTA) for 'negative staining' are employed. Flagella can also be demonstrated by the light microscope, using special staining methods which require most careful attention to details of technique. To make possible their resolution, the flagella must be thickened at least ten-fold by a superficial deposition of stain. In spite of this, their characteristic arrangement and wave form are generally distinguishable.

STAINING OF FLAGELLA BY A MODIFICATION OF LEIFSON'S METHOD

The stain, basic fuchsin with tannic acid, is deposited on the bacteria and flagella from an evaporating alcoholic solution. The degree of staining is controlled by an exact determination of the duration of exposure. Good results depend to a large extent on preliminary thorough cleaning and flaming of the glass slides.

1. Clean the glass slides with absolute alcohol, rubbing with a fine cotton cloth. Then immerse them in concentrated sulphuric acid saturated with potassium dichromate for several days at room temperature or for an hour at 90°C. (In the latter case it is advisable to place the beaker of solution in a strong metal container with sand while heating.) *During all subsequent stages until staining is complete, take care not to finger the slides, even at their edges, and do not let them touch surfaces not properly cleaned and grease-free.* Using forceps, transfer the slides to cleaned Coplin jars in which they will be kept for rinsing, drying and storing; do not overcrowd. Rinse thoroughly with tap water and finally with distilled water. Allow to drain and dry in air with the jar inverted on clean blotting-paper. Store with the jar closed to prevent contamination by air-borne dust. Just before use, flame the slide for a few seconds, passing it with each face downwards about six times through a blue Bunsen flame. Place on a clean warmed metal rack and allow to cool. Mark or number the slide with a diamond while holding with forceps.

2. Fix the broth culture, or saline suspension of an agar culture, by adding formalin to give a final formaldehyde concentration of 1–2 per cent (w/v). Sediment the bacilli by centrifuging at 2000–3000 rev/min, preferably in a horizontal centrifuge. Decant the supernatant liquid and gently resuspend the bacilli in distilled water by rotating the tube alternately in opposite directions, rolling it between the palms of the hand. Centrifuge again and gently resuspend in fresh distilled water so as to obtain a final suspension which is only slightly cloudy (e.g. equal to Brown's opacity standard No. 1, see Chap. 13). With a flamed platinum loop, place a large loopful of the suspension on the prepared slide and gently spread over an area 1–2 cm in diameter. Allow to dry in air at room temperature or in an incubator at 37°C. Do not fix film.

3. The stain is prepared as follows:

Tannic acid	10 g
Sodium chloride . .	5 g
Basic fuchsin . . .	4 g

Thoroughly mix the powdered ingredients in these proportions and store dry in a stoppered container. Prepare the solution by adding 1·9 g of the powder mixture to 33 ml of 95 per cent ethyl alcohol and, when mostly dissolved (e.g. in ten minutes), adding distilled water to make a final volume of 100 ml. Adjust the pH to 5·0 (at least within 0·2) by addition of NaOH or HCl, using a pH meter. Store the solution in a stoppered bottle in the refrigerator at 3°–5°C, where it may remain stable for several weeks.

Alternatively, prepare three stock solutions: (1) tannic acid, 3·0 per cent (w/v) in water with 0·2 per cent (w/v) phenol as preservative; (2) sodium chloride, 1·5 per cent (w/v) in water; and (3) basic fuchsin, 1·2 per cent (w/v) in 95 per cent ethyl alcohol. (The basic fuchsin must have a pH of 5·0; it may be compounded thus by mixing one part of pararosaniline hydrochloride with three parts of pararosaniline acetate. Allow several hours for solution in the alcohol.) Mix the three solutions in exactly equal proportions to prepare the stain.

4. Place the prepared slide horizontally on a carefully levelled staining rack. Pipette exactly 1 ml stain on to the slide so that it covers the whole surface. Leave at room temperature for

exactly the required time, using a stop watch. Several similar preparations should be stained for different times, e.g. for 6, 8, 10 and 12 min, so that the best may be chosen. The optimal duration of staining will vary with the batch of stain, the room temperature and other factors; the apparent thickness of the flagella increases with the duration of staining. Rinse off the stain gently by placing the slide under a slowly running water tap; do not pour off stain before rinsing. Counterstain with methylene blue, e.g. with borax methylene blue for 30 min to colour the bacterial protoplast. Wash with water, rinse with distilled water, drain, dry in air and examine by oil immersion.

STAINING OF INTRACELLULAR LIPID WITH SUDAN BLACK
BURDON'S (1946) METHOD

Sudan Black Stain

Sudan black B powder . . . 0·3 g
70 per cent ethyl alcohol . . 100 ml
Shake thoroughly at intervals and stand overnight before use. Keep in a well-stoppered bottle.

Procedure

1. Make a film, dry in air and fix by flaming.
2. Cover the entire slide with Sudan black stain and leave at room temperature for 15 min.
3. Drain off excess stain, blot, and dry in air.
4. Rinse thoroughly with xylol and again blot dry.
5. Counterstain lightly by covering with 0·5 per cent aqueous safranine or dilute carbol fuchsin for 5–10 s; rinse with tap water, blot and dry.

Lipid inclusion granules are stained blue-black or blue-grey, whilst the bacterial cytoplasm is stained light pink.

STAINING OF CELL POLYSACCHARIDES BY THE PERIODIC ACID SCHIFF (PAS) METHOD
HOTCHKISS (1948)

The polysaccharide constituents of bacteria and fungi are oxidized by periodate to form polyaldehydes which yield red-coloured compounds with Schiff's fuchsin-sulphite; the proteins and nucleic acids remain uncoloured. The method may be used to reveal fungal elements in sections of infected animal tissue; the fungi stain red, while the tissue material, except glycogen and mucin, fails to take the stain.

Periodate Solution. Dissolve 0·8 g periodic acid in 20 ml distilled water; add 10 ml of 0·2 M sodium acetate and 70 ml ethyl alcohol. The solution may be used for several days if protected from undue exposure to light.

Reducing Rinse. Dissolve 10 g potassium iodide and 10 g sodium thiosulphate pentahydrate in 200 ml distilled water. Add, with stirring, 300 ml ethyl alcohol, and then 5 ml of 2 N hydrochloric acid. The sulphur which slowly precipitates may be allowed to settle out.

Fuchsin-Sulphite Solution. Dissolve 2 g basic fuchsin in 400 ml boiling water, cool to 50°C and filter. To the filtrate add 10 ml of 2 N hydrochloric acid and 4 g potassium metabisulphite. Stopper and leave in a dark cool place overnight. Add 1 g decolourizing charcoal, mix and filter promptly. Add up to 10 ml or more 2 N hydrochloric acid until the mixture when drying in a thin film on glass does not become pink. Preserved in the dark and well stoppered, the stain remains effective for several weeks.

Sulphite Wash. Add 2 g potassium metabisulphite and 5 ml concentrated hydrochloric acid to 500 ml distilled water. This should be freshly prepared.

Procedure

1. Dry films in air and fix by flaming. For sections, fix tissue with usual fixatives; bring to 70 per cent ethyl alcohol and wash thoroughly with this.
2. Treat with periodate solution for 5 min at room temperature. Rinse with 70 per cent alcohol.
3. Treat with reducing rinse for 5 min. Rinse with 70 per cent alcohol.
4. Stain with fuchsin-sulphite for 15–45 min.
5. Wash two or three times with sulphite wash solution. Wash with water.
6. Counterstain, if desired, with dilute aqueous malachite green (e.g. 0·002 g per 100 ml).

7. Wash with water. Dehydrate and mount by the usual methods.

Control sections are prepared similarly, omitting step (2).

Unless easily soluble polysaccharides such as glycogen are to be demonstrated, the method may be simplified by substituting distilled water for the alcohol in the periodate solution and by substituting tap water for rinsing in steps (1)–(3), e.g. see below.

MODIFIED PAS STAIN FOR FUNGI IN TISSUE SECTIONS

1. Bring sections to distilled water.
2. Treat for 5 min with a freshly prepared 1 per cent solution of periodic acid in water.
3. Wash in running tap water for 15 min and rinse in distilled water.
4. Stain with fuchsin-sulphite for 15 min.
5. Wash two or three times with sulphite wash solution. Wash with water.
6. Wash in running tap water for 5 min and rinse in distilled water.
7. Counterstain with dilute aqueous malachite green or with 0·1 per cent light green in 90 per cent alcohol for 1 min.
8. Dehydrate rapidly in absolute alcohol, clear in benzol and mount in Canada balsam.

IMPRESSION PREPARATIONS
KLIENEBERGER, 1934; BISSET, 1938

These have been used in the morphological study of mycoplasma cultures and of 'rough' and 'smooth' colonies of various bacteria.

The essential part of the technique is to remove a small slab about 2 mm thick of the solid medium (e.g. serum-agar) on which the organism is growing and place it colony downwards on a coverslip. The whole is immersed in fixative, so that the fixing fluid penetrates through the agar to reach the colony. When the bacteria are fixed, the agar is removed carefully from the coverslip which is well washed for two hours in distilled water, suitably stained and mounted. As fixative Bouin's fluid (p. 55) may be used, or Flemming's solution (p. 56) For staining, methylene blue or dilute carbol fuchsin may be employed, but Giemsa's stain, applied by the slow method is the most satisfactory for mycoplasmas. The agar slabs, after

fixation, may also be embedded, and vertical sections of the colony cut with a microtome.

The 'hot-water transfer' method of Clark, Fowler and Brown (1961) is also useful for morphological studies of mycoplasma. The transferred colonies may be stained directly on the slide by Dienes' stain diluted 1 in 10 or by the slow method of Giemsa. In addition, the colonies may be used for immuno-fluorescence by the direct or indirect methods.

DEMONSTRATION OF NUCLEAR MATERIAL IN BACTERIA
ROBINOW'S (1944, 1949) METHOD

The nuclear bodies of bacteria can be differentiated from the cytoplasm if the cells are first treated with 1 N HCl at 60°C and then stained with Giemsa's solution.

Method (*Modified*)

Fixation

Cut a small square block from an agar plate on which the organisms are growing in a thin layer and immerse it, bacteria-carrying side uppermost, in a shallow layer of methyl alcohol for 5 min. Dry the block in air and then place it downwards on a clean coverslip. Remove the agar, dry the film of fixed bacteria deposited on the coverslip and fix in warm alcohol-mercuric-chloride (Schaudinn's fluid) for 5 min. Wash in water and store in 70 per cent alcohol.

Staining

Transfer films from 70 per cent alcohol to 1 N HCl at 60°C for 10 min to 'hydrolyse'. Rinse in tap water and twice in distilled water and float on a staining solution made with 2–3 drops of Giemsa stain per ml of phosphate buffer (pH 7·0). Stain for 30 min at 37°C, rinse and mount in water, and examine at once.

Feulgen staining of deoxyribonucleic acid in the nuclear bodies may be effected by staining with Schiff's fuchsin-sulphite (p. 45) for 1 h at 15–20°C instead of staining with the Giemsa stain in the above method.

To demonstrate the *cell wall*, make impression preparations fixed in Bouin's fluid, as described above. Mordant for 20–30 min with 5–10 per cent tannic acid and stain with 0·02 per cent crystal violet in water for about 1 min. Mount in water.

STAINING WITH ACRIDINE ORANGE R

This dye has a marked affinity for nucleic acid. Staining of purified virus preparations has been used as a means of determining the nature of the nucleic acid core of viruses. When combined with tests of nuclease susceptibility the method allows of the differentiation of single and double stranded forms of the molecules (Jamison and Mayor, 1965). When cells stained with this dye are viewed with UV light the RNA components fluoresce with shades of orange and red while the DNA components take on shades of green. The method is of great value in studying the growth of animal viruses and bacteriophages in their respective host cells (Anderson, Armstrong and Niven, 1959).

Method

Coverslip preparations of living cells, tissue cultures or exudates are used.

The following are required:

1. 3 per cent HCl in 95 per cent alcohol.
2. Citrate-phosphate buffer pH 3·8 (see Chap. 4).
3. Stock Acridine Orange R 0·1 per cent in distilled water.

Solutions 2 and 3 are prepared freshly each week and stored at 4°C.

Proceed as follows:

1. Dilute the stock acridine orange solution 1 in 10 with the buffer on the day of use.
2. Place the coverslip without delay in acid-alcohol for 5 min.
3. Rinse for 2 min in two changes of buffer.
4. Stain in the 0·01 per cent acridine orange for 4–10 min.
5. Wash in two changes of buffer for 2 min.
6. Mount in buffer.
7. Ring the coverslip with nail varnish.

THE ROMANOWSKY STAINS

The original Romanowsky stain was made by dissolving in methyl alcohol the compound formed by the interaction of watery solutions of eosin and zinc-free methylene blue. The original stain has now been replaced by various modifications which are easier to use and give better results; these are: Leishman's, Wright's, Jenner's and Giemsa's stains. The peculiar property of the Romanowsky stains is that they impart a reddish-purple colour to the chromatin of malaria and other parasites. This colour is due to a substance which forms when methylene blue is 'ripened', either by age, as in polychrome methylene blue, or by heating with sodium carbonate. The latter method is employed in the manufacture of Leishman's and Wright's stains. The ripened methylene blue is mixed with a solution of water-soluble eosin, when a precipitate, due to the combination of these dyes, is formed. The precipitate is washed with distilled water, dried and dissolved in pure methyl alcohol. (The methyl alcohol, i.e. methanol, must be 'pure, for analysis', and have a pH of 6·5. If too acid, the reaction must be adjusted by the addition of 0·01 N NaOH.) Each modification of the Romanowsky stain varies according to the 'ripening' and the relative proportions of methylene blue and eosin.

The Romanowsky stains are usually diluted for staining purposes with distilled water, when a precipitate is formed which is removed by subsequent washing.

LEISHMAN'S STAIN
(For protozoa in blood films)

This stain may be purchased ready for use or made by dissolving 0·15 g of Leishman's powder in 100 ml pure methyl alcohol. The powder is ground in a mortar with a little methyl alcohol ('pure for analysis', pH 6·5), the residue of undissolved stain allowed to settle and the fluid decanted into a bottle. The residue in the mortar is treated with more methyl alcohol, and the process is repeated until all the stain goes into solution. The remainder of the methyl alcohol is now added. The stain can be used within an hour or two of making.

Films

Dry unfixed films are used. The stain is first used undiluted, and the methyl alcohol fixes the film. The stain is then diluted with distilled water, and the staining proper carried out.

1. Pour the undiluted stain on the unfixed film and allow it to act for 1 min.

2. By means of a pipette and rubber teat add double the volume of distilled water to the slide, mixing the fluids by alternately sucking them up in the pipette and expelling them. Allow the diluted stain to act for 12 min.

3. Flood the slide gently with distilled water, allowing the preparation to differentiate in the distilled water until the film appears bright pink in colour—usually about 30 s.

4. Remove the excess of water with blotting paper and dry in the air.

It is important that the reaction of the distilled water be neither acid nor alkaline. Any slight variations from neutrality may alter considerably the colour of granules in white blood corpuscles, etc., and give rise to supposed 'pathological' appearances in cells which are really normal. A simple method of ensuring a suitable reaction of the distilled water is to keep large bottles of it—e.g. aspirator bottles—specially for these stains. Add 2 or 3 drops of 1 per cent aqueous neutral red solution. The usual reaction of distilled water is slightly acid, and a few drops of 1 per cent sodium carbonate solution should be added until the solution shows the faintest possible suggestion of pink colour.

Much trouble will be eliminated if a buffer solution is used instead of distilled water for diluting the stain and washing the slide. It is made as follows:

Na_2HPO_4 (anhydrous) . . . 5·447 g
KH_2PO_4 . . . . . 4·752 g

Mix together in a mortar and keep as such. The buffer mixture is quite stable.

Add 1 g of buffer mixture to 2 litres of distilled water and this gives a pH of 7·0, which is suitable for most work.

Some samples of stain may require a slightly more acid solution, of pH 6·8. For this mix

Na_2HPO_4 (anhydrous) . . . 4·539 g
KH_2PO_4 . . . . . 5·940 g

Add 1 g of the mixture to 2 litres of distilled water.

Shute (1950) maintains that fifteen seconds' fixation with the undiluted stain is sufficient and that only four drops of stain are necessary. The slide is rocked for 12–15 s and then eight to twelve drops of water are added and thoroughly mixed. Staining proceeds for 15 min and the diluted stain is flooded off in 2–3 s only. If washed for longer, Schüffner's dots will not be seen. Shute advocates a pH of 7·2 for the diluting fluid.

For demonstrating Schüffner's dots in Benign Tertian Malaria the use of Giemsa's stain following Leishman's stain has been recommended by Discombe (1945).

Fix thin blood film with Leishman's stain for 15–60 s. Dilute with twice the volume of buffer solution at pH 7·0 and stain for 15 min.

Wash off with dilute Giemsa's stain (e.g. G. T. Gurr's R66)—1 drop of stain to 1 ml buffer solution at pH 7·0—and stain with this for a further 30 min.

Wash with buffer solution.

Blot and dry.

Sections

1. Treat the section with xylol to remove the paraffin, then with alcohol and finally distilled water.

2. Drain off the excess of water and stain for 5–10 min with a mixture of 1 part Leishman's stain and 2 parts of distilled water or buffer solution.

3. Wash with distilled water.

4. Differentiate with a weak solution of acetic acid (1 : 1500), controlling the differentiation under the low power of the microscope until the protoplasm of the cells is pink and only the nuclei are blue.

5. Wash with distilled water or buffer solution.

6. Blot, dehydrate with a few drops of absolute alcohol, clear in xylol and mount in Canada balsam or preferably DPX mounting medium.

GIEMSA'S STAIN
(For protozoa and spirochaetes)

This consists of a number of compounds made by mixing different proportions of methylene blue and eosin. These have been designated Azur I, Azur II and Azur II-eosin. The preparation can be purchased made up, but batches may vary considerably.

We can recommend the following method of preparation devised by Lillie (1943), which gives consistent and reliable results. It is excellent for staining blood films for malaria parasites, and also mouse or rat blood for trypanosomes.

1. *Azure B Eosinate*. Dissolve 10 g methylene blue in 600 ml distilled water. Add 6·0 ml concentrated sulphuric acid. Bring to the boil and add 2·5 g potassium bichromate dissolved in 25 ml distilled water. Boil for 20 min. Cool to 10°C or lower (place in refrigerator overnight). When cold add 21 g dry sodium bicarbonate slowly with frequent shaking. Then add a 5 per cent solution of eosin (yellowish) and shake constantly until the margin of the fluid appears pale blue or bluish-pink. About 205 ml will be required, and 150 ml of this can be added at once. Filter immediately, preferably on a vacuum funnel with hard paper. When the fluid has been drawn through and the surface begins to crack, add 50 ml distilled water. Allow to drain, and wash again with a second 50 ml distilled water. Now wash with 40 ml alcohol (95 per cent) and repeat with a second 40 ml alcohol. Dry the precipitate at room temperature or 37°C (not higher). This constitutes Azure B eosinate.

2. *Azure A Eosinate*. Proceed exactly as above, but use 5·0 g potassium bichromate (in place of 2·5 g) and dissolve it in 50 ml distilled water.

3. *Methylene Blue Eosinate*. Dissolve 10 g methylene blue in 600 ml cold distilled water and precipitate as before with 5 per cent eosin solution, filtering and drying as above.

To make the finished stain, grind the three eosinates separately into fine powder in separate clean mortars. Then weigh out 500 mg azure B eosinate, 100 mg azure A eosinate, 400 mg methylene blue eosinate, and 200 mg finely ground methylene blue. Decant the mixed powder on to the surface of 200 ml solvent, allowing it to settle in gradually. Then shake frequently for two or three days, keeping the bottle between 50° and 60°C between shakings. The solvent consists of equal volumes of methyl alcohol (AR) and glycerol (AR). The proportion of stains given above should yield a satisfactory staining picture. The diluting fluid is buffer solution pH 7·0.

This stain may be used in a manner somewhat similar to Leishman's preparation (the 'rapid method'), or prolonged staining may be carried out, as, for example, in staining spirochaetes (the 'slow method'). In both cases the preparation must be fixed prior to staining, either with methyl alcohol (methanol) for 3 min, or with absolute alcohol (ethanol) for 15 min.

Rapid Method

1. Fix films in methyl alcohol for 3 min.
2. Stain in a mixture of 1 part stain and 10 parts buffer solution pH 7·0 for 1 h.
3. Wash with buffer solution, allowing the preparation to differentiate for about 30 s.
4. Blot and allow to dry in the air.

This method of staining gives excellent results with thin blood films for malaria parasites, Schüffner's dots being well defined. Trypanosomes are also well demonstrated.

A rapid method with the application of heat is useful for demonstrating spirochaetes.

Fix preparations with absolute alcohol (15 min) or by drawing three times through a flame. Prepare a fresh solution of 10 drops of Giemsa's solution with 10 ml of buffer solution of pH 7·0 (p. 88), shake gently and cover the fixed film with the diluted stain. Warm till steam rises, allow to cool for 15 s, then pour off and replace with fresh stain and heat again. Repeat the procedure four or five times, wash in distilled water, dry and mount.

Slow Method

This is a specially valuable method for demonstrating objects difficult to stain in the ordinary way, e.g. certain pathogenic spirochaetes. The principle is to allow the diluted stain to act for a considerable period. As the mixture of stain and water causes a fine precipitate, care has to be taken that this does not deposit on the film.

Slides. The film is fixed in methyl alcohol for 3 min. A mixture is made in a Petri dish in the proportion of 1 ml of stain to 20 ml of buffer solution, pH 7·0. A piece of thin glass rod is placed in the Petri dish, and the slides, after fixing, are laid film downwards in the fluid with one end of the slide resting on the glass rod so that there is sufficient staining fluid between the film and the bottom of the dish. After staining for 16–24 h, the slides are washed in a stream of buffer solution, allowed to dry in air and mounted. There should be no deposits of precipitated stain on the preparation.

FIELD'S (1941) RAPID METHOD OF STAINING THICK BLOOD FILMS FOR MALARIA PARASITES

This method can be recommended for routine use.

In preparing the blood films it is important to ensure that they are not too thick. Drying may be assisted by placing the film in the incubator. After the film is quite dry it may be passed very rapidly two or three times through a Bunsen or spirit flame, each passage occupying two to three seconds. When cool the film is ready for staining.

FIELD'S STAIN
(Obtainable also in tablet form)

Solution A (methylene blue)

Methylene blue . . . . 1·3 g
Na$_2$HPO$_4$ (anhydrous) . . . 5·0 g
(If Na$_2$HPO$_4$, 12 H$_2$O, is used, 12·6 g)

Dissolve in 50 ml distilled water, bring to the boil and evaporate almost to dryness in a waterbath, then add KH$_2$PO$_4$ (anhydrous) 6·25 g. Add 500 ml of freshly boiled and still warm distilled water, stir until the stain is completely dissolved and set aside for 24 h. Filter before use. If a scum forms during use, filter again.

Alternatively, if Azure I is available there is no need to carry out the polychroming of the methylene blue as outlined above, and *Solution A* can be made as follows:

Methylene blue . . . . 0·8 g
Azure I . . . . . 0·5 g
Na$_2$HPO$_4$ (anhydrous) . . . 5·0 g
(Na$_2$HPO$_4$, 12 H$_2$O, 12·6 g)
KH$_2$PO$_4$ (anhydrous) . . . 6·25 g
(KH$_2$PO$_4$, 2 H$_2$O, 8·0 g)
Distilled water . . . . 500 ml

The phosphate salts are first dissolved in freshly boiled and still warm distilled water and the stain is then added. Set aside for 24 h and filter before use.

Solution B (eosin)

Eosin . . . . . 1·3 g
Na$_2$HPO$_4$ (anhydrous) . . . 5·0 g
(Na$_2$HPO$_4$, 12 H$_2$O, 12·6 g)
KH$_2$PO$_4$ (anhydrous) . . . 6·25 g
(KH$_2$PO$_4$, 2 H$_2$O, 8·0 g)
Distilled water . . . . 500 ml

The phosphate salts are first dissolved in freshly boiled and still warm distilled water, then the stain is added. Set aside for 24 h and filter before use.

The stains are kept in covered jars, the level being maintained by the addition of fresh stain as necessary. The same solution may be used continuously for many weeks without apparent deterioration, but the eosin solution should be renewed when it becomes greenish from the slight carry-over of methylene blue. If solutions show a growth of bacteria or moulds they should be discarded and replaced from stock solutions which, if stored carefully, will remain satisfactory up to a year.

Method of Staining

1. Dip the slide into the solution A for 1–2 s only.
2. Remove slide and immediately rinse *gently* in a jar of clean distilled or tap water until the stain ceases to flow from the film and the glass of the slide is free from stain.
3. Dip the slide into solution B for 1–2 s only.
4. Rinse *gently* for 2–3 s in clean water.
5. Place *vertically* against a rack to drain and dry.

The relative times may require slight adjustment to suit different batches of stain.

Films up to 3 weeks old may benefit from immersion in phosphate buffer solution (as used for dissolving the stains) until haemoglobin begins to diffuse out. The film is stained in the ordinary way. Unduly thick films should be similarly immersed before staining to remove the greater part of the haemoglobin. The phosphate buffer solution may be used in place of water for rinsing between solutions A and B.

Another method of staining thick blood films for malaria parasites is that of Simeons (1942).

STAINING OF SPIROCHAETES
FONTANA'S METHOD FOR FILMS

Solutions required

(*a*) *Fixative:*

Acetic acid . . . . 1 ml
Formalin . . . . 2 ml
Distilled water . . . 100 ml

(b) *Mordant*:

Phenol	.	.	1 g
Tannic acid	.	.	5 g
Distilled water	.	.	100 ml

(c) *Ammoniated silver nitrate*:

Add 10 per cent ammonia to 0·5 per cent solution of silver nitrate in distilled water until the precipitate formed just dissolves. Now add more silver nitrate solution drop by drop until the precipitate returns and does not redissolve.

1. Treat the film three times, 30 s each time, with the fixative.
2. Wash off the fixative with absolute alcohol and allow the alcohol to act for 3 min.
3. Drain off the excess of alcohol and carefully burn off the remainder until the film is dry.
4. Pour on the mordant, heating till steam rises, and allow it to act for 30 s.
5. Wash well in distilled water and again dry the slide.
6. Treat with ammoniated silver nitrate, heating till steam rises, for 30 s, when the film becomes brown in colour.
7. Wash well in distilled water, dry and mount in Canada balsam.

It is essential that the specimen be mounted in balsam under a coverslip before examination, as some immersion oils cause the film to fade at once.

The spirochaetes are stained brownish-black on a brownish-yellow background.

BECKER'S METHOD (MODIFIED)

The fixative and mordant are as in Fontana's method.

Staining solution

Basic fuchsin (saturated alcoholic solution)	.	.	45 ml
Shunk's mordant B (95 or 100 per cent ethanol 16 ml and aniline oil 4 ml)	.	.	18 ml
Distilled water	.	.	100 ml

Mix the Shunk's mordant with the alcoholic fuchsin and then add the distilled water. (The glassware should be dry.)

Procedure

1. Filter stain and reagents into jars for use.
2. Make film and dry in air.

3. Place in fixative for 1–3 min.
4. Wash in water for about 30 s.
5. Treat with mordant for 3–5 min.
6. Wash in water for about 30 s.
7. Place in staining solution for 3–5 min.
8. Wash well in water and drain dry.

LEVADITI'S METHOD OF STAINING SPIROCHAETES IN TISSUES
Pyridine Modification

This method is more rapid than the original technique.

1. Fix the tissue, which must be in small pieces 1 mm thick, in 10 per cent formalin for 24 h.
2. Wash the tissue for 1 h in water and thereafter place it in 96–98 per cent alcohol for 24 h.
3. Place the tissue in a 1 per cent solution of silver nitrate (to which one-tenth of the volume of pure pyridine has been added) for 2 h at room temperature, and thereafter at about 50°C for 4–6 h. It is then rapidly washed in 10 per cent pyridine solution.
4. Transfer to the reducing fluid, which consists of:

Formalin 4 per cent	.	.	100 parts

to which are added immediately before use:

Acetone (pure)	.	.	10 parts
Pyridine (pure)	.	.	15 parts

Keep the tissue in this fluid for two days at room temperature in the dark.

5. After washing well with water, dehydrate the tissue with increasing strengths of alcohol and embed in paraffin (p. 56). Thin sections are cut and mounted in the usual way. After removing the paraffin with xylol the sections are immediately mounted in Canada balsam.

STAINING OF AMOEBAE AND OTHER INTESTINAL PROTOZOA IN FAECES
Iron Haematoxylin Stain

Fix wet smears in Schaudinn's fluid (p. 56) for 5 min or longer.

Wash the films in 50 per cent alcohol and apply Gram's iodine for 2 min to remove the mercury salt, remove the iodine with alcohol and wash the films in water.

Stain with iron haematoxylin for 10–20 min.

Iron Haematoxylin

(a) Haematoxylin   .   .   . 1 g
       Absolute alcohol .   .   . 100 ml
(b) Liquor ferri perchlor. 30 per
       cent   .   .   .   .   . 4 ml
       Concentrated hydrochloric acid 1 ml
       Distilled water   .   .   . 100 ml

Mix equal parts of (a) and (b) immediately before using.

After staining, wash films in water, pass through alcohol, clear with xylol and mount in balsam, as in the treatment of tissue sections.

Preparations may be counterstained with van Gieson's stain for 15–30 s.

Saturated aqueous solution of
acid fuchsin   .   .   .   . 1–3 parts
Saturated aqueous solution of
picric acid   .   .   .   . 100 parts

Dehydrate rapidly with absolute alcohol, clear in xylol and mount in balsam. Fixed wet preparations must be treated in the same manner as sections and never be allowed to become dry.

Dobell's (1942) Method

Fix films as above, and after washing in distilled water, mordant for 10 min in 2 per cent watery solution of ammonium molybdate.

Wash in distilled water and stain for 10 min with 0·2 per cent haematoxylin solution in water (the haematoxylin should be fresh, not 'ripened').

Wash in distilled water and transfer to tap water for about 30 min, i.e. until the film assumes a blue colour. Dehydrate with alcohol, clear with xylol and mount in balsam.

Sargeaunt's Stain

(For staining chromatoids in amoebic cysts)

Malachite green   .   .   . 0·2 g
Glacial acetic acid   .   .   . 3·0 ml
95 per cent ethanol   .   .   . 3·0 ml
Distilled water to   .   .   . 100 ml

Dissolve the Malachite green in the alcohol, add acetic acid and make up to volume with distilled water. Keeps well on bench.

STAINING OF FUNGI IN WET MOUNTS WITH LACTOPHENOL BLUE

Staining solution

Phenol crystals   .   .   .   . 20 g
Lactic acid .   .   .   .   . 20 ml
Glycerol   .   .   .   .   . 40 ml
Distilled water   .   .   .   . 20 ml
Cotton blue (or methyl blue) .   . 0·075 g

Dissolve the phenol crystals in the liquids by gentle warming and then add the dye.

Needle-mount Method

1. Place a drop of 95 per cent alcohol on the slide. Gently tease out a fragment of the culture in the alcohol with needles or straight wires. When it is satisfactorily spread, let most of the alcohol evaporate and then add a drop of stain.

2. Apply a coverslip, avoiding bubbles, and exert gentle pressure if the fungus fragments do not lie flat.

3. Remove any excess stain round the coverslip with the edge of a piece of blotting paper. Let the stain penetrate; it may be satisfactory within a few minutes but differentiation may go on improving for up to 24 hours. For permanent preparations, seal the edges with nail varnish or cellulose lacquer.

Staining Agar Block Cultures

Slides or coverslips on to which fungi have grown from the sides of the agar block can be stained without disturbing the growth by treating them as above, first with alcohol to remove air bubbles attached to the mycelium and then with stain.

Transparent self-adhesive tape (Sellotape, Scotch Tape) may be used to transfer fungel elements to a slide for examination either unstained or stained by lactophenol blue (Butler and Mann, 1959). The adhesive on the tape may be used to coat slides or coverslips to make a more permanent preparation (Shannon, 1971).

STAINING OF VIRUS INCLUSION AND ELEMENTARY BODIES, AND RICKETTSIAE
INCLUSION BODIES

For intranuclear and cytoplasmic inclusions Giemsa's stain, p. 48, is satisfactory when such forms are of a basophilic nature as in psittacosis. For acidophilic inclusion bodies other stains give more satisfactory results.

Mann's Methyl-Blue Eosin Stain

1 per cent aqueous solution of
methyl blue   .   .   .   . 35 parts
1 per cent aqueous solution of
eosin   .   .   .   .   . 45 parts
Distilled water .   .   .   . 100 parts

Fix tissues in Bouin's solution or Zenker's fluid, and cut paraffin sections in the usual way. Stain for 12 h in the incubator at 37°C. Rinse the section in water, differentiate under the microscope in 70 per cent alcohol to each ml of which has been added one drop of saturated aqueous Orange G solution, dehydrate and mount in balsam.

In Ford's modification the sections are stained for 3 h at 37°C treated with 40 per cent formaldehyde (strong formalin) for 5 s, washed in water, differentiated and mounted as above. This method is especially useful for staining the Negri bodies in rabies.

VIRUS ELEMENTARY BODIES
Giemsa's Stain

This has already been described on p. 48, and whilst satisfactory for the elementary bodies of vaccinia and psittacosis, it has been replaced by other methods that are quicker, free from deposit and give more consistent results.

Brucella Differential Stain

The method described on p. 40 is useful for staining the elementary bodies of chlamydia.

Gutstein's Method

This method is valuable for staining the elementary bodies of the variola-vaccinia group of viruses in smears made from scrapings of skin lesions and elsewhere.

Solution 1
Methyl violet   .   .   . 1 g
Distilled water   .   .   . 100 ml
Solution 2
Sodium carbonate .   .   . 2 g
Distilled water   .   .   . 100 ml

Prepare films of infected material and if much protein is present rinse first in saline and then in distilled water. Fix in methyl alcohol for 20–30 min. Place the slide, film facing downwards, supported on two pieces of capillary tubing in a Petri dish.

Mix equal volumes of solutions 1 and 2, filter, and run the stain under the slide in the Petri dish.

Cover the Petri dish, and incubate at 37°C for 20–30 min. Remove the slide, rinse in distilled water, and leave to dry in air.

Castaneda's Stain (Bedson's Modification)

This method is useful for rickettsiae as well as for virus particles.

Reagents

1. 1·0 N HCl.
2. *Formaldehyde buffer.* Add 40 ml commercial formalin (previously neutralized with 1·0 N NaOH in the presence of phenol red) to 960 ml. Sørensen's (Geigy, 1962) M/15 phosphate buffer pH 7·2.
3. *Stock Azure II.* Dissolve 1 g Azure II (Gurr) in 100 ml distilled water. Filter.
4. *Counterstain.* Dissolve 0·25 g safranine in 100 ml distilled water. Filter.

Procedure

1. Fix the film in 1·0 N HCl for 2 min.
2. Wash thoroughly with distilled water to remove acid.
3. Dilute the azure II stock solution 1 in 10 with formaldehyde buffer and use this to stain the smear for 20 min.
4. Wash thoroughly with distilled water.
5. Counterstain with 0·25 per cent safranine for 6–8 s (not longer).
6. Wash in running water, blot and dry.

The rickettsiae remain blue while the protoplasm and nuclei of the cells are red.

Nicholau's Stain

Stain

Isamine blue	.	.	.	.	1·0 g
Phenol	.	.	.	.	3·0 g
Ethanol	.	.	.	.	10·0 ml
Distilled water	.	.	.	.	100 ml

This stain keeps indefinitely, does not precipitate and, even in thick films containing much protein, shows clearly defined virus particles.

Procedure

Fix smears with gentle heat or methanol. Cover with stain and heat until the stain steams, but does *not* boil. After 5 min rinse the smear and blot dry.

Macchiavello's Method for Staining Rickettsiae

This method is very suitable for staining rickettsiae in films from tissues.

Make a film in the usual way and dry in air. Warm the slide gently and stain for 4 min with 0·25 per cent basic fuchsin (in distilled water) which has been adjusted to pH 7·2–7·4 with alkali and filtered through paper.

Then wash off the stain rapidly with 0·5 per cent citric acid and after this with tap water.

Finally, stain with 1 per cent watery methylene blue for a few seconds.

The rickettsiae are coloured red, tissue cells blue.

FIXATION AND EMBEDDING OF TISSUES; SECTION CUTTING

As the ordinary routine bacteriological investigation of tissues is carried out almost exclusively with paraffin sections, this technique only will be described.

The fixed tissue is embedded in paraffin wax to support it during the cutting of the section, and the section is held together by the wax in the process of transferring it to the slide.

The paraffin wax must completely permeate the tissue, but before it can do so, all water must be removed from the material and replaced by a fluid with which melted paraffin will mix.

Water, therefore, is first removed with several changes of alcohol; the alcohol is replaced by some fluid—such as xylol, benzol, acetone, chloroform—which is a solvent of both alcohol and paraffin wax, and the tissue is finally embedded in melted paraffin.

Before removing the water from the tissue preparatory to embedding, the tissue must be suitably fixed and hardened.

The essentials for obtaining good sections are:

1. The tissue must be fresh.

2. It must be properly fixed by using small pieces and employing a large amount of fixing fluid.

3. The appropriate fixing fluid must be employed for the particular investigation required.

4. The tissue must not remain too long in the embedding bath.

FIXATIVES
FORMALIN 10 PER CENT

Formalin is a 38–40 per cent (w/v) solution of formaldehyde (H.CHO) in water containing 10 per cent methanol to inhibit polymerization (i.e. 38–40 g H.CHO per 100 ml solution).

Ten per cent commercial formalin (4 per cent formaldehyde) in 0.85 NaCl solution is a good general fixative. It is easily prepared, has good penetrating qualities, does not shrink the tissues, and permits considerable latitude in the time during which specimens may be left in it. Moreover, the subsequent handling of the material is much easier in our experience than in the case of mercuric chloride fixatives, such as Zenker's fluid. Formalin fixation is not as good as other methods where fine detail has to be observed, as, for example, in material containing protozoa. For general routine use, however, it is the most convenient and useful of fixatives. Tissue should be cut into thin slices, about 4 mm thick, and dropped into a large bulk of fixative. The fluid may be changed at the end of 24 h, and fixation is usually complete in 48 h. Specimens are then washed in running water for an hour and transferred to 50 per cent alcohol. In the latter fluid they may be kept for a considerable time without deterioration.

Formalin tends to become acid owing to the formation of formic acid. The strong formalin should be kept neutral by the addition of an excess of magnesium carbonate. The clear supernatant fluid is decanted off when formalin dilutions are required.

ZENKER'S FLUID

Mercuric chloride	.	.	50 g
Potassium bichromate .	.	.	25 g
Sodium sulphate .	.	.	10 g
Water	.	. .	1000 ml

Immediately before use, add 5 ml of glacial acid per 100 ml of fluid.

The fluid should be warmed to body temperature and only small pieces of tissue must be placed in it. Fixation is complete in 24 h, and thereafter the pieces of tissue are washed in running water for 24 h to remove the potassium bichromate and mercuric chloride. The tissue is then transferred to 50 per cent alcohol.

It is essential that all the mercuric chloride should be removed, otherwise a deposit will appear in the sections. The bulk of it is removed by washing. The remainder can be removed with iodine during the dehydration stage in alcohol. The material after washing is transferred to 50 per cent, and later to 70 per cent alcohol to which sufficient iodine has been added to make the fluid dark brown in colour. (It is convenient to keep a saturated solution of iodine in 90 per cent alcohol in a drop-bottle, and add a few drops as required.) If the alcohol becomes clear more iodine is added until the fluid remains brown. This indicates that all the mercury salt has been dissolved out by the iodine-alcohol.

Cut sections fixed on slides can also be treated with iodine, e.g. Gram's iodine, for 3–5 min, to remove mercuric chloride.

Animal tissues fixed in Zenker's fluid are more difficult to cut, and sections are apt to float off the slide, particularly if fixation has been unduly prolonged.

ZENKER-FORMOL FLUID

This is similar to Zenker's fluid except that the acetic acid is omitted and 5 ml of formalin are added per 100 ml immediately before use. It is a useful general fixative for animal tissues.

MERCURIC-CHLORIDE-FORMALIN SOLUTION

Mercuric chloride, saturated aqueous solution .	.	.	90 ml
Formalin, commercial .	.	.	10 ml

Small portions of tissue must be used and fixation is complete in 1–12 h. Then transfer to alcohol and iodine as after Zenker's fluid. This fluid fixes with the minimum amount of distortion and the finer cytological details of the cells are retained. It is useful when staining virus inclusion bodies.

'SUSA' FIXATIVE (M. Heidenhain)

Mercuric chloride	.	.	45 g
Distilled water	.	.	800 ml
Sodium chloride .	.	.	5 g
Trichloracetic acid	.	.	20 g
Acetic acid (glacial)	.	.	40 ml
Formalin (40 per cent formaldehyde)	.	.	200 ml

This is one of the best fixatives for both normal and pathological tissues. Pieces of tissue not thicker than 1 cm should be fixed for 3–24 h, depending on the thickness. The material should be transferred *direct* to 95 per cent alcohol. Lower grades of alcohol, or water, may cause undue swelling of connective tissue. Add to the alcohol sufficient of a saturated solution of iodine in 95 per cent alcohol to give a brown colour. If the latter fades, more iodine should be added.

The advantages of 'Susa' fixative are rapid and even fixation with little shrinkage of connective tissue. The transference direct to 95 per cent alcohol shortens the time of dehydration, while tissues thus fixed are easy to cut.

BOUIN'S FLUID

This fixative is useful for the investigation of virus inclusion bodies.

Saturated aqueous solution of picric acid .	.	.	75 parts
Formalin .	.	.	25 parts
Glacial acetic acid	.	.	5 parts

This solution keeps well. Use thin pieces of tissue not exceeding 10 mm thick. Fix for 1–12 h according to thickness and density of tissue. Wash in 50 per cent alcohol (not water), then 70 per cent until the picric acid is removed.

SCHAUDINN'S FLUID

Absolute ethyl alcohol . . .	100 ml
Saturated aqueous solution of mercuric chloride	200 ml

This is an important fixative for protozoa. It may be used cold or warmed to 60°C, when it is more quickly penetrating. It is also a suitable fixative for wet films.

FLEMMING'S FLUID

Osmic acid	0·1 g
Chromic acid	0·2 g
Glacial acetic acid . . .	0·1 ml
Water	100 ml

The osmic and chromic acids, when mixed, will keep for only 3–4 weeks. The acetic acid should be added immediately before use.

EMBEDDING AND SECTION CUTTING

After fixation by any of the above-mentioned methods and transference to 50 per cent alcohol, *small pieces* of tissue are treated as follows:

1. Place in 90 per cent alcohol for 2–5 h.
2. Transfer to absolute alcohol for 2 h.
3. Complete the dehydration in fresh absolute alcohol for 2 h.
4. Transfer to a mixture of absolute alcohol and chloroform (equal parts) till tissue sinks, or overnight.
5. Place in pure chloroform for 6 h.
6. Transfer the tissue for 1 h to a mixture of equal parts of chloroform and paraffin wax, which is kept melted in the paraffin oven.
7. Place in pure melted paraffin in the oven at 55°C for 2 h, preferably in a vacuum embedding oven.

The tissue is embedded in blocks of paraffin. These are cut out, trimmed with a knife, and sections 5 μm thick are cut by means of a microtome. The sections are flattened on warm water, floated on to slides and allowed to dry. Albuminized slides are useful where the staining process involves heating, and where animal tissue is used, especially after fixation with Zenker's fluid. The slides are coated with albumin either by means of a small piece of chamois leather or by the finger tip. The albu-min solution is made by adding three parts of distilled water to one part of egg-white and shaking thoroughly. The mixture is filtered through muslin into a bottle, and a crystal of thymol is added as a preservative. It is usual to coat a number of slides and, after drying, these are stored until required. The albuminized side may be identified by breathing gently on the slide; it is not dimmed by the breath, whereas the plain side is.

For additional details, reference must be made to works on histology.

REFERENCES AND FURTHER READING

ANDERSON, E. S., ARMSTRONG, J. A. & NIVEN, J. S. F. (1959) Fluorescence microscopy: observations of virus growth with aminoacridines. *Symposium of the Society of General Microbiology*, No. IX, p. 224. Cambridge University Press.

ASHBY, G. K. (1938) Simplified Schaeffer spore stain. *Science*, **87**, 443.

BISSET, K. A. (1938) The structure of 'rough' and 'smooth' colonies. *Journal of Pathology and Bacteriology*, **47**, 223.

BURDON, K. L. (1946) Fatty material in bacteria and fungi revealed by staining dried, fixed slide preparations. *Journal of Bacteriology*, **52**, 665.

BURKE, V. (1922) Notes on the gram stain with description of a new method. *Journal of Bacteriology*, **7**, 159.

BUTLER, E. A. & MANN, M. P. (1959) The use of cellophane for mounting and photographing cytopathogenic fungi. *Phytopathology*, **49**, 231.

BUTT, E. M., BONYNGE, C. W. & JOYCE, R. L. (1936) The demonstration of capsules about haemolytic streptococci with India ink or azo blue. *Journal of Infectious Diseases*, **58**, 5.

CLARK, H. W., FOWLER, R. C. & BROWN, T. McP. (1961) Preparation of pleuropneumonia-like organisms for microscopic study. *Journal of Bacteriology*, **81**, 500.

DISCOMBE, G. (1945) The demonstration of Schüffner's dots in benign tertian malaria. *British Medical Journal*, **1**, 298.

DOBELL, C. (1942) Some new methods for studying intestinal amoebae and other protozoa. *Parasitology*, **34**, 109.

DUGUID, J. P. (1951) The demonstration of bacterial capsules and slime. *Journal of Pathology and Bacteriology*, **63**, 673.

EHRLICH, P. (1882) Aus dem Verein für innere Medizin zu Berlin. *Deutsche medizinische Wochenschrift*, **8**, 269.

FIELD, J. W. (1941) Further notes on a method of staining malarial parasites in thick blood films. *Transactions of the Royal Society of Tropical Medicine and Hygiene*, **35**, 35.

GEIGY (1962) *Documenta Geigy Scientific Tables*, 6th edn., p. 314. Edited by K. Diem. Manchester: Geigy Pharmaceuticals.

GRAM, C. (1884) Ueber die isolirte Färbung der Schizomyceten in Schnitt- und Trockenpräparaten. *Fortschritte der Medicin*, **2**, 185. See 'The differential staining of

Schizomycetes in tissue sections and in dried preparations', p. 215 in *Milestones in Microbiology*, edited by T. D. Brock (1961). London: Prentice-Hall.

HOTCHKISS, R. D. (1948) A microchemical reaction resulting in the staining of polysaccharide structures in fixed tissue preparations. *Archives of Biochemistry*, **16**, 131.

HOWIE, J. W. & KIRKPATRICK, J. (1934) Observations on bacterial capsules as demonstrated by a simple method. *Journal of Pathology and Bacteriology*, **39**, 165.

JAMISON, R. M. & MAYOR, H. D. (1965) Acridine Orange staining of purified rat virus strains X14. *Journal of Bacteriology*, **90**, 1486.

JOHNE, A. (1885) Einzweiffelöser Fall von congenitaler Tuberkulose. *Fortschritte der Medizin*, **3**, 198 (footnote p. 200).

KIRKPATRICK, J. & LENDRUM, A. C. (1939) A mounting medium for microscopical preparations giving good preservation of colour. *Journal of Pathology and Bacteriology*, **49**, 592.

KIRKPATRICK, J. & LENDRUM, A. C. (1941) Further observations on the use of synthetic resin as a substitute for Canada balsam. Precipitation of paraffin wax in the medium and an improved plasticizer. *Journal of Pathology and Bacteriology*, **53**, 441.

KLIENEBERGER, E. (1934) The colonial development of the organisms of pleuropneumonia and agalactia on serum agar and variations in the morphology under different conditions of growth. *Journal of Pathology and Bacteriology*, **39**, 409.

KOPELOFF, N. & BEERMAN, P. (1922) Modified Gram stains. *Journal of Infectious Diseases*, **31**, 480.

LAYBOURN, R. L. (1924) A modification of Albert's stain for the diphtheria bacillus. *Journal of the American Medical Association*, **83**, 121.

LILLIE, R. D. (1943) Giemsa stain of quite constant composition and performance, made in the laboratory from eosin and methylene blue. *U.S. Public Health Report*, **58**, 449.

PRESTON, N. W. & MORRELL, A. (1962) Reproducible results with the Gram stain. *Journal of Pathology and Bacteriology*, **84**, 241.

ROBINOW, C. F. (1944) Cytological observations on *Bact. coli, Proteus vulgaris*, and various aerobic spore-forming bacteria with special reference to the nuclear structures. *Journal of Hygiene* (*London*), **43**, 413.

ROBINOW, C. F. (1949) In *The Bacterial Cell*, by R. J. Dubos, Cambridge, Mass., Harvard University Press, Addendum.

SHANNON, R. (1972) A simple method of preparing fungi for microscopy. *Medical Laboratory Technology*, **29**, 210.

SHUTE, P. G. (1950) Thin and thick films showing malarial parasites on the same slide and in the same microscope field. *Transactions of the Royal Society of Tropical Medicine and Hygiene*, **43**, 364.

SIMEONS, A. T. W. (1942) Economy and simplification in staining blood slides. *Indian Medical Gazette*, **77**, 725.

3. Sterilization: Procedures and Applications

TECHNICAL PROCEDURES AND APPLICATIONS IN MEDICINE AND SURGERY

Sterilization is the freeing of an article from all living organisms including bacteria and their spores. The sterilization of culture media, containers and instruments is essential in bacteriological work for the isolation and maintenance of pure cultures.

Of the methods available—heat, filtration and radiation—heat is the most certain and should be used in the microbiology laboratory whenever possible. Most culture media, because they contain water, must be sterilized by moist heat. Dry heat is suitable for glassware, syringes, metal instruments, paper-wrapped goods which are not spoiled by the high temperature, and water-impermeable oils, waxes and powders. Filtration is often the only means of sterilizing heat-labile fluids, e.g. serum, antibiotic solutions and some culture media.

STERILIZATION BY DRY HEAT

1. Red Heat. Inoculating wires, points of forceps and searing spatulas are sterilized by holding them, as near the vertical as possible, in the flame of a Bunsen burner until they are seen to be red hot.

2. Flaming. Scalpels, needles, the mouths of culture tubes, cotton-wool stoppers, and glass slides and coverslips are sterilized by passing the article through the Bunsen flame without allowing it to become red hot. When glass is heated sufficiently for sterilization, it is apt to crack if placed at once on a cold surface. Treating needles, scalpels and basins by immersing them in methylated spirit and burning off the spirit does not produce a sufficiently high temperature for sterilization.

3. Hot-Air Oven. This allows controlled application of dry heat. The oven should be electrically heated and provided with a thermostat and a fan or blower to ensure rapid, uniform and controlled heating of the load (Darmady and Brock, 1954).

This is the best method of sterilizing dry glassware such as test-tubes, Petri dishes, flasks, pipettes and instruments such as forceps, scalpels, scissors, throat swabs and assembled *all-glass* syringes. Glassware should be perfectly dry before being placed in the sterilizing oven; wet glassware is liable to be cracked and should first be dried in a 'drying oven' at about 100°C. Before sterilization, plug test-tubes and flasks with cotton-wool stoppers. Other glassware, e.g. pipettes, may be wrapped in kraft paper, or sterilized in metal cans. (Note that during sterilization, certain brands of cotton-wool give off volatile substances that condense on the glass and may interfere with the growth of sensitive bacteria.) Slip-on metal caps may be substituted for cotton-wool. Screw-capped bottles will themselves withstand the temperature of the hot-air oven, but the ordinary rubber liners or washers in their caps may not, and bottles already capped should therefore be autoclaved unless the liners are made of silicone rubber.

The hot-air oven is also used for sterilizing dry materials in sealed containers, and powders, fats, oils and greases (e.g. petroleum jelly) that are impermeable to moisture. These materials are penetrated very slowly by heat and must therefore be sterilized in small lots, e.g. not exceeding 10 g, or shallow layers not more than 0·5 cm depth. Do not overload the sterilizing oven and leave spaces for circulation of air through the load. The oven may be cold or warm when loaded, and is then heated up to the sterilizing temperature in the course of 1–2 h. Time the *holding period* of 1 h at 160°C when the thermometer first shows that the oven air has reached 160°C. Finally, allow the oven to cool gradually during about 2 h before the door is opened, because glassware may be cracked by sudden or uneven cooling.

A holding period of 1 h at 160°C is generally considered sufficient, especially if the oven is equipped with a fan and if loads are of a kind that will heat up rapidly and reach 160°C soon after the oven air does so, e.g. loosely packed loads of simple glassware and metal instruments. Heavy loads in an oven without a fan, assembled *all-glass* syringes packed in test-tubes and slowly heating materials such as powders, oils and greases, should be exposed at 160°C for 2–2½ h.

4. Infra-red radiation. This may be employed to sterilize metal instruments and glass syringes in central sterile supply departments, but has no routine use in the microbiology laboratory.

STERILIZATION BY MOIST HEAT

Moist heat can be employed:
1. at temperatures below 100°C;
2. at a temperature of 100°C (either in boiling water or in free steam); or
3. at temperatures above 100°C (in saturated steam under increased pressure).

Only the third procedure fully ensures sterilization by killing the most highly resistant spores.

1. Moist Heat at Temperatures below 100°C

Temperatures below 100°C will not reliably effect sterilization. The best known example of their use is in the pasteurization of milk.

Microorganisms in serum or body fluids containing coagulable protein can sometimes be killed by heating for 1 h at 56°C on several successive days. It may be necessary to repeat the heating eight times to effect sterilization. Care must be taken not to allow the temperature to rise above 59°C, as inspissation may occur. The exposure to 56°C is best carried out in a waterbath, but a 56°C oven may be used. The effectiveness of this procedure should always be checked by subculture in a range of suitable media.

Vaccines prepared from cultures of non-sporing bacteria may be sterilized in a special waterbath ('vaccine bath') at a comparatively low temperature, 1 h at 60°C being *usually* sufficient. Higher temperatures may diminish the immunizing power of the vaccine. Again, test the effectiveness of the treatment by subculture.

2. Moist Heat at a Temperature of 100°C

Boiling at 100°C for a minimum of 10 min is sufficient to kill all non-sporing and many, but not all, sporing organisms. The method thus does not ensure sterility, but it has been found satisfactory for certain purposes in bacteriology where sterility is not essential or better methods are unavailable. It may be used for tubing, pipettes, measuring cylinders, rubber stoppers, instruments such as scalpels, forceps and scissors, and syringes of the metal and glass type that do not stand higher temperatures. Articles to be boiled should first be scrupulously cleaned. If the water supply is 'hard' distilled water should be used, otherwise the instruments on removal become covered with a film of calcium salts.

Boiling should be carried out in an enamel or copper bath with a removable tray provided with a raised edge to prevent cylindrical instruments from falling off. The boiled articles should be removed from the water with long-handled forceps which have been stored in 3 per cent lysol (saponated cresol) solution to a level approaching the finger grips. Before handling the newly boiled instrument, hold it by the forceps for a few moments while it dries by evaporation. If handled while still wet, its working end (e.g. scalpel blade or syringe needle) may be contaminated with skin bacteria floating down from the fingers in the film of water.

STEAMING AT 100°C. Pure steam in equilibrium with water boiling at normal atmospheric pressure (760 mm Hg) has a temperature of 100°C; at high altitudes the temperature is slightly less, e.g. 99°C at 1000 feet, 97°C at 3000 feet and 95°C at 5000 feet. Because of its convenience, 'steaming' at 100°C is commonly used for the preparation of culture media such as broth and nutrient agar, although it is not as certainly effective as autoclaving. A Koch or Arnold steam sterilizer ('steamer') heated by steam, gas or electricity is employed. In its simplest form this is a vertical metal cylinder with a removable conical lid (having a small opening for the escaping steam) and containing water which is boiled by a heater under the cylinder; but various modifications are available. A perforated tray situated above the water bears the articles to be sterilized. The apparatus is inexpensive and simple to operate. Bottles of medium may be introduced or removed while steaming is in progress, but unnecessary opening of the steamer with the consequent introduction of cool air should be avoided. Sterilization may be effected in two ways:

(a) *By a single exposure at 100°C for 90 min.* The spores of some thermophilic and rare mesophilic bacteria can survive this treatment, but in practice it seldom fails to sterilize. The steaming period of 90 min includes the time required for the tubes and bottles of media to be heated up from room temperature to 100°C. This may be about 15–20 min for tubes or bottles containing up to 100 ml, 30 min for bottles of 600 ml and 45 min for a flask of 5 litres. For larger volumes increase the total steaming period by an appropriate amount.

(b) *By intermittent exposure at 100°C, e.g. for 20–45 min on each of three successive days.* The principle of this method ('Tyndallization') is that one exposure kills vegetative organisms; between heatings the spores, being in a favourable nutrient medium, become vegetative forms which are killed during the subsequent heating. The duration of each steaming should be sufficient to heat up the medium to 100°C, i.e. 20 min for lots up to 100 ml and longer for larger volumes (see (a) above). Use this method for media containing sugars that may be decomposed at higher temperatures, and for gelatin media which after prolonged heating fail to solidify on cooling. This method may fail to kill thermophilic, anaerobic and other bacteria whose spores will not germinate in the particular medium and under the conditions of storage between the heatings.

3. Moist Heat at Temperatures above 100°C

STERILIZATION IN THE AUTOCLAVE

Water boils when its vapour pressure equals the pressure of the surrounding atmosphere. This occurs at 100°C for normal atmospheric pressure (i.e. 760 mm Hg, 14·7 lb per in^2 absolute pressure or 0 lb per in^2 'gauge pressure'). Thus, when water is boiled within a closed vessel at increased pressure, the temperature at which it boils and that of the steam it forms, will rise above 100°C.

Sterilization by steam under pressure ('autoclaving') is especially suitable for culture media and aqueous solutions, the atmosphere of steam preventing evaporation during heating. To avoid drenching of cotton-wool stoppers in a steamer or autoclave, the stoppers should be covered with kraft paper; thus a wire basket of test-tubes is covered by a single sheet of paper turned down at the edges.

In the autoclave all parts of the load to be sterilized must be permeated by steam. Once the whole of the load has been heated-up to the working temperature, there is a minimum holding time at that temperature necessary for sterilization. The minimum holding times are 2 min at not less than 134°C (30 lb per in^2 gauge pressure); 12 min at not less than 121°C (15 lb per in^2 gauge pressure) and 30 min at not less than 115°C (10 lb per in^2 gauge pressure). A 50 per cent safety period is usually added to these minimum holding times so that the recommended holding times are 3, 18 and 45 min respectively (Table 3.1).

Table 3.1

Steam pressure i.e. pressure above atmospheric (lb/in^2)	Temperature in °C	Holding time for sterilization (min)
0	100	—
10	115	45
15	121	18
30	134	3

The Importance of Air Discharge. All the air must be removed from the autoclave chamber and articles of the load, so that the latter are exposed to pure steam during the period of sterilization. There are three reasons for this: (1) the admixture of air with steam results in a lower temperature being achieved at the chosen pressure; (2) the air hinders penetration of the steam into the interstices of porous materials, surgical dressings especially, and the narrow openings of containers, syringes, etc; and (3) the air, being denser than the steam, tends to form a separate and cooler layer in the lower part of the autoclave, and so prevents adequate heating of the articles there (e.g. in an autoclave with no air discharge, a temperature of only 70°C was recorded at the bottom when that at the top was 115°C).

There is one exception to the necessity for complete air discharge from the load. Hermetically sealed bottles and ampoules of aqueous solutions and culture media are satisfactorily sterilized in spite of the presence of some air within them. The contained water provides the conditions for moist-heat sterilization, making unnecessary the entry of steam for this purpose, and the contents are heated to the same temperature as the chamber steam, though to a higher pressure, by conduction of heat through the container walls.

The Simple Non-jacketed Laboratory Autoclave

The simplest form of laboratory autoclave, the 'pressure-cooker' type (see figure), is a vertical or horizontal cylinder of gun-metal or stainless steel (up to 18 in in diameter and 30 in in length) in a supporting frame or case. The lid (or door) is fastened by screw clamps, and is rendered air-tight by means of an asbestos washer. The cylinder contains water up to a certain level (e.g. $3\frac{1}{2}$ in for a vertical autoclave of 19 in internal height) and this is heated by a gas burner or electric heater below the cylinder. The bottles, tubes, etc., to be sterilized, protected with kraft paper where necessary, are placed on a perforated tray situated above the water level. The lid or door is fitted with a discharge tap for air and steam, a pressure gauge and a safety valve that can be set to blow off at any desired pressure.

Directions for Using the Simple Autoclave. See that there is sufficient water in the cylinder. Insert material to be sterilized and turn on the heater. Place the lid in position, see that the discharge tap is *open* and then screw down the lid. Adjust the safety valve to the required pressure; in some varieties of autoclave this adjustment has to be determined previously by trial. As steam rises from the boiling water, it mixes with the air in the chamber and carries this out through the discharge tap. *Allow the steam and air mixture to escape freely until all the air has been eliminated from the autoclave.* A means of testing this is to lead a rubber tube from the discharge tap into a pail of cold water. The steam condenses within the water, while the air rises in bubbles to the surface. When the latter cease, the air discharge is seen to be as complete as is possible with this type of autoclave. After some trials it will be known what period of discharge to allow under normal operating conditions.

Now close the discharge tap. The steam pressure rises until it reaches the desired level, e.g. 15 lb per in^2 for 121°C, when the safety valve opens and allows the excess steam to escape. From exactly this point begin to time the *holding period*, continuing exposure at 15 lb pressure for the appropriate time, i.e. usually 18 min for aqueous media in lots up to 100 ml and longer for the large volumes that heat up more slowly. Then turn off the heater and allow the autoclave to cool until the pressure gauge indicates that the inside is at atmospheric pressure (0 lb per in^2). At once open the discharge tap slowly to allow the air to enter the autoclave. If the tap is opened while the chamber pressure is still high and the pressure is reduced too rapidly, liquid media will tend to boil violently and spill from their containers. On the other hand, if the tap is not opened until the pressure has fallen much below atmospheric pressure, an excessive amount of water will be evaporated and lost from the media. (When spontaneous cooling is too slow, e.g. taking about 1 h, the discharge tap may be opened very slightly so as to cause a gradual reduction to atmospheric pressure during 15–30 min.)

Deficiencies of the Simple Autoclave. The simple form of laboratory autoclave is effective when carefully operated, but has several important disadvantages. The method of air discharge is inefficient; air trapped in the chamber lowers the working temperature and this failure to achieve the proper temperature is likely to pass undetected, because these simple autoclaves are not furnished with a thermometer showing the temperature in the lowest and coolest part of the chamber. The simple autoclave also lacks means for *drying* the load after sterilization. Articles are moistened during sterilization by the condensation of the steam. When damp, paper and cloth wrappings, even in several layers, are unable to prevent the entry of contaminating bacteria. *It is therefore important to avoid placing sterilized articles in contact with unsterile objects until their wrappings are dry.*

A wide variety of autoclaves are manufactured which incorporate various devices to overcome these and other difficulties, some being specialized for particular purposes. Many autoclaves at present in hospitals and laboratories have been badly designed or wrongly installed, and cannot ensure sterilization. In recent years there has been a great increase in interest in these problems prompted particularly by the work of Bowie (1955) and Howie and Timbury (1956). In 1957 the Medical Research Council set up a working party to examine the whole question of sterilization by steam under increased pressure and their report (MRC Report 1964) is very comprehensive. The following description is given of an autoclave suitable for either laboratory or surgical purposes.

STEAM-JACKETED AUTOCLAVE WITH AUTOMATIC AIR AND CONDENSATE DISCHARGE

Most are horizontal cylinders or rectangles (e.g. 20 in diameter by 30 in) of rustless metal (e.g. Monel metal). Rectangular chambers are more conveniently loaded. At the front is a swing door fastened by a 'capstan head' which operates radial bolts and automatically remains locked while the chamber pressure is raised. A pressure-locked safety door is a valuable guard against the possibility of a dangerous explosion through premature opening by the operator.

The autoclave (Fig. 3.1) also possesses: (1) a supply of steam from an external source, e.g. an independent boiler beside the autoclave or, more usually, the main steam supply of the building; (2) a steam jacket which heats the side walls independently of the presence of steam in the chamber and so prevents undue condensation and facilitates drying of the load; (3) a channel for discharging air and condensate by gravity from the bottom of the chamber, with a 'no-return' valve and a thermostatic valve ('steam trap') to control this discharge

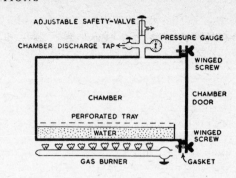

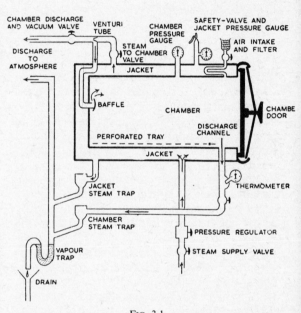

FIG. 3.1

AUTOCLAVES. *Above:* Simple non-jacketed autoclave. *Below:* Steam-jacketed autoclave with automatic gravity discharge of air and condensate, and system for drying by vacuum and intake of filtered air.

automatically; (4) a thermometer indicating the temperature in the discharge channel above the steam trap, i.e. approximately that of the lowest and coolest part of the chamber; (5) a vacuum system which may be used to assist drying of the load; (6) an air-intake with a self-sterilizing filter for introducing warm sterile air into the chamber. Sheet glass fibre provides the most reliable filter and has a working life of at least one year (MRC Report 1964); (7) a cooling system to hasten the cooling of liquids without violent boiling, and (8) an automatic control system which carries through exactly a pre-selected cycle of sterilization, including heating-up, holding, cooling and drying stages, without requiring attention from the operator.

Steam Supply. The steam supplied to the autoclave should be *dry*, and *saturated*, i.e. not superheated above the phase boundary of equilibrium with water boiling at the same temperature and pressure. Wet steam is an inefficient sterilizing agent because it soaks porous materials and the particles of water in it lack latent heat. However, mains steam (ideally at a pressure of 55 lb per in^2) passing through a reducing valve and pressure regulator so that it enters the autoclave at a pressure of 15 lb per in^2 usually becomes dried to a sufficient extent. Superheating may take place if the jacket temperature is greater than the chamber temperature, or if air remains mixed with the steam in the chamber.

The employment of saturated steam is necessary in order to maintain the conditions of 'moist heat' and prevent evaporation of condensation water from the articles of the load during the period of sterilization. Superheated steam is unsatisfactory because it abstracts water from the exposed material; by producing 'dry heat' conditions it is less lethal to micro-organisms but more destructive to the materials in the autoclave.

Starting of Autoclave and Heating of Jacket. The steam is first introduced into the jacket, which should be kept filled with steam at 121°C throughout the whole day, both during and between the successive steamings in the chamber. Steam which condenses to water on the walls of the jacket is drained away through a jacket discharge channel controlled by a thermostatic 'jacket steam trap'. Ensure that there is no obstruction to this discharge.

Loading of Chamber. When the jacket is heated, the load is placed in the chamber. Articles requiring different treatment, e.g. aqueous media in unsealed containers and wrapped goods requiring drying, should not be sterilized together. The articles must be arranged loosely enough to allow free circulation of steam and displacement of air. For further details see the section dealing with sterilization of individual articles.

Heating-up and Air-displacement Period. The door is closed and steam allowed to enter the chamber through a baffle high up at the back. The steam for the chamber is drawn from the jacket, which thus acts as a reservoir between the chamber and the supply line; the same pressure and therefore temperature, must be maintained in the chamber as in the jacket. The steam tends to float as a layer above the cooler and denser air, and as more is introduced it displaces the air downwards through the articles of the load and out through the chamber discharge channel which leads from the bottom of the chamber near the front. The condensation water formed on the cool load and chamber door also drains through this channel. The channel's thermostatic steam trap remains open while steam mixed with air and condensate passes through it to the drain, but as soon as all free air has been eliminated and the arrival of pure steam raises the trap's temperature to 121°C, it automatically closes and prevents further escape. About 5 or 10 min may be taken for this displacement of air by steam.

Holding Period of Sterilization. The holding period at 121°C begins when the thermometer in the discharge channel first shows that this temperature is reached. The exact duration of the holding period is decided according to the nature of the load, particularly the time which must be allowed for this to become heated throughout to the temperature of the steam (see pp. 71, 74). During the early part of the holding period some air will be displaced from the interior of a porous load; this collects with condensate in the discharge channel above the steam trap, cools the trap valve to 120°C or less, and so causes the trap to open momentarily and allow its escape. (A 'near-to-steam' trap is essential, i.e. one which opens when the temperature falls by only 1°C below that of pure steam.)

The working temperature must be controlled by the discharge-line thermometer to ensure that autoclaving is carried out at the correct temperature. Inferring the chamber temperature from pressure gauge readings is inaccurate and often leads to sterilization failure. Any obstruction to the discharge of air and condensate is indicated by the temperature falling below 121°C while the pressure remains at 15 lb. The discharge channel and trap must be kept clear and the removable strainer in the mouth of the discharge channel should be cleaned daily.

Cooling and Drying Period. At the end of the holding period the supply of steam to the chamber is stopped, while that to the jacket is maintained. The steam left in the chamber begins to cool by loss of heat through the unjacketed door and its pressure falls accordingly. The management of this stage depends on whether drying of the load is required, as for wrapped apparatus or surgical dressings, or must be avoided, as for aqueous media in loosely stoppered containers. Details of the methods of cooling and drying are given in the section dealing with the sterilization of these articles in detail.

HIGH PREVACUUM STERILIZERS

The most advanced surgical sterilizers are equipped with electrically driven pumps capable of exhausting the chamber almost to a perfect vacuum (e.g. to an absolute pressure of 20 mm Hg or below), thus removing more than 98 per cent of the air. (MRC, 1964.) The absence of air enables the steam to penetrate very rapidly and heat up all parts of the load making it feasible to employ a higher sterilizing temperature for a shorter time, namely 134°C for 3 minutes (i.e. jacket and chamber steam at 30 lb per in^2 gauge pressure). The total operation time is greatly shortened and damage to heat-sensitive materials through exposure to injurious air-steam mixtures or prolonged heating in the outer parts of the load, is avoided. Note, however, that the operating steam temperature need not always be as high as this. For many purposes a temperature of 121°C–126°C held for a longer period is perfectly satisfactory.

The chamber is loaded with as tight packing as desired and the vacuum drawn to remove all air from the chamber and load within 5–10 min. (Automatic control obviates the possibility of the evacuation being unduly prolonged, with resultant overdrying and superheating, *see above*.) Steam is admitted to the chamber and heats the whole load to 134°C within 2–3

min. The holding period is continued for 3 min from the time the discharge line thermometer first reaches 134°C. The load is then dried within a few minutes by exhaustion of the chamber to a high vacuum with a water-sealed pump, and the vacuum is finally broken by admission of air through a filter. A specification is detailed in *British Standard* 3970: Part 1: 1966.

AUTOCLAVE CONTROLS AND STERILIZATION INDICATORS

Automatic Process Control. It is advantageous for the sterilizer to be furnished with an automatic control system that carries through the whole sterilization cycle, including the heating-up, holding, cooling and drying stages, according to a pre-selected scheme for the duration, temperature and pressure of each stage. After the chamber has been loaded and the process started, no further attention is required until the load is ready for removal. Apart from saving the time of a skilled operator, automatic control is a valuable safeguard against error due to negligence or distraction. A monitoring system ensures that if the temperature at any time falls below that selected, the operation will be repeated.

Recording Thermometer. This desirable adjunct makes a graphic timed record of the temperature changes in the chamber discharge channel and thus, in the absence of automatic control, helps the operator to avoid errors in timing the holding period.

It has been emphasized (MRC Report, 1959) that a daily inspection of such a temperature record by a responsible person is of more value than more elaborate tests carried out at infrequent intervals.

Thermocouple Measurement of Load Temperature. This is the method of discovering the heating-up time required for a given kind of load. A thermocouple is inserted deeply inside a test article in the autoclave chamber, e.g. a bottle of liquid or a pack of dressings, and its wire leads are carried out under the chamber door or through a leak-proof port to a potentiometer. The latter indicates the temperature inside the test article during the course of autoclaving.

This means of controlling the sterilizing cycle in the autoclave is of the greatest value but it is not suitable for routine use. Two methods are available for routine use, one using chemical indicators, the other spore indicators.

Chemical indicators are placed inside the load, preferably in the centre of a fabric pack in the coolest, i.e. lowest, part of the chamber. Browne's sterilizer control tubes contain a red solution which turns green when heated at 115°C for 25 min (type 1) or 15 min (type 2), or at 160°C for 60 min (type 3). They must be stored below 20°C to avoid deterioration and premature colour change. They have the advantage of being readable immediately the sterilizing run is completed and Browne's tubes are generally accepted as being satisfactory for daily routine use.

Adhesive tape. The Bowie-Dick autoclave tape test for steam penetration used in conjunction with other tests yields valuable information (MRC Report, 1964).

Spore indicators. A preparation of dried bacterial spores is placed within the load in the autoclave and after autoclaving is tested for viability.

Bacillus stearothermophilus, a thermophile that requires to be cultivated at 55°–60°C, is a suitable test organism. Its spores are killed at 121°C in about 12 min. Commercial spore preparations are available. Otherwise a culture grown aerobically on nutrient agar for five days is suspended in sterile water to a concentration of one million spores per ml. Small strips of filter paper are soaked in the suspension, dried at room temperature and placed in paper envelopes which are then sealed. The heat-resistance of the spore strips should be tested before use by holding small sealed tubes of the spore suspension for varying periods in an oil bath at temperatures above 100°C.

The chemical or spore indicators are placed in the centre of the largest and most densely packed items of the load, and some in the coolest part, i.e. the bottom of the chamber where air tends to collect. After autoclaving, the envelope is cut with sterile scissors and the strip transferred with sterile forceps to a 'recovery medium', e.g. thioglycollate broth or cooked-meat medium; it is necessary to take rigorous precautions against contamination while making this transfer. The tube is incubated for seven days at 55°C and then examined for growth. An unautoclaved spore strip is cultured as a positive control and an uninoculated tube of medium as a negative control. The results should be reported in terms of the degree of heat-resistance of the spore preparation used. Envelopes containing about 1 g of dried earth have been used instead of spore strips but they are too variable and less satisfactory.

Recovery media. Bacteria and spores that have been damaged by heat may require special cultural conditions to allow their recovery and growth. They may lie dormant for several days when placed in a culture medium, and incubation should be continued for at least a week to give them the opportunity of growing. Moreover, certain enriched media may permit their growth when ordinary media fail. Enrichment with yeast extract, starch, glucose, blood or milk has been found beneficial. Thioglycollate broth and cooked-meat medium are suitable for recovery of both aerobic and anaerobic bacteria.

The results of chemical and spore tests reveal that some parts of the load are not adequately heated and thus will draw attention to a fault in the construction, loading or operation of the sterilizer. Successful tests, on the other hand, give no assurance that the sterilizer and technique are reliable, because heating might yet be inadequate in other parts of the load or under different conditions of loading. The essential guarantee of sterilization is that a properly designed and properly loaded autoclave be operated so as to show the correct sterilizing temperature on an accurate discharge-channel thermometer for the appropriate time.

STERILIZATION BY RADIATION

Ultra-Violet Radiation

The ability of sunlight to kill bacteria is mainly due to the ultra-violet rays that it contains. Visible light at the violet end of the spectrum has a wave-length of 400 nm and ultra-violet radiation is not markedly bactericidal until 250 nm is reached. Thereafter the effectiveness of ultra-violet light as a sterilizing agent increases with decrease in wave-length. The shortest ultra-violet rays in sunlight that reach the earth's surface in quantity have a wave-length of some 290 nm, but even more effective radiations, 240–280 nm can be produced by mercury vapour lamps.

Ultra-violet radiation is equally effective against Gram-positive and Gram-negative cells; bacterial spores are up to ten times, and viruses up to 200 times, more resistant.

Bactericidal ultra-violet rays are, however, of low energy and are unable to penetrate more than a few millimetres into fluids and scarcely, if at all, into solids. Their use is therefore best restricted to the disinfection of clean surfaces, and possibly also to disinfect particles suspended in air, as when they are used as 'curtains' at the entrance to isolation cubicles.

Ultra-violet rays are used in the microbiology laboratory to disinfect the internal surfaces of safety cabinets. The surfaces should be kept as clean as possible; the ultra-violet source must be shielded to prevent injury to the eyes and skin of staff in the vicinity and the lamp must be switched off when the cabinet is being used. Ultra-violet lamps have a limited 'working life' during which the amount of bactericidal ultra-violet radiation emitted falls off, eventually to an insignificant level.

In an attempt to reduce post-operative sepsis high intensity ultra-violet radiation has been applied to the operation area but elaborate precautions have to be taken to protect the skin and cornea from the highly irritant rays (Hart, 1942). Ultra-violet rays from suitably shielded lamps have been used to reduce the number of bacteria in the atmosphere but for safety their intensity has to be restricted (Wells and Wells, 1942).

STERILIZATION BY FILTRATION

It is possible to remove bacteria from fluids, including bacterial cultures, by passing them through filters with pores so small that bacteria are arrested. The method is especially useful in making preparations of the soluble products of bacterial growth, such as toxins, and in sterilizing liquids that would be damaged by heat, such as serum and antibiotic solutions. The British Pharmaceutical Codex test for bacteria-proof filters requires that efficient filters should be able to retain *Serratia marcescens*. This indicates an average pore diameter of 0·75 μm or less. It is possible to produce some types of filter with a smaller pore diameter and they are able to retain smaller microorganisms including many viruses. In fact, it is possible to estimate the size of viral particles by using filters of different pore diameter although this technique has been replaced by others. In general, however, 'sterilizing' filters may be regarded as rendering a liquid bacteria-free but *not* virus-free; for many laboratory purposes this is perfectly satisfactory but such fluids, e.g. serum 'sterilized' by Seitz filtration, must *not* be regarded as safe for clinical use.

Types of Filter

The various types of filter used in bacteriological work are considered here, but some are clarifying filters and do not remove bacteria.

1. Earthenware candles, e.g. Berkefeld, Chamberland.
2. Asbestos and asbestos-paper disks, e.g. Seitz.
3. Sintered glass filters.
4. Cellulose membrane filters.

Berkefeld Filters

These are made from kieselguhr, a fossil diatomaceous earth found in deposits in Germany and other parts of the world. Filters made from this material are coarse—that is, have relatively large pores owing to the size of the granules forming the substance of the filter. They are made in three grades of porosity—namely V (viel) the coarsest, W (wenig) the finest, and N (normal) intermediate. Of these, the Berkefeld V is the one usually employed, and it should not allow a small organism, such as *Serratia marcescens*, to pass.

A similar type to the Berkefeld is the Mandler filter, manufactured in the United States.

These filters can be sterilized by steaming or

autoclaving. After use they should be brushed with a stiff nail-brush and then boiled in distilled water. Before sterilizing again, distilled water should be run through them to show that they are pervious. When earthenware or porcelain filters become clogged with organic matter they should be heated to redness in a muffle furnace and allowed to cool slowly.

Chamberland Filters

These are made of unglazed porcelain and are produced in various grades of porosity. The finer grades will pass only certain very small viruses such as the viruses of foot-and-mouth disease and of fowl plague. The most porous, L_{1a}, L_2 and L_3, are comparable with the Berkefeld V, N and W candles respectively. Porcelain filters may be used for the removal of organisms from fluid cultures in order to obtain the bacterial toxin.

Seitz Filters

These consist of a disk of an asbestos composition through which the fluid is passed. The disk is inserted into a metal holder that ensures a tight joint being made. After use the asbestos disk is discarded. Various sizes are available for laboratory work. The large size of Seitz filter, with 14 cm diameter disk, can be recommended for the filtration of large amounts of serum to be used in the preparation of media. The disks are supplied in three grades—termed clarifying (K), normal and 'special EK'. The normal and EK grades of disk do not allow the ordinary test bacteria, e.g. *Serratia marcescens*, to pass.

Similar disks are made in Britain, and are as reliable and efficient as the foreign ones. The grade GS corresponds to the EK, and the FCB to the K disks. These are supplied by A. Gallenkamp & Co. Ltd., London, and John C. Carlson, Ltd., Weir Mills, Mossley, Lancs.

The filter is loosely assembled with the asbestos disk in position and the delivery tube passed through a rubber bung when a filtering flask is used. The whole is wrapped in kraft paper and sterilized in the steamer or autoclave. The filtering flask is plugged and the side-arm fitted with an air filter. When using Seitz filters it is advisable to flush the disk with sterile saline and after this to screw down tightly the upper part of the metal holder on the softened asbestos before pouring in the liquid to be filtered.

Sintered Glass Filters

These are made of finely ground glass fused sufficiently to make the small particles adhere. A special grade for sterilization purposes is manufactured by supporting a specially fine ('grade 5') filter on a coarser ('grade 3') layer, and is known as the '5/3' type. These filters are attached to the filtering apparatus and sterilized in the same way as the Seitz filter, but care must be taken that extremes of temperature are avoided. After use they are washed with running water in the reverse direction. They should be cleaned with warm sulphuric acid to which has been added a quantity of potassium nitrate, and not with sulphuric-acid-bichromate mixture.

Cellulose Membrane Filters

Two types of cellulose membrane filters are available: the older type (gradocol membranes) are composed of cellulose nitrate whereas the modern membrane filters consist of cellulose acetate.

Gradocol membranes (Elford, 1931) may be made in different grades with average pore diameter ranging from 3 μm down to 10 nm. They have been used to determine the size of many viruses.

Modern membrane filters. These filters were first developed by the Millipore Filter Corporation in America and are often referred to as 'millipore' filters (Millipore (UK) Ltd., Millipore House, Abbey Road, London NW10 75P). They can be obtained in diameters 13–293 mm and in porosities of 8 μm to 0·01 μm. Similar filters made by Courtaulds Limited and marketed by Oxo Limited as 'Oxoid' membrane filters have been available in this country since 1955. The filters consist of cellulose acetate and are composed of two layers, a basal layer with pores of 3–5 μm and an upper layer with pores of 0·5–1·0 μm in diameter. This structure gives a remarkable degree of porosity yet ensures that bacteria are trapped on the upper surface. The filters are effective in retaining *Serratia marcescens*. They withstand sterilization by autoclaving for 35–45 min at 121°C and may be stored indefinitely in a dry condition. They are made in a variety of sizes from 1·7 cm to 14 cm and can be fitted into metal or glass holders.

Cellulose membrane filters have several advantages over the widely used Seitz asbestos filters. They are much less adsorptive and the rate of filtration is much greater. Also, bacteria retained on the surface of a membrane filter can be subsequently grown by placing the filter in contact with culture media when, after suitable incubation, visible colonies will develop. This technique, which can be made quantitative, has many varied applications (see Chap. 12).

Technique of Filtration

As fluids do not readily pass through filters by gravity, it is necessary to use positive or negative pressure. Suction is the most convenient method of filtration, the fluid being drawn through the filter into a sterile container, usually a 'filtering flask', which is a conical flask of thick glass with a side-arm. It is wise to include a similar flask distally in the vacuum line to prevent contamination of the filtrate by back-flow. The use of positive pressure carries a smaller risk of transmitting bacterial contamination. Note, however, that negative pressure is unsuitable for filtering bicarbonate-buffered solutions.

The smallest negative pressure that produces satisfactory filtration should be used, commencing with a small pressure and gradually increasing it. A negative pressure of 100–200 mm of mercury is usually sufficient.

When a filter of the Berkefeld type is used, the earthenware 'candle' is fitted by means of a screw and washers into a cylindrical glass mantle, and the metal tube of the filter passes through a rubber stopper which is fitted into the neck of the flask. The side-arm of the flask which is fitted with an air filter is connected with an exhaust pump via a 'trap' flask by pressure tubing. The fluid is poured into the mantle and after filtration is collected into the flask. The necessary suction is obtained by the usual form of water pump or by a mechanical air pump. The negative pressure is estimated by means of an attached mercury or other type of manometer.

Similarly, when other filters are used, the metal tube may be inserted into a rubber bung which fits into a filtering flask.

A disadvantage of the filtering flask is that the filtered fluid has to be transferred later to another container, and where it is desired to store filtered fluids, e.g. serum or culture media, contamination may occur in the process. It has also been observed that rubber bungs are not resilient after one autoclaving and do not again fit satisfactorily so that it is necessary to tie the bung to the filter flask and seal the joints with wax.

As an alternative to a filtering flask a simple fitting attached to a screw-capped bottle can be recommended. It consists of a straight piece of metal tubing, 6–7 mm external diameter, surrounded by a wider piece of tubing to which is fitted a side-arm. The tubes are fitted into a metal screw-cap furnished with a washer to secure an air-tight joint (Fig. 3.2). The fitting is made preferably of stainless steel. Any of the screw-capped bottles can be used according to the amount of fluid to be filtered. As several sizes of bottles may fit one size of screw-cap, a few different sizes of cap will cover a·range from a few ml to four litres. The filter employed is connected to the top of the fitting by rubber pressure tubing.

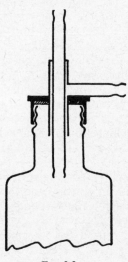

FIG. 3.2

One of the advantages of the metal screw-cap fitting is that when the filtrate has to be stored, e.g. toxin, serum, etc., it need not be removed from the container. An ordinary screw-cap for the bottle is wrapped in kraft paper and sterilized with the remainder of the apparatus. After filtration the filter and screw attachment are removed, the ordinary cap is taken from its sterile wrapper and screwed on. Where the filtrate is to be kept for some time a viskap over the screw-cap is recommended.

Filtration of Small Amounts of Fluid

With the smaller sizes of filters, a small test-tube may be arranged inside the filtering flask so that the delivery tube of the filter projects into the open end of the tube and the filtered fluid is collected directly in the small tube instead of the flask itself.

Centrifugal filter. A small amount of fluid may be conveniently filtered with a simple holder (supplied by H. A. Jones, Beaumaris, Anglesey) carrying a sterile screw-topped $\frac{1}{4}$-oz or 1-oz bottle at either end. The fluid is placed in one bottle and the holder, which is fitted with either a Seitz filter pad (1·8 cm), or an 'Oxoid' membrane filter (1·7 cm) is screwed on to the top of the bottle. The second bottle is screwed on to the other end of the holder and the assembly then placed in a bucket of a centrifuge so that the empty bottle will be outermost. Filter holders are now available that fit on to the end of a syringe so that the fluid to be sterilized is forced through the membrane by the syringe piston. They are fitted with a prefiltration pad and a millipore membrane.

The Whatman (Gamma 12) In-Line filter unit (03) is very useful for filtration sterilization of small or medium volumes of fluids in virology. It can be used with positive or negative pressure. (W. & R. Balston, Ltd., Springfield Mill, Maidstone, Kent, England.)

CHEMICAL METHODS OF DISINFECTION

Chemical substances are widely used to kill bacteria but few of them have any effect on spores. The terms *disinfectant* and *antiseptic* have been applied to different types of substance but the distinction is not clear-cut.

Both are antibacterial chemicals, often with a narrow spectrum of activity, effective principally on non-acid fast vegetative bacteria and with an uncertain action on bacterial endospores. It is reasonable to refer to all substances with these properties as disinfectants. The mass of available data concerning these agents is often contradictory and it may be difficult to be dogmatic regarding the best preparation for a particular purpose. A few disinfectants with their particular uses are mentioned here and elsewhere in this chapter. They receive further attention in Chapter 8 and for comprehensive treatment of the clinical aspects of this subject the reader is referred to Williams *et al.* (1966).

The main use of disinfectants *in the laboratory* is to render infected materials safe to handle, e.g. in discard jars. Depending on the discarded materials, a phenolic disinfectant, e.g. Hycolin 2 per cent or hypochlorite solution yielding 10000 parts per million of available chlorine is suitable. Hypochlorite solution should be made up freshly each day in carefully cleansed containers. Disinfectants are used for many purposes *in hospitals*, but often incorrectly and ineffectively. Each hospital should have a carefully planned policy for the use of disinfectants, known to all staff concerned. Steps to be taken in setting up such a policy are described by Kelsey and Maurer (1972).

1. Volatile disinfectants, e.g. chloroform. Chloroform is sometimes used in the 'sterilization' and preservation of serum (for culture media). The chloroform, added in the proportion of 0·25 per cent, can later be removed by heating at 56°C. If the serum is to be used for making a coagulated serum medium (e.g. Löffler's medium) the chloroform will be removed by the heating applied for coagulation. Chloroform is used also for preserving culture media in bulk. Vegetative bacteria are killed by exposure to chloroform liquid or strong vapour within a minute or so. Plate cultures of vegetative bacteria are sometimes killed by exposure for a few minutes to the vapour of a little chloroform placed in the lid of the plate (which must be of glass).

2. Disinfectants of the phenol group. Liquor cresolis saponatus (lysol) and cresol are powerful disinfectants formerly used in laboratories for disinfecting surgical instruments and discarded and split cultures, but now largely replaced by Hycolin (see above). Lysol is used as a 3 per cent solution. Phenol, 0·5 per cent, or *p*-chloro-*m*-cresol, 0·1 per cent, is used for preserving sera and vaccines.

3. Metallic salts or organic compounds of metals, e.g. mercuric chloride (perchloride of mercury) is sometimes used as a disinfectant in a 1 in 1000 solution. 'Merthiolate', a proprietary name for sodium ethylmercurithiosalicylate, is used as a dilution of 1 in 10000 for the preservation of antitoxic and other sera.

4. Formaldehyde. This irritant water-soluble gas is highly lethal to all kinds of microbes and spores, killing bacterial spores almost as readily as the vegetative forms. It is cheap, and non-injurious to cloth-fabrics, wood, leather, rubber, paints and metals, and can thus be used to disinfect rooms, furniture and a wide variety of articles liable to damage by heat (e.g. woollen blankets and clothing, shoes, respirators, hairbrushes, gum-elastic catheters). It is applied as an aqueous solution or in gaseous form (Ministry of Health, 1958).

Disinfection with aqueous formaldehyde solution. Commercial 'formalin' is a 40 per cent (w/v) solution of formaldehyde in water containing 10 per cent methanol to inhibit polymerization. A solution containing 5 or 10 per cent (w/v) formaldehyde in water is a powerful and rapid disinfectant when applied directly to a contaminated surface.

Bacterial cultures and suspensions are commonly killed and fixed by addition of formaldehyde to a concentration of 0·04–1·0 per cent, e.g. for preservation prior to counting or other measurements, and in preparation of a killed vaccine or agglutinable suspension.

Cleaned metal instruments may be disinfected by overnight immersion in a borax-formaldehyde solution (sodium tetraborate, 50 g, formaldehyde, 4 per cent in water, 1000 ml).

Disinfection by formaldehyde gas. Gaseous disinfection is required for articles that cannot be wetted completely with solution, or are damaged by wetting, but care is required to provide the proper conditions for action of the gas. Thus, the atmosphere must have a high relative humidity, over 60 per cent and preferably 80–90 per cent, and a temperature of at least 18°C. Moreover, the materials must be arranged to allow free access of the gas to all infected surfaces, since its penetration into porous fabrics is slow.

The gas is liberated by spraying or heating formalin, or by heating solid paraformaldehyde. When spraying cold formalin, an equal volume of industrial spirit (ethanol) may be added to prevent polymerization. The best method is by boiling 1 part formalin diluted with 2 parts of water (Beeby, Kingston and Whitehouse, 1967). Because of the tendency of the gas to polymerize to paraformaldehyde, the maximal vapour concentration attainable at 20°C is about 2·0 mg per litre of air; it is desirable to achieve this concentration. Higher concentrations, which may be potentially explosive, are attainable at higher temperatures. After disinfection, the article may contain sufficient paraformaldehyde to give off irritant vapour over a long period; this paraformaldehyde can be neutralized by exposure to ammonia vapour.

Small articles, such as instruments, shoes and hair-brushes, are disinfected by exposure for at least 3 h to formaldehyde gas in an airtight cabinet of metal or painted wood. The gas is introduced into the air in the cabinet by boiling formalin in an electric boiler using 50 ml of 40 per cent formaldehyde per 100 ft^3 of air space.

Blankets and the surfaces of mattresses are disinfected similarly in a large cabinet, where they are hung unfolded; to allow for absorption by the fabric, a much greater amount of formalin is used, namely 500 ml per 100 lb of fabrics. The vapour is finally vented to the open air.

An efficient process of sterilizing articles using formaldehyde and steam at 80°C (i.e. at subatmospheric pressures) has been described (Alder, Brown and Gillespie, 1967). Penetration is good and most fabrics, plastics and instruments are unharmed.

5. Ethylene oxide. This gaseous disinfectant is also highly lethal to all kinds of microbes and spores, but is capable of much more rapid diffusion into dry, porous materials. It is of particular value for sterilizing articles liable to damage by heat, e.g. plastic and rubber articles, blankets, pharmaceutical products and complex apparatus such as heart-lung machines (Kelsey, 1961). It is a colourless liquid, boiling point 10·7°C. Above this temperature it is a moderately toxic gas which forms an explosive mixture when more than 3 per cent is present in air. A non-explosive mixture, however, of 10 per cent ethylene oxide in carbon dioxide, or in halogenated hydrocarbon can be employed for sterilization. It is lethal to bacteria and viruses, and kills spores almost as easily as vegetative cells. The sterilization time depends, among other factors, on the temperature of the reaction and the relative humidity, which ideally should be between 20 and 40 per cent. The test organism commonly used is *Bacillus subtilis* var. *globigii*. Desiccated organisms are difficult to kill especially if they have been dried on to a hard surface such as glass or plastic. Objects to be sterilized are placed in a cabinet from which the air has been removed by drawing a high vacuum, and a non-explosive mixture containing ethylene oxide is then introduced to a pressure of 5–30 lb per in² above atmospheric pressure. The cabinet should be maintained at 45°–55°C and water introduced, if necessary, to give a relative humidity of 30 per cent. After exposure for several hours or overnight, the gas is removed by drawing a high vacuum.

An alternative system using pure ethylene oxide at subatmospheric pressure has been described (Weymes, 1966). Ethylene oxide sterilization should be undertaken only in a room specially set aside for that purpose and specially equipped to minimize the dangers of explosion and toxicity.

SOME SPECIAL APPLICATIONS OF STERILIZING METHODS IN LABORATORY AND MEDICAL PRACTICE

AUTOCLAVING OF AQUEOUS SOLUTIONS AND CULTURE MEDIA

The autoclaving of aqueous solutions and culture media must be managed in such a way that the exposure to heat is sufficient for sterilization, but not so excessive or prolonged as to damage heat-sensitive ingredients. Culture media vary in heat sensitivity. Some, such as gelatin media, will not stand autoclaving and are sterilized by intermittent steaming at 100°C. Many other media can withstand autoclaving at 121°C for 15 min, but are spoiled if heated at this temperature for 30–45 min, or if, after a 15-min exposure, they are cooled so slowly as to be maintained above 100°C for a further 30–60 min. Thus, sugars such as glucose, maltose and lactose may be partially decomposed to form acids, peptones may be broken down, and agar, especially in acid media, may lose its ability to form a firm gel. The media should therefore be autoclaved for the minimum period sufficient for sterilization and then cooled as rapidly as possible (see above). Bottles of media should be of such a size that their whole contents are used on one occasion, so as to avoid the need for repeated sterilization or melting. Agar medium should be sterilized when first made and melted, to avoid the extra heating needed to melt it on another occasion.

An exposure of 121°C for 12 min is generally thought sufficient for sterilization. The holding period of sterilization, which is timed to begin when the chamber steam first reaches 121°C at 15 lb pressure, must include not only this 10–12 min but also a time sufficient for the bottles, tubes, etc., and their contents to become heated up to the same temperature as the steam. The length of the heating-up period depends on the nature of the container, the volume of its contents and the mode of operation of the autoclave. Thus, it might be only 1–2 min for 10-ml volumes in test-tubes loosely placed to allow free circulation of steam, and as much as 45 min for a flask of 9 litres. Ideally, the exact time should be determined by trial for the particular kind of container and volume of contents, e.g. by the autoclave with a thermocouple inserted in a test container to reveal its temperature throughout the course of autoclaving. In general, the following are recommended as the total holding periods in steam at 121°C; 12 min for 10-ml volumes in loosely packed test-tubes, 15 min for 10-ml volumes in tubes tightly packed in wire baskets, 15 min for volumes up to 100 ml in bottles or flasks, 20–25 min for 500-ml volumes, 25–30 min for 1000-ml volumes and 35–45 min for 2000-ml volumes. It is a bad practice to autoclave large and small volumes in the same load, because with the same holding period (e.g. 20 min) the large may not be sterilized, while the small may be damaged by overheating.

The bottles, tubes, etc., should not be filled to more than 75–80 per cent of their capacity lest the contents overflow on expansion during heating. The containers may be loosely stoppered, e.g. with cotton-wool plugs or loosely applied screw-caps, or else hermetically sealed, e.g. sealed ampoules and bottles with tightly applied screw-caps. In sealed containers the aqueous content provides the conditions for moist-heat sterilization and the presence of some air does not interfere with this. Hermetic sealing is an advantage in preventing loss of water from the contents by evaporation or violent boiling during the cooling period when the steam pressure is being reduced. It also makes possible the autoclaving of solidified egg medium without disruption by bubble formation. However, except for the smallest bottles, the tight application of a screw-cap increases the liability to breakage during autoclaving and slows down cooling.

For these reasons, it is usual to autoclave aqueous media in containers stoppered with cotton-wool, with loose metal caps or with screw-caps which are loosened slightly. This practice necessitates careful management of the cooling period. When the steam supply to the chamber is stopped at the end of the holding period, the steam already in the chamber gradually cools and diminishes in pressure. This induces evaporation of water from the medium in the container and escape of the vapour through the loose stopper. The evaporation is the main means of cooling of the containers and contents. With correct management the loss of water from the medium is only 3–5 per cent. It is therefore usual to prepare aqueous media and solutions for autoclaving by adding an extra 5 per cent of distilled water, so that their concentration will be correct after the autoclaving. The cooling process should be managed in such a way that the chamber pressure diminishes gradually from 15 lb per in^2 to atmospheric pressure in the course of 10–30 min, the

optimal time varying with the volume of medium per container (15–20 min is usually most satisfactory). The rate at which the chamber steam spontaneously cools and loses pressure, i.e. without opening of the chamber discharge valve, varies with the type of autoclave, the load and other conditions. The reduction to atmospheric pressure may occur in the desired time (e.g. 15–20 min), or may take up to an hour or longer. The slower cooling is undesirable since it may result in damage to heat-sensitive materials. If necessary, therefore, the chamber discharge valve should be opened slightly so as to bring about a gradual reduction to atmospheric pressure over the proper period of time. Too rapid a reduction must be avoided, because the media would then boil explosively. Some modern autoclaves, specially designed for sterilizing aqueous media, incorporate a device which effects rapid cooling without violent boiling; this may involve the replacement of chamber steam with air at the same pressure, or spraying of the load with condensate at a temperature slightly below that of the steam.

When the pressure gauge shows that the steam in the chamber has reached 0 lb per in^2 (atmospheric pressure), air is at once admitted into the chamber, through the air inlet and filter if available, or through the chamber discharge tap, or by opening the chamber door slightly. If this is not done until the pressure has fallen below atmospheric, more water will be lost by evaporation from the containers. When sufficiently cool, e.g. below 70°C the containers are removed from the autoclave and their screw-caps tightened firmly.

Autoclaving in 'free steam'. When a Koch or Arnold steamer is not available, an autoclave may be used to sterilize culture media at a temperature of 100°C, or just over. The door of the chamber is tightly closed, the steam supply turned on and the air expelled through the open discharge tap. After expulsion of the air, the steam supply is adjusted so that an adequate amount continues to escape through the open tap, and a pressure of 1–2 lb (above atmospheric) is maintained in the chamber during the holding period; this may be less than in the ordinary steamer (e.g. 60 instead of 90 min).

Sterilization of Bottled Fluids

Intravenous infusion fluids can be sterilized in a relatively simple manner because any contaminating bacteria will already be moist and their destruction merely necessitates heating the fluid in each container to the appropriate temperature and holding it there for the appropriate time viz. 121°C for 12 min or 115°C for 30 min (MRC Report, 1964). Unduly prolonged heating is to be avoided because deterioration of the solutions may result. Water itself should be sterilized in this way as it is the only safe method of preparing and handling sterile water for use in operating theatres and elsewhere. For sterilizing bottled fluids a gravity displacement autoclave is satisfactory. It does not need to be jacketed and it does not require a vacuum-producing apparatus. The autoclaves employed are often large and heat 'layering' may be present. The rate and evenness of heating can be improved by introducing steam through a number of inlets so that turbulence of the steam/air mixture is produced (Wilkinson and Peacock, 1961). Excessive breakage, the result of heating or cooling the bottles too quickly, has to be avoided and the process is a slow one. However, devices are being developed to give more rapid cooling and shorten the whole cycle of sterilization (*British Standard* 3970: Part 2: 1966).

Sterilization of Empty Bottles and Impervious Containers

If empty and dry containers are to be autoclaved, they must not be tightly stoppered, because steam would be excluded and sterilization by moist heat impossible. They should be placed on their sides in the autoclave to allow a horizontal path for the entry of steam and escape of air. If unstoppered, they will be sterilized quickly, but if stoppered even loosely, as with cotton-wool or a loosened screw-cap, the displacement of air is slow and the holding period at 121°C should be extended to at least 30 min. Because of the uncertainty of air displacement from stoppered empty containers, it is better to sterilize them in the hot-air oven.

The disadvantage of dry heat sterilization, however, is that rubber liners inside the screw-cap perish at the high temperatures (160°C) employed. This problem can be overcome by using liners made of silicone rubber (available from ESCO (Rubber) Ltd., Seal Street, London, E.8). Although expensive, silicone rubber is able to withstand repeated exposures in the hot air oven and being more porous than ordinary rubber the caps may be screwed down tightly without the risk of the bottle exploding during sterilization.

Sterilization of Wrapped Dry Goods and Surgical Dressings

Dry goods such as paper- or cloth-wrapped apparatus, and surgical linen and dressings, require special attention in autoclaving, firstly to ensure the complete displacement of air from their interior by steam, and secondly to dry them before removal from the autoclave (for much detailed information consult the MRC Report, 1964).

In conventional sterilizers the air is removed by the *gravity displacement method*, being driven downwards through the load by the lighter steam accumulating above it. This method requires that the load be loosely packed so that adequate spaces are left for circulation of steam between the packs and that a free downward movement of air is possible through the materials of each pack. Dry materials must not be enclosed in sealed impervious containers which prevent the entry of steam and escape of air. Glass and metal containers are left open or covered only loosely, and placed on their sides. For surgical packs, a wrapping of at least two layers of cloth or paper is recommended. A single layer is not satisfactory because dust on the outside can contaminate the contents when the pack is opened. A paper wrapping is commonly used for small articles of laboratory apparatus (see Maintenance of Sterility).

Surgical dressings and other cloth articles should be arranged in packs no bigger than 12 × 12 × 20 inches, and these should be placed on edge in the autoclave so that the layers of cloth are vertical. Rubber gloves are powdered and packed loosely in muslin wraps, with pads of muslin in the palm and folds to allow access of steam to all parts. In an attempt to minimize deterioration it used to be customary to autoclave rubber gloves at 5 to 10 lb pressure for a short period of time. Such exposures do *not* quarantee sterility and gloves should be autoclaved at the same temperature as other packaged goods. Treatment in a high-pressure, high-vacuum sterilizer requires only a brief exposure at 130°–134°C and this probably combines safety with minimum deterioration (MRC Report, 1964). Tubing is wetted inside with sterile water just before placing in the autoclave. Jointed instruments must be open, and syringes free from oil and grease and either disassembled or else moistened internally with water. The auto-clave chamber must not be overloaded nor the perforated tray removed to make more room.

Metal drums and caskets must be provided with air ports and these must not be obstructed by the contents being packed against them. The ports must always be fully open during sterilization and the containers so positioned in the autoclave that steam can flow through freely from top to bottom via the open vents. Formerly, dressing drums were round, but rectangular caskets are much more easy to pack and handle. It must be stressed that a drum which can only be closed with difficulty is grossly overpacked. In many ways it is prefer-able to pack materials in a wrapper of porous cloth or paper, since this allows a much freer passage of air and steam.

Vacuum removal of air. The venturi vacuum device that is commonly incorporated in auto-claves to assist drying is relative inefficient and removes no more than a third to a half of the air from the chamber. This vacuum is some-times applied before the admission of steam, but the partial evacuation of air is of little value. Sometimes this vacuum is drawn two or more times, steam being admitted between each vacuum. In the case of textiles such repeated evacuation merely produces a 'breath-ing' motion of the same air inside the material. In fact, if prolonged, the result of this type of vacuum may be overdrying and injurious super-heating of the load. On the other hand, efficient removal of more than 98 per cent of the air is employed to great advantage in modern 'high pre-vacuum' sterilizers. The high pre-vacuum contributes to the efficient steam sterilization of dressings, helping to produce a dry sterile load in the shortest possible time without causing damage (Fallon, 1961). It should be emphasized that this method is the only one which overcomes the effects of bad packing and overloading.

Avoidance of damage by superheating. Cloth and rubber articles are liable to be damaged by excessive heating. When very dry cloth is first exposed to steam, it adsorbs and con-denses an excessive amount of it and receives the corresponding excess of latent heat; this may raise its temperature to 25°–100°C above that of the autoclave. Freshly laundered fabrics contain sufficient moisture to prevent this and so should not be stored overlong in a place of low humidity before being sterilized, nor be subjected to drying by pre-heating in the sterilizer or a prolonged application of vacuum. Heating in steam mixed with some air is more damaging than heating in pure steam, especially in the case of rubber articles.

The duration of the holding period at 121°C. The holding period is timed as beginning when the discharge-channel thermometer first indi-cates 121°C. All free air has then been dis-placed from the chamber, but some still remains trapped in the interior of the porous load. The further time required for the steam to penetrate all parts, displace the air and heat the load throughout to 121°C, may extend to 30 min or even longer. This 'steam penetration time' must be added to the 'sterilizing time' of 12 min in computing the holding period. The following are generally recommended as the total holding times at 121°C: 15–20 min for muslin- or paper-wrapped instruments, rubber gloves and open metal or glass con-tainers; 30 min for muslin- or paper-wrapped packs of surgical linen and dressings, wrapped syringes, and loosely stoppered metal or glass containers; 45 min for metal surgical dressing drums with muslin liners. The holding period is much shorter when a high pre-vacuum sterilizer is employed. Once the pre-sterilization vacuum has been drawn, heating up and full penetration by steam of a load of textiles firmly packed in dressing drums will be accomplished in 3 min and the sterilization time is also shorter, e.g. 3 min at 134°C (see Table 3.2).

Drying of the load. The load is dried during the cooling period. The supply of steam at 121°C is maintained in the jacket, while that to the chamber is cut off. The chamber steam is allowed to escape rapidly through the discharge tap until zero gauge pressure is reached. The moisture of the load is then evaporated by the residual heat of the articles and radiant heat from the jacketed walls of the chamber. The drying is assisted to completion by the removal of vapour from the chamber. The venturi device is used to suck warmed, filtered air into and through the chamber; this carries away the vapour and dries the load in 15–25 min. The air allowed into the chamber must be drawn through an efficient filter to free it from dust-borne bacteria which otherwise might enter the sterilized packages.

Without the concurrent admission of air, the application of the partial vacuum (15 mm Hg or less) obtainable by the venturi device is quite inadequate to effect drying. Alternatively as long as the load is not wet from inadequately dried steam the attaining of a vacuum of 20 mm Hg or more should be sufficient to achieve drying since water retained in the load will 'boil off' more rapidly at this reduced chamber pressure. Filtered air is still required, however,

to break the vacuum before the sterilizer is opened. Thus in a modern high pre-vacuum autoclave the drying period is very short. Table 3.2 shows how the overall process time for a load of surgical dressings is greatly reduced by employing a high pre-vacuum autoclave (Bowie, 1958).

STERILIZATION OF SURGICAL INSTRUMENTS

Boiling is not an effective or dependable sterilizing process; the use of small pressure sterilizers that will ensure the safety of un-wrapped instruments and bowls is to be preferred. Such autoclaves can be of simple design and because heating up and penetration are instantaneous the process time is short, especially if the sterilizer can be operated at 132°–134°C or at 150°C.

Heat is said to blunt sharp instruments but this effect is mainly due to oxidation and damage should not be caused by pure steam. The only established chemical sterilizing agents are ethylene oxide and formaldehyde and they can be used to sterilize instruments such as scalpels. Complex pieces of apparatus like cystoscopes, which cannot withstand heat even at 100°C, may often be rendered safe for their particular purposes by ethylene oxide steriliza-

Table 3.2 Comparison of process times in a gravity displacement and a high pre-vacuum sterilizer (after Bowie, 1958)

Process time in a 9 ft³ gravity displacement sterilizer (Load—*dressings packed loosely in caskets*)		Process time in a 9 ft³ high pre-vacuum sterilizer (Load—*dressings firmly packed in caskets*)	
Stage	*Time (min)*	Stage	*Time (min)*
Time for thermometer to indicate 121°	10	Time to draw pre-sterilization vacuum . . .	7
Estimated penetrating and heating up time . . .	27	Time for thermometer to indicate 134°C . . .	3
		(includes steam penetration and heating-up time)	
Sterilization holding period .	12	Sterilization holding period .	2
Safety margin . . .	6	Safety margin . . .	1
Vacuum drying period . .	25	Vacuum drying period . .	3
		Breaking vacuum . .	1
Total . .	80	Total . .	17

tion. For some purposes pasteurization at 75°C, treatment with chlorhexidine preferably in 75 per cent ethanol, or total immersion of a thoroughly clean endoscope in 2 per cent buffered glutaraldehyde (e.g. 'Cidex') may be satisfactory.

STERILIZATION OF SYRINGES

Syringes play an important part in the work of bacteriological laboratories and hospital wards. Nowadays, disposable sterile plastic syringes are widely used; where these are not available, particular attention must be given to the use, care and sterilization of substitutes. Sterilization by heat is the method of choice; chemical agents are unsatisfactory.

It is recommended that all-glass syringes should be used in preference to the glass-metal syringe, over which they have many advantages. The glass-metal type is more difficult to clean, and is more likely to break on heating owing to the difference of expansion of glass and metal. It cannot be sterilized when assembled and is more difficult to keep sterile until ready for use. The solder uniting the glass and metal parts may melt in the hot-air oven, and may even do so in the autoclave. Syringes are now available, however, with cement at the glass-metal junction that will withstand 200°C. Syringes of 5 ml capacity and upwards should have eccentric nozzles. The needles should be of stainless steel of the best quality. The mounts of the needles must fit accurately to the nozzle of the syringe.

All-glass syringes. Before being put into use, new syringes must be well washed in soap and water with a test-tube brush or burette brush according to size. After washing in clean, warm water, both barrel and piston are dried. It is convenient to have the syringes assembled, wrapped and sterilized, ready for use and to have a supply of these sterilized syringes always on hand.

Dry heat. All-glass syringes are best sterilized in the hot-air oven as follows. New syringes are cleaned as above in soap and water, washed and dried. The piston is lightly smeared with liquid paraffin or silicone fluid, the lubricant being well rubbed into the ground glass, inserted into the barrel, and moved backwards and forwards several times so that the syringe works evenly and smoothly. Excess of lubricant is to be avoided. The syringe may be packed in a metal tube, usually made of aluminium and sealed with a foil cap. Alternatively, the assembled syringe is placed in a stout glass tube of such diameter that the barrel of the syringe fits loosely and the flange rests on the top of the tube. The tube should be of such length that it accommodates the syringe with needle fitted. The tube containing the syringe is then wrapped in clear transparent cellophane or similar material, a strip of material of the following sizes being used: for 1-ml and 2-ml syringes 3 in × 9 in, for 5-ml, 4 in × 11 in, for 10-ml and 20-ml 5 in × 14 in. The cellophane is rolled in a spiral fashion round the tube, commencing at the bottom with a fold and turn-in, and finishing above the piston of the syringe with a firm twist. If cellophane is not available, kraft paper can be used, but the disadvantage of this is that the syringe cannot be seen, and relevant information, e.g. size of syringes, etc., must be written in pencil on the paper.

The assembled and wrapped syringe is sterilized in the hot-air oven at 160°C (± 2°C) for not less than 1 h. Under these conditions the cellophane turns slightly brown, indicating to the user that the syringe has been sterilized.

Needles are sterilized in 3 in × $\frac{1}{2}$ in test-tubes plugged with cotton-wool. In order to protect the point of the needle, a piece of 5-mm glass tubing 2 in long is placed in the tube and the point of the needle passed down it so that the mount of the needle rests on the tubing. The cotton-wool plug keeps the needle in place. The tubes with contained needles are individually wrapped in cellophane and sterilized as above at 160°C for 1 h.

Moist heat. Sterilization in the autoclave is possible only if steam is able to penetrate to every surface of the syringe. In practice this means that the piston must not be smeared with lubricant and if packed in an impervious container this must not be sealed until *after* the syringe has been sterilized. Assembled syringes may be sterilized in a high pre-vacuum autoclave, but in a gravity-displacement sterilizer the syringe must be dismantled otherwise air discharge would be inefficient.

Boiling. When the above methods are not available, all-glass syringes may be disinfected just before use by boiling in a fish kettle or saucepan. If the tap water is hard it is best to use distilled water. The syringe is dismantled and the barrel and piston are placed in cold water, which is brought to the boil and kept boiling continuously for not less than 10 min. The perforated tray is removed from the sterilizer and the water poured off. When *dry* and cool enough, the barrel and piston are assembled with sterile forceps or clean, dry fingers, touching only the outside of the barrel and the top of the piston. The sterile syringe should be used immediately and not placed in stock 'sterile' water or alcohol. The needle should be boiled at the same time, and it is an advantage to thread it through a piece of lint to protect the point. The needle is affixed to the nozzle by means of sterile forceps.

Cleaning. After the syringe has been used, e.g. for blood culture, aspiration, etc., it is *immediately* washed out in a cold solution of 2 per cent lysol, which should always be ready for the purpose. Blood must never be allowed to clot in the syringe, otherwise it will be difficult to remove the piston. Hot fluid must not be used otherwise it will coagulate the protein and the piston will stick. If the needle has been removed before the blood, etc., is expelled, it must immediately be cleaned after the syringe has been washed out by affixing it to the syringe again and washing it through with the lysol solution. After washing, syringe and needle are returned to the tube in which they were sterilized.

Before re-sterilizing, the syringe is thoroughly cleaned in soapy water, a brush being used, then washed in clean, warm water and dried. If it is to be sterilized by dry heat it is finally lubricated with liquid paraffin, before assembly.

The needle is washed in warm water, the bore of the needle cleared with a stilette, and the mount of the needle cleaned with a piece of cotton-wool on a swab-stick to remove any blood, etc. After washing it with warm water it is run through with alcohol and allowed to dry. Before being sterilized the point is touched up on a fine Arkansas slip-stone (size 4 in $\times$ 1$\frac{1}{4}$ in), lubricated with thin machine oil or liquid paraffin, and examined with an 8 $\times$ hand-lens to see that the point is really sharp. It is then run through with the stilette, washed in alcohol and dried.

Glass-metal ('Record') syringes. These cannot be sterilized as above described because the solder-cement joining the glass and metal parts together may melt in the hot-air oven. Moreover, they cannot be sterilized, while assembled, by any heat method as the unequal expansion of glass and metal causes cracking of the barrel. In order to sterilize Record type syringes they must be taken apart. The Record type syringe is usually disinfected by boiling for 5 min as described above for all-glass syringes. Alternatively, the piston and barrel can be wrapped separately in kraft paper and sterilized in the autoclave, although it should be noted that the solder-cement in some makes may melt even at this temperature.

Glass-metal syringes are washed out immediately after use as described above, and the needles are cleaned and sharpened as for all-glass syringes.

DISINFECTION OF ROOMS

Fumigation with gaseous disinfectants was at one time commonly performed after a room had been occupied by a patient with an infectious disease. Sulphur dioxide, generated by burning sulphur, was the popular agent for this purpose but it is effective only if the relative humidity is 60 per cent or more.

Terminal disinfection is now practised only if the environment has been contaminated with the organisms of a serious infectious disease such as anthrax, smallpox or tuberculosis and formaldehyde is generally used.

Disinfection of rooms by spraying formalin (Jack, 1952, 1954). This is probably the most effective means of disinfecting the interior and furniture of a room. The room is first well sealed by covering cracks, ventilators, fireplaces, etc., with brown paper and adhesive tape. An operator protected by an efficient anti-gas respirator thoroughly moistens all surfaces of the walls, floor and furniture with a spray of 10 per cent formaldehyde solution (1 volume of formalin and 3 volumes of water), and finally saturates the atmosphere by spraying undiluted formalin to the extent of

1 litre per 1000 ft³. The room is closed by sealing the door and left for 24 h. A basin of ammonia solution is then introduced and left to evaporate for several hours (1 litre SG 880 ammonia solution mixed with 1 litre of water per litre of 40 per cent formaldehyde used). This neutralizes the formaldehyde and paraformaldehyde, and the excess ammonia is readily removed by ventilation.

Disinfection of rooms with formaldehyde vapour. The room is sealed as described above and heated, if necessary, to above 18°C. Formalin is boiled within the room in an electric boiler having a safety plug which kicks out when the vessel boils dry and a time switch set to cut off the current just prior to this; 500 ml of 40 per cent formaldehyde plus 1000 ml water are boiled per 1000 ft³ of air space. The room is kept sealed for 4–24 h and an operator wearing a respirator then introduces a cloth soaked in ammonia solution (250 ml per litre of formalin used). This is left for 2 h to neutralize the formaldehyde.

DISINFECTION OF BEDCLOTHES

The bedding of a patient or carrier is liable to become heavily contaminated with pathogenic bacteria such as *Staph. aureus* and *Strept. pyogenes*, and, when disturbed, liberates large numbers of these into the air. Cotton and linen sheets, and blankets made from cotton or some synthetic fibres (Calnan, 1959), may be sterilized by boiling during laundering and it has been recommended that these blankets replace the conventional woollen ones which shrink on boiling. High temperature laundering of woollen blankets sufficient to destroy vegetative bacteria is feasible, however, if a slightly acid detergent mixture is used. Alternatively, steam at subatmospheric pressure may be used to disinfect bedding (Alder, *et al.*, 1966). Woollen blankets can be rendered safe by exposure to suitable chemical agents. Treatment with gaseous disinfectants such as formaldehyde vapour or ethylene oxide is effective but requires special equipment. Simpler methods include impregnation of the blankets with either quaternary ammonium disinfectants or synthetic phenolic compounds (Larkin *et al.*, 1961). Application of oil to the blankets

in the last stage of the laundering process reduces the subsequent scatter of organisms.

DISINFECTION OF SKIN

The normal commensal bacterial flora of the skin is made up of a few species of resident organisms, mainly coagulase-negative staphylococci and corynebacteria, which grow in the glands and hair follicles and cannot be removed entirely; and a potentially large number of species of transient organisms deposited on the skin from the environment. Skin disinfection may be directed mainly towards the removal of harmful transients, as in removing accidental contaminants from laboratory cultures, or to removing transients and as many of the resident organisms as possible, as in disinfection of the skin before operation.

In the laboratory, a regular routine of thorough handwashing with warm water and soap, drying of the hands on disposable paper towels and the use thereafter of 70 per cent isopropyl or ethyl alcohol containing 1 per cent glycerine, is a sensible and useful precaution, especially if carried out at the end of work periods, before leaving the laboratory, and before eating or drinking. If the skin is knowingly contaminated with pathogens from cultures or specimens, more powerful disinfectants, such as 1 to 5 per cent aqueous sodium hypochlorite solution or 1 per cent Hycolin (or equivalent clear soluble phenolic) should be applied first, and carefully removed thereafter by washing.

A prolonged reduction in the resident skin flora can be achieved by the exclusive use of a detergent containing 2 to 3 per cent hexachlorophane.

The first step in skin disinfection is thorough washing. After the skin is washed, it may be rinsed in 70 per cent ethanol, which dries rapidly and has a transient bactericidal effect. The action of the alcohol is slightly improved by the addition of 0·5 per cent chlorhexidine.

Where strict asepsis is required, as in surgery, it is necessary to wear sterile rubber gloves which are impervious to the organisms on the skin. As there is always a danger of the gloves being perforated during use, it is important before donning them to remove as many of the bacteria from the hands as possible. This may be done as above. Since the operator's hands may have to be disinfected repeatedly it is essential that non-irritant agents are employed, but when only a single application is required, as in preparing the skin of a patient or animal for incision or puncture, stronger disinfectants may be used. Recently however, it has been shown that 0·5 per cent chlorhexidine in 70 per cent ethanol is as effective a disinfectant as 1 per cent iodine in alcohol and its use is free from the risks of sensitization and irritation. Iodine compounds have some sporicidal action and this is of special value when cleansing sites which may have been contaminated with clostridia; an iodophor (e.g. 'Betadine') may be used for this purpose. For further details see Lowbury (1961).

Maintenance of Sterility

Once articles have been rendered sterile it is essential that they are handled and stored in such a way as to prevent recontamination before they are used.

Test-tubes and flasks. The interiors of test-tubes, flasks, bottles, etc., must be carefully protected from bacterial contamination due to access of air, dust, etc., before and after the addition of medium and during the subsequent cultivation of organisms. This has usually been done by means of cotton-wool stoppers. These should be $1\frac{1}{4}$ to $1\frac{1}{2}$ in long, $\frac{3}{4}$ to 1 in being inserted into the mouth of the tube, etc., and the remainder projecting. They should fit firmly, but not so tightly as to render their removal difficult.

The stoppers should be made from long-fibre cotton-wool which is free from short broken fibres and dust. Non-absorbent cotton is preferable, because, after steaming, plugs tend to remain moist, and if the medium is to be kept for any length of time and absorbent wool is used, moulds will grow through the stopper and contaminate the medium. A sufficient amount of cotton-wool (see above) should be forced into the tube with a rod or pair of forceps, but should not be twisted in, as creases are formed along the sides of the glass and create channels for contaminating organisms.

Instead of the ordinary roll of cotton-wool being used, it is recommended that the non-absorbent wool be obtained in the form of a long thin ribbon known as 'rope wool' or 'neck wool' of the type used by hairdressers. It is kept in a tin container with a hole in the lid, and the appropriate amount of wool for the stopper is easily obtained without waste.

When tubes or flasks have to be stored for some time the stoppers or tops of the crates or boxes should be covered with sterile kraft paper, kept in place by means of fine string or a rubber band. Sterile rubber stoppers may, in some cases, be used instead of cotton-wool, particularly where the contents of the flask or tube have to be kept a considerable time, as in the case of immune sera; this also applies to vessels that have to be transported by post or by messenger.

Slip-on aluminium caps of various patterns are available for use instead of cotton-wool plugs, for the stoppering of test-tubes. They have the advantage of protecting the rim of the tube from airborne dust and their use thus makes unnecessary the conventional 'flaming' of the mouth of the tube on each occasion of its opening. These caps should be used for cultures of delicate organisms that are affected by toxic volatile substances liberated from cotton-wool during the process of sterilization.

Screw-capped bottles. Flasks for storing culture media have now been replaced by screw-capped bottles of 3-, 5- and 10-oz capacity, while the smaller bottles of $\frac{1}{4}$-, $\frac{1}{2}$- and 1-oz capacity may be employed instead of test-tubes.

Petri dishes. Each individual dish should be wrapped in kraft paper before sterilization, and kept in the paper until used. For a 4-in dish the size of paper should be 12 in square. The dishes may also be sterilized (unwrapped) and kept in metal boxes.

Pipettes. 1-ml and 10-ml graduated pipettes should be wrapped in a long strip of kraft paper, which is wound round them in a spiral manner before sterilizing in the hot-air oven. Bulb pipettes (10 ml, 50 ml, etc.) are also covered with kraft paper. Under these conditions pipettes remain sterile in their wrappers for considerable periods of time. Alternatively they may be sterilized and stored in suitable canisters.

Capillary pipettes are sterilized in large test-tubes 15 in × 2½ in, having a gauze or cotton-wool stopper, or in metal boxes. The former method is preferable. Alternatively, 8-in lengths of 5-mm glass tubing are plugged with cotton-wool at both ends, wrapped in batches of a dozen in kraft paper, sterilized and stored. When capillary pipettes are required, the middle of the tubing is heated in a Bunsen or blowpipe and pulled out, the ends of the two pipettes being sealed in the making.

Ampoules are sterilized in the hot-air oven with the necks sealed, and are kept in metal boxes. If unsealed ampoules are used, they should be plugged with cotton-wool before sterilization.

It must be emphasized that a wrapping of kraft paper or double-thickness muslin is effective in excluding contaminating bacteria *only when it is dry*. If the wrapped articles are sterilized in an autoclave instead of a hot-air oven, they must be dried before placing on an unsterile surface.

Surgical dressings. The MRC Report (1964) points out that a load sterilized in the auto-clave may become contaminated during removal from the sterilizer, in transport or during subsequent storage. It is essential that metal dressing drums should have tightly fitting lids and a protective lining that will cover the ports inside the drums. Wrapped packs on removal from the autoclave should not at once be placed on a cold flat surface, since residual moisture will condense on this, make damp the fabric or paper wrapping, and so permit the entry of contaminating bacteria. Alder and Alder (1961) measured the recon-tamination rate of dressings wrapped in different materials. They concluded that paper was more efficient than either calico or balloon cloth and that one layer of any of these materials was better than two layers of muslin. Crepe paper is usually preferred to kraft paper because it drapes better and it is always advisable to use a double layer in case the outer covering becomes torn. As an extra precaution the double-wrapped packs may be enclosed in rigid or semi-rigid containers such as cardboard cartons. The shelf life after sterilization of dressings packaged in this way is several weeks and this period can be pro-longed if storage conditions are good.

Pre-sterilized materials. Disposable syringes, catheters and needles sterilized by gamma radiation or ethylene oxide gas are usually marketed in plastic or paper envelopes. It must be emphasized that a high standard of packag-ing is necessary if such pre-sterilized products are to remain sterile. Particular attention must be paid to the sealing of the container.

FURTHER READING

RUBBO, S. D. & GARDNER, J. D. (1965) *A Review of Sterilisation and Disinfection* London: Lloyd-Luke Ltd.

REFERENCES

ALDER, V. G. & ALDER, F. I. (1961) Preserving the sterility of surgical dressings wrapped in paper and other materials. *Journal of Clinical Pathology*, **14**, 76.

ALDER, V. G., BROWN, A. M. & GILLESPIE, W. A. (1966) Disinfection of heat-sensitive material by low-tempera-ture steam and formaldehyde. *Journal of Clinical Pathology*, **19**, 83.

BEEBY, M. M., KINGSTON, D. & WHITEHOUSE, C. E. (1967) Experiments on terminal disinfection of cubicles with formaldehyde. *Journal of Hygiene (Cambridge)*, **65**, 115.

BOWIE, J. H. (1955) Modern apparatus for sterilisation. *Pharmaceutical Journal*, **174**, 473.

BOWIE, J. H. (1958) The nurse, steam and the engineer. *Hospital Engineer*, **12**, 158, 182.

CALNAN, J. S. (1959) Clean blankets, new boilable bed-cover. *Lancet*, **i**, 300.

DARMADY, E. M. & BROCK, R. B. (1954) Temperature levels in hot-air ovens. *Journal of Clinical Pathology*, **7**, 290.

ELFORD, W. J. (1931) A new series of graded collodion membranes suitable for general bacteriological use, especially in filterable virus studies. *Journal of Pathology and Bacteriology*, **34**, 505.

FALLON, R. J. (1961) Factors concerned in the efficient steam sterilisation of surgical dressings. *Journal of Clinical Pathology*, **14**, 505.

HART, D. (1942) The importance of air-borne pathogenic bacteria in the operating room: a method of control by sterilisation of the air with ultra-violet radiation. In *Aerobiology*, p. 186, edited by F. R. Moulton. Washing-ton D.C.: American Association for Advancement of Science.

HOWIE, J. W. & TIMBURY, M. C. (1956). Laboratory tests of operating-theatre sterilisers. *Lancet*, **ii**, 669.

JACK, R. P. (1952 & 1954) *City of Edinburgh Public Health Reports*.

KELSEY, J. C. (1961) Sterilisation by ethylene oxide. *Journal of Clinical Pathology*, **14**, 59.

KELSEY, J. C. & MAURER, ISOBEL M. (1972) *The Use of Chemical Disinfectants in Hospitals*. Public Health Laboratory Service Monograph Series No. 2. London: HMSO.

LARKIN, I. M., BRIDSON, E. Y., GRIEVE, W. S. M. & GIBSON, J. W. (1961) Disinfection of hospital blankets with synthetic phenolic compounds. *Journal of Clinical Pathology*, **14**, 80.

LOWBURY, E. J. L. (1961) Skin· disinfection. *Journal of Clinical Pathology*, **14**, 85.

MEDICAL RESEARCH COUNCIL (1964) Working party's report on sterilisation by steam under increased pressure. *Lancet*, **ii**, 193.

MINISTRY OF HEALTH (1958) The practical aspects of formaldehyde fumigation. *Monthly Bulletin of the Ministry of Health Laboratory Service*, **17**, 270.

WELLS, W. F. & WELLS, M. W. (1942) Air-borne infection as a basis for a theory of contagion. In *Aerobiology*, p. 99. American Association for Advancement of Science.

WEYMES, C. (1966) Sterilisation with Ethylene Oxide at Sub-Atmospheric Pressure. *British Hospital Journal and Social Science Review*, 1745.

WILKINSON, G. R. & PEACOCK, F. G. (1961) Improvement of heating of bottled fluids during autoclave sterilisation using low pressure steam. *Journal of Pharmacy and Pharmacology*, 13 (Supplement) 72 T.

WILLIAMS, R. E. O., BLOWERS, R., GARROD, L. P. & SHOOTER, R. A. (1966) Chapter XIX. Sterilisation or disinfection by chemicals. In *Hospital Infection*, p. 311. London: Lloyd-Luke Ltd.

4. pH Measurements and Buffers, Oxidation-Reduction Potentials, Suspension Fluids, Preparation of Glassware

pH in Microbiology

Microorganisms, in common with other living organisms, are very susceptible to changes in the acidity or alkalinity of the surrounding medium. This is true with regard to both growth and survival. Whilst many bacteria show vigorous growth within a fairly wide range of acidity or alkalinity, there are others that require the 'reaction' of the medium to be adjusted within narrow limits before multiplication takes place. Moreover, all microorganisms have a particular 'reaction' at which growth is optimal. In order, therefore, to secure the best growth, particularly of highly parasitic organisms, it is necessary that the adjustment of the 'reaction' should be made as accurately as possible. For this purpose, it is necessary to become familiar with the factors determining this 'reaction', with the mode of its expression and with the methods used for its estimation.

The Meaning of the pH Scale

Pure water is very slightly dissociated into an equal number of hydrogen ions and hydroxyl ions.

$$H_2O \rightleftharpoons H^+ + OH^-.$$

According to the law of mass action, the following formula will hold at equilibrium (the square brackets refer to the molar concentrations):

$$K = \frac{[H^+][OH^-]}{[H_2O]}.$$

But the amount of water ionized will be extremely small, so that the concentration of unionized water, $[H_2O]$, is virtually constant. Therefore, at equilibrium, the product of the concentration of hydrogen ions and hydroxyl ions will be a constant, which is termed the ion product of water K_w, i.e.

$$K_w = [H^+][OH^-].$$

From conductivity measurements, it has been found that the concentration of hydrogen ions and hydroxyl ions in pure water at 22°C is 10^{-7} gram ions per litre. Therefore K_w at 22°C will be 1.0×10^{-14}. At a given temperature and in dilute aqueous solutions, the product of the molar concentrations of hydrogen ions and hydroxyl ions will always be the same, *no matter what other substances are present*.

Consider what happens when an acid is added to water. The acid will dissociate, liberating hydrogen ions, the amount of which depends on the amount of acid added and on the degree of dissociation of the acid. A strong acid will be largely dissociated in dilute solutions while a weak acid will be largely undissociated, e.g.

$$HCl \rightleftharpoons H^+ + Cl^-$$
$$CH_3COOH \rightleftharpoons H^+ + CH_3COO^-$$

As a result of the liberation of hydrogen ions caused by dissociation of the acid, the number of hydroxyl ions must be decreased in order to maintain the ion product of water at a constant value. Similarly, when an alkali is dissolved in water, it also undergoes dissociation and ionization with the liberation of hydroxyl ions, the amount of these being proportional to the amount of alkali and its degree of ionization, e.g.

$$NaOH \rightleftharpoons Na^+ + OH^-$$
$$NH_4OH \rightleftharpoons NH_4^+ + OH^-$$

As a result of the liberation of hydroxyl ions, there must be a corresponding decrease in the number of hydrogen ions to keep the ionic product of water constant. It will be seen, therefore, that in spite of the fact that a solution may be alkaline, its reaction can still be expressed in terms of the hydrogen ions present, the stronger the alkali the smaller the concentration of hydrogen ions. A solution is *neutral* if $[H^+] = 10^{-7}$, a solution is *acid* if $[H^+]$ is greater than 10^{-7} and is *alkaline* if $[H^+]$ is less than 10^{-7}. Since $[H^+]$ can be measured with considerable accuracy, it is convenient to express acidity and alkalinity in terms of [H$^+$]. For reasons of practical convenience, [H$^+$] is usually expressed as a logarithmic or pH scale.

The pH value of a liquid is defined as the logarithm of the reciprocal of the hydrogen-ion concentration, i.e.

$$pH = \log \frac{1}{[H^+]}$$

For neutral water, $pH = \log \dfrac{1}{10^{-7}} = 7$

Two points should be borne in mind about the pH scale.

1. Since it is a *logarithmic* scale, a change in one unit of pH is equivalent to a tenfold change in hydrogen-ion concentration, that is a tenfold change in acidity; thus a liquid of pH 5 is ten times more acid than one at pH 6, while a liquid of pH 9 is ten times more alkaline than one of pH 8.

2. Since it is a *reciprocal* scale, the lower the pH, the greater will be the acidity. A pH value of less than 7 indicates an acid solution*, and greater than 7 indicates an alkaline solution.

IMPORTANCE OF pH MEASUREMENTS IN MICROBIOLOGY

Microorganisms are sensitive in varying degrees to the pH of the external environment. Although this is important for survival, it is even more important for growth, where there is an optimum, a maximum and a minimum pH. Media should be adjusted as far as possible to the pH optimal for the growth of the organism concerned. Most pathogenic bacteria have a fairly restricted pH range and grow best around pH 7·5, that is, at a slightly alkaline reaction. This may be a reflection of the fact that the pH of mammalian blood and tissues is of this order. For example, the pneumococcus has an optimum pH of 7·8, and a growth range between pH 7·3–8·3. On the other hand, commensal and saprophytic bacteria have a wider pH growth range. *Escherichia coli* has an optimum pH of 6·5, and a growth range

between pH 4·4–7·8. Yeasts and fungi generally have an acid optimum and may grow at a pH of 2·0 or even lower. Not only should growth media be adjusted to the optimum pH, but all suspending fluids should be at a reaction giving the largest survival time (usually of the same order as the optimum pH).

METHODS USED IN pH MEASUREMENT

Two types of methods are generally employed for the measurement of pH in the laboratory. These depend either upon the use of pH indicator dyes or upon the use of electric pH meters.

Methods Depending Upon the Use of pH Indicator Dyes

Indicator dyes are substances that will change in colour with variations in the pH of the solution in which they are dissolved. For example, phenol sulphone-phthalein (phenol red) is yellow in acid solution and red in alkaline solution. If alkali be gradually added to an acid solution containing phenol red, the change in colour will commence at pH 6·8, the yellow becoming redder until the final red is reached at pH 8·4; thus the 'range' of the indicator is pH 6·8–8·4. Within this range, phenol red will have different colours for different pHs and this can be used to determine pH. The range of phenol red is particularly suitable for the adjustment of the pH of bacterial culture media. It must be emphasized that outside the range at which the colour is changing, an indicator can show only whether the solution is more acid or more alkaline than the indicator range. For example, phenol red is yellow at all pHs below 6·8 and is red at all pHs above 8·4. However, other dyes have their own different ranges in which colour change occurs, and there is now available a series of indicators which will cover the range from pH 1 to 11. The following (shown overleaf) are examples:

---

*1 N HCl has an approximate pH value of 0.

0·1 N HCl has an approximate pH value of 1.

0·01 N HCl has an approximate pH value of 2.

Table 4.1

Indicator	Range of pH	Colour change
Thymol blue (acid range)	1·2–2·8	red to yellow
Bromophenol blue	2·8–4·6	yellow to violet
Bromocresol green	3·6–5·2	yellow to blue
Methyl red	4·4–6·2	red to yellow
Litmus	4·5–8·3	red to blue
Bromocresol purple	5·2–6·8	yellow to violet
Bromothymol blue	6·0–7·6	yellow to blue
Neutral red	6·8–8·0	red to yellow
Phenol red	6·8–8·4	yellow to purple-pink
Cresol red	7·2–8·8	yellow to violet-red
Thymol blue (alkaline range)	8·0–9·6	yellow to blue
Phenolphthalein	8·3–10·0	colourless to red
Thymolphthalein	9·3–10·5	colourless to blue
B.D.H. 'Universal'	3·0–11·0	red—orange—yellow—green—blue—reddish violet

The simplest method of determining the pH of a solution is to use commercially available pH indicator papers. These papers are impregnated with an indicator that gives a change of colour over a specific or general range of pH. The paper can simply be dipped in the solution to be tested or, alternatively, a drop of the solution can be withdrawn by a wire loop or Pasteur pipette and placed on the paper. The resulting colour is compared with the chart supplied with the papers. One example of a good wide-range indicator is the 'Universal Indicator' contained in test-papers supplied by Messrs. Johnson & Sons, Hendon, London NW4. It must be emphasized, however, that these test-papers will only give, at the best, an approximate idea of the pH and the results should always be checked by a more accurate method.

The Comparator Method

The most convincing instrument of this type is the Lovibond Comparator (obtainable from British Drug Houses, Ltd.) (see Fig. 4.1).

The comparator normally consists of a bakelite case with two holes at the top for tubes of standard bore and of colourless glass. Tube A contains water if the untreated 'unknown' solution is colourless, but some of the untreated 'unknown' if it is coloured. The hinged door of the case holds a rotatable disk containing a series of standard coloured glasses corresponding to various pH values and each glass can be brought in front of tube A in turn and viewed through aperture A.

It is possible to obtain disks for various indicators and the appropriate one can be inserted in the comparator. A solution of the indicator is added to tube B, which contains the unknown solution, and the disk is rotated until a match is obtained. The pH is then read in the aperture at the bottom of the apparatus. If the 'unknown' is in the middle of the range of the indicator selected, it is possible to obtain a value accurate to within 0·1–0·2 pH units.

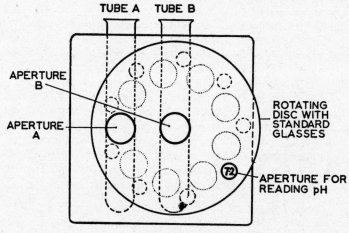

FIG. 4.1

Adjustment of pH of Nutrient Media

One of the commonest uses for a comparator in a bacteriological laboratory is in the adjustment of the pH of standard culture media. As an example, the adjustment of nutrient broth to pH 7·5 using phenol red will be considered. For this purpose, the following are required in addition to the Lovibond comparator with a phenol red disk.

1. A solution of phenol red, 0·01 per cent*, in distilled water.

2. 0·05 N NaOH made up as follows:
    500 ml 0·1 N NaOH
    91 ml 0·01 per cent phenol red
    distilled water to 1 litre

The indicator is incorporated into the standard alkali solution, so that when the medium is titrated, the actual concentration of the dye always remains constant.

3. A burette, preferably a microburette, measuring to 0·01 ml.

To tube A is added 5 ml nutrient broth and to tube B 5 ml nutrient broth + 0·5 ml of 0·01 per cent phenol red solution. The 0·05 N NaOH solution is run into tube B until the tint produced is midway between the standard glasses of pH 7·4 and 7·6. The average of the two readings is taken and this gives the amount of 0·05 N NaOH required to bring 5 ml of broth to the correct pH. From this, one can calculate the amount of 1 N NaOH required to bring the total amount of broth to the correct pH.

When media adjusted in this way by the addition of alkali are sterilized, it is common to obtain a precipitate of phosphates so that the medium has to be filtered again before use. It may be preferable, therefore, when making media in bulk to have the reaction slightly alkaline and to adjust it for use by the addition of acid. The medium is first adjusted to a pH of about 8·0 with NaOH and steamed for thirty minutes. The precipitated phosphates are filtered off. The medium is then adjusted back to pH 7·5, using acid. The titration is carried out in exactly the same way as described previously except that, instead of NaOH solution, 0·05 N HCl containing phenol red is employed, and the calculated amount of normal hydrochloric acid is added per litre to obtain the desired reaction.

The standardization of a solid medium such as nutrient agar presents greater difficulty than in the case of fluid media. The medium may be titrated when liquid, but the exact determination is not easy to obtain with any degree of accuracy. It has been found that agar of good quality has very little effect on the reaction of the broth to which it is added, but the reaction of the finished agar should be controlled by titrating the melted medium and then comparing the colour *when cold*. We have found the following method satisfactory. Mix together 0·5 ml of the melted agar, 4·5 ml of hot (neutral) distilled water and 0·5 ml of 0·01 per cent phenol red solution; cool and compare with the standard tubes. Gelatin may conveniently be adjusted if the medium is liquefied and kept at about 37°C.

The Capillator Method

A knowledge of the pH of bacterial cultures and of the pH changes which they undergo is often of importance and is sometimes of practical value (e.g. in the differentiation of *Streptococcus agalactiae* from *Streptococcus pyogenes*). When only small quantities of culture are available, one of the best methods of pH determination is the use of the capillator. The 'B.D.H. Capillator Outfit'† is available with indicators and cards to cover the range from pH 1·2–11·0. Alternatively, separate sets can be obtained for each indicator.

The technique is as follows. The pH is first approximately determined by the use of a universal indicator. This can be done in two ways.

1. A small quantity of the microbial culture is withdrawn with a sterile Pasteur pipette and transferred to a white tile and an equal amount of indicator added. From the resulting colour of the mixture, the approximate pH can be obtained by comparison with the standard

---

* First prepare a stock 0·02 per cent solution as follows. Weigh out 0·1 g phenol red, add to this 10 ml (accurately) of 0·1 N NaOH and 20 ml of distilled water. Dissolve by gentle heat. Transfer the contents to a 500 ml volumetric flask, washing out all the indicator into the flask. Now add accurately 10 ml 0·1 N HCl, and fill up to the mark. The 0·01 per cent solution of phenol red is made by diluting the stock solution with an equal part of distilled water.

† For full details see catalogue, British Drug Houses, Ltd.

set of colours supplied with the indicator. The tile is appropriately sterilized after use with 3 per cent v/v lysol solution.

2. A universal pH test-paper can be used (see previously). After use the test-paper is destroyed by burning or is placed in disinfectant solution.

The pH is then determined more accurately, using a capillator and choosing an indicator that acts over the desired range. The capillator consists of a series of standard-sized capillary tubes filled with buffer solutions and indicator. These tubes show the colours corresponding to different pH values over the whole range of the indicator, and the pH value corresponding to each colour is marked on the card. The capillator set is used as follows:

(a) A capillary tube, identical in diameter with those in the capillator, is fitted with a rubber teat and is used for withdrawing a tube full of indicator (supplied with the caplator set and of double the concentration occurring in the standard tubes). The indicator is then pipetted on to the small watch-glass provided.

(b) After washing, the same 'pipette' is used to withdraw an equal volume of the microbial culture or unknown solution which is pipetted on to the same watch glass. If the culture is to remain uncontaminated, a sterile capillator pipette must be used.

(c) The two fluids are mixed on the watch-glass by sucking in and out of the pipette, and finally the tube is filled with the mixture.

(d) The prepared tube is compared in colour with the standards and the pH value thus obtained.

Errors due to the colour of the culture or fluid itself can be corrected by using a compensation cell. Care should be taken when working with pathogenic cultures, and the used capillary tubes should be dropped into lysol solution.

The pH Meter

The methods described above, although simple and requiring relatively cheap apparatus, are generally not accurate. They are also very laborious if large numbers of estimations have to be carried out. Further, they all assume that the colour of an indicator is influenced only by the pH of the solution. This is not always so, since the dissociation of an indicator can be influenced by substances such as salts, ethanol and proteins in solution. These errors may be quite appreciable, although in the choice of indicators listed previously those with large errors have been discarded. The only accurate method of measuring pH is by using a pH meter, and in laboratories where numerous routine determinations of pH are required, this apparatus is a necessary piece of laboratory equipment. It is easy and quick to use although care must be taken in its maintenance.

A pH meter consists of an electrode pair which is sensitive to hydrogen-ion concentration and an electrical circuit which measures the e.m.f. developed across the electrode pair. Almost all modern pH meters employ a glass electrode as it is easy to use and maintain, together with a calomel electrode as a standard. Only a brief description of the instrument and basic directions for its use can be given here. More detailed descriptions of theory can be found in appropriate textbooks and instructions are provided in the makers' pamphlets.

The e.m.f. developed between the glass electrode and the calomel electrode will depend upon the concentration of hydrogen ions and, hence, the pH. In order to measure this e.m.f., no current must flow in the electrode pair or the resultant chemical reactions at the cell boundaries will result in a 'polarization' of the electrodes so that the observed e.m.f. will be due to a combination of phenomena. For this reason, a high impedance circuit is used to detect the potential developed and a vacuum tube is used to drive the measuring meter. This meter can be a microammeter in a vacuum tube circuit as in most line-operated meters, or a null-type bridge circuit may be used as with battery-operated meters.

The following precautions should be observed in the use and maintenance of a pH meter to avoid damaging the instrument and to get an accurate pH value.

1. Always exercise extreme care in handling the electrodes, particularly the glass electrodes

which usually have a very thin glass bulb. Do not allow this glass bulb to touch the beaker in which the measurements are taking place, or any other hard surface.

2. Before a series of pH measurements, ensure that the calomel electrode is filled with a solution of saturated KCl.

3. Make sure the instrument has been given sufficient time to warm up as specified by the manufacturers.

4. Make frequent standardizations of the meter against a standard buffer solution of known pH as near as possible to the pH to be measured.

5. Between measurements, wash the electrodes with a stream of distilled water using a wash bottle.

6. When a 'drift' in the reading occurs, give the electrodes time to reach equilibrium. Gently stirring the solution often hastens equilibrium.

7. Never remove the electrodes from the solution when the measuring circuit is closed.

8. When the instrument is not in use, keep the electrodes immersed in water.

BUFFERS AND THEIR USES

Not only is it important to have the suspending fluids for microorganisms within a certain pH range, it is also important to keep the pH within the same range. Most microorganisms produce acids or alkalis as a result of their metabolic activities and these must be prevented from altering the pH of the environment too radically. For example, bacteria when grown on a medium containing a sugar generally produce acid intermediates or end-products (e.g. formic, acetic, propionic, butyric, or lactic acids). This is particularly true of fermentation under relatively anaerobic conditions. If these acidic products were allowed to accumulate in an unbuffered medium, the organism would soon be killed by the low pH produced.

It is, therefore, preferable and often essential to include buffers in culture media and in suspending fluids. These buffers tend to resist changes in hydrogen-ion concentration. They are usually formed by mixing a weak acid with its salt, although a weak alkali and its salt can also be used. Buffering action is due to the fact that a weak acid is only weakly dissociated while its salt with an alkali metal is strongly dissociated. Thus, whereas 0·1 N acetic acid is only 1·35 per cent dissociated, 0·1 N sodium acetate is 97 per cent dissociated. If hydrogen ions are added to such a buffer solution, they will react with the high concentration of salt anions to form unionized acids. This weak acid, once formed, does not tend to ionize appreciably and, at the same time, its ionization is opposed by the high concentration of anions present. Therefore hydrogen ions have been added, but have been removed leaving the pH of the solution only slightly altered.

Generally speaking, the buffering power of a mixture of a weak acid and its salt is greatest when the two are present in equimolar proportions. From such mixtures, buffers can be prepared covering a range of about 1 pH unit on each side of the pH given by an equivalent mixture (the pK of a buffer). Outside this range, the buffering capacity falls off very rapidly. Although the concentration of the buffer determines its ability to resist changes in hydrogen-ion concentration, the actual pH given by a certain mixture is only slightly affected by dilution.

Buffers suitable for use with biological material should have a pK around the optimal for this material and ideally they should also be non-toxic and non-physiological, i.e. not react with or affect the living organism or the component of the living organism to be studied. In practice, however, most buffers with useful pKs around 7 are physiologically active, and allowance must be made for this.

The following is a list of suitable buffer systems for use in microbiology. It should also be noted that some components of the complex organic growth media commonly used in microbiology are also buffers. This is particularly true of amino acids and peptides which, as well as providing nutrients, act as important buffers.

PREPARATION OF BUFFERS

1. Citrate Buffer

Stock Solutions

   A: 0·1 M solution of citric acid (19·21 g in 1000 ml).

B: 0·1 M solution of sodium citrate (29·41 g $C_6H_5O_7Na_3.2H_2O$ in 1000 ml).

x ml of $A + y$ ml of B, diluted to a total of 100 ml

x	y	pH
46·5	3·5	3·0
43·7	6·3	3·2
40·0	10·0	3·4
37·0	13·0	3·6
35·0	15·0	3·8
33·0	17·0	4·0
31·5	18·5	4·2
28·0	22·0	4·4
25·5	24·5	4·6
23·0	27·0	4·8
20·5	29·5	5·0
18·0	32·0	5·2
16·0	34·0	5·4
13·7	36·3	5·6
11·8	38·2	5·8
9·5	40·5	6·0
7·2	42·8	6·2

2. Acetate Buffer

Stock Solutions

A: 0·2 M solution of acetic acid (11·55 ml in 1000 ml).

B: 0·2 M solution of sodium acetate (16·4 g of $C_2H_3O_2Na$ or 27·2 g of $C_2H_3O_2Na.3H_2O$ in 1000 ml).

x ml of $A + y$ ml of B, diluted to a total of 100 ml

x	y	pH
46·3	3·7	3·6
44·0	6·0	3·8
41·0	9·0	4·0
36·8	13·2	4·2
30·5	19·5	4·4
25·5	24·5	4·6
20·0	30·0	4·8
14·8	35·2	5·0
10·5	39·5	5·2
8·8	41·2	5·4
4·8	45·2	5·6

3. Citrate-Phosphate Buffer

Stock Solutions

A: 0·1 M solution of citric acid (19·21 g in 1000 ml).

B: 0·2 M solution of dibasic sodium phosphate (28·39 g of Na_2HPO_4 or 71·7 g of $Na_2HPO_4.12H_2O$ in 1000 ml).

x ml of $A + y$ ml of B, diluted to a total of 100 ml

x	y	pH
44·6	5·4	2·6
42·2	7·8	2·8
39·8	10·2	3·0
37·7	12·3	3·2
35·9	14·1	3·4
33·9	16·1	3·6
32·3	17·7	3·8
30·7	19·3	4·0
29·4	20·6	4·2
27·8	22·2	4·4
26·7	23·3	4·6
25·2	24·8	4·8
24·3	25·7	5·0
23·3	26·7	5·2
22·2	27·8	5·4
21·0	29·0	5·6
19·7	30·3	5·8
17·9	32·1	6·0
16·9	33·1	6·2
15·4	34·6	6·4
13·6	36·4	6·6
9·1	40·9	6·8
6·4	43·6	7·0

4. Phosphate Buffer

Stock Solutions

A: 0·2 M solution of monobasic sodium phosphate (31·2 g NaH_2PO_4, 2 H_2O in 1000 ml).

B: 0·2 M solution of dibasic sodium phosphate (28·39 g of Na_2HPO_4 or 71·7 g of $Na_2HPO_4.12H_2O$ in 1000 ml).

x ml of $A + y$ ml of B, diluted to a total of 200 ml

x	y	pH
92·0	8·0	5·8
87·7	12·3	6·0
81·5	18·5	6·2
73·5	26·5	6·4
62·5	37·5	6·6
51·0	49·0	6·8
39·0	61·0	7·0
28·0	72·0	7·2
19·0	81·0	7·4

x	y	pH
13·0	87·0	7·6
8·5	91·5	7·8
5·3	94·7	8·0

5. Barbitone (Veronal) Buffer

Stock Solutions

    A: 0·2 M solution of sodium barbitone (sodium diethyl barbiturate).

    B: 0·2 M HCl.

        50 ml of *A* + *x* ml of *B*, diluted to a total of 200 ml

x	pH
1·5	9·2
2·5	9·0
4·0	8·8
6·0	8·6
9·0	8·4
12·7	8·2
17·5	8·0
22·5	7·8
27·5	7·6
32·5	7·4
39·0	7·2
43·0	7·0
45·0	6·8

Solutions more concentrated than 0·05 M may crystallize on standing, especially in the cold.

6. Tris (hydroxymethyl) aminomethane HCl (Tris HCl) Buffer

Stock Solutions

    A: 0·2 M solution of tris (hydroxymethyl) aminomethane (24·2 g in 1000 ml).

    B: 0·2 M HCl.

        50 ml of *A* + *x* ml of *B*, diluted to a total of 200 ml

x	pH
5·0	9·0
8·1	8·8
12·2	8·6
16·5	8·4
21·9	8·2
26·8	8·0
32·5	7·8
38·4	7·6
41·4	7·4
44·2	7·2

7. Boric Acid-Borax Buffer

Stock Solutions

    A: 0·2 M solution of boric acid (12·4 g in 1000 ml).

    B: 0·05 M solution of borax (19·05 g in 1000 ml; 0·2 M in terms of sodium borate).

        50 ml of *A* + *x* ml of *B*, diluted to a total of 200 ml

x	pH
2·0	7·6
3·1	7·8
4·9	8·0
7·3	8·2
11·5	8·4
17·5	8·6
30·0	8·8
59·0	9·0
115·0	9·2

8. Bicarbonate—CO_2 Buffer

The pH of these buffers is markedly dependent on temperature. The following examples are for a temperature of 37°C.

	Concentration of CO_2 in gaseous phase		
	5%	10%	20%
Concentration 0·02 M	7·4	7·1	6·8
of $NaHCO_3$ 0·05 M	7·8	7·5	7·2

9. Carbonate-Bicarbonate Buffer

Stock Solutions

    A: 0·2 M solution of anhydrous sodium carbonate (21·2 g in 1000 ml).

    B: 0·2 M solution of sodium bicarbonate (16·8 g in 1000 ml).

        x ml of *A* + *y* ml of *B*, diluted to a total of 200 ml

x	y	pH
4·0	46·0	9·2
9·5	40·5	9·4
16·0	34·0	9·6
22·0	28·0	9·8
27·5	22·5	10·0
33·0	17·0	10·2
38·5	11·5	10·4
42·5	7·5	10·6

Note. These buffers are all made up to a final concentration of 0·1 M (with the exception of the bicarbonate-CO_2 buffers). The pH will not change appreciably on dilution. It should be noted, however, that there will be variation in the ionic strengths of the different buffers and of the same buffer at different pHs. If isotonic solutions are required, the concentration should be adjusted accordingly. All the buffers are given as a mixture of the sodium salts with the acid. Potassium salts may also be used.

For fuller discussion of pH measurements in microbiology, see Munro (1970).

OXIDATION-REDUCTION (REDOX) POTENTIALS

It has been stated previously that the oxidation-reduction conditions in a medium are very important in the growth of certain bacteria. Strict aerobes are able to grow only in presence of dissolved oxygen while strict anaerobes require reducing conditions and hence absence of dissolved oxygen. This may be related to the metabolic character of the organism, a strict aerobe obtaining its energy and intermediates only through oxidation involving oxygen as the ultimate hydrogen acceptor, a strict anaerobe utilising hydrogen acceptors other than oxygen while a facultative anaerobe can act in both ways. However, strict anaerobes may be actually poisoned by the presence of oxygen, possibly due to the production of toxic hydrogen peroxide which cannot be removed by catalase, or possibly due to the oxidation of certain essential groupings in the organism, e.g. the sulphydryl groups of proteins.

We may consider oxidising agents as substances capable of taking up electrons and reducing agents as substances able to part with electrons. It is therefore possible to determine the intensity level of oxidizing or reducing conditions in a system by the net readiness of all the components in that system to take up, or part with, electrons. This ability is usually expressed as the oxidation-reduction (redox) potential of the system.

Redox potentials can be best measured by virtue of the fact that when an 'unattackable' electrode is immersed in a solution, an elec-trical potential difference is set up between the electrode and the solution, and the magnitude of this potential depends on the state of oxidation or reduction of the solution. This electrode potential (or, more shortly E_h) can be measured in millivolts, and the more oxidized a system, the higher (or more positive) is the potential; in more reduced systems the potential is lower (or more negative). By measuring the electrode potential it is possible to determine and follow the reducing conditions in cultures at different periods and to grade different systems in order according to their state of oxidation or reduction. This measurement can usually be carried out by coupling up a potentiometer with an electrode pair of platinum electrode (the 'unattackable' electrode) and a standard calomel electrode. The redox potential can then be measured by the millivolt scale provided on most commercial pH meters. It should be borne in mind that the redox potential of a system indicates the oxidation-reduction *intensity* of the system itself, and not its *capacity* to oxidize or reduce some other component or system. Further, it must be emphasized that for a microorganism, not only is the redox potential of the system important, but the factors contributing to this redox potential may be equally critical. Thus a substance capable of giving up or taking in electrons may not necessarily affect a microorganism unless it can spatially reach certain essential components of the cell. Further, a substance, like oxygen, which can actually be metabolized by the catalytic action of enzymes in the cell, may be important through this metabolism as well as through its direct contribution to the redox potential.

Although the redox potential of a bacterial culture may be measured accurately by electrical methods, an approximate idea of the state of reduction may sometimes be obtained by adding various special dyes (oxidation-reduction indicators) and observing by the colour changes how much they are reduced. Such changes are in intensity of colour, not changes from one colour to another, as is the case with the indicators used for the measurement of pH. It is found that the state of oxidation or reduction of any particular dye depends on the electrode potential, so that at any given pH value, if we know the electrode potential of the solution, we can calculate the degree of reduction of the dye. Conversely, and this is more important practically, if the percentage reduction of the dye has been observed colorimetrically the corresponding electrode potential can be determined. Different dyes are reduced over different ranges of potential; for instance, methylene blue at pH 7 is 95 per cent in the oxidized condition at $E_h + 50$ mv, and 99 per cent reduced at $E_h - 50$ mv, whilst neutral red is still 87 per cent oxidized at -300 mv, and 87 per cent reduced at -350 mv. Theoretically it should be possible by suitable choice of indicators to measure any range of E_h, but in practice experimental difficulties arise due to poising (this corresponds to the buffering effect in pH estimation), catalytic effects and the toxicity of the dyes used towards bacteria, etc. Colorimetric E_h determinations do not reach the degree of accuracy and convenience attained in the case of pH indicators.

A few examples will suffice to illustrate the results obtained when the electrode potential of growing bacteria cultures are measured. In a culture of *C. diphtheriae* the initial E_h of the medium, about $+300$ mv, falls gradually and reaches -200 mv after some 48 hours' incubation, and the potential remains at this low level for some considerable time. With haemolytic streptococci, on the other hand, the potential falls from $+300$ mv to -150 mv in 12 hours, but then rises fairly rapidly, probably owing to the formation of hydrogen peroxide. In a dextrose broth culture of *Esch. coli*, in which gas formation occurs, the potential falls extremely rapidly, reaching -370 mv after about one hour's incubation. The behaviour of staphylococci is roughly similar to that of *C. diphtheriae*, whilst pneumococci behave similarly to haemolytic streptococci. Strict anaerobes are unable to proliferate in ordinary aerobic culture media unless the E_h is lowered to some extent. This lowering of the E_h, or establishment of reducing conditions, may be effected in a variety of ways, such as removal of oxygen in an anaerobic jar or by means of a pyrogallol seal, or reduction may be effected by adding a reducing agent, e.g. thioglycollate.

Oxidation-reduction potentials and oxidation-reduction indicators are employed in the testing of sewage and sewage effluents, in cheese-making, in the keeping qualities of beer, etc. The metabolic activities of bacteria and other cells and tissues and the functioning of enzymes are followed by observing the reduction of methylene blue in Thunberg tubes. A commonly used application of this technique is in the grading of milk and testing the hygienic quality of milk samples. The milk samples are incubated under standard conditions with methylene blue, and the time of reduction is noted. Heavily contaminated milks show a rapid decolourization, whilst with good quality milk there is a long lag period and reduction is slow.

For fuller discussion on redox potentials in microbiology, see Jacob (1970).

WATER

Tap water contains many impurities and is unsuitable for the preparation of defined culture media, for chemical solutions and for many other uses in the laboratory. These impurities can be largely removed by distillation or demineralization.

DISTILLED WATER

Normally distilled water is prepared in a commercial metal-lined still which will deliver it at the rate of $\frac{1}{2}$-50 gallons per hour, depending on size. However, for some purposes this water is insufficiently pure, and it may be necessary to use an all-glass distillation apparatus which should be fitted with an efficient spray tap. It is often advisable to add a knife point of potassium permanganate and a few pellets of sodium hydroxide to the tap water before commencing distillation in order to oxidize steam volatile organic compounds which might otherwise be carried over into the distillate. For some experimental methods such as tissue culture it may be necessary to repeat the distillation in a glass still to give doubly glass distilled water.

It is useful to check the purity of distilled water at times by simple conductivity testers. Satisfactory distilled water should have a conductivity no greater than that given by 1·5 parts/10^6 of NaCl, and preferably below 1·0 parts/10^6.

DEMINERALIZED WATER

Ion-exchange resins may be used to demineralize water. A simple apparatus consists of an anion and a cation-exchanger in two columns of glass tubing about 2 m tall and 3 cm in diameter. A variety of resins are available for the purpose, e.g. Amberlite 120 (H) as the cation-exchange resin followed by Amberlite IRA 400 (OH) as the anion-exchange resin.* Tap water or distilled water is passed over each of the resins in turn. The columns must be periodically regenerated by rinsing with 10 per cent aqueous HC1 for the cation-exchanger and 10 per cent aqueous NaOH for the anion-exchanger. After regeneration, the columns are rinsed with distilled water until the final product has a neutral reaction. Commercial demineralizers are available,† which have the advantage of being transportable and of requiring no external source of heat or electricity. Demineralized water should be equivalent to double glass-distilled water and should have a very low conductivity. However, it may carry dissolved organic compounds derived from the resins.

FLUIDS FOR CELL SUSPENSION AND DILUTION

A variety of fluids are used for the suspension of microorganisms, blood cells or tissue culture cells. These fluids should preserve, as far as possible, the cells in their original condition. The following points should be noted.

1. They should have an osmotic pressure nearly isotonic with the cell to be suspended. This is particularly true of mammalian cells (e.g. red blood corpuscles) where lysis readily occurs in non-isotonic media. Microorganisms are generally more resistant to changes in the external osmotic pressure, but suspension in water or very dilute salt solutions may cause loss of viability.

2. Suspension fluids should preferably contain a buffer to keep the cells at their optimum pH.

3. Certain ions may be necessary for the optimal maintenance of cells, particularly with mammalian cells. Moreover, they may be required for certain in-vitro reactions, e.g. agglutination, complement fixation, etc. In some cases a source of energy such as glucose may be required.

4. Other additions may be made for specific purposes.

The following suspension and diluent fluids are commonly used. In all cases analytical grade reagents (when available) should be made up in distilled or demineralized water.

PHYSIOLOGICAL SALINE

A solution of 0·85 per cent NaCl in water. This solution is sometimes called normal saline, a term which should be discarded because of its chemical connotation. It is also often referred to as 'saline'. The solution has an osmotic pressure roughly equivalent to that of mammalian blood serum and can therefore be used for the suspension of blood cells as well as most microorganisms. However, the solution has no buffer present and it is recommended that phosphate-buffered saline be used as a general suspension fluid in the laboratory.

BUFFERED SALINES

As stated previously, it is preferable to have a buffer present in a suspending fluid or diluent and a variety of solutions containing basically NaCl but with a buffer added have been proposed. They should all have a final osmotic pressure roughly equivalent to that of physiological saline. A series of solutions can be prepared by diluting standard buffer solutions of the required pH with physiological saline to a strength of 0·01 M. If a greater buffering power is required, the concentration of buffer must be increased and of saline decreased.

The following types of buffered saline are recommended for various purposes:

(a) *Phosphate buffered saline:*

NaCl	8·00 g/l
K_2HPO_4	1·21 g/l
KH_2PO_4	0·34 g/l

This solution gives a pH of about 7·3 and also provides potassium and phosphate ions. It is a very useful general diluent and suspending fluid.

---

* Obtainable from British Drug Houses, Ltd.

† For example, the 'Portable Deminrolits' produced by the Permutit Co. Ltd., Gunnersbury Avenue, London W4.

(b) *Azide saline.* Sodium azide at a concentration of 0·08 per cent is added to physiological saline or buffered saline. The azide acts as a preservative preventing microbial decomposition and is often used for the dilution of serum, etc.

(c) *Borate-calcium saline:*

NaCl	8·0	g/l
$CaCl_2$	1·0	g/l
H_3BO_3	1·2	g/l
$Na_2B_4O_7.10H_2O$	0·052	g/l

This solution gives a pH of about 7·3 and is used for haemagglutination experiments where calcium is required and phosphate should be absent.

(d) *Veronal-NaCl diluent:*

NaCl	8·5	g/l
Barbitone	0·575	g/l
(diethyl-barbituric acid)		
Sodium barbitone	0·20	g/l
$MgCl_2.6H_2O$	0·168	g/l
$CaCl_2$	0·028	g/l

A stock solution concentrated ×5 is made up by dissolving 5·75 g barbitone in 500 ml hot distilled water. Add 85 g NaCl and make up the volume to about 1400 ml. Dissolve 2·0 g sodium barbitone in 500 ml distilled water and add it to the NaCl-barbitone solution. Make up to 2000 ml. Add 1·68 g $MgCl_2.6H_2O$ and 0·28 g $CaCl_2$. For use dilute 1 in 5 with distilled water.

This saline may be used for complement-fixation tests and gives more reproducible results than physiological saline. If glass tubes are used to contain the reaction mixtures, there may be some absorption of complement on to the glass surfaces. To reduce this absorption, add 0·1 per cent inactivated rabbit serum, 0·1 per cent gelatin or 0·1 per cent bovine serum albumin.

COMPLEX SUSPENDING MEDIA

More complex media are required for the suspension and dilution of microorganisms and other cells where optimum viability must be maintained. For example, in viable counts of many bacteria, physiological saline may be to some extent bactericidal and must be replaced by solutions containing other ions as well as a buffer. For these fluids, prepare the following solutions which are all isotonic with mammalian serum and can be mixed in any proportions. The mixtures, although of different composition, will remain isotonic.

To simplify preparation and handling, the first five solutions can be made up in concentrations five times those listed. They are stable for months when stored in the cold.

The Krebs-Ringer solutions seem to be the most generally useful for the suspension of mammalian cells and are also valuable for many bacteria. It is also possible to use Davis's minimal medium for bacterial suspension. If growth is to be avoided, leave out the nitrogen source (ammonium sulphate) or the carbon and energy sources (glucose and citric acid).

Suspending media for tissue culture work are described in Chapter 9.

Table 4.2

	g/l	Ringer	Locke	Plain	Krebs-Ringer Bicarbonate†	Phosphate
NaCl	9·0	100	100	100	100	100
KCl	11·5	4	4	4	4	4
		3	3	3	3	3
KH_2PO_4	21·1	—	—	1	1	—
$MgSO_4.7H_2O$	38·2	—	—	1	1	1
$NaHCO_3$	13·0	—	3	—	21	—
0·1 M phosphate buffer* pH 7·4	—	—	—	—	—	20

* 17·8 g $Na_2HPO_4.2H_2O$ + 20 ml 1 N HCl diluted to 1 litre.
† The solution should be gassed with 5 per cent v/v CO_2 in O_2, air or N_2.

PREPARATION AND CLEANSING OF GLASSWARE

NEW GLASSWARE

New glassware requires special attention because of the resistant spores which may be present in the straw and other packing material and also because it tends to give off free alkali which may be sufficient to interfere with the growth of certain organisms. Consequently it should be placed in 1 per cent HCl overnight, washed in tap water and distilled water and autoclaved.

Screw-capped bottles (described later) are subjected to a special cleansing process by the makers whereby surface alkali is removed, and the above treatment is unnecessary. The bottles may be used without further treatment, as received from the manufacturers.

CLEANSING OF GLASSWARE FOR GENERAL LABORATORY USE

Glass containers with discarded cultures can be placed in 3 per cent lysol after use or transferred directly to boiling soap solutions. Containers with tubercle bacilli or spore-bearing organisms such as *B. anthracis*, *B. subtilis* or *Cl. tetani* must be autoclaved. The discarded cultures and their containers are then boiled for one hour in a 5 per cent solution of a good quality soft soap in either tap water (if it is sufficiently soft) or distilled or demineralized water (if the tap water is hard). The glassware is cleansed with a test-tube brush (or other suitable brush) and well rinsed in hot and cold water. Again, if the tap water is hard and contains a considerable amount of calcium salts, rinsing in distilled or demineralized water is necessary. The glassware is then allowed to drain and is dried in a hot-air oven or cabinet.

WASHING OF TISSUE CULTURE TUBES

Since tissue cells are particularly sensitive to minute traces of toxic substances, meticulous care is essential in cleaning glassware for tissue cultures and it is preferable to use hard glass (e.g. Pyrex) tubes, flasks and containers. The following cleaning method has been found satisfactory.

1. Autoclave with rubber bungs *in situ* after use.

2. Remove bungs and rinse tubes in hot running tap water.

3. Boil for twenty minutes in demineralized water in a boiler with soapflakes (one handful to about five gallons). Small tubes are boiled in an enamel basin on a gas-ring. (Rinse water from the demineralizer may be used for this purpose.)

4. Brush the tubes as removed from boiler (preferably with a motor-driven nylon brush). Do this *while the tubes are hot* or serum remains.

5. Rinse in hot running tap water or in demineralized water if the local water is hard.

6. Transfer tubes into hot demineralized water containing an inorganic detergent. Thoroughly wash in this by emptying and filling. The following solution can be used:

Sodium hexametaphosphate .   . 40 g
Sodium metasilicate (technical)   . 360 g
Demineralized water   .   .   . 1 gallon

Dissolve and allow to stand overnight. Dilute 1 in 100 before use.

7. Rinse in hot running tap water at least four times.

Rinse three times in demineralized water.

8. Drain and dry in drying cabinet.

9. Dry-sterilize at 160°C for three hours in racks with the tubes either metal-capped or covered with aluminium foil.

Rubber bungs should be treated as follows after autoclaving:

1. Rinse in hot tap water.
2. Boil for 20 min in 20 per cent $NaHCO_3$.
3. Rinse in hot tap water.
4. Boil for 20 min in 20 per cent HCl.
5. Rinse in hot tap water.
6. Pack in layers separated by lint in tins or glass containers and autoclave.

CLEANING OF GLASSWARE FOR BIOCHEMICAL WORK

1. Remove any grease with petroleum. Wash with warm tap water.

2. Place in dichromate-sulphuric acid cleaning solution for 12–24 hours.

3. Remove, washing by rinsing in hot tap water at least four times and in distilled water twice.

4. Dry in oven if the glassware is not used for accurate volumetric purposes.

DICHROMATE-SULPHURIC ACID CLEANING SOLUTION

Dissolve 63 g of sodium (or potassium) dichromate by heating with 35 ml water. Cool and add concentrated H_2SO_4 to 1 litre. Technical grade reagents may be used.

This fluid should be handled with care. Preferably rubber gloves and an apron should be worn. If clothes or skin are splashed with the fluid, they should be immediately washed in water, and any residual acid neutralized with sodium carbonate solution. This, in time, is washed off with water.

CLEANING OF PIPETTES

1. If contaminated with infective material, discard the used pipette into a 3 per cent v/v lysol solution and leave until convenient to wash. (The lysol solution is best contained in a rubber cylinder about 15 in high and 4 in in diameter. The points of the pipettes are not liable to be broken when dropped to the rubber bottom of the cylinder.)

2. Rinse in tap water.

3. If necessary, steep overnight in dichromate-sulphuric acid cleaning fluid.

4. Wash with tap water in an automatic pipette washer.

5. Connect the pipette to a water pump by rubber tubing and draw through distilled or demineralized water followed by acetone. Finally, suck through air until the internal surface is quite dry.

6. If required, the top end of the pipette is plugged with cotton-wool; this is pressed entirely within the end of the pipette so that there are no protruding strands of cotton to prevent close fitting of a rubber teat or mouthpiece tube which may be later attached to operate the pipette.

7. To sterilize the pipettes, pack them in copper cylinders with slip-on lids or in lengths of wide-bore glass tubing stoppered with cotton-wool. Place in a hot air oven at 160°C for 60 min.

Note. Accurately calibrated volumetric glassware should never be heated in an oven, since the expansion and contraction of the glass makes the graduations inaccurate. Such glassware should be kept separate from that intended for sterilization.

REFERENCES

JACOB, H. E. (1970) In *Methods in Microbiology,* Vol. 2, p. 91. London: Academic Press.
MUNRO, A. L. S. (1970) In *Methods in Microbiology,* Vol. 2, p. 39. London: Academic Press.

5. Cultivation of Bacteria, Fungi and Protozoa: Culture Media

Only in exceptional cases can the identity of a microorganism be established by its morphological characters. It is therefore essential to obtain a culture by growing the organism in an artificial culture medium, and if more than one species or type of organism are present, each requires to be carefully separated or isolated in pure culture. In this process there are three distinct operations:

1. The preparation of a suitable culture medium.

2. The initial removal of other organisms from the medium and its containers by sterilization. Bacteria are ubiquitous and are present in the material and on the articles used for making media. These contaminating organisms must be destroyed or removed so that the culture medium is rendered sterile.

3. The cultivation of the organism and its isolation from others present in the material to be examined. Techniques for the separation of mixed cultures are described in the next chapter and the general subject of bacterial nutrition and conditions for growth has been dealt with in Vol. I, Chapter 3.

LIQUID AND SOLID MEDIA

There are two broad groups of media, liquid and solid. Many liquid media containing different nutrients have been devised and most bacteria will grow in at least one of them. However, liquid media have two disadvantages. Growths usually do not exhibit specially characteristic appearances in them and, except when they are designed for a particular biochemical test, they are of only limited use in identifying species. Also, organisms cannot be separated with certainty from mixtures by growth in liquid media. If liquid media are made solid (gelatinous) these disadvantages are overcome. On solid media the appearances exhibited by the colonies of different bacteria are useful in identification; and solid media are almost indispensable for the isolation of pure cultures. It is only occasionally that organisms can be grown directly from the body in pure culture so that solid media are almost always needed for the examination of pathological specimens.

Gelatin was used by the early bacteriologists to make the first solid media; pieces of potato impregnated with nutrient solutions can be used as solid media; serum or egg can be coagulated by heating in an inspissator to make media solid; but agar is most commonly used for this purpose.

Agar-agar, or 'agar' for short, is derived from certain seaweeds. In watery solutions it gives a firm gel that remains unmelted at all incubation temperatures and that is generally bacteriologically inert, being decomposed or liquefied only by a few varieties of marine bacteria. In these respects it is more suitable than gelatin; a 15 per cent solution of gelatin melts at 24°C and gelatin is decomposed by many proteolytic bacteria. Agar does not add to the nutritive properties of a medium and a suitable agar should be free from growth-promoting as well as growth-inhibiting substances.

The melting and solidifying points of agar solutions are not the same. At the concentrations normally used, most bacteriological agars melt at about 95°C and solidify only when cooled to about 42°C. The ability of agar to be melted is an advantage compared with the inability of serum or egg to be melted, and the low solidifying point of agar allows heat-sensitive nutrients to be mixed with it in the molten state at temperatures as low as 45°C.

CONTAINERS FOR MEDIA AND CULTURES

Flasks stoppered with cotton-wool, test-tubes stoppered with cotton-wool or with slip-on metal caps, and screw-capped bottles of different capacity and shape can be used as containers for media and cultures. Metal caps are satisfactory provided the medium is stored for only a few weeks and they are economical because they can be used repeatedly. Cotton-wool plugs must be discarded after each use. Air passing into the tubes as a result of changes in temperature or pressure, as when cultures are incubated anaerobically, is filtered through the wool; such protection is not provided by metal caps. Screw-capped bottles are air-tight and thus do not allow their contents to dry out during storage. Media in bottles need not be stored in a cold room and can be kept almost indefinitely. Bottles are particularly valuable in large laboratories where culture media are prepared in quantity for distribution.

Screw-capped bottles are made of clear white flint glass, the neck having an external screw thread. The caps are made of aluminium and each has a rubber washer 3 mm thick, of special rubber that is not inhibitory to bacterial growth. A list of bottles that covers practically all needs is given in Table 5.1. With the exception of the 2-oz squat bottle, these are made by United Glass, Ltd., and may be bought only from retailers. The 4-oz is the standard blood culture bottle and perforated caps may be obtained for these. The 2-oz squat is suitable for specimens of sputum. The 40- and 20-oz

rounds are also used for intravenous solutions such as saline and glucose saline.

Glassware must be thoroughly cleaned before use for culture media and new glassware requires special treatment to remove free alkali. Most of the bottles listed are supplied cleaned and washed by a special process. The rubber washers have been well boiled and the caps already fitted. No further treatment is necessary before they are used. This saving of time is of especial value where large quantities of culture media are produced. The cardboard cartons in which the bottles are supplied keep them clean during storage, either empty or containing medium, and are useful for dispatching medium. When bottles are cleaned for re-use the old caps and washers should be discarded and replaced with new caps and washers. If undamaged caps are to be re-used they should be thoroughly washed and dried, care being taken to see that there is no moisture between the washer and the cap, since this can interfere with sterilization.

The use of plastic Petri dishes, e.g. Sterilin, Dyos, Falcon, is a substantial saving of labour. They are supplied sterile by the manufacturer

Table 5.1

Bottle	Capacity in ml	Cap	Washer
1 gallon, narrow mouth	4600	Special, to fit	'Compo' cork and 'resistol'
80 oz round	2400	KN 31	
40 oz round	1190	KN 31	
20 oz round	600	KN 31	
10 oz round	290	KN 350	
5 oz round	140	KN 350	
1 oz round (H 53), McCartney	28	KN 135	
$\frac{1}{2}$ oz round	15	KN 132	Rubber
$\frac{1}{4}$ oz round, bijou	6	KN 132	
1 oz Universal container	28	KN 86	
8 oz medical flat	236	KN 350	
6 oz medical flat	180	KN 349	
4 oz medical flat	125	KN 349	
3 oz medical flat	85	KN 359	
2 oz medical flat	60	KN 359	
1 oz medical flat	33	KN 347	
2 oz squat (J1/2)*	65	2 in	Cardboard or rubber

* The 2-oz squat bottle, and a range of squat forms from 1–16 oz capacity with aluminium screw-caps, are obtainable from Solmedia Ltd., 31, Orford Road, London, E.17.

and are disposable after one use. Care must be taken to ensure that plastic used for Petri dishes is not inhibitory to microorganisms, especially mycoplasmas, and also to tissue cultures for which specially treated dishes are available. Some plastics are oxidising and unsuitable for anaerobic media.

Copper salts are inimical to the growth of many organisms and copper utensils should not be used for the preparation of media. Heavily tinned copper articles are safe to use, but if the tinning shows signs of wear the article must be re-tinned.

Forms in which Liquid and Solid Media are used

Tubing and Bottling of Liquid Media

Liquid media may be distributed in test-tubes with slip-on metal caps or cotton-wool plugs, the tubes being about half-filled. If bottles are to be used, broth or peptone water in 2·5 ml amounts and fermentation media in 3 ml amounts may be distributed in bijou bottles. Media required in 5 or 10 ml amounts may be put in 1-oz bottles and 50 to 100 ml amounts of media in 3- or 5-oz bottles. It is convenient to store liquid media in 250 ml amounts in 10-oz bottles but larger amounts in larger bottles may be desired.

Tubing, Bottling and Pouring Plates of Solid Media

Solid media may be distributed in test-tubes with slip-on metal caps or cotton-wool plugs. The shape in which the medium is allowed to solidify depends on the method of inoculation for which it is to be used. The commonest shape is the 'slope' or 'slant', which provides a large surface area of medium for inoculation. For $6 \times \frac{5}{8}$ in test-tubes, 5 ml of medium is sufficient and it is allowed to set at such an angle that there is a thick butt at the bottom (Fig. 5.1). When a large number of tubes of agar have to be sloped, special trays that allow the tubes to be laid at the correct angle are useful and, moreover, the tubes can be stacked one upon another so that very little bench space is required during solidification. After cooling, fresh agar slopes contain 'water of

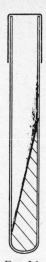

FIG. 5.1
Slope of solid medium in test-tube. A cotton-wool plug may be used instead of the slip-on metal cap illustrated here.

condensation' at the foot of the tube, and the tubes should be stored and handled in the vertical position to prevent the liquid from flowing over the surface of the medium or entering the cotton-wool plug or metal cap.

If the medium is to be used for a 'stab' or 'shake' culture the test-tube is half filled with the medium, which is allowed to solidify in the upright position. The most frequent use of media solidified with gelatin is as a stab culture.

Screw-capped bottles can be substituted for test-tubes. The amounts of medium for slopes in 1-oz and bijou bottles are 5 ml and 2·5 ml respectively. The medium may be allowed to set at an angle to form a butt as in test-tubes, but it is easier to inoculate with a loop if it is parallel to the side of the bottle (Fig. 5.2). For stab or shake cultures 1-oz bottles are half-filled with medium.

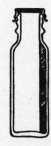

FIG. 5.2
Slope of solid medium in screw-capped bottle.

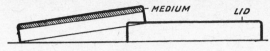

FIG. 5.3
The drying of an agar plate before inoculation.

Agar media stored in 4-, 6- or 8-oz medical flat bottles melt much more quickly than agar in 3-, 5- or 10-oz round bottles.

Where a large surface is necessary as in the separation of organisms from mixtures the medium is allowed to solidify in the form of a thin layer in a Petri dish. Solid media in Petri dishes are often called 'plates'. For a dish of $3\frac{1}{2}$ in (88 mm) diameter, 14 ml of medium is usually ample and it is convenient to store 100 ml amounts in 4- or 5-oz screw-capped bottles, sufficient for seven plates. The melted medium is poured into the dishes on a flat surface and the dishes are left undisturbed until the medium has set. In separating organisms from mixed cultures by plating, it is essential that the surface of the medium should be dry. When plates have been poured, the steam from the hot liquid condenses on the surface of the medium and this moisture is undesirable. It is removed by drying the poured and set plates in a warming or drying cabinet at 37°C for 1 h, or at 60°C for 15 to 30 min, depending on the medium. Suitable cabinets are available from manufacturers of food catering equipment. A bacteriological incubator may be used, but this is less efficient since it is not provided with a means of escape for the moist air. The lid of the dish is first laid down; the portion containing the medium is then inverted, so that the surface of the medium is downwards and placed in the incubator with the free edge resting on the lid (Fig. 5.3). If care is taken to avoid disturbing dust, there is very little risk of contamination of the medium by air organisms.

DISTRIBUTION OF MEDIA INTO TUBES, BOTTLES AND PLATES

Tubing and Bottling of Media Without Sterile Precautions

All media are distributed as liquids, gelatin and agar media being melted, and serum and egg media being distributed before they are solidified by heat. For safety it is usual to cool melted agar media to 55°C before distribution.

Most media are tubed or bottled without sterile precautions being taken. Clean but un-sterile glassware is used, and the medium and container together are subsequently sterilized by heat. A suitable apparatus is a 6-in glass funnel, fixed in a burette stand, with a short length of rubber tubing and a glass delivery nozzle fitted to the stem and controlled by a pinchcock.

However, an automatic filler devised by T. H. Ayling and supplied by R. B. Turner & Co., London, can be recommended. It consists of a glass funnel 7 in in diameter, connected by rubber tubing to a metal 3-way stopcock which in turn is connected to an all-glass syringe of 15 ml capacity (Fig. 5.4). The syringe is of the three-piece type, but without the nozzle, and the plunger is hollow, as the head of liquid will not lift a solid glass piston. The barrel is graduated to 15 ml by 0·5 ml, and the numbers are so engraved as to be readable when the syringe is vertical. The syringe is connected to the stopcock by means of a metal screw fitting. A clamp secures the lower end of the syringe. The amount of fluid delivered is determined by the adjustable screw. The action of the filler is simple. The head of medium in the funnel forces up the plunger until it is stopped by the adjustable screw. The handle of the stopcock is then turned and the syringe empties itself under the weight of the plunger. Air bubbles in the syringe are removed by first filling the apparatus, and emptying and filling the syringe two or three times, manipulating the piston by hand while this is being done. The adjustable screw is then turned to deliver the correct amount. If a smoothly working syringe is used, very little head of pressure is necessary, and the height need not be greater than 18 inches. Once set, the accuracy of the filler is much greater than that of an ordinary pipette, and media can be tubed with great rapidity. It works equally well with melted agar or gelatin, provided that fresh hot supplies are available, and the syringe and stopcock are washed out immediately after use.

An electrically driven automatic dispenser designed by Struer can be obtained from Camlab (Glass) Ltd., Cambridge. With it, measured volumes from 0·2 to 20 ml can be

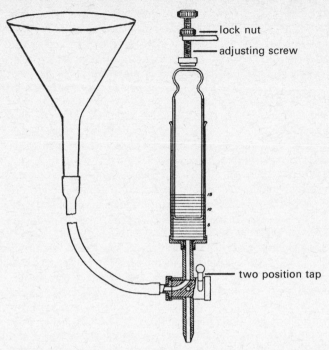

lock nut

adjusting screw

two position tap

FIG. 5.4 Automatic filler for dispensing media without sterile precautions.

delivered at any chosen rate, or individually at the touch of a foot pedal, and media may be dispensed under sterile conditions.

Pouring of Plates, and Tubing and Bottling of Media with Sterile Precautions

Plates are always poured with sterile precautions. Bulk medium is prepared sterile and is poured into sterile Petri dishes. Care must be taken to avoid contamination from the air during pouring. It is desirable to pour plates on a bench in a small room free from draughts and preferably with ultraviolet radiation to reduce the number of bacteria in the air. Alternatively, an inoculation hood or cabinet, may be used. To reduce water of condensation on the Petri dish lids, the medium should be cooled to 52°C before pouring.

Sterile precautions for tubing and bottling media are necessary if an ingredient of the medium is heat-labile, for example, certain sugars used in fermentation test media. The ingredients that are stable to heat are prepared and sterilized, the unstable ingredient (previously sterilized in a suitable way) is added

with sterile precautions and the medium is distributed with sterile precautions into sterile containers. An apparatus (Fig. 5.5) suitable for

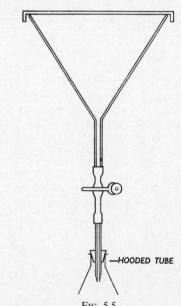

—HOODED TUBE

FIG. 5.5
Apparatus for dispensing media with sterile precautions.

distributing medium with sterile precautions is a hooded tube attached by means of rubber tubing and a pinchcock to a funnel covered with a large Petri dish lid. The whole apparatus is wrapped in paper and sterilized. The Petri dish lid protects sterile medium in the funnel and the hood protects the medium as it is distributed to sterile tubes or bottles.

Alternatively the heat-stable part of the medium may be distributed into clean glass-ware without sterile precautions and then be sterilized. The sterile unstable ingredient, for example, a sugar, can later be added from a sterile graduated pipette or an apparatus in-corporating a filter, a siphon and a hooded pipette (Fig. 5.6).

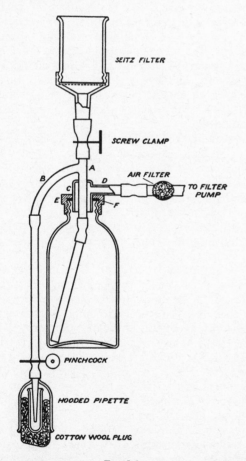

FIG. 5.6
Apparatus for adding small quantities of sterile ingredients to media.

A special stainless-steel metal fitting is adapted to a 10-oz bottle with a screw neck. It consists of a straight piece of tube (A), with a curved side-arm (B); around this is a slightly wider tube (C), with a side-arm (D), fitted to a screw-cap (E) which screws on to the bottle, a rubber washer (F) ensuring an air-tight joint. To the upper end of tube A is connected a bacterial filter such as a Seitz filter by means of a short piece of pressure tubing furnished with a screw-clamp, and attached to the lower end by means of a short piece of rubber tubing is a glass tube, 5 mm in diameter, reaching to the bottom of the bottle. To the side-arm B is connected a piece of rubber tubing furnished at the other end with a pinchcock and hooded pipette. The hooded pipette is covered with a small glass tube and closed with a cotton-wool stopper. The side-arm D is connected with pressure tubing to a cotton-wool air filter, the other end of which is to be attached to a filter pump. The joints are bound with tinned copper wire and the whole apparatus, as figured, is wrapped in kraft paper. If silicone rubber is used for all the fittings it can be sterilized in the hot air oven. Otherwise it must be auto-claved with a little water (a few drops) in the bottle to provide steam to drive out air from the interior.

The unstable ingredient is sterilized by Seitz filtration and, before the pressure is released, the tubing to the filter is closed with the screw-clamp. The filter is then removed and the end of the rubber tubing plugged with a piece of glass rod. The filter pump is now disconnected; the air pressure forces the solution down the siphon tube as far as the pinchcock so that the siphon is in operation as soon as the pinchcock is opened. Alternatively, air may be forced through the cotton-wool filter on D by means of a rubber blowball to start the siphon action. In use, the neck of the bottle is held by a clamp at the top of a tall retort stand. The stem of the hooded pipette is held below the bottle by means of another clamp, at a height convenient for placing a test-tube (or bottle) under it to receive the sterile solution. The cotton-wool stopper and small glass tube are removed and the pipette flamed. After use, the stopper and glass tube are replaced and the hooded pipette fastened to the neck of the bottle with a piece of copper wire. The number of drops per ml delivered from the pipette is determined, so that the amount required is easily estimated. Thus, if a pipette delivers 18 drops per ml, then 9 drops (0·5 ml) of 10 per cent sugar solution per tube of 4·5 ml peptone water gives a final concentration of 1 per cent sugar.

ADJUSTMENT OF pH OF CULTURE MEDIA

The pH of a culture medium should always be checked and adjusted if necessary, methods being given in Chapter 4. It should be noted that the pH always rises as the temperature falls and allowance for this rise must be made if the pH is tested when the medium is hot, as is the case with agar which must be melted for the adjustment of pH. During autoclaving, solutions that have been adjusted to be a little on the alkaline side of neutrality tend to fall about 0·1 unit.

STERILIZATION OF PREPARED MEDIA

The choice of method to be used to sterilize a medium depends on whether or not the ingredients are decomposed by heat. If autoclaving will not damage the medium, it is the best method of sterilization, and its application was discussed in Chapter 3.

The sterilization time at a particular temperature is the sum of the heat penetration time, which is variable, and the holding time, which is constant for media prepared under clean conditions for each temperature. The heat penetration time, and consequently the sterilization time, varies greatly with the volume of medium and also with the container. For test tubes containing 10 ml of medium, a sterilization time of 15 min at 121°C, or 35 min at 115°C, is required. McCartney bottles containing 10 ml of medium require 20 min at 121°C. Larger amounts of medium require longer sterilization times and so do small amounts of medium in large containers. Sterilization times at 121°C given in this chapter are based on the following table. Molten agar requires the same sterilization time as liquid media; but if agar is solid, 5 to 10 min must be added for melting (Table 5.2).

Tubes and bottles of medium must be put in the autoclave so that steam has free access to

Table 5.2 Sterilization times at 121°C.

Volume of medium	Container	
	Flask	Bottle
10 ml	15 min	20 min
100 ml	20 min	25 min
500 ml	25 min	30 min
1 l	30 min	40 min

them. Wire crates are suitable holders, but tins are unsuitable unless holes have been punched in them. Care must be taken that bottles of medium are not packed tightly in a holder, otherwise breakages will occur.

Sometimes lower temperatures, such as 115°C, for times ranging from 10 to 20 min are recommended for 'sterilization' of media containing ingredients that are not very stable to heat. These conditions are not strictly reliable for sterilization and should be used only for media distributed in small quantities. They are usually satisfactory because it is unlikely that many heat-resistant spores would be present in media prepared under clean conditions.

Steaming at 100°C, either for a long time, e.g. 90 min on one occasion or for shorter times on several occasions, is not a sure way of sterilizing media. Spores are not invariably destroyed at 100°C and will not be destroyed by successive heatings at 100°C unless they are incubated in the intervening periods under conditions in which they will germinate to yield heat-sensitive vegetative organisms.

If any of the ingredients of a medium are liable to be spoiled by autoclaving, the complete medium should not be sterilized by heat. In such cases, it is usual to autoclave the heat-resistant ingredients of the medium and to add the sterile heat-sensitive ingredients with sterile precautions. Some heat-sensitive ingredients such as blood, serum or egg-yolk can be obtained sterile from natural sources. Others must be sterilized by filtration through a bacterial filter (Chapter 3).

Some media that cannot be autoclaved contain ingredients that are inhibitory to the most probable contaminants. These media are sometimes prepared without the sterilization of some ingredients, reliance being placed on the inhibitors to suppress contaminants. The method is usually successful but must always be regarded as less than ideal.

INSPISSATION OF SERUM AND EGG MEDIA

The serum in Löffler's medium and the egg in media such as Löwenstein-Jensen medium are usually solidified in an apparatus called an inspissator. It consists of a water-jacketed copper box, the temperature of which can be regulated automatically. The serum or egg medium is tubed and placed in special racks, so that the tubes are at the correct angle for forming slopes. The temperature used is between 75° and 85°C. At this temperature the protein is completely solidified, but the temperature is not so high as to cause bubbles of steam to disrupt the surface of the medium. As medium in tubes is apt to dry if kept in the inspissator for any time, a small opening should be present in the inner wall communicating with the top of the water-chamber above the level of the water. Water vapour can enter the interior of the inspissator and the medium is kept moist. If an electric inspissator without a water-jacket is to be used, it is better to dispense media in bottles rather than in tubes with cotton-wool stoppers.

VARIETIES OF CULTURE MEDIA

1. *Defined synthetic media.* Chemically defined media are used for various experimental purposes. They are prepared exclusively from pure chemical substances and their exact composition is known. The ingredients should be of analytical reagent quality and are dissolved in distilled or demineralized water.

Simple synthetic media contain a carbon and energy source such as glucose or lactate; an inorganic source of nitrogen, usually in the form of ammonium chloride, phosphate or sulphate; and various inorganic salts in a buffered aqueous solution. They provide the basic essentials for the growth of many non-parasitic heterotrophs, but they will not support growth of most kinds of parasitic bacteria. *Complex synthetic media* incorporate, in addition, certain amino acids, purines, pyrimidines

and other growth factors. They can therefore be used for the growth of more exacting bacteria.

2. *Routine laboratory media.* The majority of organisms to be studied in medical bacteriology are either pathogens or commensals of the human body, and in order to obtain suitable growths the artificial culture medium should provide nutrients and a pH (about 7·2) approximating to those of the tissues and body fluids. For routine purposes many of these nutrients are supplied by aqueous extracts of meat and peptone which is a product of the digestion of protein.

Basal media such as nutrient broth and peptone water are simple routine laboratory media. *Enriched media* are prepared to meet the nutritional requirements of more exacting bacteria by the addition of substances such as blood, serum and egg to a basal medium. *Selective media* contain substances that inhibit or poison all but a few types of bacteria. They facilitate the isolation of particular species from a mixed inoculum. If a liquid medium favours the multiplication of a particular species, either by containing enrichments that selectively favour it or inhibitory substances that suppress competitors, cultures from mixed inocula are called *enrichment* cultures. These cultures fail to indicate the proportion of the species present in the inoculum. *Indicator media* incorporate some substance that is changed visibly as a result of the metabolic activities of particular organisms. Combinations of enriched media with selective agents and indicator systems are frequently used in the diagnostic laboratory.

COMMON INGREDIENTS OF CULTURE MEDIA

Information on the preparation and composition of commercial products used in culture media is given in a report edited by Sykes (1956).

WATER. Tap water is often suitable for culture media, particularly if it has a low mineral content, but if the local supply is found unsuitable, glass-distilled or demineralized water must be used instead. Small amounts of copper are highly inhibitory to bacterial growth so that copper-distilled water cannot be used for media. Suitable demineralizers are manufactured by the Permutit Co. Ltd., Chiswick, London.

AGAR. Agar is prepared in several countries from a variety of seaweeds, *Gelidium, Eucheuma, Pterocladia* and others, by extraction from the dried weed by hot-water processes; the product is clarified, dried and finally supplied as the dried strands or as a powder. There are considerable differences in the properties of the agars manufactured in different places, and even between different batches from the same source. Japanese and New Zealand agars are well known and were formerly predominant. Japanese agar yields a gel of suitable firmness at a concentration of about 2 per cent, and New Zealand agar at about 1·2 per cent. Now, Spanish and Portuguese agars are widely used in Europe and also supplement American supplies taken from the American coasts, and Mexican and South American coasts (see Bridson and Brecker, 1970). The exact concentration to be used may require some adjustment according to the batch of agar and also according to the other constituents of the medium. The manufacturer's instructions should be followed.

The chief component of agar is a long-chain polysaccharide, mainly composed of d-galactopyranose units. It also contains a variety of impurities including inorganic salts, a small amount of protein-like material and sometimes traces of long-chain fatty acids which are inhibitory to growth. The minerals present are mainly magnesium and calcium, and agar is thought to exist as the magnesium or calcium sulphate esters of the polysaccharide.

In preparing agar media, the appropriate amount of agar powder or fibre is added to the liquid medium and dissolved by placing the mixture in a steamer at 100°C for 1 h.

Most agars dissolve to give a clear solution but sometimes it is necessary to filter off particulate impurities and, possibly, excess phosphates from the nutrient liquid. The hot agar solution, preferably first adjusted to pH 8·0 and held at 100°C for 30 min to precipitate phosphates, is filtered before it can cool and is re-adjusted to pH 7·4. For smaller amounts a hardened filter paper that is rapid in passing fluid and strong when wet, is used. A recommended grade is 'Hyduro' 904½, supplied by J. Barcham Green, Ltd., Maidstone, England. For larger amounts, paper pulp or cellulose wadding enclosed in muslin is better, a fresh filter being prepared on each occasion. A suitable paper pulp is 'White Heather' brand or T. B. Ford's filter pulp, both of which are sold in slabs. A suitable cellulose wadding is 'Cellosene' supplied in sheet form by Robinson & Sons, Ltd., Chesterfield. A porcelain Buchner-type filter funnel with a flat perforated platform about 10 in in diameter is convenient for 5–10 litre quantities. Place two 10 in disks of cellulose wadding, one on top of the other, on a 24-in square of muslin and fold over the excess muslin to enclose them completely. Invert the disk-like bundle and press it into position on the platform of the filter, ensuring a good fit at the edges. Pour some hot water through the filter and then heat it at 100°C in the steamer at the same time as the agar solution, so that it is hot at the time of its use. Without allowing any time for cooling, pour the whole of the hot agar solution quickly through the filter without assistance by suction. If a large Buchner funnel is not available, quantities up to five litres may be filtered using a 10-in conical glass funnel, the lower third of which is filled with pebbles or glass beads to form a supporting platform for the filter material. Paper pulp or cellulose wadding wrapped in muslin to form a bundle about 2 in deep is pressed into position on the platform and fitted closely to all sides of the filter funnel. Moist pulp may be superimposed to ensure that the filter is not leaky.

Agar can be added to any nutrient liquid medium if the advantages of a solid medium are desired. Nutrients that are not damaged by autoclaving may be added to the medium before dissolving the agar. Such media can be sterilized and allowed to set for storage, being remelted in the steamer before use. However, nutrients that are damaged by autoclaving must be prepared sterile, separately from the agar base. The sterilized agar base can be melted in the steamer and cooled to about 45–50°C before adding any heat-labile ingredients, but once these are added the medium must at once be distributed for its final use because it cannot be remelted without damaging the heat-sensitive ingredients.

Agar is hydrolyzed to products that do not solidify on cooling if it is heated at a low pH. Agar usually does not alter the pH of the medium to which it is added but if it contains free acid this must be neutralized before it is autoclaved. For media whose pH is about 5, such as those for lactobacilli and fungi, heating should be reduced to a minimum after the agar is in an acid solution. After autoclaving, the medium may be allowed to solidify in bulk but it should be remelted with as little heating as possible and then be wholly distributed for its final use; it should not be partly used, allowed to solidify and later heated a third time.

PEPTONE. Peptone consists of water-soluble products obtained from lean meat or other protein material, such as heart muscle, casein, fibrin or soya flour, by digestion with, mainly, the proteolytic enzymes, pepsin, trypsin or papain. The important constituents are peptones, proteoses, amino acids, a variety of inorganic salts, including phosphates, potassium and magnesium, and certain accessory growth factors, including nicotinic acid and riboflavin. Peptone is supplied as a golden granular powder with a low moisture content, preferably under 5 per cent and usually a slightly acid reaction, giving a pH between 5 and 7 in a 1 per cent solution. It is hygroscopic and soon becomes sticky when exposed to air; stock bottles should therefore be kept firmly closed and weighing of loose powder rapidly completed. According to the starting materials and mode of preparation, the brands of peptone supplied by different manufacturers show appreciable differences in composition and growth-promoting properties; moreover, variations may occur between different batches of one brand.

The essential requirements of a good peptone have not yet been fully defined, but include the ability to support the growth of moderately exacting bacteria from small inocula (e.g. *Staph. aureus Strept. pyogenes* and *Sh. dysenteriae* type 1), the absence of fermentable carbohydrates, a low content of contaminating bacteria and a very low content of copper. Apart from the standard grades of bacteriological peptone, some manufacturers supply special grades of peptone recommended for particular purposes, e.g. 'Neopeptone', 'Proteose peptone', mycological peptone, etc.

The analysis of a suitable bacteriological peptone (Oxoid) has been supplied by the makers as follows:

Total nitrogen	14·5 per cent
Total proteose nitrogen (sat. $ZnSO_4$)	1·9 per cent
Primary proteose nitrogen (half-sat. $ZnSO_4$)	0·14 per cent
Amino acid nitrogen (formol titration)	1·7 per cent
Tryptophane	1·2 per cent
Ash	5·5 per cent
Chloride	1·0 per cent
Phosphate (as P_2O_5)	1·3 per cent
Calcium	0·13 per cent
Magnesium	0·07 per cent
Copper	0·0010 per cent
Iron	0·0075 per cent
Zinc	0·0025 per cent
Sulphur (total)	0·68 per cent
Ether-soluble extract	0·03 per cent
Nicotinic acid	75 μg per g
Riboflavin	50 μg per g
Carbohydrate (fermentation test)	nil
Moisture	less than 5 per cent
pH of a 1 per cent solution	5·9 to 6·1

(Indole production test, good reaction)

CASEIN HYDROLYSATE. This consists largely of the amino acids obtained by hydrolysis of the milk protein, 'casein'. It also contains phosphate and other salts, and certain growth factors. Hydrolysis is effected either with hydrochloric acid, when the product is neutralized with sodium carbonate and so becomes very rich in sodium chloride, or with a proteolytic enzyme (trypsin). The acid hydrolysate is the poorer nutritionally because tryptophane is largely destroyed during the hydrolysis and some other amino acids are reduced in amount; tryptophane must therefore be added to the medium to make it suitable for tryptophane-requiring bacteria. The more expensive enzymic hydrolysate contains abundant tryptophane and the full range of amino acids, and does not require such supplementation. Casein hydrolysate may be substituted for peptone in broth and other media. It is of particular use in experimental work where a nearly defined medium is required, since its composition is more constant and more fully known than that of other peptones. Thus it may be added to a minimal synthetic medium to render it suitable for growth of exacting bacteria.

MEAT EXTRACT. A commercially prepared meat extract known as Lab-Lemco is used as a substitute for an infusion of fresh meat. Meat extract is manufactured by a method derived from that invented by Liebig. Finely divided lean beef is held in boiling water for a short time while its readily soluble constituents pass into solution and form the unconcentrated extract. After removal of excess fat it is concentrated by evaporation to a dark viscid paste containing 70–80 per cent of solids. The product contains a wide variety of water-soluble compounds, including protein degradation products, e.g. gelatin, albumoses, peptones, proteoses and amino acids and other nitrogen compounds such as creatine, creatinine, carnosine, anserine, purines and glutathione (total N about 10 per cent); it also contains many mineral salts (KH_2PO_4 and $NaCl$ most abundantly), accessory growth factors (e.g. thiamine, nicotinic acid, riboflavine, pyridoxine, pantothenic acid and choline) and some carbohydrates. The required quantity of the sticky extract is conveniently weighed on a piece of clean paper and put with the paper into the water for solution; the paper is subsequently removed from the broth. Meat extract is now available in powder form and this is more easily handled.

YEAST EXTRACT. Commercial yeast extract is prepared from washed cells of brewers' or bakers' yeast. These are allowed to undergo autolysis, which is initiated by mild heating (e.g. at 55°C) or, in some cases, are hydrolysed with hydrochloric acid or a proteolytic enzyme. After removal of the cell walls by filtration or centrifugation, the extract is evaporated to a thick dark paste containing about 70 per cent of solids. It contains a wide range of amino acids (amounting to nearly 50 per cent of its mass), growth factors (especially of the vitamin B group) and inorganic salts (particularly potassium and phosphate); over 10 per cent of carbohydrates are present, including glycogen, trehalose and pentoses. Yeast extract is used mainly as a comprehensive source of growth factors and may be substituted for meat extract in culture media. Yeast extract is also now available in powder form.

BLOOD. Blood for use in media must be collected with aseptic precautions adequate to exclude bacterial contamination and preserve the blood in its original sterile condition. Any attempt to sterilize blood by heat would lead to disintegration of the cells, coagulation of cell and serum proteins, and denaturation of the red haemoglobin to brown derivatives. It must be rendered non-coagulating by defibrination or by the addition of citrate or oxalate; the former is recommended because it involves no additive that might alter the nutritive properties of the medium.

Sterile horse blood can be obtained commercially from Evans Medical Supplies Ltd., Liverpool; Wellcome Reagents Ltd., Beckenham; or Oxoid Ltd., London. Alternatively blood may be collected from rabbits and other laboratory animals, sheep, oxen and horses at the abattoir, or from man.

Human or animal blood may contain antibiotics. These can be detected by testing with a bacterium sensitive to a wide range of antibiotics. Donor blood sometimes contains glucose and is unsuitable for some purposes. Even screened human blood may contain hepatitis viruses and strict precautions should be taken when handling it (Marmion and Tonkin, 1972).

Small amounts of blood may be obtained from rabbits, up to 20–30 ml from the ear vein and about 50 ml per kg body weight by cardiac puncture. The procedures for withdrawing blood aseptically in these ways are described in Chapter 3.

Very large quantities of sterile blood are obtained from sheep or horses. A cannula or wide-bore needle is inserted into the external jugular vein. If a sheep is selected, the wool is clipped from the side of the neck and the part shaved. Contamination can be minimized by placing a bag made of waterproof material over the head of the animal. It is best to use a cannula connected with rubber tubing to a screw-capped bottle containing glass beads or anticoagulant, the whole being enclosed in kraft paper and sterilized. The vein may be made prominent by pressure on the lower part of the side of the neck. The skin over the vein is carefully disinfected with soap and water and then alcohol. The cannula is inserted into the vein and the requisite amount of blood removed. Horses are treated similarly except that it is advisable to make a small incision with a sharp knife in the skin over the vein. The cannula is then more easily introduced.

For defibrination, a bottle containing glass beads is half filled with the blood, stoppered at once and shaken continuously for 5 min. Oxalated blood is prepared by bleeding the animals into bottles containing 10 ml of a 10 per cent solution of neutral potassium oxalate per litre of blood. For citrated blood, which is often preferred to oxalated blood, the blood is collected and gently but thoroughly shaken in a bottle containing sodium citrate 60 mg per 10 ml of blood, e.g. 0·3 ml of a 20 per cent solution of sodium citrate.

The sterile blood is immediately distributed in 5 or 10 ml amounts in sterile $\frac{1}{2}$-oz screw-capped bottles and stored in the refrigerator. It will keep for up to two months. It must not be allowed to freeze or the corpuscles may be lysed.

FILDES' PEPTIC DIGEST OF BLOOD. Peptic digestion of blood liberates nutrients from red cells. Fildes' digest is prepared as follows:

Sodium chloride, NaCl,
    0·85 per cent aqueous   150 ml
Hydrochloric acid,
    HCl, pure . . 6 ml
Defibrinated sheep
    blood . . . 50 ml
Pepsin (B.P. granulated) 1 g
Sodium hydroxide,
    NaOH, 20 per cent,
    aqueous . . About 12 ml
Chloroform . . 0·5 ml

In a stoppered bottle, mix the saline, acid, blood and pepsin. Heat at 55°C for 2–24 h. Add sodium hydroxide until a sample of the mixture diluted with water gives a permanganate red colour with cresol red indicator. Add pure hydrochloric acid drop by drop until a sample of the mixture shows almost no change of colour with cresol red but a definite red tint with phenol red. It is important to avoid excess of acid. Add chloroform and shake the mixture vigorously.

This peptic digest of blood keeps well for months.

SERUM. Serum for use in media need not be collected with aseptic precautions because it can be Seitz-filtered to sterilize it. Sterile horse serum can be obtained commercially.

If serum is to be collected without aseptic precautions, a wide-mouthed stoppered bottle is taken to the abattoir at a time when animals, preferably sheep, are being killed. After the neck vessels have been severed, the blood is allowed to flow for a short time and then the stream from the carotid artery is allowed to spurt directly into the bottle. When filled, the bottle is stoppered and returned carefully to the laboratory. The clot is then separated from the sides of the bottle by means of a stiff wire. The blood is kept overnight in the refrigerator and the clear serum is then pipetted off. At some abattoirs serum is prepared in bulk from blood allowed to coagulate in open trays; this is liable to greater bacterial contamination, but may be used when large quantities are required.

Serum may also be prepared from unsterile defibrinated or oxalated blood which does not clot on standing. It is stored overnight in the cold to allow settling of the corpuscles, and the serum or plasma is siphoned off into a Winchester quart bottle. Plasma requires warming to about 37°C, the addition of 22·5 ml of a 4 per cent solution of calcium chloride per litre and shaking, preferably on a machine, until the fibrin has separated.

Serum is sterilized by filtration through a Seitz filter using a sterilizing grade of Ford's Sterimat asbestos-cellulose disk, and may be stored at 3–5°C in the refrigerator until required for use. It is convenient to store serum in a large sterile screw-capped bottle of 1–5 litres capacity, fitted with siphon delivery tube and hooded pipette.

Small quantities of serum may be prepared without filtration from sterile rabbit blood.

The blood is collected into a sterile container and allowed to clot. Free contraction of the clot is assisted if the container is lined with agar; 10 ml of melted 1·5 per cent agar in physiological saline (0·85 per cent NaCl) is spread inside an 8 × 1 in boiling tube by rotating the tube until the agar sets as a thin layer. When the blood is fully coagulated the serum is removed with a sterile pipette. It may require centrifuging to remove any remaining red cells. It can be stored in sterile screw-capped bottles, preferably fresh but it can be heated at 56°C for 1 h without being coagulated.

Serum, like blood, may contain antibiotics or hepatitis viruses.

FORMULAE FOR THE PREPARATION OF CULTURE MEDIA

DEHYDRATED CULTURE MEDIA

Several manufacturers (e.g. Oxoid, Wellcome Reagents Ltd., Difco, Baltimore Biological Laboratories) prepare numerous culture media in dehydrated form. These are especially convenient for small laboratories where facilities for media-making are limited but they are also coming into wide use in larger laboratories. Although in general they are not equal in quality to freshly made media they are significantly labour-saving, being easy to reconstitute for use. However claims that dehydrated media are absolutely constant and reliable cannot be substantiated. Microbiologists who have used dehydrated media have had problems due to variations between batches even from a single manufacturer. Nevertheless the advantages of dehydrated media make it desirable that their use should be extended provided that the quality of microbiology does not suffer. Microbiologists who use dehydrated media must be constantly vigilant, rejecting media whose performance falls below standards that have already been achieved and also encouraging improvements. As a minimum a small batch from every bottle of medium should be tested before it is taken into use, noting colony size and germination rate as well as the ability of the medium to perform any special function. More stringent tests such as those recommended by Stokes (1968) or Cowan and Steel

(1965) are advisable. Anderson and Faine (1971) quote tables showing the likelihood of error if a given size of sample fails to show a fault in a batch with a given incidence of fault, such as contamination.

Dehydrated media tend to deteriorate during storage. They should be bought in amounts small enough to be used within a few months. Storage should comply with manufacturer's instructions or, if unspecified, should be somewhere cool and dry. Media that show physical signs of deterioration should be discarded but deterioration can occur without physical change. Quality control by the exchange of simulated clinical specimens (Stokes and Whitby, 1971) though aimed primarily at evaluating the standard of laboratory methods will also tend to sustain the standard of dehydrated media.

The selection of a range of media suitable for a routine diagnostic laboratory can be confused by the enormous number that are available. Generally the fewer the kinds of media a laboratory uses, the better. This is especially true when they are in dehydrated form because rate of turnover is correspondingly faster and the laboratory's more extensive experience of each medium will tend to improve judgements as to when it is unsatisfactory. It is a false economy to use any but a first-class basal medium. Enrichment with natural products, such as blood, does not compensate for a poor base. The basal medium should be suitable for enrichment for special purposes such as to show haemolysis, particularly of streptococci, and· to grow fastidious species. A suggested minimum of five dehydrated culture media for primary cultivation of specimens in a diagnostic laboratory is:

1. Nutrient broth – a broth base from which nutrient broth, cooked meat broth, Löffler's medium, etc., can be made, e.g., Nutrient Broth No. 2 (Oxoid).

2. Nutrient agar – used to make blood agar, heated blood agar, etc., e.g. Columbia Agar (Oxoid).

3. MacConkey Agar – a medium without added sodium chloride is chosen as this inhibits the spreading of *Proteus spp.*; sodium chloride can be added if especially desired, e.g., MacConkey agar without salt (Oxoid).

4. Sensitivity Test Agar – an 'ordinary' nutrient agar is not suitable for antibiotic sensitivity testing as various inhibitors may be present, e.g., Sensitivity Test Agar (Wellcome Reagents Ltd.).

5. Deoxycholate–citrate agar (Oxoid).

The dehydrated media listed are those with which the authors are familiar. Additional special media can be added to suit local conditions. There must be adequate mixing and solubilization of dehydrated ingredients.

The formulae that follow are for the use of laboratories that still prefer to prepare their own media from fresh ingredients, a practice that one hopes will continue long enough to ensure that dehydrated media are as good as, if not better than, the freshly made media that they replace. Dehydrated cooked meat broth tends to be particularly defective in that the meat particles are insufficient for a column 2·5 cm in depth.

Synthetic Media

Minimal Medium of Davis and Mingioli and its Variants

This medium is suitable for growth of a wide variety of bacteria for research purposes.

Basal medium

Glucose, sterile 10 per cent solution	20 ml
Dipotassium hydrogen phosphate, K_2HPO_4 . .	7 g
Potassium dihydrogen phosphate, KH_2PO_4 . .	3 g
Sodium citrate, $Na_3C_6H_5O_7.2H_2O$ . .	0·5 g
Magnesium sulphate, $MgSO_4.7H_2O$ . .	0·1 g
Ammonium sulphate, $(NH_4)_2SO_4$ . . .	1 g
Agar, if required . .	20 g
Distilled water to . .	1 l

Trace element solution

Ferrous sulphate, $FeSO_4.7H_2O$.	0·5 g
Zinc sulphate, $ZnSO_4.7H_2O$.	0·5 g
Manganese sulphate, $MnSO_4.3H_2O$ . .	0·5 g

Sulphuric acid, H_2SO_4, 0·1 N .	10 ml
Distilled water	1 l

Since glucose is partly decomposed when autoclaved in the presence of phosphate, it is added as a sterile solution after the remainder of the medium has been autoclaved.

Essential minerals other than those in the basal medium are likely to be present in sufficient amounts contaminating agar, water and other ingredients. If necessary, 5 ml of the trace element solution and also 1 ml of a 1 per cent calcium chloride solution may be added per litre of medium.

The large phosphate content is required to buffer the acid that is formed by fermentation of glucose, the mixture shown giving a pH of 7·1. If it is required that the phosphate content of the medium should be low, a citrate or bicarbonate buffer may be used. Thus a pH of 7·1 is obtained by incorporation of 0·3 per cent of $NaHCO_3$ in the medium and incubation of the culture in an atmosphere containing 20 per cent (v/v) of carbon dioxide.

Other sugars may be substituted for the glucose. The citrate may be omitted. Particular amino acids or growth factors may be added, or a mixture of the essential amino acids in the form of a vitamin-free casein hydrolysate, to give a nearly defined medium.

Nutrient Broth

This is the basis of most media used in the study of the common pathogenic bacteria. It should be of the best quality possible, because enrichment does not fully compensate for a poor basal medium. There are three types of nutrient broth; meat infusion broth consisting of a watery extract of lean meat to which peptone is added; meat extract broth prepared as a mixture of commercial peptone and meat extract; and digest broth consisting of a watery extract of lean meat that has been digested with a proteolytic enzyme so that additional peptone need not be added.

Meat Infusion Broths

These are good broths but the amount of peptone in them makes them expensive compared with digest broths.

Standard Meat Infusion Broth

Lean meat, ox heart or beef	500 g
Water	1 l
Peptone	10 to 20 g
Sodium chloride, NaCl	5 g

The type of meat used is an important factor in determining the quality of the broth. It should be fresh, not frozen. Horse flesh is cheap, but is usually not so fresh, and, coming from older animals, is more fibrous than beef. In addition it contains a higher percentage of fermentable sugar which may make the broth unsuitable for many purposes, such as the preparation of toxins.

Carefully remove all fat from the meat and mince it as finely as possible. Add the minced meat to the water and extract for 24 h in the cold, for example in the refrigerator, then strain through muslin and express the meat residue. The extract is bright red and often has a thin surface layer of fat which can be removed by skimming with a piece of filter paper. Boil for 15 min or steam at 100°C for 2 h. The extract becomes brown and turbid because haemoglobin is altered and soluble proteins are coagulated. Filter through a Whatman No. 1 paper. If filtration is done when the medium is hot, it may be necessary to use a hardened filter paper such as 'Hyduro 904½' supplied by J. Barcham Green Ltd., Maidstone, England. The extract should be clear and light yellow in colour. Make the volume up to 1 litre with water, add the peptone and salt and dissolve by heat. Filter. The reaction of the broth will be acid because of lactic acid from the meat. Adjust to the desired pH, usually 7·5, which will give a final pH of 7·4, distribute to tubes or bottles and sterilize by autoclaving at 121°C for 15 min.

Wright's (1933) Meat Infusion Broth

This differs from ordinary meat infusion broth in that veal is used and the peptone and salt are present when the meat is extracted. A little (0·15 per cent) glucose is added and the medium is especially good for the cultivation of the pneumococcus, although anaerobes such as the tetanus bacillus do not grow well in it.

MEAT EXTRACT BROTHS

These broths are the easiest and quickest to prepare. They can be varied widely but are usually less nutritive than infusion or digest broths. They are good for the preservation of stock cultures.

Standard Meat Extract Broth

Peptone	10 g
Meat extract (Lab-Lemco)	10 g
Sodium chloride, NaCl	5 g
Water	1 l

Mix the ingredients and dissolve them by heating briefly in the steamer. When cool, adjust the pH to 7·5–7·6. A precipitate of phosphates may appear and this may be removed by filtration through filter paper. If clarity of the broth is essential, the mixture should be adjusted to pH 8·0, heated at 100°C for 30 min to precipitate most of the phosphates, cooled, filtered and finally adjusted to pH 7·5. Distribute in tubes or bottles and sterilize by autoclaving at 121°C for 15 min.

The medium should be clear. The presence of a deposit, generally of phosphates, does not interfere with the nutrient value of the medium, but it may hinder the recognition of slight bacterial growth indicated by a developing turbidity.

Modifications of Meat Extract Broth

The formula for meat extract broth may be varied. With less exacting bacteria, 0·5 per cent of peptone and 0·3 per cent of meat extract are sufficient, and if the peptone is of high quality it may be possible to omit the meat extract. Sodium chloride can be omitted without reducing the nutritive value of the medium, but then the broth is hypotonic enough to lyse red cells and is unsuitable as a base for blood agar.

Sometimes meat extract is replaced by yeast extract, or peptone is replaced by either casein hydrolysate or soya hydrolysate.

DIGEST BROTHS

Digest broths are economical and are good for obtaining luxuriant growths of exacting organisms. However, cultures tend to die out rapidly in them. The proteolytic enzyme used may be varied. Trypsin obtained from pancreas, and papain (Asheshov, 1941) obtained from paw-paw may be used, attention being paid to the optimum temperature and pH for activity of the enzyme.

Hartley's Broth (Hartley, 1922)

Trypsin is the proteolytic enzyme used to prepare this medium.

Pancreatic extract (Cole and Onslow, 1916)

Fresh pig pancreas . .	500 g
Water . . .	1500 ml
Absolute alcohol or methylated spirit . .	500 ml
Concentrated hydrochloric acid, HCl . .	About 2 ml

Remove fat, mince the pancreas and mix it with the water and alcohol. Shake the mixture thoroughly in a large stoppered bottle and allow it to stand for three days at room temperature, shaking occasionally. Strain through muslin and filter through paper. Measure the volume of the filtrate and add 0·1 per cent hydrochloric acid. This causes a cloudy precipitate which settles in a few days and can be filtered off, although this is not essential.

This extract keeps for about two months in stoppered bottles in the cold. If used at once there is no need to add acid, whose action is to retard the slow deterioration of the trypsin.

Preparation of complete medium

Lean meat, ox heart, or beef .	1500 g
Water	2500 ml
Sodium carbonate, Na_2CO_3, 0·8 per cent solution .	2500 ml
Pancreatic extract . .	50 ml
Chloroform . .	50 ml
Concentrated hydrochloric acid, HCl . . .	40 ml

Mix the minced meat and water and heat them in the steam sterilizer until a temperature of 80°C is reached. Add the sodium carbonate, cool to 45°C and add the pancreatic extract and chloroform. Incubate the mixture at 37°C for 6 h or 45°C for 3 h, stirring frequently. When digestion is complete, add the acid, steam at 100°C for 30 min and filter. The broth is stored in an acid condition in one-gallon screw-capped bottles with 0·25 per cent of chloroform. Shake vigorously and frequently in the next two or three days. Store in a cool, dark place.

For use, adjust to pH 8·0 with normal caustic soda and steam at 100°C for 1 h to precipitate phosphates. Filter while hot and allow to cool. Adjust the reaction to pH 7·6, distribute, and autoclave at 115°C for 20 min.

Horse Flesh Digest Medium

This medium is a pancreatic digest of horse meat enriched by the addition of peptone and sterilized by Seitz filtration to preserve heat-sensitive substances. It is specially suitable for cultivating haemolytic streptococci when an abundant growth is required.

Horse flesh . . .	900 g
Water	3500 ml
Sodium carbonate, Na_2CO_3 .	12 g
Pancreatin . . .	17·5 g
Concentrated hydrochloric acid, HCl . . .	20 ml
Peptone, high quality .	35 g
Calcium chloride, $CaCl_2$ . .	4·4 g
Sodium bicarbonate, Na_2HCO_3 . . .	7 g

Mince the meat and mix it with 1500 ml of cold water, raising the temperature to 80°C. Add the remainder of the cold water and the sodium carbonate. Adjust the pH to 8·0, add the pancreatin and keep the mixture at 56°C for 6 h. Add the acid, boil at 100°C for 30 min to arrest digestion and filter. Add the peptone, adjust the pH to 8·0, add the calcium chloride, steam and filter when cold. Add the sodium bicarbonate and filter through a Seitz filter.

Store in bottles, first incubated at 37°C to test for sterility.

NUTRIENT AGAR

Standard Nutrient Agar

Nutrient agar is nutrient broth solidified by the addition of agar (see p. 104). It should be noted that nutrient agar is frequently referred to as 'agar', the context making clear that the agar-broth mixture is meant and not the pure, non-nutritive agar itself. Japanese agar yields a gel of suitable firmness at a concentration of about 2 per cent and New Zealand agar at about 1·2 per cent.

Semi-Solid Agar

For special purposes agar is added to media in concentrations that are too low to solidify them. At 0·2–0·5 per cent it yields a semi-solid medium through which motile, but not non-motile, bacteria may spread. At 0·05–0·1 per cent it prevents convection currents and retards the diffusion of air into media used for anaerobic and micro-aerophilic organisms.

Firm Agar

If agar is added to media in concentrations greater than that necessary for solidification, 'spreading' bacteria such as *Pr. vulgaris* and *Cl. tetani* will grow as discrete colonies. The necessary concentration must be determined by experiment but 6 per cent of Japanese agar and 4 per cent of New Zealand agar are usually satisfactory.

Firm agar takes longer to dissolve and to cool and is more difficult to handle than agar at ordinary concentrations.

STANDARD BASAL MEDIUM

CYLG Medium

In this modification (Marshall and Kelsey, 1960) of the CCY medium of Gladstone and Fildes (1940) yeast autolysate and casein digest replace the meat extract and peptone of broth. It is a good nutrient medium, cheap and easy to prepare, versatile in use and as fully defined as possible in terms of known nutritional factors.

Inorganic salt solution

Magnesium sulphate,
$MgSO_4.7H_2O$ . . . 4 g
Manganese sulphate,
$MnSO_4.4H_2O$ . . . 0·4 g
Ferrous sulphate,
$FeSO_4.7H_2O$ . . . 0·4 g
Water . . . . . 100 ml
Sulphuric acid, 10 N H_2SO_4 . 2 drops
Dissolve the salts and acidify them.

Concentrate for storage

Casein digest (Oxoid Tryptone) 10 g
Yeast autolysate (Marmite) . 5 g
Sodium glycerophosphate,
$Na_2C_3H_7O_6P.5H_2O$ . . 10 g
Potassium lactate, 50 per cent
w/v . . . . . 10 ml
Inorganic salt solution . . 5 ml
Water to . . . . 100 ml
Dissolve the ingredients. Filter. The concentrate can be stored in this form at room temperature without autoclaving provided a volatile preservative is added; 3–4 ml per litre of carbon tetrachloride/toluene (1:1, v/v) is recommended.

Sterile glucose solution

Glucose . . . . 20 g
Water . . . . 100 ml
Dissolve and autoclave at 121°C for 20 min at a pH not greater than 7. Adding a drop of phosphoric acid ensures that the solution is not alkaline.

Double strength agar

Agar . . . . . 40 g
Water . . . . . 1 l
Dissolve the agar, filter if necessary and distribute 100 ml amounts in 200 ml bottles. Autoclave at 121°C for 25 min.

Preparation of complete CYLG liquid medium

Concentrate . . . . 100 ml
Water . . . . . 900 ml
Sterile glucose solution . . 10 ml
Dilute the concentrate with water, autoclave it at 121°C for 30 min and add the glucose with sterile precautions.

Preparation of complete solid medium

Concentrate . . . . 20 ml
Water . . . . . 80 ml
Double strength agar . . 100 ml
Sterile glucose solution . . 2 ml
Melt the agar, add the concentrate and water, autoclave at 121°C for 20 min and add the glucose with sterile precautions.

Preparation of supplemented CYLG media. Additional ingredients such as blood or serum can replace part of the water when the concentrate is diluted. For MacConkey-type media, solutions of ingredients such as lactose, bile salts and neutral red replace some of the water, and glucose is omitted.

CARBOHYDRATE-FREE BASAL MEDIUM

Peptone Water

This medium is used chiefly as the basis for carbohydrate fermentation media (see Chap. 7). Broth may contain a small amount of sugar derived from meat and it is essential that the basal medium to which various carbohydrates are added for fermentation tests should be free from natural sugars. It is also used to test the formation of indole.

Peptone	.	.	.	10 g
Sodium chloride, NaCl	.	.	5 g
Water	.	.	.	.	1 l

Dissolve the ingredients in warm water, adjust the pH to 7·4–7·5 and filter. Distribute as required and autoclave at 121°C for 15 min.

ENRICHED CULTURE MEDIA FOR GENERAL USE

Any additional enrichment may be added to nutrient broth or nutrient agar. Some of these enriched media are described here.

Blood Agar and Broth

Blood agar is widely used in medical bacteriology. It is especially suitable for the gonococcus, the haemophilic group of bacteria and other delicate pathogens. In addition to being an enriched medium, it is an indicator medium showing the haemolytic properties of bacteria such as *Strept. pyogenes*. It is generally poured as plates.

The medium is prepared by adding sterile blood to sterile nutrient agar that has been melted and cooled to 50°C. The appropriate amount of blood can be poured from a screw-capped bottle. No pipette is necessary as the screw cap keeps the lip of the bottle sterile.

The concentration of blood may be varied from 5 per cent up to 50 per cent for special purposes. Ten per cent is the most usual concentration. Either human or animal blood may be used. Horse blood is the commonest.

A fairly thick layer of medium is required to prevent excessive drying during incubation and if this consists entirely of 10 per cent blood agar, the medium is almost opaque when viewed by transmitted light and haemolysis is difficult to see. Double-layer blood agar overcomes this difficulty. A thin layer of melted nutrient agar, about 7 ml for a 4-in Petri dish, is poured and allowed to set. Then a similar thin layer of 10 per cent blood agar is poured on top of the first layer. Any bubbles caused by the mixing of the blood and agar can easily be removed by drawing a Bunsen flame quickly across the surface of the medium in the dish.

Nutrient broth to which 5 to 10 per cent of blood has been added with sterile precautions is occasionally used as an enriched liquid medium.

Heated Blood Agar ('Chocolate Agar')

This medium is suitable for *H. influenzae* and other organisms such as the pneumococcus. During heating the red cells are ruptured and nutrients are liberated.

It is prepared by heating 10 per cent of sterile blood in sterile nutrient agar. Melt the agar, cool it in a waterbath at 75°C, add the blood and allow the medium to remain at 75°C, mixing the blood and agar by gentle agitation from time to time until the blood becomes chocolate-brown in colour, within about 10 min. Then pour as slopes or plates.

An alternative method of preparing plates of heated blood agar (Naylor, 1961) involves the heating of already poured and set plates of ordinary blood agar. The blood agar plates are held in an incubator or hot-air oven at 55°C for 1–2 h. The exact time of heating required for 'chocolating' depends on the conditions of heating and is determined by trial. Colonies of *H. influenzae* on this medium are larger than on medium heated at 75°C and it is more conveniently prepared.

Serum Agar and Broth

Serum agar can be used to grow the more highly exacting pathogens. It is generally used as slopes.

It is prepared by adding 10 per cent of sterile serum to sterile nutrient agar that has been melted and cooled to 55°C. In an emergency, a useful but less satisfactory serum medium can be made by running a few drops of sterile serum over the surface of a nutrient agar slope or plate.

Serum broth is frequently used for liquid medium cultures of the more highly exacting pathogens. It is prepared by adding 10 per cent of sterile serum to sterile nutrient broth.

Sterile hydrocele fluid or ascitic fluid may be used instead of serum.

Fildes' Agar and Broth

Fildes' peptic digest of blood is added to nutrient broth or agar in the proportion of 2 to 5 per cent after heating at 55°C for 30 min to remove the chloroform. It stimulates the growth of *Haemophilus* and *Cl. tetani* and the toxin production of *Cl. welchii*.

Glucose Agar and Broth

Glucose added to nutrient media promotes luxuriant growth of many organisms. It also acts as a reducing agent, and glucose agar is used for deep stab and shake cultures of anaerobes.

If glucose is added before autoclaving the medium, some darkening of it may occur. It is better to prepare a 20 per cent solution of glucose separately, add a drop of phosphoric acid to ensure that the pH is not more than 7·0, and autoclave at 115°C for 20 min. The sterile glucose can then be added with sterile precautions to the sterile basal medium.

Concentrations of 0·1, 0·25 and 1·0 per cent glucose are used. One per cent is the commonest.

p-Aminobenzoic Acid or Penicillinase in Culture Media

There may be enough sulphonamide in the blood stream or other body fluids of patients treated with sulphonamide compounds to prevent the growth of bacteria when culture is carried out. Sulphonamides are antagonized by *p*-aminobenzoic acid and its addition to the medium will prevent the bacteriostatic action of the sulphonamide. It has also been found valuable in media for the isolation of pathogenic cocci and even if no sulphonamide has been administered, *p*-aminobenzoic acid improves the nutritive qualities of the medium.

p-Aminobenzoic acid is stable and withstands autoclaving. It is added in the proportion of 5 to 10 mg per 100 ml of medium.

Penicillin may be present in specimens from patients treated with penicillin. It can be destroyed by penicillinase. 1 ml of the penicillinase solution supplied by Burroughs Wellcome inactivates 100,000 units of penicillin but proportionately more of it is required for less penicillin. A suitable dilution containing 0·01 ml of the solution should be added with aseptic precautions to 100 ml sterile broth for blood culture.

MEDIA FOR THE CULTIVATION OF STAPHYLOCOCCI

Milk Agar

On this medium (Christie and Keogh, 1940) large characteristic colonies of staphylococci appear within 24 h. Pigmentation is particularly marked and easily recognized against the opaque white background; this facilitates recognition of weakly golden colonies.

Fresh milk   .   .   .   . 100 ml
Sterile nutrient agar, containing
    3 per cent agar   .   .   . 200 ml

Heat the milk to 60°C, shake it, then sterilize it by autoclaving at 121°C for 20 min. Repeated sterilization should be avoided as this causes caramelization with alteration of colour. Suitable sterilized milk may be obtained commercially.

Melt the agar, cool to 56°C, mix with the milk and pour plates or make slopes.

Glycerol Monoacetate Agar

This medium (Jacobs, Willis and Goodburn, 1964) is an alternative to milk agar for the examination of clinical specimens, particularly nose swabs, for staphylococci. On it, colonies of coagulase-positive staphylococci are always orange, yellow or buff whereas coagulase-negative strains are usually porcelain-white. There is maximum differentiation after 48 hours' incubation. Colonies from this medium give brisk and coarse clumping in the slide coagulase test.

Heart infusion broth (Difco)   . 100 ml
Glycerol monoacetate (BDH)   .   1 g
Agar   .   .   .   .   .   2 g

Dissolve the agar in the broth by steaming at 100°C, add the glyceride and autoclave at

121°C for 15 min. Cool to 50–55°C, mix thoroughly to ensure even distribution of the glyceride and pour plates immediately.

The use of heart infusion base is essential. Overheating of the medium must be avoided; it cannot be allowed to solidify and then be remelted.

Salt Media

Staphylococci grow in sodium chloride concentrations that are high enough to be inhibitory to many other bacteria (Hill and White, 1929; Fairbrother and Southall, 1950). Salt has been used in selective media for isolating *Staph. aureus* when these organisms are likely to be present in small numbers, as in faeces.

Salt cooked meat broth. This is the most satisfactory salt liquid medium. It is less inhibitory to staphylococci than meat extract or digest broth containing increased salt and enables very small numbers to be detected. It is prepared in the same way as cooked meat broth except that 10 per cent of sodium chloride is added to the peptone infusion broth.

Salt milk agar. Besides being selective, salt in this medium has been thought to increase chromogenesis. The medium is prepared in the same way as milk agar excepting that 7–10 per cent of sodium chloride is added.

Salt glycerol monoacetate agar. For isolating staphylococci from sources such as blankets and dust, 5 per cent of sodium chloride may be added before the glyceride.

Polymyxin Agar

Lithium chloride and tellurite (Ludlam, 1949) have been used in a selective medium for *Staph. aureus.* More recently it has been found that coagulase-positive strains of staphylococci grow well on nutrient agar containing concentrations of polymyxin that inhibit coagulase-negative strains and most coliform bacilli (Finegold and Sweeney, 1961). Growth and pigment production by *Staph. aureus* are optimal after 24 hours' incubation and at this time growth of other organisms is minimal. Cycloheximide (Actidione), 400 μg per ml may be added to inhibit fungi in cultures from air, dust and clothes.

Nutrient agar . . . 1 l
Polymyxin B (Wellcome
  Reagents Ltd.) . . . 75 units
Melt the agar, add the polymyxin and autoclave at 121°C for 30 min. Pour plates.

Phenolphthalein Phosphate Agar

On this medium colonies of bacteria that produce sufficient phosphatase to liberate free phenolphthalein become bright pink when held over an open bottle of ammonia (Barber and Kuper, 1951).

Nutrient agar, pH 7·4 . . 98 ml
Sodium phenolphthalein
  phosphate solution, 0·6
  per cent . . . . 2 ml
A stock solution of sodium phenolphthalein phosphate can be prepared, sterilized by filtration and stored at 4°C. For use it is added to melted nutrient agar and plates are poured. Also the complete medium can be stored and remelted for use.

MEDIA FOR THE CULTIVATION OF STREPT. PYOGENES

Crystal Violet Blood Agar

The addition of a low concentration (1 in 500,000, i.e. 0·0002 per cent) of crystal violet to blood agar inhibits the growth of some bacteria, notably staphylococci, while allowing the growth of *Strept. pyogenes.* Crystal violet blood agar is therefore a selective medium for *Strept. pyogenes.*

Sterile nutrient agar . . 90 ml
Sterile horse blood . . . 10 ml
Crystal violet, 1 in 1000
  aqueous solution . . 0·2 ml
Melt the agar, cool to 50°C, add the blood and crystal violet and pour plates.

Todd-Hewitt Meat Infusion Broth

This glucose broth is used for grouping and typing *Strept. pyogenes* (Diagnostic Procedures and Reagents, 1950). The pH of the medium is high (7·8) and it contains 0·2 per cent glucose.

MEDIA FOR THE CULTIVATION OF NEISSERIA

Thayer and Martin Medium

Thayer and Martin (1966) medium is the best known selective medium for isolating gonococci from contaminated specimens. It is also suitable for meningococci. It consists of a special basal medium enriched with haemoglobin and yeast supplement and made selective with vancomycin, colistin and nystatin. Trimethoprim (5 μg per ml) to inhibit *Proteus* species is also added, particularly for cultures of rectal swabs, by Phillips, Humphrey, Middleton and Nicol (1972) who use a saponin-lysed blood agar as their basal medium.

In the modification described here, lysed blood agar is prepared using Columbia agar base (Ellner *et al.*, 1966) and then made selective with vancomycin (3 μg per ml), colistin (7·5 μg per ml) and nystatin (12·5 units per ml) as an optional supplement.

Basal nutrient medium (Columbia agar base)

Microbiotone (Oxoid)	.	23 g
Starch . . .	.	1 g
Sodium chloride, NaCl	.	5 g
Agar (Oxoid, No. 1)	.	10 g
Distilled water .	.	900 ml

Suspend the solids in the water. Bring to the boil to dissolve them completely. Boil for 1 min, adjust the pH to 7·4, dispense in 90 ml aliquots in flasks and autoclave at 121°C for 20 min.

Antibiotic solution

Vancomycin solution, 3 mg per ml in sterile water .	.	1 ml
Colistin methane sulphonate, 1·5 mg per ml in sterile water . . .	.	5 ml

Aliquots of 0·6 ml of the mixture are stored at −20°C. A mixture of antibiotics sufficient for 1 litre of medium is available commercially (Difco or Baltimore Biological Laboratories). It contains colistimethate 7,500 μg, vancomycin 3,000 μg and nystatin 12,500 units.

Preparation of complete medium

Basal nutrient medium	.	90 ml
Blood (lysed by heating at 55–56°C for at least 1 h)	.	10 ml
Antibiotic solution .	.	0·6 ml

Prepare lysed blood agar, add the antibiotics and pour plates.

Lysed Blood Agar

This medium is suitable for subculture of gonococci.

Basal nutrient medium. As for Thayer and Martin medium, dispensed in 15 ml aliquots in tubes and autoclaved at 121°C for 15 min.

Lysed blood. Human blood, lysed by heating at 55–56°C for approximately 1 h.

Preparation of complete medium

Basal nutrient medium .	.	15 ml
Lysed blood . . .	.	2·5 ml

Melt the basal medium, cool to 50°C, add the lysed blood and pour plates.

Mueller Hinton Agar

This medium was originally formulated for the isolation of pathogenic *Neisseria* species (Mueller and Hinton, 1941). Nowadays it is more commonly used in conjunction with high potency antibiotic disks, for the determination of antibiotic sensitivity patterns by the Kirby-Bauer Technique (Bauer *et al.*, 1966).

Beef infusion . .	.	300 ml
Casein hydrolysate .	.	17·5 g
Starch . . .	.	1·5 g
Agar . . .	.	10 g
Distilled water to .	.	1 l

Emulsify the starch in a small amount of cold water, pour into the beef infusion and add the casein hydrolysate and the agar. Make up the volume to 1 litre with distilled water. Dissolve the constituents by heating gently at 100°C with agitation. Filter if necessary. Adjust the pH to 7·4. Dispense in screw-capped bottles and sterilize by autoclaving at 121°C for 20 min. Pour plates.

MEDIA FOR THE CULTIVATION OF CORYNEBACTERIA

Hoyle's Medium

This medium (Hoyle, 1941) is satisfactory for routine examination of throat swabs for the diphtheria bacillus. Type differentiation on colonial morphology is not as good as on other media. It is a medium for isolation rather than typing of diphtheria bacilli.

Agar base

Meat extract (Lab-Lemco)	.	10 g
Peptone (Difco proteose, or Evans) . . .	.	10 g
Sodium chloride, NaCl .	.	5 g
Agar	.	20 g
Water	.	1 l

Dissolve the ingredients and adjust the pH to 7·8. Distribute in 100 ml quantities in screw-capped bottles and autoclave at 121°C for 25 min.

Laked horse blood. Sterile horse blood may be laked by freezing and thawing four times and then stored in the cold, preferably frozen.

It is more simple and convenient to lake with saponin (Young, 1942). Prepare 10 per cent saponin (white) in water and sterilize it in the autoclave at 115°C for 30 min. Incubate the blood for 15 min, add 0·5 ml saponin solution for each 10 ml blood and invert the bottle gently several times to ensure thorough mixing, avoiding the formation of bubbles. Replace the blood in the incubator for a further 15 min when it should have an 'inky' black appearance. It will keep for several months in the refrigerator.

Tellurite solution

Potassium tellurite, K$_2$TeO$_3$	.	0·7 g
Water	.	20 ml

Dissolve, autoclave at 115°C for 20 min and store in a tightly stoppered bottle in the dark.

Preparation of complete medium

Agar base	. .	200 ml
Laked blood .	. .	10 ml
Tellurite solution	. .	2 ml

Melt the agar and cool it to 55°C, add the blood and tellurite and pour plates.

Anderson's Medium

This medium can be recommended for the provisional detection of *C. diphtheriae* from throat swabs in 24 h (Anderson, 1944). It is selective and preserves the microscopic morphology of *C. diphtheriae* but type-specific colonial morphology is not elicited.

Agar base

Meat extract (Lab-Lemco)	.	5 g
Peptone (Parke, Davis & Co.)	.	10 g
Sodium chloride, NaCl .	.	5 g
Agar	.	25 g
Water	.	1 l

Dissolve the ingredients and adjust the pH to 7·6. Distribute in 100 ml quantities in bottles and autoclave at 121°C for 25 min.

Glycerolated blood tellurite mixture

Sterile defibrinated sheep blood	14 ml
Sterile glycerol . .	.	6 ml
Sterile potassium tellurite solution, 1 per cent aqueous	.	4 ml

Sterilize the glycerol in a hot-air oven at 160°C for 60 min and the tellurite solution by autoclaving at 115°C for 20 min. Mix the ingredients in a sterile flask, incubate for 1–2 h at 37°C, then refrigerate. Haemolysis is complete after 24 h. The mixture keeps well in the refrigerator.

A 1 per cent solution of good quality tellurite is sufficient but up to 2 per cent of some batches is necessary.

Preparation of complete medium

Agar base	. . .	100 ml
Glycerolated blood tellurite mixture	. . .	24 ml

Melt the agar, cool to 45°C, add the blood and tellurite and pour plates.

Downie's Medium

The classical medium for the typing of *C. diphtheriae* is McLeod's medium (Anderson *et al.*, 1931) which is a chocolate agar medium made from a meat infusion broth sterilized by filtration to avoid heating, rabbit blood and tellurite. Downie's medium is easier to prepare and has been used to give good differentiation of the types of *C. diphtheriae* on colonial morphology without interfering with microscopic morphology.

Nutrient agar	. .	100 ml
Sterile defibrinated blood	.	10 ml
Sterile potassium tellurite solution, 4 per cent aqueous	.	1 ml

The effectiveness of the medium depends on the quality of the nutrient agar. A digest broth agar may be satisfactory or may require the addition of 1 per cent peptone.

The potassium tellurite solution is prepared as for Hoyle's medium. Double layer plates are poured, a layer of nutrient agar being covered by a layer of blood tellurite agar.

Löffler's Serum Medium

This medium is especially useful for cultivation of the diphtheria bacillus, producing luxuriant growth in 12 to 18 h with characteristic staining of the organism by Neisser's and Albert's methods. It is also used to show proteolytic properties particularly of *Clostridium* species.

Sterile ox, sheep or horse serum 300 ml
Nutrient broth   .   .   . 100 ml
Glucose   .   .   .   .   1 g

Dissolve the glucose in the broth and autoclave at 115°C for 20 min. Add the glucose broth to the serum with sterile precautions and distribute in sterile test tubes or in 2·5 ml amounts in sterile ¼-oz bottles. To inspissate, tubes are laid on a sloped tray but bottles are laid flat with the caps tightly screwed on. The temperature is then slowly raised to 80–85°C and maintained for 2 h, when the serum coagulates to a yellowish-white solid.

If an inspissator is not available, the serum may be coagulated by placing the slanted tubes at the top of a steam sterilizer, where the temperature is a little below 100°C, for 5–7 min. Overheating causes expansion of air bubbles and the formation of steam from the fluid droplets in the partially solidified material, leading to disruption of the medium.

Inspissated medium should be allowed to cool before being handled. Medium in screw-capped bottles can be stored for a long period of time.

MEDIA FOR THE CULTIVATION OF LACTOBACILLI

DeMan, Rogosa and Sharpe's (1960) Medium

This is a non-selective medium that supports good growth of lactobacilli. By replacing the glucose with 2 per cent of test substrate, omitting the meat extract and adding 0·004 per cent chlorophenol red, this medium can be amended for fermentation tests.

Peptone (Oxoid)   .   .   . 10 g
Meat extract (Lab-Lemco)   . 10 g
Yeast extract .   .   .   .   5 g
Glucose   .   .   .   . 20 g
Tween 80 (Polyoxyethylene
  sorbitan mono-oleate) .   .   1 ml
Dipotassium hydrogen
  phosphate, K_2HPO_4 .   .   2 g

Sodium acetate,
  $CH_3COONa.3H_2O$.   .   5 g
Triammonium citrate   .   .   2 g
Magnesium sulphate,
  $MgSO_4.7H_2O$.   .   . 200 mg
Manganese sulphate,
  $MnSO_4.4H_2O$.   .   . 50 mg
Water .   .   .   .   . 1 l

Dissolve the ingredients, distribute and autoclave at 121°C for 15 min. The pH lies between 6·0 and 6·5 after sterilization. A solid medium can be prepared by the addition of agar.

Tomato Juice Agar

Hadley's Modification of Kulp and White's Medium. In the formula given here, Hadley's (1933) medium is further modified by replacing peptonized milk with casein hydrolysate. Tomato juice provides growth factors and a pH of 5·0 makes the medium selective for lactobacilli. The medium can be used for counts of lactobacilli in saliva.

Peptone   .   .   .   .   1 g
Casein hydrolysate .   .   .   1 g
Tomato juice   .   .   . 40 ml
Agar   .   .   .   .   2 g
Water .   .   .   .   . 60 ml

The tomato juice sold as a beverage is not suitable. Juice must be expressed from canned whole tomatoes.

Dissolve the peptone and casein hydrolysate in the tomato juice, heating gently and taking care to avoid overheating. Adjust to pH 5·0 with lactic acid. Dissolve the agar in the water and mix both solutions while they are hot. Filter through a thin layer of absorbent cotton-wool, distribute in 100-ml amounts and autoclave at 115°C for 10 min.

On cooling, the tomato tends to flocculate. On remelting the medium the bottle must be inverted several times until the tomato goes into suspension. At pH 5·0, agar tends to be hydrolysed on heating and repeated melting of a batch of this medium should be avoided.

Glucose–Yeast Extract–Acetic Acid Agar

This medium is more selective and better defined than tomato juice agar for oral, vaginal and faecal lactobacilli (Rogosa, Mitchell and Wiseman, 1951).

Salt solution

    Magnesium sulphate,
        $MgSO_4.7H_2O$ . . . 11·5 g
    Manganese sulphate,
        $MnSO_4.2H_2O$ . . . 2·4 g
    Ferrous sulphate,
        $FeSO_4.7H_2O$ . . . 0·68 g
    Distilled water . . . 100 ml

Preparation of complete medium

    Trypticase . . . 10 g
    Yeast extract . . 5 g
    Potassium dihydrogen
        phosphate, KH_2PO_4 . . 6 g
    Ammonium citrate,
        $C_6H_{14}N_2O_7$ . . . 2 g
    Glucose . . . 20 g
    Sorbitan mono-oleate . . 1 g
    Sodium acetate,
        $C_2H_3NaO_2.3H_2O$ . . 25 g
    Acetic acid, glacial . . 1·32 ml
    Salt solution . . . 5 ml
    Agar . . . . 15 g
    Distilled water . . . 1 l

Heat sufficiently to dissolve the agar and distribute. The medium does not require autoclave sterilization because the final pH is 5·4.

MEDIA FOR THE CULTIVATION OF MYCOBACTERIA

Detailed instructions for the preparation of media for optimal growth of clinically important mycobacteria are given by Stonebrink *et al.* (1969).

Löwenstein-Jensen Medium

As prescribed by the International Union against Tuberculosis (IUT).

This medium (Jensen, 1955) has been modified from the original Löwenstein-Jensen medium by omitting starch, which makes it more difficult to prepare and is unnecessary for the growth of tubercle bacilli. Malachite green suppresses the growth of organisms other than mycobacteria. The medium is recommended for the isolation of the human type of the tubercle bacillus whose growth is enhanced by glycerol, and for drug sensitivity tests. Colonial morphology on this medium allows the differentiation of human and bovine types.

Mineral salt solution

    Potassium dihydrogen
        phosphate, KH_2PO_4
        anhydrous . . . . 2·4 g
    Magnesium sulphate, $MgSO_4$. 0·24 g
    Magnesium citrate,
        $Mg_3(C_6H_5O_7)_2.14H_2O$. 0·6 g
    Asparagine . . . . 3·6 g
    Glycerol . . . 12 ml
    Water . . . . . 600 ml

Dissolve the ingredients by heating. Autoclave at 121°C for 25 min to sterilize. This solution keeps indefinitely and may be stored in suitable amounts.

Malachite green solution. Prepare a 2 per cent solution of malachite green in sterile water with sterile precautions by dissolving the dye in the incubator for 1–2 h. This solution can be stored indefinitely and should be shaken before use.

Preparation of complete medium

    Mineral salt solution . . 600 ml
    Malachite green solution . 20 ml
    Beaten egg (20 to 22 hens'
        eggs, depending on size) . 1 l

All utensils used to prepare the complete medium must be sterile. The eggs must be fresh, i.e. not more than four days old. Wash them thoroughly in warm water with a brush and a plain alkaline soap, such as Windsor soap, and rinse in running water for 30 min. Drain off the water and allow the eggs to dry covered with paper until the following day. Alternatively, to save time, the washed and rinsed eggs may be dried by sprinkling them with methylated spirit and burning it off. The risk is that wet shells lead to contamination of the egg. Before handling the clean, dry eggs, scrub the hands and dry them. Crack the eggs with a sterile knife into a sterile beaker and beat them with a sterile egg whisk. There is no need to filter the beaten egg. Mix the complete medium, distribute it in 5 ml amounts in sterile 1 oz (McCartney) bottles and screw the caps tightly on. Lay the bottles horizontally in the inspissator and heat at 75–80°C for 1 h. Since the medium has been prepared with sterile precautions this heating is to solidify the medium, not to sterilize it.

The medium will keep for some months in screw-capped bottles, but if slopes are made in test tubes they must be stored in the cold and used within a month.

Stonebrink's Medium

This medium (Stonebrink, 1957) is particularly suitable for the isolation of bovine strains of the tubercle bacillus. It does not contain glycerol, which has no effect on or may even be inhibitory to the growth of the bovine type. The medium may also be used for the isolation of human strains that are drug-resistant and difficult to grow. It should be used for specimens other than sputa and for sputa if the tubercle bacillus is highly resistant. It is unsuitable for drug sensitivity tests.

Mineral salt solution

Potassium dihydrogen phosphate, KH_2PO_4 anhydrous	. . .	7 g
Disodium hydrogen phosphate, $Na_2HPO_4.2H_2O$		4 g
Sodium pyruvate	. . .	12·5 g
Water	. . . .	1 l

Dissolve the salts and autoclave at 121°C for 30 min. This solution keeps indefinitely.

Malachite green solution. This is a 2 per cent solution prepared as for Löwenstein-Jensen medium.

Preparation of complete medium

Mineral salt solution	. .	1 l
Malachite green solution	.	40 ml
Beaten egg	. . .	2 l

Prepare the beaten egg, mix and dispense the medium with sterile precautions and inspissate it as for Löwenstein-Jensen medium.

Dorset's Egg Medium

This simple egg medium is suitable for the growth of laboratory strains of tubercle bacilli. In an emergency it may be used for isolations, when it would be advisable to add malachite green, but the more enriched media yield the greatest number of positive cultures from primary inoculations of specimens from human and animal infections.

Beaten egg (2 or 3 hens' eggs, depending on size)	.	75 ml
Sterile broth	. . .	25 ml

Malachite green solution, 2 per cent (if for isolation of tubercle bacilli)	. . .	1·25 ml

Prepare the beaten egg, mix and dispense the medium with sterile precautions as for Löwenstein-Jensen. If an inspissator is not available the medium may be solidified in about 20 min on the top of the steam sterilizer but it is better to heat at a lower temperature for a longer time.

Liquid Media for M. tuberculosis

Various liquid media such as those of Kirchner (1932) and Youmans (1944) may be used for growing tubercle bacilli for special purposes. The medium of Dubos and Davis and that of Šula are described here.

Dubos and Davis Medium

The composition described by the Medical Research Council (1948) is given for this medium.

Bovine albumin solution, 9 per cent

Bovine albumin (fraction V, Armour & Co.)	. .	4·5 ml
Water	. . . .	45·5 ml

Mix and sterilize by filtration.

Preparation of complete medium

Potassium dihydrogen phosphate, KH_2PO_4	. .	1 g
Disodium hydrogen phosphate $Na_2HPO_4.12H_2O$	. .	6·25 g
Sodium citrate, $C_6H_5Na_3O_7.2H_2O$	. .	1·5 g
Magnesium sulphate, $MgSO_4.7H_2O$	. .	0·6 g
Tween 80, 10 per cent solution		5 ml
Casein hydrolysate, 20 per cent solution	. .	10 ml
Distilled water	. .	1145 ml
Bovine albumin solution	.	40 ml

Dissolve each salt separately and mix the solutions with the Tween, casein hydrolysate and remaining water. The medium should be at pH 7·2. Distribute, autoclave at 115°C for 10 min and add the bovine albumin with sterile precautions.

Sula's Medium

This medium is recommended by Ives and McCormick (1956) for culturing tubercle bacilli from pleural fluid. It is double the strength of the original medium (Šula, 1947) so that an equal volume of pleural fluid can be added as inoculum.

Disodium hydrogen phosphate, Na_2HPO_4 .	2·5 g
Potassium dihydrogen phosphate, KH_2PO_4 .	1·5 g
Sodium citrate, $Na_3C_6H_5O_7.2H_2O$ . .	1·5 g
Magnesium sulphate, $MgSO_4$	0·5 g
Asparagine . . .	2·0 g
Alanine . . .	0·15 g
Glycerol . . .	25 ml
Ferric ammonium citrate, green scales . . .	0·05 g
Malachite green (0·2 per cent aqueous)	1 ml
Distilled water . . .	500 ml
Ascitic fluid, sterile . .	50 ml
Penicillin solution, 2,000 units per ml, sterile . . .	5 ml

Dissolve the salts, amino acids, glycerol and malachite green in water, distribute in 100 ml amounts in 10 oz bottles and autoclave at 121°C for 15 min. Add the ascitic fluid with sterile precautions. Add the penicillin at time of inoculation with pleural fluid.

Smith's Medium

This medium (Smith, 1953) is suitable for the growth of Jöhne's bacillus. Essentially it is Dubos's medium with the addition of an alcoholic extract of *Mycobacterium phlei* and solidified with agar. For isolations from the intestinal mucosa cycloheximide and chloramphenicol may be added to inhibit contaminants (Brotherston, Gilmour and Samuel, 1961).

MEDIA FOR THE CULTIVATION OF CLOSTRIDIA

Freshly steamed media that have been cooled rapidly without shaking are at least temporarily anaerobic. This principle is used when deep agar, to which 0·5 per cent glucose may be added to act as a reducing agent and an additional nutrient, is inoculated with minimal shaking and solidified rapidly by placing the tube in cold water. Colonies of anaerobes develop best in the depth of the tube, becoming fewer and smaller towards the surface. Usually there is no growth of anaerobes in the top centimetre of medium.

Liquid media soon become aerobic unless a reducing agent is added. Reducing agents include 0·5–1 per cent glucose, 0·1 per cent ascorbic acid, up to 0·1 per cent cysteine, 0·1 per cent sodium thioglycollate (Brewer, 1940) and the particles of meat in cooked meat broth. Iron strips about 25×3 mm in size, cut from 26 gauge or other thin sheet iron (a mild steel containing less than 0·25 per cent carbon) or ordinary iron nails, sterilized by flaming and dropped while hot into the medium, are a convenient method of providing anaerobic broth, peptone water media, gelatin and milk for immediate use in identification tests. The results should be read before the heavy deposit of iron hydroxide masks the reaction but this is minimal if the iron is completely immersed in the medium.

The effectiveness of reducing agents can be increased by making the liquid medium into an 0·05 to 0·1 per cent semi-solid agar. This can be done at short notice by melting a nutrient agar slope in boiling water and adding about 10 per cent of it to the warmed liquid medium. Another method is to cover the surface with petroleum jelly, used particularly with glucose broth. Long tubes, 20×1 cm are half-filled with medium and are steamed or heated in boiling water for 30 min. Melted petroleum jelly, which has been sterilized by dry heat, is then poured on the surface of the medium and the tubes are rapidly cooled so that the jelly effectively seals the medium from air. Inoculation is made with a capillary pipette after warming the jelly to soften it. This method is unsuitable for gas-producing anaerobes because the gas will force out the petroleum jelly seal.

Liquid media for the cultivation of anaerobes may be stored for periods up to a few weeks, but are most effective if they are steamed or heated in boiling water for 30 min and cooled rapidly in cold water immediately before use.

The preparation of two of them, cooked meat broth and thioglycollate broth will be described in detail.

Cooked Meat Broth

The original medium is known as 'Robertson's bullock-heart medium', but the following modification of Martin and Lepper is recommended. It is suitable for growing anaerobes in air and also for the preservation of stock cultures of aerobic organisms. The inoculum is introduced deep in the medium in contact with the meat.

When cooked meat broth is to be used as a *recovery medium* for spores, following heat resistance tests, or prolonged storage of cultures, the incorporation of a little soluble starch or serum in the medium is an improvement, presumably because the inhibitory effect of fatty acids is thus neutralized.

Cooked Meat

Fresh bullock's heart	.	500 g
Water .	.	500 ml
Sodium hydroxide, 1 *N* NaOH		1·5 ml

Mince the heart, place in the alkaline boiling water and simmer for 20 min to neutralize the lactic acid. Drain off the liquid through a muslin filter and, while still hot, press the minced meat in a cloth and dry partially by spreading it on a cloth or filter paper. In this condition it can be introduced into bottles without soiling them.

Peptone Infusion Broth

Liquid filtered from cooked meat	.	500 ml
Peptone	.	2·5 g
Sodium chloride, NaCl .	.	1·25 g

Steam at 100°C for 20 min, add 1 ml pure hydrochloric acid and filter. Bring the reaction of the filtrate to pH 8·2, steam at 100°C for 30 min and adjust reaction to pH 7·8.

Preparation of complete medium. Place meat in 1-oz bottles to a depth of about 2·5 cm and cover with about 10 ml broth. Extra nutrient broth is necessary if all the meat is to be used. Autoclave at 121°C for 20 min. After sterilization, the pH of the broth over the meat is about 7·5. If test-tubes are used the surface of the medium may be covered with a 1-cm layer of sterile liquid paraffin, but this is not essential.

A tall column of meat is essential because conditions are anaerobic only where there are meat particles. There need be only sufficient broth to extend about 1 cm above the meat.

Thioglycollate Broth

In addition to a reducing agent and semi-solid agar, this medium contains methylene blue or resazurin to act as an oxidation-reduction potential indicator which should show that the medium is anaerobic except in the surface layer.

Any nutrient broth can be made anaerobic in this way. The formula given here is that prescribed in the Pharmacopeia (1970) for sterility tests. It contains only half (0·05 per cent) the usual concentration of sodium thioglycollate (0·1 per cent).

Yeast extract, water soluble	.	5·0 g
Casein hydrolysate, pancreatic digest	.	15·0 g
Glucose	.	5·5 g
L-cystine	.	0·5 g
Agar	.	0·75 g
Sodium chloride, NaCl .		2·5 g
Sodium thioglycollate	.	0·5 g
Resazurin sodium solution, 1 in 1000, freshly prepared .		1·0 ml
Water .	.	1 l

Dissolve the ingredients other than thioglycollate and resazurin by steaming at 100°C. Add the thioglycollate and adjust the pH to 7·3. If there is a precipitate, heat without boiling and filter hot through moistened filter paper. Add the resazurin solution, mix thoroughly, distribute and sterilize at 121°C for 15 min. Cool at once to 25°C and store in the dark, preferably between 20° and 30°C. Do not use the medium if it has evaporated enough to affect its fluidity. If more than the upper third is pink in colour, anaerobic conditions may be restored once only by steaming at 100°C for a few minutes.

Lowbury and Lilly's (1955) Medium

An indicator medium for *Cl. welchii* containing Fildes' peptic digest of blood to stimulate the production of lecithinase, human serum or egg yolk to show lecithinase production and *welchii* antitoxin spread over the surface of half the plate to show neutralization of the lecithinase was devised by Hayward (1943) who named it the Nagler plate. Nagler (1944) observed the lipase in addition to the lecithinase reaction in egg yolk and proposed an egg yolk medium as indicator of the lecithinase and lipase of *Cl. oedematiens*. Lowbury and Lilly (1955) modified the human serum medium by increasing the concentration of agar to prevent the swarming of *Proteus*, making a double layer medium to allow a clearer demonstration of lecithinase reactions and adding neomycin (100 μg per ml) to inhibit lecithinase-producing aerobic sporing bacilli. However in the description given here the concentration of neomycin is only 70 μg per ml, the maximum that is not markedly inhibitory to many clostridia (Collee and Watt, 1971).

Agar base

    Agar, New Zealand (Davis) . 50 g
    Peptone water (Evans peptone) 1 l

This agar base autoclaved at 121°C for 30 min is used for the lower layer of the medium and as basal medium for the upper layer.

Preparation of complete medium

    Agar base . . . . 100 ml
    Fildes' peptic digest of sheep
      blood . . . . 6·5 ml
    Human serum, sterile . . 40 ml
    Neomycin sulphate (Upjohn),
      sterile aqueous solution:
      10,000 μg per ml . . 1·0 ml

The serum may be prepared by treating plasma with 5 per cent of sterile 10 per cent calcium chloride at 37°C. Heat the Fildes' digest at 55°C for 30 min, melt the agar base and cool it to 56°C. Add the remaining ingredients and pour the medium as the upper layer of double layer plates on a layer of agar base.

Spread 250 international units of *Cl. welchii* antitoxin over half of the agar surface.

Willis and Hobbs' (1959) Medium

This medium for the isolation of clostridia is a lactose egg-yolk milk agar made selective for various clostridia, particularly *Cl. welchii*, by the addition of neomycin. The recommended concentration of 250 μg neomycin sulphate per ml inhibits some clostridia, usually inhibits strains of *Bacillus* and *Staphylococcus*, and greatly reduces the growth of coliform bacilli.

Lecithinase-positive organisms produce zones of opalescence that can be specifically inhibited by the appropriate antiserum spread over half the medium in a plate and dried-in before inoculation. Some clostridia produce a lipase that causes the development of a 'pearly layer' on the surface of the medium. Lactose fermentation is indicated by a pink halo in the medium around the colony and proteolysis by a clearing of the milk in the medium.

Egg yolk suspension. Break eggs with precautions to keep their contents sterile, as described for Löwenstein medium, at the same time separating the yolks from the whites. Discard the whites and dilute the yolks with an equal volume of sterile 0·9 per cent sodium chloride solution.

Sterile stock milk. Remove the cream from ordinary milk by centrifuging. Sterilize the skimmed milk by autoclaving at 121°C for 15 min.

Basal medium

    Agar (New Zealand) . . 4·8 g
    Lactose . . . . 4·8 g
    Neutral red, 1 per cent
      solution . . . . 1·3 ml
    Meat infusion broth, pH 7 . 400 ml
    Egg yolk suspension . . 15 ml
    Milk . . . . . 60 ml

Dissolve the agar and lactose in the neutral red and broth by steaming, and sterilize at 121°C for 25 min. Cool to 50–55°C and add the egg yolk and milk. Pour plates.

Possible additions to basal medium

    Neomycin sulphate
      (Upjohn) . . . 250 μg per ml
    Sodium thioglycollate . 0·1 per cent

Stock sterile solutions of neomycin may be stored in the refrigerator with little loss of potency. The antibiotic is not decomposed by heating at 60°C for 20 min. Thioglycollate may assist the growth of the stricter anaerobes.

Either or both of these reagents may be added at the same time as the egg yolk and milk.

Reinforced Clostridial Agar

This medium is specially enriched with substances that might promote the growth of clostridia. Its preparation involves the heating of cystine in the absence of any chemical that could protect it substantially against prompt oxidation, but the medium is nevertheless widely used for the culture of various anaerobes in the following form (modified from Reinforced Clostridial Medium of Hirsch and Grinsted, 1954).

Peptone	.	.	.	10 g
Yeast extract	.	.	.	3 g
Meat extract	.	.	.	10 g
Glucose	.	.	.	5 g
Sodium acetate	.	.	.	3 g
Sodium chloride	.	.	.	5 g
L-Cysteine hydrochloride		.	.	0·5 g
Soluble starch	.	.	.	1 g
Distilled water to	.	.	.	1 l

Steam the ingredients in a flask; filter when dissolved. Adjust pH to 7·4. Add agar 10 g and sterilize by autoclaving at 115°C for 20 min.

Cysteine Dithiothreitol Blood Agar

Moore (1968) described the use of the reducing agents, cysteine and dithiothreitol, to improve solid media for *Cl. oedematiens*, particularly of the more fastidious types B and D. Collee, Rutter and Watt (1971) modified Moore's medium by increasing the concentrations of cysteine to 1 mg per ml, dithiothreitol to 0·09 mg per ml and of human blood to 33 per cent and later (Watt, 1972) substituted 10 per cent horse blood for the human blood. This latest modification is described here.

Solid media that contain the reducing agent, cysteine, are recommended for non-sporing anaerobes (Barnes, 1969). In a limited trial Watt (1972) did not find any improvement in the growth of non-sporing anaerobes on his medium compared with blood agar. Barnes and Watt emphasize the importance of using freshly prepared media and incubation immediately after inoculation, and these precautions together with a strictly controlled anaerobic procedure (Chap. 6) are probably more important than reducing agents in the medium.

Cysteine–dithiothreitol solution

Cysteine (Koch-Light)	.	.	150 mg
Dithiothreitol (Koch-Light)	.	13·5 mg
Distilled water	.	.	3 ml

Prepare the solution immediately before use and sterilize by Millipore filtration.

Preparation of complete medium

Nutrient agar (Oxoid blood agar base, No. 2)	.	.	88 ml
Cysteine–dithiothreitol solution	.	.	2 ml
Horse blood	.	.	10 ml

Melt the nutrient agar, cool to 45–55°C and add the remaining ingredients, mixing carefully before pouring plates. Dry the plates quickly at 60°C for 10 min to protect the reducing agents. *Inoculate and incubate them immediately.*

Ellner's (1956) Medium

This medium is used to induce spore formation in *Cl. welchii*. Anaerobiosis may be ensured by heating at 100°C for 10 min and cooling just prior to inoculation. It is important that the inoculum should be adequate; 0·5 ml of an actively growing 4–12 h meat broth culture should be introduced with a pipette into the bottom of the tube of medium. Incubation is in an anaerobic jar at 37°C.

Peptone (e.g. Proteose peptone, Difco)	.	.	10 g
Yeast extract	.	.	3 g
Soluble starch	.	.	3 g
Magnesium sulphate, $MgSO_4$			0·1 g
Potassium dihydrogen phosphate, KH_2PO_4	.	.	1·5 g
Disodium hydrogen phosphate, $Na_2HPO_4.12H_2O$	.	.	67 g
Water	.	.	.	1 l

Steam briefly at 100°C to dissolve, adjust to pH 7·8 with $1N$ sodium hydroxide, dispense in tubes and autoclave at 121°C for 15 min. Tubes should be half to two-thirds full.

Alkaline Egg Medium

This medium promotes spore formation by clostridia. Clostridia remain viable in it for years.

Egg yolk	.	.	.	1
Egg whites	.	.	.	2
Sodium hydroxide, $1N$ NaOH		6 ml
Water to	.	.	.	500 ml

Beat the yolk and whites, add the sodium hydroxide and water. Heat slowly to 95°C for

1½ h, filter through cotton-wool and distribute. Sterilize by autoclaving at 121°C for 15 min.

MEDIA FOR THE CULTIVATION OF ENTEROBACTERIA

MacConkey's Agar

This is a useful medium for the cultivation of enteric bacteria. It contains a bile salt to inhibit non-intestinal bacteria and lactose with neutral red to distinguish the lactose-fermenting coliforms from the lactose non-fermenting salmonella and dysentery groups. The omission of sodium chloride from the medium prevents the spreading of *Proteus* colonies.

Peptone . . .	20 g
Sodium taurocholate, commercial . . .	5 g
Water	1 l
Agar	20 g
Neutral red solution, 2 per cent in 50 per cent ethanol	About 3·5 ml
Lactose, 10 per cent aqueous solution	100 ml

Dissolve the peptone and taurocholate (bile salt) in the water by heating. Add the agar and dissolve it in the steamer or autoclave. If necessary, clear by filtration. Adjust the pH to 7·5. Add the lactose and the neutral red, which should be well shaken before use, and mix. Heat in the autoclave with 'free steam' (*c.* 100°C) for 1 h, then at 115°C for 15 min. Pour plates.

The medium should be a distinct reddish-brown colour. If it is acid, it assumes a rose-pink colour. When the medium is stored for any length of time the neutral red indicator tends to fade. To overcome this the medium is made up and stored without neutral red, indicator being added and thoroughly mixed before pouring plates.

Teepol Lactose Agar

Jameson and Emberley (1956) described this medium as a substitute for MacConkey's agar. Teepol (Shell Chemicals Ltd.), which is a detergent containing sodium and potassium salts of alkyl sulphates with chains of 8–18 C atoms, is used in place of sodium taurocholate as the selective agent for enterobacteria; it has the advantages of being much cheaper and more reliable in its properties. Bromothymol blue replaces neutral red as the indicator of lactose fermentation.

Eupeptone No. 2 (Allen & Hanburys) . . .	20 g
Lactose	10 g
Sodium chloride, NaCl . .	5 g
Teepol	1 g
Bromothymol blue (1 in 500 solution)	25 ml
Agar (New Zealand, Davis) .	9 g
Water	1 l

Adjust to pH 7·5 and heat at 115°C for 15 min.

Colonies of lactose-fermenting *Esch. coli* organisms are *pale cream* in colour and are usually large and opaque. Colonies of salmonellae and shigellae are *pale green* and less opaque.

Brilliant Green MacConkey Agar

Brilliant green is inhibitory to *Esch. coli* and renders the medium selective for salmonella organisms.

The medium is prepared as MacConkey's agar but with the addition of 0·04 g brilliant green per litre.

Deoxycholate Citrate Agar (DCA)

Hynes' (1942) modification of Leifson's (1935) medium is particularly suitable for the isolation of the dysentery bacilli, the salmonella food-poisoning group and *S. paratyphi B*. It is not quite so selective for *S. typhi*, though superior to MacConkey's medium. In the medium described here, Hynes' change to ferric citrate from the ferric ammonium citrate of Leifson's medium is not adopted because there is less precipitation of solution A and the medium is slightly less inhibitory, providing the best chance of recovering scanty pathogens at the expense of some growth of *E. coli*.

Neutral red lactose agar

Meat extract (Lab-Lemco) .	20 g
Peptone (Difco proteose or Evans)	20 g
Agar	90 g

Neutral red solution, 2 per
    cent in 50 per cent ethanol .   5 ml
Lactose   .   .   .   40 g
Water .   .   .   .   4 l

Dissolve the meat extract in 200 ml water over the flame. Make just alkaline to phenolphthalein with 50 per cent sodium hydroxide, boil at 100°C and filter. Adjust the pH to 7·4, make up the volume to 200 ml and add the peptone. Dissolve the agar in 3800 ml water by steaming at 100°C for 1 h. Filter if necessary. Add the meat extract and peptone solution and mix. Add the neutral red and lactose, mixing again. Bottle in accurate 100 ml lots and heat in the autoclave with 'free steam' at 100°C for 1 h and then at 115°C for 15 min.

Solution A

Sodium citrate, Analar,
    $Na_3C_6H_5O_7.2H_2O$.   .   17 g
Sodium thiosulphate, Analar,
    $Na_2S_2O_3.5H_2O$.   .   17 g
Ferric ammonium citrate,
    green scales   .   .   4 g
Sterile water   .   .   100 ml

Solution B (*bile salt*)

Sodium deoxycholate   .   10 g
Sterile water   .   .   100 ml

Prepare these solutions with sterile precautions, heating at 60°C for 1 h to facilitate solution.

Preparation of complete medium

Neutral red lactose agar   .   100 ml
Solution A   .   .   .   5 ml
Solution B   .   .   .   5 ml

Melt the agar and add solutions A and B in this order, using separate sterile pipettes and mixing well between. Pour plates *immediately* and dry the surface. The medium is pale pink in colour and should be quite clear.

The medium should be poured and cooled as soon as possible after the addition of the deoxycholate, otherwise it tends to become very soft. The deoxycholate must be pure and samples should be tested with known positive specimens before purchase is made because batches vary in their inhibitory capacity.

Wilson and Blair's Medium

The use of this medium (Wilson, 1938) depends on the reduction of sulphite to sulphide in the presence of glucose by *S. typhi* and *S. paratyphi*

B, yielding black colonies, and the inhibition of *Esch. coli* by brilliant green and by bismuth sulphite in the presence of an excess of sodium sulphite.

Bismuth sulphite glucose phosphate mixture

Bismuth ammonio-citrate,
    scales   .   .   .   30 g
Sodium sulphite, Na_2SO_3 .   100 g
Disodium hydrogen
    phosphate,
    $Na_2HPO_4.12H_2O$.   .   100 g
Glucose, commercial   .   .   50 g
Sterile water   .   .   .   1 l

With sterile precautions dissolve the bismuth ammonio-citrate in 250 ml boiling water, and the sodium sulphite in 500 ml boiling water. Mix the solutions and while the mixture is boiling add the sodium phosphate crystals. When this mixture is cool add the glucose dissolved in 250 ml boiling water and cooled. This mixture will keep for months.

Iron citrate brilliant green mixture

Ferric citrate, brown scales   .   2 g
Brilliant green   .   .   .   0·25 g
Sterile water   .   .   .   225 ml

With sterile precautions mix solutions of the ferric citrate in 200 ml water and the brilliant green in 25 ml water. This mixture will keep for months.

Preparation of complete medium

Sterile 3 per cent nutrient agar   100 ml
Bismuth sulphite glucose
    phosphate mixture   .   20 ml
Iron citrate-brilliant green
    mixture   .   .   .   4·5 ml

Melt the agar and cool to 60°C. Add the other ingredients with sterile precautions and pour plates.

Tetrathionate Broth

The tetrathionate in this liquid medium inhibits coliform bacilli while permitting bacilli of the typhoid-paratyphoid group to grow freely; thus, an enriched culture of the latter can be obtained from faeces and sometimes an almost pure growth. However it permits the growth of *Proteus* spp.

Thiosulphate solution

Sodium thiosulphate,
    $Na_2S_2O_3.5H_2O$.   .   24·8 g
Sterile water to   .   .   100 ml

Mix the salt and water with sterile precautions and steam at 100°C for 30 min. It is a 1 M solution.

Iodine solution

Potassium iodide, KI	.	20 g
Iodine, I	.	12·7 g
Sterile water to	.	100 ml

With sterile precautions dissolve the potassium iodide in about 50 ml of warm water, add the iodine and make up to a final volume of 100 ml. This gives a normal or 0·5 M solution.

Preparation of complete medium

Calcium carbonate, CaCO₃	.	2·5 g
Nutrient broth	.	78 ml
Thiosulphate solution	.	15 ml
Iodine solution	.	4 ml
Phenol red, 0·02 per cent in 20 per cent ethanol	.	3 ml

Add the calcium carbonate to the broth and sterilize it by autoclaving at 121°C for 20 min. When cool, add the thiosulphate, iodine and phenol red solutions with sterile precautions. Distribute in 10 ml amounts in sterile screw-capped bottles. Even in the refrigerator, tetrathionate broth does not keep for more than a few weeks. It is convenient to keep stock solutions and prepare the complete medium as required (Knox, Gell and Pollock, 1942).

Kauffmann-Müller Tetrathionate Broth

This medium is more selective than the original tetrathionate broth because the brilliant green in it checks the growth of *Proteus* spp.

Thiosulphate solution

Sodium thiosulphate, Na₂S₂O₃.5H₂O	.	50 g
Sterile water	.	100 ml

Mix the salt and water with sterile precautions and steam at 100°C for 30 min.

Iodine solution

Potassium iodide, KI	.	25 g
Iodine, I	.	20 g
Sterile water	.	100 ml

With sterile precautions dissolve the potassium iodide and add the iodine.

Ox bile solution

Desiccated ox bile	.	0·5 g
Water .	.	5 ml

Dissolve with sterile precautions.

Preparation of complete medium

Nutrient broth, pH 7·4 .	.	90 ml
Calcium carbonate, CaCO₃	.	5 g
Brilliant green, 1 in 1000 aqueous	.	1 ml
Thiosulphate solution	.	10 ml
Iodine solution	.	2 ml
Ox bile solution	.	5 ml

Add the calcium carbonate to the broth and sterilize it by autoclaving at 121°C for 20 min. When cool, add the other solutions and distribute aseptically in approximately 10 ml amounts. Heat once in the steamer at 100°C for 10 min.

Selenite F Broth

The selenite in this medium (Leifson, 1936) serves the same purpose as tetrathionate in tetrathionate broth and has been preferred to it (Hobbs and Allison, 1945).

Sodium acid selenite, NaHSeO₃	.	4 g
Peptone	.	5 g
Lactose	.	4 g
Disodium hydrogen phosphate, Na₂HPO₄.12H₂O	.	9·5 g
Sodium dihydrogen phosphate, NaH₂PO₄.2H₂O	.	0·5 g
Sterile water	.	1 l

Dissolve the ingredients with sterile precautions and distribute the yellowish solution in 10 ml amounts in sterile screw-capped bottles. Steam at 100°C for 30 min. Excessive heat is detrimental to the medium and autoclaving must not be used to sterilize it. The amount of red precipitate should be very slight. The pH of the medium should be 7·1 and the phosphates may be varied slightly if necessary to attain this.

Salts of selenium are very toxic for animals and man and must be handled with some care.

Some organic compounds of selenium and hydrogen selenide are volatile and toxic if inhaled (Robertson, 1970).

MEDIA FOR THE CULTIVATION OF PSEUDOMONAS AERUGINOSA (PYOCYANEA)

King, Ward and Raney's Medium

Identification of the organism *Pseudomonas aeruginosa* (*pyocyanea*) may be facilitated by the use of synthetic media that enhance the production of the characteristic pigments – pyocyanin (blue) and fluorescein (yellow) (King, Ward and Raney, 1954).

Medium A – Pyocyanin

Bacto-peptone (Difco)	.	20 g
Glycerol	.	10 ml
$MgCl_2$ (anhydrous)	.	1·4 g
K_2SO_4 (anhydrous)	.	10 g
Agar	.	15 g
Distilled water to	.	1 l

Medium B – Fluorescein

Proteose peptone No. 3 (Difco)	.	20 g
Glycerol	.	10 ml
K_2HPO_4 (anhydrous)	.	1·5 g
$MgSO_4.7H_2O$	.	1·5 g
Agar	.	15 g
Distilled water to	.	1 l

Dissolve the ingredients by heating at 100°C. Adjust pH to 7·2. Dispense 10-ml amounts in tubes and sterilize by autoclaving at 121°C for 15 min. Allow the medium to solidify in a sloped position to give a butt approximately 1 inch long. Alternatively, plates may be poured.

Incubate the inoculated media as follows:

Medium A – 37°C for 48 h or longer;

Medium B – 37°C for 24 h and then 2–3 days at room temperature.

Cetrimide Agar

Cetrimide at 0·03 per cent in Lemco agar has proved to be a useful selective agent for the isolation of *P. pyocyanea* from pus, sputum, drains, etc. (Lowbury and Collins, 1955).

An improved medium (Brown and Lowbury, 1965) combines the selective property of cetrimide with the fluorescein-enhancing property of the medium of King, Ward and Raney (1954).

Basal medium

Proteose peptone No. 3 (Difco)	.	20 g
Glycerol	.	10 ml
Agar	.	15 g
Distilled water to	.	1 l

Dissolve the ingredients by heating at 100°C. Adjust pH to 7·2. Sterilize by autoclaving at 121°C for 30 min.

Complete medium

To 1 l of melted basal medium add the following Seitz-filtered solutions:

10 ml of 15 per cent K_2HPO_4 (anhydrous)

10 ml of 15 per cent $MgSO_4.7H_2O$

15 ml of 2 per cent solution of Cetrimide (BP)

The yellow fluorescence of the colonies of *Pseudomonas* may be enhanced by examining the culture plates in a dark box fitted with a source of ultra-violet irradiation.

MEDIA FOR THE CULTIVATION OF VIBRIOS

The classical vibrio media are Dieudonné's (1909) alkaline blood agar and Aronson's (1915) sucrose dextrin agar. New media utilize the ability of cholera vibrios to hydrolyse gelatin with the production of haloes around colonies on solid agar media containing gelatin.

Monsur's Medium

This medium is for the isolation of cholera and other vibrios either from rectal swabs and stool specimens or from other contaminated sources. A similar fluid medium is used for enrichment or preservative purposes (see Monsur, 1963); this is the 'Bile peptone transport medium'. The potassium tellurite in these media is highly inhibitory to most coliform bacilli although *Proteus* species grow as small colonies.

Bile salt gelatin agar

Trypticase (Baltimore Biological Laboratories) or Bactotryptone	.	1 g
Sodium chloride, NaCl	.	1 g
Sodium taurocholate	.	0·5 g
Sodium carbonate, Na_2CO_3	.	0·1 g
Gelatin (Difco)	.	3 g

Agar . . . . . 1·5 g
Water . . . . . 100 ml

It is thought essential to use the Difco brand of gelatin. Dissolve the ingredients by steaming and adjust the pH to 8·5 with 1N sodium hydroxide. Sterilize by autoclaving at 121°C for 20 min.

Potassium tellurite solution. Prepare a 0·5 per cent solution in water and autoclave at 115°C for 20 min. This solution keeps indefinitely.

Preparation of complete medium

Bile salt gelatin agar . . 100 ml
Potassium tellurite solution,
    K_2TeO_3, 0·05 per cent . 1 ml

Make a 1 in 10 dilution of the stock potassium tellurite solution with sterile precautions and add it to the melted and cooled agar medium. The final pH of the medium must be 8·5 to 9·2. Pour plates.

This medium should be used when fresh because its pH tends to fall on keeping.

Gelatin Agar

This medium is complementary to Monsur's medium. It is unsuitable as the sole medium for primary isolation of cholera vibrios because it is not inhibitory to coliform bacilli. It is used to provide a semi-quantitative assessment of the numbers of vibrios that are being excreted.

Trypticase (Baltimore
    Biological Laboratories) . 1 g
Sodium chloride, NaCl . . 1 g
Gelatin (Difco) . . . 3 g
Agar . . . . . 1·5 g
Water . . . . . 100 ml

It is thought essential to use the correct brands of trypticase and of gelatin. Dissolve the ingredients by steaming. The pH should be 7·2–7·4. Autoclave at 121°C for 20 min to sterilize, and pour plates.

Thiosulphate Citrate Bile Sucrose Agar (T.C.B.S.)

This medium (Sakazaki, 1969 modified) is highly selective for *V. parahaemolyticus* and is satisfactory for the isolation of cholera vibrios. It is inhibitory to Gram-positive organisms, most coliforms and many strains of *Proteus*. *V. parahaemolyticus* does not ferment sucrose and has colonies with green or blue centres.

Enrichment cultures for *V. parahaemolyticus* from sources such as food can be made in 5 per cent sodium chloride cooked meat broth.

T.C.B.S. agar resembles deoxycholate citrate agar except that it contains additional salt, it is at the high pH of 8·6 and sucrose replaces lactose. Part of the function of the salt is probably to supply traces of minerals found in sea water and therefore a relatively impure salt is to be preferred to a purified analytical reagent. The high pH is typical of media for vibrios and necessitates the use of indicators that show colour changes on the alkaline side of neutrality to detect acid formed by sucrose fermentation.

Precautions in preparing the medium are similar to those required for deoxycholate citrate agar. In addition, the medium will not remain at pH 8·6 unless it is protected from atmospheric carbon dioxide. Plates should either be used fresh, or be stored at 4°C in airtight plastic bags fitting closely to the plates to exclude as much air as possible.

Indicator sucrose agar

Yeast extract . . . 5 g
Peptone . . . . 10 g
Sodium chloride, kitchen salt 10 g
Agar . . . . . 20 g
Thymol blue solution, 2 per
    cent, in 50 per cent ethanol 2 ml
Bromothymol blue solution,
    2 per cent, in 50 per cent
    ethanol . . . . 2 ml
Sucrose . . . . 10 g
Water . . . . . 800 ml

Dissolve the yeast extract, peptone and salt in 200 ml water and adjust the pH to 8·6. Dissolve the agar in 600 ml water by steaming. Add the yeast extract and peptone solution and mix. Add the indicators and sucrose, mixing again. Bottle in accurate 80 ml lots and heat in the autoclave with 'free steam' at about 100°C for 1 h then at 115°C for 15 min.

Solution A

Sodium citrate,
    $Na_3C_6H_5O_7.2H_2O$ . . 10 g
Sodium thiosulphate,
    $Na_2S_2O_3.5H_2O$ . . 10 g
Ferric citrate . . . 1 g
Water . . . . . 100 ml

Solution B

| Ox bile, desiccated | . | . | 8 g |
| Water . | . | . | . | 100 ml |

Prepare these solutions with sterile precautions, heating at 60°C for 1 h to facilitate solution.

Preparation of complete medium

Indicator sucrose agar	.	.	80 ml
Solution A	.	.	.	10 ml
Solution B	.	.	.	10 ml

Melt the agar and add solutions A and B in this order, using separate sterile pipettes and mixing well between. Pour plates *immediately*.

Batches of ox bile differ in inhibitory capacity and must be tested before they are brought into use.

MEDIA FOR THE CULTIVATION OF BRUCELLA

Liver infusion agar (Huddleson, 1939) has been used to grow brucellae but some infusions can be inhibitory and lead to differences in the quality of different batches of medium. Glucose serum agar or Albimi agar are to be preferred.

Glucose Serum Agar with Added Antibiotics

This medium (Jones and Morgan, 1958) containing antimicrobial agents is good for isolating even very fastidious strains of *Br. abortus*. The antimicrobial substances may be omitted if cultures are being made from uncontaminated sources.

Bacitracin solution (2000 units per ml). Bacitracin (Sigma) is supplied in vials containing 500,000 units. Dissolve the contents of one vial in 250 ml of sterile water. Store at 4°C, but this solution will not keep for more than one week.

Polymyxin B solution (5000 units per ml). Polymyxin B (Burroughs-Wellcome) is supplied in bottles containing 500,000 units. Dissolve the contents of one bottle in 100 ml of sterile water. Store in a deep freeze at −20°C or in the ice chamber of a refrigerator.

Cycloheximide solution (10 mg per ml). Cycloheximide (Actidione Upjohn) is supplied in 4 g bottles. It is important to dissolve this amount of powder in 20 ml of acetone and dilute to 400 ml with sterile water. Store at 4°C.

Glucose solution (25 per cent)

| Glucose | . | . | . | . | 12·5 g |
| Water . | . | . | . | . | 50 ml |

Prepare the solution and sterilize it by Seitz filtration.

Preparation of complete medium

Agar .	.	.	.	.	15 g
Peptone	.	.	.	.	10 g
Sodium chloride, NaCl .	.	5 g
Meat extract	.	.	.	5 g
Water .	.	.	.	.	1 l
Sterile inactivated horse serum	50 ml
Glucose solution, 25 per cent	40 ml
Bacitracin solution, 2000 units per ml	.	.	.	12·5 ml
Polymyxin B solution, 5000 units per ml	.	.	.	1·2 ml
Cycloheximide solution, 10 mg per ml	.	.	.	10 ml

Dissolve the first four ingredients by gentle heating, adjust to pH 7·5 and autoclave at 121°C for 30 min. Cool to 52°C and add the remaining ingredients, mixing well to ensure even distribution of the antimicrobial agents. Pour plates, this amount of medium making about 50 plates. Cooling to 52°C will reduce water of condensation on the lids.

It is best to use freshly prepared medium because Cycloheximide is unstable. However plates can be stored for a week in the refrigerator with the lids uppermost, either in a container with a lid or in a wire tray covered with a sheet of polythene. Before use, plates should be incubated overnight with the medium uppermost, but in an emergency plates with lids partly opened may be dried for 1 h in the incubator. It is important that the surface of the medium be dry to discourage dissociation.

Albimi Agar (*Joint FAO/WHO, 1958*)

This selective medium is an alternative to glucose serum agar for isolating brucellae but is not so suitable for fastidious strains. By raising the agar concentration to 2·5 or 3 per cent of the final medium its selectivity is increased and the possibility of overgrowth by *Proteus* is reduced. Albimi agar is manufactured by Albimi Laboratories, Brooklyn, N.Y. It has the advantage of not requiring the addition of serum.

Ethyl violet solution (1 in 1000). The concentration is calculated on the basis of the pure dyestuff and not on the weight of the product as supplied.

Bacitracin, polymyxin B and Cycloheximide solutions are prepared as for glucose serum agar.

Preparation of complete medium

Albimi agar	1 l
Ethyl violet solution, 1 in 1000	1·25 ml
Bacitracin solution, 2000 units per ml	12·5 ml
Polymyxin B solution, 5000 units per ml . . .	1·2 ml
Cycloheximide solution, 10 mg per ml	10 ml

Prepare and sterilize the Albimi agar in accordance with the manufacturer's instructions. Cool to 52°C and add the remaining ingredients. Mix the medium, pour, store and dry plates as for glucose serum agar.

MEDIUM FOR THE CULTIVATION OF *FRANCISELLA TULARENSIS*

A solid medium containing 2·5 per cent glucose and 0·1 per cent cystine hydrochloride is described. Growth in liquid culture may be obtained using a casein partial hydrolysate with added thiamine and cystine, but no blood.

Glucose cystine solution

Glucose	12·5 g
Cystine hydrochloride . .	0·5 g
Water	50 ml

Prepare the solution and sterilize it by Seitz filtration.

Preparation of complete medium

Nutrient agar . . .	85 ml
Glucose cystine solution .	10 ml
Human blood, fresh . .	5 ml

Melt the agar, cool to 50°C and add the remaining ingredients.

MEDIA FOR THE CULTIVATION OF BORDETELLA

Bordet-Gengou Medium

This modification has given good growth of *Bord. pertussis*. Peptone was not included in the original Bordet-Gengou medium and may be omitted. Some brands of peptone are markedly inhibitory to the growth of *Bord. pertussis* probably due to their content of colloidal sulphur or sulphide. The medium can be made more selective for *Bord. pertussis* by adding 0·25 units penicillin per ml. Lacey (1954) has described an even more selective medium containing a diamidine, sodium fluoride and penicillin.

Glycerol potato agar

Potato slices . . .	250 g
Sodium chloride, NaCl . .	9 g
Water	2 l
Agar	45 g
Glycerol	20 ml
Proteose peptone (Difco) .	20 g

Clean and pare potatoes, and cut them into thin slices. Boil the slices with the salt in 500 ml of water until they fall to pieces. Make up the water lost in boiling, filter through linen and adjust to pH 7·0. Dissolve the agar in 1500 ml of water by heat and add the potato extract, glycerol and peptone. Distribute in bottles and heat in the autoclave with 'free steam' at about 100°C for 1 h, then at 115°C for 10 min. Store until required.

Preparation of complete medium

Glycerol potato agar . .	2 volumes
Sterile defibrinated horse blood	1 volume

Melt the agar in the steamer for 1 h, inverting the bottle several times. Place in the water bath at 55°C for about 5 min until the temperature of the agar has dropped to about 65°C. Warm the blood slightly by placing it in the 55°C bath for 2–3 min. Mix the blood and the agar thoroughly and pour plates. The layer of agar should be thick, about 30 ml of medium per 4 in Petri dish. The plates should not be dried in the incubator, but should be stored at once in the refrigerator, and may be used up to two or three days after preparation.

Colindale Modification of Bordet-Gengou Medium

This medium is easier to prepare than the original Bordet-Gengou medium because starch is used in place of a preparation from potato slices. Also the brand of peptone used appears to be better for growth of *Bordetella*. The penicillin and diamidine (M & B 938) make it more selective for *Bordetella*.

Glycerol starch agar

Peptone (Bengers or Evans)	.	10 g
Sodium chloride, NaCl	. .	5 g
Glycerol	. . .	10 ml
Starch (Soluble, BDH)	. .	2·5 g
Water	. . . .	1 l
Agar (Davis)	. . .	11 g

Dissolve the ingredients, except the agar, in the water and adjust to pH 7·8. Add the agar. Check the pH which should be 7·5–7·6. Distribute in 200 ml quantities and autoclave at 115°C for 10 min.

Preparation of complete medium

Glycerol starch agar	.	200 ml
Penicillin (50 units per ml)	.	1·5 ml
M & B 938 (0·1 per cent solution)	. . .	0·9 ml
Sterile defibrinated horse blood		100 ml

Melt the agar in the steamer at 100°C, cool to 40–45°C. Warm the blood to 37°C and add all the ingredients. Mix thoroughly and pour not more than 10 plates from this quantity of medium. Store in the refrigerator. A short (10–15 min) period of drying *may* be necessary but only when the plates are freshly poured.

M & B 938 is 4:4 diamido-diphenylamine-hydrochloride (May and Baker).

Charcoal Blood Agar

This recipe is basically that of Mishulow *et al.* (1953) who used the medium for the culture of *Bordetella pertussis* for vaccine production and found it as good as Bordet-Gengou medium.

Charcoal Agar Base

Beef extract ('Lab-Lemco', Oxoid).	.	10 g
Starch	. . .	10 g
Peptone	. . .	10 g
Sodium chloride, NaCl	.	5 g
Charcoal – Bacteriological grade	.	4 g
Yeast extract	. .	3·5 g
Agar	. . .	12 g
Water	. . . .	1 l

Dissolve the ingredients, except the charcoal, in the water by heating gently. Adjust to pH 7·5–7·6 and add the charcoal. Dispense into suitable containers, shaking the medium oc-casionally to keep the charcoal in suspension. Autoclave at 121°C for 30 min.

Preparation of complete medium

Charcoal agar base	.	100 ml
Sterile defibrinated horse blood		10 ml
Penicillin (100 i.u./ml)	. .	0·3 ml
M & B 938 (0·1 per cent solution)	. . .	0·3 ml

Cool the molten agar to 45–50°C. Add the blood (previously warmed to 37°C), the penicillin and M & B 938. Pour 4–5 plates from this volume. Do not dry the poured plates unless they are for immediate use.

The medium may also be dispensed in 5–10 ml amounts in screw-capped bottles and 'sloped'. In this form the medium is useful for the maintenance of stock cultures of *Bordetella pertussis*, with weekly subcultures.

MEDIA FOR THE CULTIVATION OF HAEMOPHILUS

The nutrients required by *Haemophilus* species, additional to those provided by blood agar, can be supplied by heating red cells to liberate their contents. Heated blood agar is usually best for this purpose but if a clear medium is needed Levinthal's is an alternative.

Levinthal's Medium

Sterile nutrient agar	.	100 ml
Sterile rabbit or human blood		5 ml

Melt the agar, add the blood and heat the mixture in boiling water. Allow the deposit to settle and distribute the clear supernatant.

Bacitracin Heated Blood Agar

Bacitracin (Sigma) may be added to heated blood agar ('chocolate blood agar') when attempting isolation of *Haemophilus* spp. from heavily contaminated specimens, e.g. sputum (Baber, 1969). The concentration recommended is 10 i.u. per ml medium. A similar result may be obtained by placing a filter paper disk impregnated with 8 i.u. bacitracin at the edge of the 'well' on a heated blood agar plate seeded with sputum. The haemophilus colonies grow in the zone immediately around the disk.

Media for the Cultivation of *Mycoplasma pneumoniae* and other Mycoplasmas

(Lemcke, 1965; Marmion, 1967; Shepard, 1969).

Media for mycoplasmas contain horse serum. Some batches may contain inhibitors and each batch should be tested for inhibitory activity before use. Burroughs-Wellcome Horse Serum No. 3 (not inactivated) is suitable.

Standard Solid Medium

Yeast Extract

Baker's yeast	1·0 kg
Deionized water	1·0 l
Hydrochloric acid, HCl, Analar grade	About 6·5 ml

Add the yeast to 500 ml water at 50°C, in a large beaker. Mix and knead well (this is particularly important). Add the remaining water, warm to 80°C and add acid until the pH reaches 4·5, checked with pH papers. Mix well and heat at 80°C for 20 min. Allow the yeast cells to settle and clarify by centrifugation. Filter the supernatant through Green's Hyduro 995 filter paper (38·5 cm diameter) and then through a Seitz EK filter or other bacterium-tight grade. Check for sterility by adding 5 ml filtrate to 10 ml nutrient broth, incubating 24 h and subculturing on blood agar. Dispense in convenient amounts and store at -20°C or -40°C. Adjust the pH to 7·0 immediately before use.

Preparation of complete medium

PPLO agar base without crystal violet (Difco) pH 7·8	70·0 ml
Yeast extract, pH 7·0	10·0 ml
Horse serum (unheated)	20·0 ml
Sodium deoxyribonucleate (calf thymus) solution, 0·2 per cent w/v	1·0 ml
Thallous acetate solution, $TlC_2H_3O_2$, 1 in 80 w/v	1·0 ml
Dipotassium hydrogen phosphate solution, K_2HPO_4, 1M	2·0 ml
Penicillin solution, 50,000 units per ml	0·2 ml

The solutions are sterilized by filtration. The agar is dissolved, sterilized and cooled to 48°C before adding the remaining ingredients which should be at room temperature. The final pH should be 7·8 to 8·0. It is convenient to dispense 10-ml amounts in disposable 5-cm Petri dishes (Sterilin, Falcon, Esco, etc.). The poured plates are stored in closed containers at 4°C. Plates should not be used if more than one week old, as mycoplasmas require a soft agar for growth.

Liquid Medium

This medium, with or without glucose, may be used for primary isolation of mycoplasmas but it is not so good as diphasic medium. It can be used for antigen production.

PPLO broth without crystal violet (Difco) pH 7·8	70·0 ml
Yeast extract, pH 7·0, see above	10·0 ml
Horse serum (unheated)	20·0 ml
Glucose solution, 10 per cent w/v	10·0 ml
Sodium deoxyribonucleate (calf thymus) solution, 0·2 per cent w/v	1·0 ml
Thallous acetate solution, $TlC_2H_3O_2$, 1 in 80 w/v	1·0 ml
Dipotassium hydrogen phosphate solution, K_2HPO_4, 1M	2·0 ml
Penicillin solution, 50,000 units per ml	0·2 ml
Phenol red solution, 0·2 per cent w/v	1·0 ml
Methylene blue solution, 0·1 per cent w/v	1·0 ml

Methylene blue is omitted unless the examination is only for *M. pneumoniae*. It inhibits the growth of human commensal mycoplasmas. Sometimes it contains inhibitors for *M. pneumoniae* and each batch should be tested for inhibitory activity before use.

Sterilize the solutions by filtration and add them to the sterile broth. Dispense with sterile precautions.

Diphasic Medium

For the primary isolation of mycoplasmas.
Solid phase. Standard solid medium, above.
Liquid phase. Liquid medium, above.

Preparation of complete medium. Dispense the solid phase in approximately 5-ml quantities in 1-oz sterile screw-capped bottles and allow it to set. Overlay with 10 ml of the liquid phase.

T-strain Mycoplasma Medium

PPLO broth *or* PPLO agar without violet (Difco) pH 6·0	70·0 ml
Yeast extract, pH 7·0, see p. 133 . . .	10·0 ml
Horse serum (unheated) .	20·0 ml
Urea solution, 20 per cent w/v	5·0 ml
Phenol red solution, 0·2 per cent w/v	1·0 ml
Penicillin solution, 200,000 units per ml . . .	0·25 ml

The solutions are sterilized by filtration and added to the sterile broth or agar. The pH of the medium is adjusted to 6·0 before dispensing it with sterile precautions.

Sloppy Agar Medium

This medium is useful for primary isolation of mycoplasmas.

PPLO broth without crystal violet w/o cv (Difco) pH 7·8	70·0 ml
PPLO agar base without crystal violet (Difco) pH 7·8	10·0 ml
Yeast extract pH 7·0, see p. 133 . . .	10·0 ml
Horse serum (unheated) .	20·0 ml
Sodium deoxyribonucleate (calf thymus) solution 0·2 per cent w/v . .	1·0 ml
Thallous acetate solution, $TlC_2H_3O_2$, 1 in 80 w/v .	1·0 ml
Dipotassium hydrogen phosphate solution, K_2HPO_4, 1M . . .	2·0 ml
Penicillin solution, 50,000 units per ml . . .	0·2 ml

Sterilize the solutions by filtration and add them to the sterile broth. Add the 10 ml molten agar base. Mix gently. Dispense aseptically in 4-ml amounts in small screw-capped bottles (bijoux).

MEDIA FOR THE CULTIVATION OF SPIROCHAETES

Of the three genera of spirochaetes, *Leptospira*, *Treponema* and *Borrelia*, only *Leptospira* will grow readily in culture media. Noguchi's (1912) medium is chiefly of historical interest but it has been used for isolating some pathogenic borreliae and for growing strains of *Treponema* that are probably non-pathogenic.

Other better media are available for cultivating *Leptospira*. These are usually liquid because the organisms do not grow readily on the surface of solid media. A semi-solid medium is less readily evaporated and may be of special value in the tropics. A good serum-free synthetic medium has been devised by Ellingha sen and McCullough (1965).

LEPTOSPIRA MEDIA
Modified Korthof's Medium

This modified medium (Alston and Broom, 1958) is good for the cultivation of *Leptospira*. Blood serum is an essential constituent of all leptospira media and a source of suitable serum must be established. Choice of a suitable peptone is also necessary for Korthof's medium because different batches, even of the same brand of peptone, vary in their growth-promoting abilities. Witte peptone and Difco neopeptone are recommended but any good brand is likely to be suitable. A preliminary test should be made of each new batch before taking it into use.

All glassware must be perfectly clean and free from any trace of soap or other detergent since these are lethal to spirochaetes. After the usual cleaning glass should be thoroughly rinsed, preferably by soaking for 24 h in a phosphate buffer solution at pH 7·6 (see Stuart's medium) and then rinsing in distilled water.

Peptone salt solution

Peptone	0·8 g
Sodium chloride, NaCl .	1·4 g
Sodium bicarbonate, $NaHCO_3$ . . .	0·02 g

Potassium chloride, KCl . 0·04 g
Calcium chloride, CaCl$_2$. 0·04 g
Potassium dihydrogen
    phosphate, KH$_2$PO$_4$ . . 0·24 g
Disodium hydrogen
    phosphate,
    Na$_2$HPO$_4$.2H$_2$O . . 0·88 g
Distilled water . . . 1 l

Steam the ingredients at 100°C for 20 min and filter through Chardin-type or double thickness Whatman No. 1 paper. The pH should be approximately 7·2. Bottle in 100 ml amounts and autoclave at 115°C for 15 min.

Blood serum. Rabbit serum is generally found the most satisfactory though the sera of some larger animals such as sheep, horse or new-born calf have been used successfully. Individual rabbit sera may be inhibitory to leptospires because of agglutinins or other agents. For this reason the sera of several rabbits should be tested individually for agglutinins or by making separate trial batches of medium from each serum. The suitable animals are retained to supply serum as required. Blood is collected from an ear vein or, preferably, by cardiac puncture and allowed to clot. The serum is pipetted off, inactivated by heating at 56°C for 30 min and sterilized by Seitz filtration.

'Haemoglobin' solution. To the blood clot after removal of the serum add an equal volume of distilled water and freeze and thaw repeatedly to haemolyse the corpuscles. Sterilize by Seitz filtration.

Preparation of complete medium
    Peptone salt solution . . 100 ml
    Sterile blood serum . . 8 ml
    Sterile 'haemoglobin' solution 0·8 ml

Mix the ingredients with sterile precautions. Distribute the medium in 2–3 ml amounts in sterile screw-capped bijou bottles. Test for sterility by incubating at 37°C for two days and at 22°C for three days.

Modified Stuart's Medium

Stuart's (1946) medium does not contain peptone and therefore is not subject to variations in peptones. It contains phenol red to confirm the pH of the medium and as an indicator of contaminants which tend to increase the acidity. Bryan's (1957) modification is described here.

All glassware must be specially cleaned as for Korthof's medium.

Stock solutions
    L-asparagine
        (dextro-rotatory) . 1·3 per cent
    Ammonium chloride,
        NH$_4$Cl . . . 0·54 per cent
    Magnesium chloride,
        MgCl$_2$.6H$_2$O . . 2·03 per cent
    Sodium chloride, NaCl . 0·58 per cent
    Thiamine hydrochloride 0·1 per cent
    Phenol red . . . 0·02 per cent

Prepare the stock solutions with distilled water and sterilize them by autoclaving at 115°C for 15 min. The salt solutions are 0·1 M.

Phosphate buffer solutions
    Potassium dihydrogen
        phosphate,
        KH$_2$PO$_4$ (A) . . 9·078 g per l
    Disodium hydrogen
        phosphate,
        Na$_2$HPO$_4$.2H$_2$O (B) . 11·876 g per l

Prepare the solutions in distilled water and sterilize them by autoclaving at 121°C for 30 min. A buffer solution of pH 7·6 contains the solutions in the proportion of 2·6 ml of A to 17·4 ml of B.

Blood serum. Serum is prepared as for Korthof's medium (see above).

Preparation of complete medium
    L-asparagine solution . . 2 ml
    Ammonium chloride solution 10 ml
    Magnesium chloride solution . 4 ml
    Sodium chloride solution . 66 ml
    Thiamine hydrochloride
        solution . . . . 0·4 ml
    Phenol red solution . . 10 ml
    Distilled water . . . 91 ml
    Phosphate buffer, pH 7·6 . 16 ml
    Sterile inactivated rabbit serum 20 ml

Mix all ingredients except the rabbit serum and steam at 100°C for 30 min to drive off dissolved carbon dioxide. Autoclave at 115°C for 15 min. Add the serum with sterile precautions, distribute and test for sterility as for Korthof's medium. If the pH is correct the medium is an amber colour.

To obtain satisfactory results a large inoculum, about 10 per cent of a previous culture introduced with a Pasteur pipette, is used.

Dinger's Modification of Noguchi's Medium

This semi-solid medium (Wolff, 1954) is slower to evaporate than liquid media, especially in the tropics. Subcultures can be made less frequently so that virulence is maintained longer.

Nutrient agar, 3 per cent	6 ml
Distilled water	100 ml
Sterile inactivated serum	10 ml

Mix the agar and water and sterilize by autoclaving at 121°C for 20 min. Cool and add the serum with sterile precautions, distribute and test for sterility as for Korthof's medium.
Solid Medium for Colonial Growth of Leptospires (Cox and Larson, 1957).

Tryptose-phosphate broth dehydrated (Difco)	0·2 g
Agar (Difco)	1·0 g
Distilled water	90 ml

Adjust pH to 7·5 and sterilize mixture by autoclaving, at 121°C for 15 min. After cooling, add 10 ml sterile rabbit serum and 1 ml haemoglobin solution prepared by lysing washed and packed sheep erythrocytes in 20 vol cold distilled water. Remove stroma by centrifugation and sterilize by Seitz filtration.

Heat mixture at 56°C for 30 min and pour into Petri dishes to give depth of medium 6 to 8 mm.

Inoculate by spreading 0·1-ml volumes of decimal dilutions of fluid culture evenly over the surface of separate plates to permit distribution of individual organisms at a suitable dilution.
Fletcher's semi-solid agar for Leptospires (Fletcher, 1928).

Tap or distilled water	5–7 ml
Nutrient agar (2·5 per cent)	0·5 ml
Rabbit serum	1·0 ml

Sterilize the above ingredients separately and mix in tubes.

This semi-solid (sloppy) agar is suitable for isolating strains of leptospires and for maintaining them for several months. They multiply within the upper part of the tube forming zones of turbidity at varying depths (Dinger's disks).

MEDIA FOR THE CULTIVATION OF FUNGI

Media for the isolation of pathogenic fungi are designed to be inhibitory to bacteria and in certain cases to other fungi as well.

Agar is hydrolysed by heat at a low pH and acid media for fungi are not heated above 115°C. After autoclaving, the medium may be allowed to solidify in bulk but it should be remelted only once and then with a minimum of heating. The high concentration of sugar in some media for fungi is another reason for avoiding overheating and repeated heating, because heat tends to char sugar.

Sabouraud's Glucose Agar and Broth

The low pH and high sugar content of these media make them particularly selective for fungi and inhibitory to bacteria. The agar medium is suitable for the primary isolation of fungi from clinical material.

In Emmons, Binford and Utz's (1970) modification of Sabouraud's medium the sugar content is reduced to 2 per cent and the pH raised to 6·8. Chloramphenicol (40 mg per l suspended in 10 ml of 95 per cent ethanol) may be added to make it selective for fungi.

It is useful to add cycloheximide (500 mg per l dissolved in 10 ml of acetone) for the isolation of dermatophytes but cycloheximide is unsuitable for general mycological use because it inhibits many other moulds and yeasts (Georg, Ajello and Papageorge, 1954).

Glucose	40 g
Peptone	10 g
Agar	20 g
Water	1 l

A suitable peptone is Oxoid mycological peptone. For broth, the agar is omitted.

Dissolve the ingredients in the steamer or autoclave. Filter through cotton gauze and adjust to pH 5·4. Dispense in stock bottles or in tubes. Autoclave at 115°C for 15 min.

Tellurite Malt Agar

Like Sabouraud's medium, this has a low pH and high sugar content. In addition it contains tellurite to inhibit bacteria.

Malt extract is prepared commercially by extracting the soluble materials from sprouted barley in water at about 55°C. The liquor is strained and concentrated by evaporation at a temperature below 55°C to yield a brown viscous material. It consists mainly of maltose (about 50 per cent), starch, dextrins and glucose, and contains about 5 per cent of proteins and protein breakdown products, and a wide range of mineral salts and growth factors, such as thiamine, nicotinic acid, riboflavine, biotin, pantothenic acid, pyridoxine, folic acid and inositol. For use in mycological media it must not contain added sugar or cod-liver oil.

Basal medium

Malt extract	.	.	.	40 g
Agar	.	.	.	20 g
Water	.	.	.	1 l

Dissolve the malt extract and agar by steaming, filter through cotton gauze, adjust to pH 5·4 and distribute in 100 ml amounts in stock bottles. Autoclave at 115°C for 15 min.

Potassium tellurite solution

Potassium tellurite, K_2TeO_3	.	0·5 g
Water	.	.	.	25 ml

Dissolve the salt, autoclave at 115°C for 20 min and store in a tightly stoppered bottle in the dark.

Preparation of complete medium

Basal medium	.	.	100 ml
Potassium tellurite solution	.	1·8 ml

Melt the basal medium, cool to 55°C, add the tellurite solution and distribute as desired.

The final concentration of tellurite is 0·036 per cent.

Dermatophyte Test Medium

This medium (Taplin et al., 1969) is highly selective for dermatophytes because the antibiotics inhibit most bacteria and cycloheximide restrains many other moulds and yeasts. Dermatophytes produce enough alkali to turn the medium red within 2 weeks at 28°C.

Phenol red solution

Phenol red (Difco)	.	.	0·5 g
Sodium hydroxide, NaOH, 0·1 N	.	.	.	15 ml
Distilled water	.	.	85 ml

Preparation of complete medium

Phytone (Baltimore Biological Laboratory)	.	.	10 g
Glucose	.	.	.	10 g
Agar	.	.	.	20 g
Phenol red solution	.	40 ml
Hydrochloric acid, HCl, 0·8 N	.	.	.	6 ml
Cycloheximide (Actidione, Upjohn), 25 per cent w/v in acetone	.	.	2 ml
Gentamicin sulphate (Garamycin, Schering), 5 per cent w/v aqueous	.	2 ml
Chlortetracycline (Aureomycin, Lederle), 0·4 per cent w/v in sterile water	.	.	25 ml
Distilled water	.	.	1 l

Ingredients must be obtained from the sources indicated. Substitution with other brands changes the specificity and effectiveness of the medium. The Garamycin powder may need assaying for specific gentamicin activity. Phytone is a papaic digest of soya meal.

Dissolve the phytone, glucose and agar in the water by boiling. Add the phenol red solution, acid, cycloheximide and gentamicin to the hot medium while stirring. Autoclave at 115°C for 15 min and cool to about 47°C. Add the chlortetracycline while stirring. Dispense in 8 ml aliquots in sterile 1 oz screw-capped bottles and cool as slopes. The medium has a pH of 5·5 ± 0·1 and should be yellow in colour. For maximum shelf life, store at 4°C.

Penicillin Streptomycin Blood Agar

This medium is used for selective cultivation of yeasts and certain dimorphic fungi.

Nutrient agar	.	.	90 ml
Blood	.	.	.	10 ml
Penicillin	.	.	.	300 units
Streptomycin	.	.	300 μg

Prepare solutions of penicillin and of streptomycin from sterile antibiotics with sterile precautions. Melt the sterile nutrient agar, cool it to 55°C and add the sterile blood and the appropriate amounts of the antibiotic solutions. Distribute as desired.

Cystine Glucose Blood Agar

This medium is useful for cultivating the yeast forms of dimorphic fungi.

Cystine solution

Cystine	.	.	.	150 mg
Distilled water	.	.	.	3 ml

Prepare the solution immediately before use and sterilize by Millipore filtration.

Preparation of complete medium

Nutrient agar, 2·5 per cent agar, sterile . . .		83 ml
Glucose, 20 per cent, sterile .		5 ml
Cystine solution . . .		2 ml
Blood (sheep or rabbit) . .		10 ml

Melt the agar, cool to 50°C, add the remaining ingredients and pour plates.

Malt Agar

This medium is extensively used for the cultivation of saprophytic as well as parasitic yeasts and fungi, its high sugar content making it very suitable for this purpose. It is the best medium for highly exacting strains of fungi.

It is the basal medium described for tellurite malt agar.

Corn Meal Agar

This medium (Benham, 1931) is used to investigate a yeast-like culture for the production of mycelium and chlamydospores. In the case of *Candida albicans* the appearance of the chlamydospores is diagnostic. Their production is favoured because the medium is poor in nutrients.

Corn meal (ground yellow maize) . . .				40 g
Agar				20 g
Water				1 l

Heat the corn meal in the water at about 60°C for one h. Filter through filter paper or gauze. Add water to bring the volume back to one litre. Add the agar and steam or autoclave to dissolve it. Filter. Autoclave at 121°C for 30 min. The pH is about 6·8, requiring no adjustment.

Zein Agar

Zein is the basic protein of corn meal and is a very effective substitute for corn meal in inducing the formation of chlamydospores by *Candida albicans*. Zein agar (Reid, Jones and Carter, 1953) has the advantage over corn meal agar of being clear, thus facilitating the search for the spores, and in giving more rapid and profuse formation of chlamydospores (within 24 h) because of the absence of reducing sugar. Zein may be obtained from Brown and Polson, Ltd., London.

Zein	.	.	.	40 g
Agar .	.	.	.	15 g
Water .	.	.	.	1 l

Heat the zein in the water at 60°C for 1 h. Filter through gauze and coarse filter paper, and make up to original volume with distilled water. Add agar and steam at 100°C for 30 min. If necessary, adjust pH to 7·3–7·6 (adjustment is usually unnecessary). Sterilize by autoclaving at 121°C for 15 min.

Rice Starch Agar

Like corn meal agar, this medium (Taschdjian, 1957) is used to stimulate mycelium and chlamydospore formation by *Candida albicans*. Rice flour is more easily obtained than American household yellow corn meal.

Rice flour	.	.	.	10 g
Agar	.	.	.	15 g
Tween 80	.	.	.	10 ml
Water .	.	.	.	1 l

Bring the water to the boil and sprinkle in the rice flour. Boil for 30 sec, stand for a few seconds and filter through cotton gauze. Add water to re-adjust the volume to one litre. Add the agar and Tween 80 and autoclave at 121°C for 30 min.

Malt Extract Broth

Malt extract	.	.	17 g
Peptone (Oxoid mycological peptone) . . .			3 g
Water .	.	.	1 l

Dissolve the ingredients, adjust to pH 5·4, distribute and autoclave at 115°C for 15 min.

MEDIA FOR THE CULTIVATION OF PROTOZOA

ENTAMOEBA

The standard medium for the isolation of *Entamoeba histolytica* from faeces is that of Dobell and Laidlaw (1926) but Balamuth's (1946) medium is an improvement on it and is suitable for the cultivation of all other entamoebae from faeces.

Balamuth's Medium

1 M *phosphate buffer, pH* 7·5
  Dipotassium hydrogen
    phosphate, K_2HPO_4,
    174 g per l   .   .   .   8·6 ml
  Potassium dihydrogen
    phosphate, KH_2PO_4,
    136 g per l   .   .   .   1·4 ml

It is convenient to keep separate stock solutions of the two salts and to mix them before use.

Stock solution of liver extract
  Liver extract   .   .   .   5 g
  Water .   .   .   .   . 100 ml

Dissolve by boiling, filter and autoclave at 121°C for 20 min.

Preparation of complete medium
  Dehydrated egg yolk   .   . 36 g
  Sodium chloride, NaCl,
    0·8 per cent aqueous .   About 150 ml
  Phosphate buffer, M/15 at
    pH 7·5   .   .   .   . 125 ml
  Liver extract, 5 per cent
    aqueous   .   .   .   25 ml
  Rice starch, sterile
                    (1 loopful per 7–10 ml)

Mix the egg yolk with an equal volume of water and add 125 ml of saline. Stir vigorously with a rotary beater or in a Waring blender. Heat in a covered double boiler for 20 min after the temperature of the infusion reaches 80°C. Make up the evaporation loss with water, about 20 ml being required. Express the extract through a double layer of muslin to yield about 100 ml of yellowish fluid. Make up the volume to 125 ml with saline. Autoclave at 121°C for 20 min. The yellowish sediment may be removed by cooling below 10°C and filtering but this is not essential.

Add phosphate buffer diluted from 1 M to M/15. Add liver extract, dispense in tall test tubes and autoclave. Make sure that the rice starch is thoroughly dry and sterilize it by dry heat at 160°C for 1½ h. Dispense the medium in 7 to 10 ml amounts in ordinary tubes and add a loopful of sterile rice just before use. The final pH is 7·3.

Robinson's Medium

Robinson (1968) has described a very sensitive method for the culture of *Entamoeba histolytica*. It involves a medium for growing *Escherichia coli*, the bacteria then being the substrate for the growth of amoebae; saline agar slopes; and various solutions, either inhibitory or nutrient, which are added in different combinations during amoebic growth. The preparation of the requirements for this method is described here.

Defined medium for growing E. coli
Concentrated stock
  Sodium chloride, NaCl .   . 125 g
  Citric acid, $C_6H_8O_7.H_2O$. 50 g
  Potassium dihydrogen
    phosphate, KH_2PO_4 .   . 12·5 g
  Ammonium sulphate,
    $(NH_4)_2SO_4$.   .   . 25 g
  Magnesium sulphate,
    $MgSO_4.7H_2O$.   .   . 1·25 g
  Lactic acid (British Drug
    Houses, 90·08 per cent)   . 100 ml
  Water .   .   .   .   . 2·5 l

This can be kept without sterilization. It should be more than 4 weeks old to avoid change of pH on autoclaving.

Medium diluted for use
  Concentrated stock   .   . 100 ml
  Sodium hydroxide, NaOH,
    40 per cent in water .   . 7·5 ml
  Bromothymol blue, 0·04 per
    cent solution   .   .   . 2·5 ml
  Water .   .   .   .   . 890 ml

Adjust to pH 7, dispense in 25 ml volumes in screw-capped 100 ml medical flat bottles and autoclave at 121°C for 20 min. For use *Escherichia coli* strain B is inoculated into the medium; the bottle is then incubated in the horizontal position at 37°C for two days. The medium prepared in this way can be stored at room temperature for two months.

Saline agar slopes

Sodium chloride, NaCl .	. 7 g
Agar	. 15 g
Water	. 1 l

Dissolve, distribute in 2·5 ml aliquots in ¼ oz screw-capped bottles, autoclave at 121°C for 15 min and allow to set as slopes. The concentration of agar may require to be increased to 2·5 per cent, depending upon its quality. '

Erythromycin solution (0·5 per cent)

Erythromycin base	. . 0·5 g
Ethanol, 70 per cent in water	. 2·5 ml
Water, sterile	. . 97·5 ml

Suspend the erythromycin in the ethanol in a sterile vessel, allow to stand for 2 h, add the water and store at 4°C.

Phthalate solution, 0·5 M

Potassium phthalate, $C_6H_4(COOK)_2$	. . 204 g
Sodium hydroxide, NaOH, 40 per cent, in water	. . 100 ml
Water	. 1·9 l

Dissolve the salt in the liquids, adjust the pH to 6·3, distribute in 1 ml aliquots and autoclave at 121°C for 10 min.

For use, add 9 ml sterile water to give 0·05 M phthalate at pH 6·5.

Sheep serum. Serum from the slaughter-house, cleared with paper pulp on a Buchner filter, is sterilized by filtration, heated at 56°C on three successive days and stored at 4°C. Horse, rabbit, ox or human serum can replace sheep serum.

Bactopeptone solution (20 per cent). This brand of peptone must be used.

Bactopeptone (Difco)	. . 20 g
Water	. 100 ml

Dissolve the peptone and autoclave in a flask at 121°C for 20 min.

Rice starch powder (British Drug Houses) is also required (as for Balamuth's medium, p. 139).

TRICHOMONAS

Modified CPLM Medium

Media for *T. vaginalis* must provide a carbohydrate energy source; inorganic phosphate; proteolysed tissue to provide the so-called pancreatic 's' factor, amino acids, nucleic bases and possibly B vitamins; and serum to provide pantothenic acid, linoleic acid and other less well-defined nutrients. Johnson and Trussell (1943) recommended CPLM (cysteine-peptone-liver infusion-maltose) medium and the following modification of it (Smith, 1964) has been found satisfactory. Agar has been omitted from this modification because it complicates handling of the medium and of cultures in it. Methylene blue is omitted also. Phosphate as such is not added because there is sufficient of it in other ingredients.

This medium supports growth from a single protozoon under strictly anaerobic conditions, the maximum population of $1–3 \times 10^6$ organisms per ml being reached in 5–7 days at 37°C. Under aerobic conditions, massive inocula are required. *T. vaginalis* is an anaerobe and contains no catalase.

Basal Medium

Peptone . . .	. 32 g
Maltose . . .	. 1·6 g
Liver digest (Panmede) .	. 20 g
Cysteine hydrochloride .	. 2·4 g
Ringer's solution, ¼ strength .	1 l
Sodium hydroxide, NaOH, 1N	. About 9 ml

The brand of peptone is not important. Panmede ox liver digest obtainable from Paines and Byrne Ltd., Greenford, Middlesex, can be replaced by 32 per cent of any brand of liver infusion made according to the manufacturer's instructions. Cysteine is not essential when cultures are incubated anaerobically but it assists the maintenance of anaerobiosis.

Dissolve the ingredients by shaking. Adjust the pH to 6·0 with sodium hydroxide, steam at 100°C for 30 min and filter off the fine grey precipitate with Whatman's No. 1 or coarse paper. Bottle in 90 ml lots and autoclave at 115°C for 10 min.

This medium keeps for several weeks.

Penicillin streptomycin solution

Penicillin . . .	1×10^5 units
Streptomycin . .	. 0·1 g
Sterile water . .	. 10 ml

Dissolve the sterile antibiotics with sterile precautions. The solution contains 10^4 units of penicillin and 10^4 μg streptomycin per ml. It will keep up to 10 days in the refrigerator.

Nystatin solution
Nystatin . . . 5×10^4 units
Sterile water . . . 10 ml
Suspend the sterile antibiotic in the water. The suspension contains 5×10^3 units per ml. It keeps in the refrigerator at less than 10°C but is rapidly destroyed at 37°C.

Preparation of complete medium
Basal medium . . . 90 ml
Sterile inactivated horse serum 10 ml
Penicillin streptomycin
solution . . . . 1 ml
Nystatin solution . . . 1 ml
Before use, add the serum and antibiotics and distribute in suitable aliquots with sterile precautions. Serum from human, calf, ox, sheep or rabbit may be used. The addition of antibiotics is unnecessary for routine subcultures but is essential for clinical diagnostic cultures and for isolating axenic cultures. Nystatin can be omitted unless yeast or fungal contaminants are suspected.

Isotonic Trichomonas Medium

All the major constituents of this medium (Lumsden, Robertson and McNeillage, 1966) are prepared as solutions that are nearly isotonic with blood plasma. This makes the medium flexible and easily modified if differences, such as in pH, are desired.

Salts solution
Sodium chloride, NaCl,
0·154 M . . . . 1 l
Potassium chloride, KCl,
0·154 M . . . . 40 ml
Magnesium chloride, $MgCl_2$,
0·103 M . . . . 30 ml
Calcium chloride, $CaCl_2$,
0·103 M . . . . 10 ml
Dissolve and autoclave in a flask at 121°C for 30 min. Store at 4°C.

Buffer solution pH 7·4
Sodium dihydrogen
phosphate, NaH_2PO_4,
0·154 M . . . . 13·6 ml
Disodium hydrogen
phosphate, Na_2HPO_4,
0·103 M . . . . 86·4 ml

Bromocresol purple (Hopkin
and Williams) . . . 15 mg
Dissolve the indicator in the buffer and autoclave in a flask at 121°C for 20 min. Store at 4°C.

Antibiotic solutions
Benzyl penicillin (Glaxo): 1 mega unit dissolved in 5 ml sterile salts solution.
Streptomycin sulphate (Glaxo): 0·5 g (potency 745 units per mg) dissolved in 2·5 ml sterile salts solution.

Preparation of complete medium
Liver digest (Oxoid), 4 per
cent solution . . . 300 ml
Glucose, 0·308 M . . . 100 ml
Salts solution . . . 392·5 ml
Buffer solution . . . 100 ml
Benzyl penicillin solution . 5 ml
Streptomycin sulphate solution 2·5 ml
Calf serum (Oxoid) . . 100 ml
Sodium thioglycollate
(British Drug Houses) . 1 g
Mix the ingredients at room temperature. The final pH is 6·1 to 6·4. Sterilize by filtration and distribute to sterile bottles in amounts that nearly fill them (6 ml to bijou bottles, 15 ml to $\frac{1}{2}$ oz round bottles). The screw caps of the bottles should be perforated like those of blood culture bottles. Medium can be stored at 4°C for two weeks, or longer at -20°C.

MEDIUM FOR THE CULTIVATION OF LEISHMANIAE AND TRYPANOSOMES

The classical medium for the cultivation of trypanosomes and leishmaniae is NNN medium, a solid medium devised by Novy and MacNeal (1904) and modified by Nicolle (1908). The following medium (Tobie, von Brand and Mehlman, 1950) differs from it in that it consists of two phases, blood agar and Locke's solution. Trypanosomes incubated at 26°C grow dispersed in the liquid and reach 20×10^6 per ml in 10 to 14 days. They develop only to the proventricular stage. If the uninoculated medium is kept for six days the overlying liquid can be drawn off and used as a liquid medium. In it trypanosomes reach 9×10^6 per ml in 8–10 days.

Solid Phase

Basal medium

Meat extract (Bacto-beef, Difco) . . .	1·5 g
Peptone (Bacto-peptone, Difco) . . .	2·5 g
Sodium chloride, NaCl . .	4 g
Agar (Bacto-agar, Difco) .	7·5 g
Water	500 ml

Dissolve the ingredients, adjust the pH to 7·2–7·4 with 1N sodium hydroxide and autoclave at 121°C for 25 min.

Citrated blood. Whole rabbit blood containing 0·5 per cent of sterile sodium citrate is inactivated at 56°C for 30 min. Human blood can be used, but the blood of different donors varies in suitability.

Preparation of complete medium

Basal medium . .	75 ml
Blood	25 ml

Melt the basal medium, cool to 45°C, add the blood and distribute in 5 ml amounts in sterile test-tubes or 25 ml amounts in sterile flasks. Keep test-tubes in a slanted position and flasks upright until the medium has solidified.

Liquid Phase

Sodium chloride, NaCl . .	8 g
Potassium chloride, KCl .	0·2 g
Calcium chloride, $CaCl_2$.	0·2 g
Potassium dihydrogen phosphate, KH_2PO_4 .	0·3 g
Glucose . . .	2·5 g
Water	1 l

Dissolve the ingredients and autoclave at 121°C for 15 min. With sterile precautions add 2 ml to test-tubes and 10–15 ml to flasks containing the solid medium.

MEDIA FOR BLOOD CULTURES

Liquoid Broth

'Liquoid' (sodium polyanethol sulphonate) is a good anticoagulant because it is generally not inhibitory and it has the added advantage of annulling the natural bactericidal action of blood. It is obtainable from Hoffmann la Roche or Koch-Light Laboratories.

Liquoid solution, 5 per cent in 0·85 per cent saline .	10 ml
Nutrient broth . . .	1 l

Mix the ingredients and check that the pH is 7·6. Distribute and sterilize at 121°C for 15 min.

The final concentration of liquoid is 0·05 per cent.

Saponin Broth

This is a special medium for *viridans* streptococci which may be slightly sensitive to Liquoid. Citrate prevents clotting and saponin causes immediate lysis of the patient's blood.

Sodium citrate, $Na_3C_6H_5O_7.2H_2O$.	2 g
Saponin, white, B.D.H. .	1 g
Nutrient broth, sterile .	1 l

This medium cannot be heated above 100°C and care should be taken in making it to reduce contamination to a minimum. Dissolve the ingredients and check that the pH is 7·6. Distribute and heat in steam at 100°C for 20 min on each of three successive days.

Castaneda's Method of Blood Culture

This method provides both solid and liquid media in the blood culture bottle. It was devised for *Brucella* and the glucose serum media described here are for them, but the technique is applicable to any blood culture. The concentration of agar is high to prevent the column of solid medium disintegrating in the broth.

Solid medium. Glucose serum agar (p. 130) with the agar concentration doubled and without bacitracin, polymyxin or cycloheximide.

4 oz 'medical flat' bottles are used. 30 ml molten agar is allowed to set on one of the narrow sides as a slope extending up to the shoulder of the bottle.

Liquid medium. Glucose serum agar without agar or antimicrobial substances.

20 ml medium is added to each bottle.

Bile Salt Streptokinase Broth

This medium is used to culture blood clots from patients with suspected enteric fever.

Nutrient broth, sterile .	1 l
Sodium taurocholate .	5 g

Streptokinase solution
(Calbiochem Ltd., London),
100,000 units per ml, sterile   1 ml

Adjust the pH of the broth to 7·6 and dissolve the bile salt in it. Autoclave at 108°C for 15 min. Cool and add streptokinase aseptically. Distribute in 15 ml amounts with sterile precautions.

MEDIA FOR PRESERVATION OF CULTURES

Egg Saline Medium

This modification of Dorset's egg medium, in which the broth is replaced by saline and no malachite green is added, is good for preserving cultures of Gram-negative bacilli.

Beaten egg   .   .   .   .   75 ml
Sodium chloride, NaCl, sterile
0·85 per cent solution   .   25 ml

Prepare the beaten egg, mix and dispense the medium with sterile precautions as for Löwenstein-Jensen medium. Bijou bottles containing 2–3 ml of medium may be used. Inspissate in a slanted position at 75–80°C for 1 h.

If the medium has been prepared without sterile precautions it can be allowed to cool for a few hours after inspissation and then autoclaved at 121°C for 15 min with the screw-caps tightened. If the screw-caps are loose, some of the slants may be disrupted by bubbles of steam.

Chalk Cooked Meat Broth

This modification of cooked meat broth is intended for the preservation of stock cultures of clostridia.

0·1 g calcium carbonate, $CaCO_3$, and possibly also some minced cooked egg white is added to each bottle of cooked meat broth before the final autoclaving.

Fungus Preservation Medium

This is used to prevent pleomorphic variation in stock cultures of ringworm fungi.

Peptone   .   .   .   .   30 g
Agar   .   .   .   .   .   20 g
Water .   .   .   .   .   1 l

Dissolve the ingredients, filter through cotton gauze, adjust to pH 5·4, distribute and autoclave at 115°C for 15 min.

TRANSPORT MEDIA

When the patient is not close to the bacteriological laboratory there is a risk that the pathogen in a bacteriological specimen may not survive or may be overgrown by non-pathogens during the time it takes to transport the specimen to the laboratory. Some media have been devised to protect pathogens during such a delay.

Pike's Medium

This medium (Pike, 1944) is used to preserve *Strept. pyogenes*, pneumococci and *H. influenzae* in nose and throat swabs (Holmes and Lermit, 1955; Masters *et al.*, 1958). It is blood agar containing 1 in 1,000,000 crystal violet and 1 in 16,000 sodium azide distributed as for stab cultures in tubes or bottles.

Stuart's (1959) Transport Medium

This soft agar medium is used to maintain the viability of gonococci on swabs during their transmission through the post to a laboratory.

It is essential that the distilled water used in the medium be free from chlorine. To ensure this, it should be passed through an ion-exchange resin column before use.

Anaerobic salt solution
Thioglycollic acid (Difco)   .   2 ml
Sodium hydroxide, 1N
NaOH   .   .   .   12–15 ml
Sodium glycerophosphate,
20 per cent aqueous .   . 100 ml
Calcium chloride, $CaCl_2$,
1 per cent aqueous   .   . 20 ml
Distilled water   .   .   . 900 ml

Mix the ingredients, adding sufficient sodium hydroxide to bring the pH to 7·2.

Agar solution
Agar .   .   .   .   .   6 g
Distilled water   .   .   .   1 l

Dissolve by steaming.

Preparation of complete medium
Anaerobic salt solution .   . 900 ml
Agar solution   .   .   .   1 l
Methylene blue, 0·1 per cent
aqueous   .   .   .   4 ml

Melt the agar and add the salt solution. Adjust the pH to 7·3–7·4. Add the methylene blue and distribute in bijou bottles, filling nearly to capacity. Autoclave at 121°C for 15 min and immediately tighten caps. When cool, the medium should be colourless.

Preparation of swabs. Make neat swabs of absorbent cotton-wool on applicator sticks and boil 5 min in 0·07 M phosphate buffer at pH 7·4. Shake off excess moisture and immerse in a 1 per cent watery suspension of *finely powdered* charcoal, such as BDH activated charcoal, twirling until the cotton-wool is black. Shake off excess moisture, place in test-tubes, plug these with cotton-wool, dry in oven and sterilize in oven at 160°C for 1½ h.

Glycerol Saline Transport Medium for Enteric Bacilli

If there is likely to be a delay of some hours before specimens of faeces for culture reach the laboratory this transport medium prevents other intestinal organisms from overgrowing the enteric fever bacilli.

Glycerol	300 ml
Sodium chloride, NaCl	4·2 g
Disodium hydrogen phosphate, Na_2HPO_4, anhydrous	10 g
Phenol red, 0·02 per cent, aqueous	About 15 ml
Water	700 ml

Dissolve the sodium chloride in the water and add the glycerol. Add the phosphate and steam to dissolve it. Then add enough phenol red to give a purple-pink colour, judged by pouring a small quantity of the solution into a Universal container. Distribute in 6 ml amounts in Universal containers and autoclave at 115°C for 20 min.

The fluid should not be used if it becomes acid, indicated by a change in colour to yellow.

Preserving Fluid for Vibrio cholerae

This fluid is valuable for maintaining the viability of *V. cholerae* and preventing overgrowth by other organisms when there may be delay in the transmission of stools to a laboratory. One to 3 g of the stool is emulsified in 10 ml preserving fluid.

Boric acid, H_3BO_3	3·101 g
Potassium chloride, KCl	3·728 g
Sodium hydroxide, NaOH 0·2 M solution	133·5 ml
Dried sea-salt	200 g
Distilled water	About 867 ml

Dissolve the boric acid and potassium chloride in 20 ml hot water. Cool and make up the volume to 250 ml. Add the sodium hydroxide, make up the volume to 1 litre and add the salt. Filter the solution through paper, distribute in 10 ml amounts in screw-capped bottles and autoclave at 121°C for 20 min.

Substitute for sea-salt

Sodium chloride, NaCl	180 g
Potassium chloride, KCl	6·7 g
Magnesium chloride, $MgCl_2.6H_2O$	20 g
Magnesium sulphate, $MgSO_4.7H_2O$	11·7 g

Bile Peptone Transport Medium

This medium is useful for field work in hot climates where cholera may occur. Rectal swabs or faeces may be inoculated into the medium which is then returned to the base laboratory. Subcultures to Monsur's medium should be made within 6 h if possible. If this is impracticable it should be subcultured to Monsur's medium immediately on return to the base laboratory and then incubated at 37°C overnight and subcultured again the next day.

Trypticase or any good peptone	1 g
Sodium chloride, NaCl	1 g
Sodium taurocholate	0·5 g
Water	100 ml

Dissolve the ingredients, adjust to pH 8·5 with 1N sodium hydroxide, distribute into bottles and autoclave at 121°C for 15 min.

In order to make this medium more selective for the vibrios, sterile potassium tellurite solution may be added after autoclaving to give a final concentration of 1 in 200,000 as for Monsur's medium. The medium is slightly turbid. It should not be kept longer than two weeks.

MEDIA FOR THE EXAMINATION OF MILK AND WATER

Yeast Extract Agar

This is a nutrient agar in which yeast extract replaces meat extract. It is employed particularly for making plate counts of the viable bacteria in drinking water. The formula given is that prescribed by the Department of Health in a Report on Public Health and Medical Subjects (1970).

Yeast extract . . .	3 g
Peptone	5 g
Agar, shredded or powdered .	15 g
Water	1 l

The recommended brand of yeast extract is 'Yeastrel', supplied by the Brewer's Food Supply Co. Ltd., Edinburgh. Dissolve the yeast extract and peptone in the water at 100°C, cool to room temperature and adjust to pH 7·4. Place the agar if shredded in a muslin bag, wash in running water for 15 min and express excess moisture before adding it to the broth. Autoclave at 121°C for 20 min and filter hot through paper pulp. Test the pH of the filtrate at 50°C and adjust to pH 7·0 to give a final pH of 7·2 when cool. Distribute in 10 ml amounts and sterilize by autoclaving at 121°C for 20 min.

Yeast Extract Milk Agar

This medium is used for making plate counts of viable bacteria in milk supplies and rinse waters from dairy and food utensils. It is the medium specified by the Secretary of State for the examination of milk supplies in Scotland under the Milk (Special Designations) (Scotland) Order, 1965. The medium is prepared in the same way as yeast extract agar, but 10 ml of fresh or spray-dried, skim or whole milk is added per litre of broth at the same time as the washed agar is added.

MacConkey Bile-Salt Lactose Peptone Water

This medium is used for detecting the presence of coliform organisms in water and milk.

Single strength

Sodium taurocholate (commercial) . . .	5 g
Peptone (any good make) .	20 g
Sodium chloride, NaCl . .	5 g
Lactose	10 g
Bromocresol purple, 1 per cent solution in ethanol . .	1 ml
or Neutral red, 1 per cent aqueous solution . .	5 ml
Water	1 l

Dissolve the bile salt, peptone and sodium chloride, steam for 2 h, cool and transfer to the refrigerator overnight. Add the lactose and when dissolved filter cold through Chardin filter paper. Adjust the reaction to pH 7·4 and add the indicator. Distribute in 5 ml amounts in 1-oz bottles or $6 \times \frac{5}{8}$ in test-tubes with Durham tubes and autoclave at 115°C for 15 min.

Double strength. Make as above, but with double the amounts of the ingredients, except water. Distribute in 50 ml amounts in 5-oz bottles using $3 \times \frac{3}{8}$ in test-tubes as Durham tubes, and in 10 ml amounts in 1-oz bottles using $2 \times \frac{1}{4}$ in Durham tubes.

Brilliant Green Bile Broth

This medium is used in the differential coliform test of water supplies to eliminate false positives due to anaerobes.

Ox bile. Fresh ox bile may be used. Otherwise dissolve 20 g dehydrated ox bile in 200 ml water and adjust the pH to 7·0–7·5.

Preparation of medium

Peptone	10 g
Ox bile	200 ml
Lactose	10 g
Brilliant green, 0·1 per cent aqueous solution . .	13 ml
Water to	1 l

Dissolve the peptone in 500 ml water, add the ox bile and lactose. Adjust the pH to 7·4. Add the brilliant green solution and water to make up 1 l. Distribute in 5 ml quantities in $6 \times \frac{5}{8}$ in tubes with Durham fermentation tubes. Autoclave at 115°C for 15 min.

Sodium Azide Medium

This medium (Hannay and Norton, 1947) is used for the isolation of *Strept. faecalis* from water.

Peptone	10 g
Sodium chloride, NaCl . .	5 g
Dipotassium hydrogen phosphate, K_2HPO_4 . .	5 g
Potassium dihydrogen phosphate, KH_2PO_4 . .	2 g
Glucose	5 g
Yeast extract (Yeastrel) .	3 g
Sodium azide, NaN_3 . .	0·25 g
Bromocresol purple, 1·6 per cent solution in ethanol .	2 ml
Water	1 l

Dissolve the ingredients. The medium has a pH of 6·6–6·8 and no adjustment is necessary. Distribute in 5 ml quantities in tubes. For use with inocula of 10 or 50 ml of water, a medium of double this strength is prepared and distributed in 10 and 50 ml quantities. Sterilize in the autoclave at 121°C for 15 min.

IDENTIFICATION OF MEDIA

It is necessary to identify a culture medium after it has been made and, as media such as the kinds of nutrient agar and the different fermentation test media are similar in appearance, it is essential to have some simple but reliable system of marking. Gummed labels are generally unsatisfactory especially as they become detached in the steamer when solid media are melted. Colours, either alone or in combination, are good for distinguishing media. It is better to use a few outstanding colours alone or in combination if necessary, rather than different shades of a colour; thus, green, irrespective of the shade, whether it be light or dark, yellowish green or bluish green, always indicates glucose. The colour may be indicated with coloured cotton-wool for tubes and flasks. It is better to dye cotton-wool in bulk than to colour white cotton-wool stoppers with various stains. Coloured beads in media or cellulose paint applied to the caps of tubes or of screw-capped bottles or as a small patch on glassware are other alternatives. The cotton-wool colour range does not include gold and silver for which there are paints.

Cellulose paint on the caps is the best method for small screw-capped bottles and tubes with metal caps. Coloured beads are good for large bottles. Ordinary opaque glass beads, 6–7 mm in diameter are suitable, but clear glass beads are not. Before use the beads are boiled twice in distilled water and dried in the incubator. The appropriate bead is dropped into the bottle before it is filled. Owing to the convexity of the bottom of the bottle, the bead remains to one side and is very easily recognized no matter what type of culture medium is used. On tilting the bottle for pouring, the bead comes to rest on the shoulder and remains in this position, even when the bottle is almost completely inverted.

It is recommended that a standard colour scheme be adopted and the following system is suggested, as it is already widely used.

Nutrient broth and agar from dehydrated stock	White
Infusion broth and agar	Yellow
Meat extract broth and agar . .	Brown
Digest broth and agar .	Black
Fildes' broth and agar .	Black/white
Casein yeast lactate (CYL) concentrate (Marshall and Kelsey)	Brown/white
Complete CYLG medium (Marshall and Kelsey) .	Brown/green
Peptone water . .	White
Salt cooked meat broth	Orange
Serum broth and agar .	Blue/white
Glucose broth and agar	Green
Crystal violet blood agar	Red/blue
MacConkey's liquid medium. Single strength . .	1 red spot
MacConkey's liquid medium. Double strength . .	2 red spots
MacConkey's agar medium . .	Red
Deoxycholate citrate agar (DCA) .	Red/orange
Tomato juice agar .	Red/yellow
Sabouraud's medium .	Light blue
Distilled water .	White
Normal saline (0·85 per cent) . .	Dark blue
Glucose in saline .	Blue/green
Saline agar bleeding tubes . .	White

Media for Biochemical Tests

Citrate . . .	Orange/white
Craigie tubes . .	White
Decarboxylase –	
Arginine . . .	Pink
Lysine . . .	White
Ornithine . . .	Blue
Control . . .	Black
Gillies' I and II . .	White
Gluconate . .	Green/yellow
Glucose phosphate for	
V.P. test . .	Green/orange
H$_2$S broth . .	Blue/brown
Malonate – Phenyl-alanine (combined medium of Shaw and Clarke) . . .	Blue/green
Nitrate broth . .	Brown/red
Nitrite broth . .	Brown/yellow
Nutrient gelatin .	Blue
Organic acids – Citrate .	Orange/white
Mucate . . .	Mauve
Dextro-tartrate . .	Red/black
Laevo-tartrate . .	Brown/black
Meso-tartrate . .	Mauve/black
Phenylalanine agar .	Pink
Plasma broth . .	Green/white
Urea broth and agar .	Mauve

Fermentation Media ('*Sugars*')

Where colours are mentioned for which there is no coloured cotton-wool, a small patch of cellulose paint is placed on the tube itself.

Adonitol	Silver
Aesculin	Brown
Arabinose	Black and yellow
Dextrin	Red and mauve
Dextrose	(see Glucose)
Dulcitol	Pink
Erythritol	Black and red
Fructose (laevulose)	Yellow
Galactose	Mauve and white
Glucose	Green
Glycerol	Brown and white
Glycogen	Blue and yellow
Inositol	Gold
Inulin	Yellow and white
Lactose	Red
Maltose	Blue and white
Mannitol	Mauve
Mannose	Black and green
Raffinose	Red and white
Rhamnose	Black and pink
Salicin	Pink and white
Sorbitol	Black and blue
Starch	Yellow and mauve
Sucrose (saccharose)	Blue
Trehalose	Mauve and green
Xylose	Red and green

REFERENCES

ALSTON, J. H. & BROOM, J. C. (1958) *Leptospirosis in Man and Animals.* p. 303. Edinburgh: Livingstone.

ANDERSON, K. F. & FAINE, S. (1971) Quality control of culture media. *College of Pathologists of Australia.* Broadsheet No. 10.

ANDERSON, J. S., HAPPOLD, F. C., McLEOD, J. W. & THOMSON, J. G. (1931) On the existence of two forms of diphtheria bacillus – *B. diphtheriae gravis* and *B. diphtheriae mitis* – and a new medium for their differentiation and for the bacteriological diagnosis of diphtheria. *Journal of Pathology and Bacteriology*, **34**, 667.

ANDERSON, P. M. (1944) A simple medium for the detection of *Corynebacterium diphtheriae*. *Medical Journal of Australia*, **1**, 213.

ARONSON, H. (1915) Eine neue Methode der bakteriologischen Choleradiagnose. *Deutsche medizinische Wochenschrift*, **41**, 1027.

ASHESHOV, I. N. (1941) Papain digest media and standardisation of media in general. *Canadian Journal of Public Health*, **32**, 468.

BABER, K. G. (1969) A selective medium for the isolation of Haemophilus from sputum. *Journal of Medical Laboratory Technology*, **26**, 391.

BALAMUTH, W. (1946) Improved egg yolk infusion for cultivation of *Entamoeba histolytica* and other intestinal protozoa. *American Journal of Clinical Pathology*, **16**, 380.

BARBER, M. & KUPER, S. W. A. (1951) Identification of *Staphylococcus pyogenes* by the phosphatase reaction. *Journal of Pathology and Bacteriology*, **63**, 65.

BARNES, E. M. (1969) Methods for the Gram-negative non-sporing anaerobes. In *Methods in Microbiology*, vol. 3B, edited by J. R. Norris & D. W. Ribbons, p. 151. London: Academic Press.

BAUER, A. W., KIRBY, W. M. M., SHERRIS, K. C. & TURCK, M. (1966) Antibiotic susceptibility testing by a standardised single disc method. *American Journal of Clinical Pathology*, **45**, 493.

BENHAM, RHODA W. (1931) Certain monilias parasitic on man. Their identification by morphology and by agglutination. *Journal of Infectious Diseases*, **49**, 183.

BREWER, J. H. (1940) Clear liquid mediums for the 'aerobic' culture of anaerobes. *Journal of the American Medical Association*, **115**, 598.

BRIDSON, E. Y. & BRECKER, A. (1970) Design and formulation of microbial culture media. In *Methods in Microbiology*, Vol. 3A, p. 229, edited by J. R. Norris and D. W. Ribbons. New York and London: Academic Press.

BROTHERSTON, J. G., GILMOUR, N. J. L. & SAMUEL, J. McA. (1961) Quantitative studies of *Mycobacterium johnei* in the tissues of sheep. *Journal of Comparative Pathology and Therapeutics*, **71**, 286.

BROWN, V. I. & LOWBURY, E. J. L. (1965) Use of an improved agar medium and other culture methods for *Pseudomonas aeruginosa*. *Journal of Clinical Pathology*, **18**, 752.

BRYAN, H. S. (1957) Studies on leptospirosis in domestic animals. *Veterinary Medicine*, **52**, 111.

CHRISTIE, R. & KEOGH, E. V. (1940) Physiological and serological characteristics of staphylococci of human origin. *Journal of Pathology and Bacteriology*, **51**, 189.

COLE S. W. & ONSLOW, H. (1916) On a substitute for peptone and a standard nutrient medium for bacteriological purposes. *Lancet*, **ii**, 9.

COLLEE, J. G., RUTTER, J. M. & WATT, B. (1971) The significantly viable particle: a study of the subculture of an exacting sporing anaerobe. *Journal of Medical Microbiology*, **4**, 271.

COLLEE, J. G. & WATT, B. (1971) Changing approaches to the sporing anaerobes in medical microbiology. In *Spore Research*, edited by A. N. Barker, G. W. Gould & J. Wolf, p. 39 London and New York: Academic Press.

COWAN, S. T. & STEEL, K. J. (1965) *Manual for the Identification of Medical Bacteria.* p. 127. Cambridge University Press.

COX, C. D. & LARSON, A. D. (1957) Colonial growth of leptospirae. *Journal of Bacteriology*, **73**, 587.

DE MAN, J. C., ROGOSA, M. & SHARPE, M. E. (1960) A medium for the cultivation of lactobacilli. *Journal of Applied Bacteriology*, **23**, 130.

Diagnostic Procedures and Reagents (1950) 3rd edn, p. 44. New York: American Public Health Association.

DIEUDONNÉ, A. (1909) Blutalkaliagar, ein Elektivnährboden für Choleravibrionen. *Zentralblatt für Bakteriologie, Abt. I Originale*, **50**, 107.

DOBELL, C. & LAIDLAW, P. P. (1926) On the cultivation of *Entamoeba histolytica* and some other entozoic amoebae. *Parasitology*, **18**, 283.

ELLINGHAUSEN, H. C. & McCULLOUGH, W. G. (1965) Nutrition of *Leptospira pomona* and growth of 13 other serotypes: fractionation of oleic albumin complex and a medium of bovine albumin and polysorbate 80. *American Journal of Veterinary Research*, **26**, 45.

ELLNER, P. D. (1956) A medium promoting rapid quantitative sporulation in *Clostridium perfringens*. *Journal of Bacteriology*, **71**, 495.

ELLNER, P. D., STOESSEL, C. J., DRAKEFORD, E. & VASI, F. (1966) A new culture medium for medical bacteriology. *American Journal of Clinical Pathology*, **45**, 502.

EMMONS, C. W., BINFORD, C. H. & UTZ, J. P. (1970) *Medical Mycology*, p. 464, 2nd end. London: Henry Kimpton.

FAIRBROTHER, R. W. & SOUTHALL, J. E. (1950) The isolation of *Staphylococcus pyogenes* from faeces. *Monthly Bulletin of the Ministry of Health Laboratory Service*, **9**, 170.

FINEGOLD, S. M. & SWEENEY, E. E. (1961) New selective and differential medium for coagulase-positive staphylococci allowing rapid growth and strain differentiation. *Journal of Bacteriology*, **81**, 636.

FLETCHER, W. (1928) Recent work on leptospirosis, tsutsugamushi disease and tropical typhus in the Federated Malay States. *Transactions of the Royal Society of Tropical Medicine and Hygiene*, **21**, 265.

GEORG, L. K., AJELLO, L. & PAPAGEORGE, C. (1954) Use of cycloheximide in the selective isolation of fungi pathogenic to man. *Journal of Laboratory and Clinical Medicine*, **44**, 422.

GLADSTONE, G. P. & FILDES, P. (1940) A simple culture medium for general use without meat extract or peptone. *British Journal of Experimental Pathology*, **21**, 161.

HADLEY, F. P. (1933) A quantitative method for estimating *Bacillus acidophilus* in saliva. *Journal of Dental Research*, **13**, 415.

HANNAY, C. L. & NORTON, I. L. (1947) Enumeration, isolation and study of faecal streptococci from river water. *Proceedings of the Society of Applied Bacteriology*, **1**, 39.

HARTLEY, P. (1922) The value of Douglas's medium for the production of diphtheria toxin. *Journal of Pathology and Bacteriology*, **25**, 479.

HAYWARD, NANCY J. (1943) The rapid identification of *Cl. welchii* by Nagler tests in plate cultures. *Journal of Pathology and Bacteriology*, **55**, 285.

HILL, J. H. & WHITE, E. C. (1929) Sodium chloride media for the separation of certain Gram-positive cocci and Gram-negative bacilli. *Journal of Bacteriology*, **18**, 43.

HIRSCH, A. & GRINSTED, E. (1954) Methods for the growth and enumeration of anaerobic spore-formers from cheese, with observations on the effect of nisin. *Journal of Dairy Research*, **21**, 101.

HOBBS, BETTY C. & ALLISON, V. D. (1945) Studies on the isolation of *Bact. typhosum* and *Bact. paratyphosum B. Monthly Bulletin of the Ministry of Health Laboratory Service*, **4**, 12 and 63.

HOLMES, M. C. & LERMIT, A. (1955) Transport and enrichment media in the isolation of haemolytic streptococci from the upper respiratory tract. *Monthly Bulletin of the Ministry of Health Laboratory Service*, **14**, 97.

HOYLE, L. (1941) A tellurite blood-agar medium for the rapid diagnosis of diphtheria. *Lancet*, **i**, 175.

HUDDLESON, I. F. (1939) *Brucelloses in Man and Animals.* p. 13. New York: Commonwealth Fund.

HYNES, M. (1942) The isolation of intestinal pathogens by selective media. *Journal of Pathology and Bacteriology*, **54**, 193.

IVES, J. C. J. & McCORMICK, W. (1956) A modification of Šula's method for the cultivation of tubercle bacilli from pleural fluid. *Journal of Clinical Pathology*, **9**, 177.

JACOBS, S. I., WILLIS, A. T. & GOODBURN, G. M. (1964) Pigment production and enzymatic activity of staphylococci: the differentiation of pathogens from commensals. *Journal of Pathology and Bacteriology*, **87**, 151.

JAMESON, J. E. & EMBERLEY, N. W. (1956) A substitute for bile salts in culture media. *Journal of General Microbiology*, **15**, 198.

JENSEN, K. A. (1955) Second Report of the Sub-Committee of Laboratory Methods of the International Union against Tuberculosis. *Bulletin of the International Union against Tuberculosis*, **25**, 89.

JOHNSON, G. & TRUSSELL, R. E. (1943) Experimental basis for the chemotherapy of *Trichomonas vaginalis* infestations I. *Proceedings of the Society of Experimental Biology (New York)*, **54**, 245.

Joint FAO/WHO Expert Committee on Brucellosis. Third Report (1958). Annex 10. Selective media for the culture of *Brucella* from potentially contaminated samples. *World Health Organization Technical Report Series*, No. 148, 50.

JONES, L. M. & MORGAN, W. J. B. (1958) A preliminary report on a selective medium for the culture of *Brucella*, including fastidious types. *Bulletin of the World Health Organization*, **19**, 200.

KING, ELIZABETH O., WARD, MARTHA K. & RANEY, D. E. (1954) Two simple media for the demonstration of pyocyanin and fluorescin. *Journal of Laboratory and Clinical Medicine*, **44**, 301.

KIRCHNER, O. (1932) Die Leistungsfähigkeit der Tiefenkultur des Tuberkelbazillus bei Verwendung besonders geeingneter flüssiger Nährboden. *Zentralblatt für Bakteriologie, Abt I Originale*, **124**, 403.

KNOX, R., GELL, P. G. H. & POLLOCK, M. R. (1942) Selective media for organisms of the Salmonella group. *Journal of Pathology and Bacteriology*, **54**, 469.

LACEY, B. W. (1954) A new selective medium for *Haemophilus pertussis*, containing a diamidine, sodium fluoride and penicillin. *Journal of Hygiene (London)*, **52**, 273.

LEIFSON, E. (1935) New culture media based on sodium desoxycholate for the isolation of intestinal pathogens and for the enumeration of colon bacilli in milk and water. *Journal of Pathology and Bacteriology*, **40**, 581.

LEIFSON, E. (1936) New selenite enrichment media for the isolation of typhoid and paratyphoid (Salmonella) bacilli. *American Journal of Hygiene*, **24**, 423.

LEMCKE, RUTH M. (1965) Media for the Mycoplasmataceae. *Laboratory Practice*, **14**, 712.

LOWBURY, E. J. L. & COLLINS, A. G. (1955) The use of a new cetrimide product in a selective medium for *Pseudomonas pyocyanea*. *Journal of Clinical Pathology*, **8**, 47.

LOWBURY, E. J. L. & LILLY, H. A. (1955) A selective plate medium for *Cl. welchii*. *Journal of Pathology and Bacteriology*, **70**, 105.

LUDLAM, G. B. (1949) A selective medium for the isolation of *Staph. aureus* from heavily contaminated material. *Monthly Bulletin of the Ministry of Health Laboratory Service*, **8**, 15.

LUMSDEN, W. H. R., ROBERTSON, D. H. H. & McNEILLAGE, G. J. C. (1966) Isolation, cultivation, low temperature preservation and infectivity titration of *Trichomonas vaginalis*. *British Journal of Venereal Diseases*, **42**, 145.

MARMION, B. P. (1967) The Mycoplasmas. New information on their properties and their pathogenicity for man. In *Recent Advances in Medical Microbiology*. p. 170. Edited by A. P. Waterson. London: Churchill.

MARMION, B. P. & TONKIN, R. W. (1972) Control of hepatitis in dialysis units. *British Medical Bulletin*, **28**, 169.

MARSHALL, J. H. & KELSEY, J. C. (1960) A standard culture medium for general bacteriology. *Journal of Hygiene (London)*, **58**, 367.

MASTERS, P. L., BRUMFITT, W., MENDEZ, R. L. & LIKAR, M. (1958) Bacterial flora of the upper respiratory tract in Paddington families, 1952–4. *British Medical Journal*, **i**, 1200.

MEDICAL RESEARCH COUNCIL (1948) Specific laboratory tests in streptomycin therapy of tuberculosis. *Lancet*, **ii**, 862.

MISHULOW, LUCY, SHARPE, L. S. & COHEN, LILLIAN L. (1953) Beef-heart charcoal agar for the preparation of pertussis vaccines. *American Journal of Public Health*, **43**, 1466.

MONSUR, K. A. (1963) Bacteriological diagnosis of cholera under field conditions. *Bulletin of the World Health Organization*, **28**, 387.

MOORE, W. B. (1968) Solidified media suitable for the cultivation of *Clostridium novyi* type B. *Journal of General Microbiology*, **53**, 415.

MUELLER, J. H. & HINTON, JANE (1941) A protein-free medium for primary isolation of the gonococcus and meningococcus. *Proceedings of the Society of Experimental Biology and Medicine*, **48**, 330.

NAGLER, F. P. O. (1944) Bacteriological diagnosis of gas gangrene due to *Clostridium oedematiens*. *Nature (London)*, **153**, 496.

NAYLOR, P. G. D. (1961) An improved method for the preparation of 'chocolate' agar. *Journal of Medical Laboratory Technology*, **18**, 275.

NICOLLE, C. (1908) Culture du parasite du bouton d'Orient. *Comptes Rendu de l'Academie des Sciences (Paris)*, **146**, 842.

NOGUCHI, H. (1912) The pure cultivation of *Spirochaeta duttoni*, *Spirochaeta kochi*, *Spirochaeta obermeieri* and *Spirochaeta novyi*. *Journal of Experimental Medicine*, **16**, 199.

NOVY, F. G. & MACNEAL, W. J. (1904) On the cultivation of *Trypanosoma brucei*. *Journal of Infectious Diseases*, **1**, 1.

Pharmacopeia of the United States of America (1970) 18th edition, Sterility tests, p. 851.

PHILLIPS, I., HUMPHREY, D., MIDDLETON, A. & NICOL, C. S. (1972) Diagnosis of gonorrhoea by culture on a selective medium containing vancomycin, colistin, nystatin and trimethoprim (VCNT). *British Journal of Venereal Diseases*, **48**, 287.

PIKE, R. M. (1944) An enrichment broth for isolating haemolytic streptococci from throat swabs. *Proceedings of the Society of Experimental Biology (New York)*, **57**, 186.

REID, J. D., JONES, MURIEL M. & CARTER, EVELYN B. (1953) A simple, clear medium for demonstration of chlamydospores of *Candida albicans*. *American Journal of Clinical Pathology*, **23**, 938.

Reports on Public Health and Medical Subjects, No. 71 (1970) The bacteriological examination of water supplies, reprint; p. 45. London: H.M. Stationery Office.

ROBERTSON, D. S. F. (1970) Selenium – a possible teratogen? *Lancet*, **i**, 518.

ROBINSON, G. L. (1968) The laboratory diagnosis of human parasitic amoebae. *Transactions of the Royal Society of Tropical Medicine and Hygiene*, **62**, 285.

ROGOSA, M., MITCHELL, J. A. & WISEMAN, R. F. (1951) A selective medium for the isolation and enumeration of oral and faecal lactobacilli. *Journal of Bacteriology*, **62**, 132.

SAKAZAKI, R. (1969) Halophilic Vibrio infections. In *Food-borne Infections and Intoxications.* p. 115. Edited by H. Riemann, New York and London: Academic Press.

SHEPARD, M. C. (1969) Fundamental biology of the T-strains. In *The Mycoplasmatales and the L-phase of Bacteria.* p. 49. Edited by L. Hayflick, Amsterdam: North-Holland Publishing Company.

SMITH, H. W. (1953) Modifications of Dubos's media for the cultivation of *Mycobacterium johnei. Journal of Pathology and Bacteriology*, **66**, 375.

SMITH, K. (1964) Personal communication.

STOKES, E. JOAN (1968a) *Clinical Bacteriology.* p. 300. London: Edward Arnold.

STOKES, E. JOAN (1968b) Quality control in diagnostic bacteriology. *Proceedings of the Royal Society of Medicine*, **61**, 457.

STOKES, E. JOAN & WHITBY, J. L. (1971) Quality control in bacteriology: preliminary trials. *Journal of Clinical Pathology*, **24**, 790.

STONEBRINK, B. (1957) Tubercle bacilli and pyruvic acid. *Proceedings of the Tuberculosis Research Council*, **44**, 67.

STONEBRINK, B., DOUMA, J., MANTEN, A. & MULDER, R. J. (1969) A comparative investigation of the quality of various culture media as used in the Netherlands for the isolation of Mycobacteria. Selected papers. *Royal Netherlands Tuberculosis Association*, **12**, 5.

STUART, R. D. (1946) The preparation and use of a simple culture medium for leptospirae. *Journal of Pathology and Bacteriology*, **58**, 343.

STUART, R. D. (1959) Transport medium for specimens in Public Health bacteriology. *Public Health Report (Washington)*, **74**, 431.

ŠULA, L. (1947) Die Fibrinspinngewebshäutchen-Kultur von Tuberkelbazillen aus Exsudaten bei sog. idiopathischen Pleuritiden. *Schweizerische Zeitschrift für allgemeine Pathologie und Bakteriologie*, **10**, 125.

SYKES, G. (1956) Constituents of Bacteriological Culture Media. *Report of the Society for General Microbiology.* Cambridge University Press.

TAPLIN, D., ZAIAS, N., REBELL, G. & BLANK, H. (1969) Isolation and recognition of dermatophytes on a new medium (D.T.M.). *Archives of Dermatology*, **99**, 203.

TASCHDJIAN, CLAIRE L. (1957) Routine identification of *Candida albicans*: current methods and a new medium. *Mycologia*, **49**, 332.

THAYER, J. D. & MARTIN, J. E. (1966) Improved medium selective for cultivation of *N. gonorrhoeae* and *N. meningitidis. Public Health Report (Washington)*, **81**, 559.

The Milk (Special Designations) (Scotland) Order 1965. p. 21. London: H.M. Stationery Office.

TOBIE, E. J., VON BRAND, T. & MEHLMAN, B. (1950) Cultural and physiological observations on *Trypanosoma rhodesiense* and *Trypanosoma gambiense. Journal of Parasitology*, **36**, 48.

WATT B. (1972) The recovery of clinically important anaerobes on solid media. *Journal of Medical Microbiology*, **5**, 211.

WILLIS, A. T. & HOBBS, G. (1959) Some new media for the isolation and identification of clostridia. *Journal of Pathology and Bacteriology*, **77**, 511.

WILSON, W. J. (1938) Isolation of *Bact. typhosum* by means of bismuth sulphite medium in water- and milk-borne epidemics. *Journal of Hygiene (London)*, **38**, 507.

WOLFF, J. W. (1954) *The Laboratory Diagnosis of Leptospirosis.* p. 23. Springfield: Thomas.

WRIGHT, H. D. (1933) The importance of adequate reduction of peptone in the preparation of media for the pneumococcus and other organisms. *Journal of Pathology and Bacteriology*, **37**, 257.

YOUMANS, G. P. (1944) Subsurface growth of virulent human tubercle bacilli in a synthetic medium. *Proceedings of the Society of Experimental Biology (New York)*, **57**, 122.

YOUNG, M. Y. (1942) Diphtheria diagnosis with Hoyle's medium. Saponin and sodium-dioctyl-sulpho-succinate as haemolysing agents in the preparation of the medium. *Journal of Pathology and Bacteriology*, **54**, 253.

6. Cultivation of Bacteria and Fungi

General methods of culture and preservation of microorganisms are described here. Special methods applicable for particular purposes are referred to elsewhere, in the appropriate chapters. Personal safety precautions are described in Chapter 16.

INSTRUMENTS USED TO INOCULATE CULTURE MEDIA

The instrument is chosen according to the nature of the medium and inoculum. Inoculating wires are widely used. The original type of inoculating wire was of platinum, No. 23 SWG, $2\frac{1}{2}$ in (6·4 cm) long, but owing to the high cost of platinum, 'Nichrome' or 'Eureka' resistance wire, No. 24 SWG, is now generally used. However, nichrome is oxidizing and either stainless steel or platinum-iridium is a better choice for work with anaerobes. One end of the wire is fused into a glass rod, or inserted into a special aluminium holder.

The wire is sterilized by holding it vertically in a Bunsen flame so that the whole length becomes red-hot at the same time. A wire charged with particulate growth, such as that of the tubercle bacillus, should be sterilized slowly in the cooler part of the flame, or a loop incinerator (Darlow, 1959), or a hooded Bunsen burner (Fig. 6.1), to avoid spurting

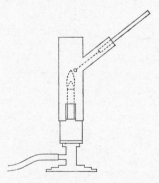

FIG. 6.1
A bunsen burner hooded with a metal tube to avoid spurting of unsterile particles during flaming of a charged wire loop.

of particles of unsterilized culture from the wire on to the bench.

Wire loop. The free end is bent in the form of a loop of 2–4 mm internal diameter, care being taken that the loop is flat, circular and completely closed. This is the most useful of the inoculating wires. It takes up a considerable amount of solid culture or a large drop of liquid.

Straight wire. This is used for stab cultures and also for picking off single colonies.

Thick wire (c. No. 60 SWG). Used as a loop, this is more rigid and is very useful for lifting thick viscid sputum; as an L-shaped wire, it is used to handle tenacious growths such as fungal colonies.

Scalpel. A sterile scalpel is used for making inoculations with scrapings from tissues and ulcers.

Sterile pipettes. Bulb pipettes (10–100 ml) are used when large amounts of liquid inoculum have to be added to a medium, and graduated 1-ml or 10-ml pipettes when the inoculum is between 0·1 and 10 ml. These pipettes are stoppered with a cotton-wool plug in their upper end to guard against contamination of their interior or accidental aspiration of their contents. They are wrapped in paper or placed in a container and sterilized in the hot-air oven. Because of the danger of infection, pipettes should not be placed directly in the mouth.

Sterile capillary pipettes. These are made by heating the middle of a piece of glass tubing, 5 mm bore and 20 cm long in a Bunsen flame; when the glass has softened, the two ends are pulled out and a thin capillary is produced in the middle. This is broken after cooling and two pipettes are obtained. The capillary ends are cut to a convenient length with a file or carborundum disk and the other ends are plugged with cotton-wool. They are placed in a container such as a large test-tube (e.g. $8 \times 1\frac{1}{2}$ in, $20·3 \times 3·8$ cm) which is then stoppered with cotton-wool, or covered with paper or aluminium foil and sterilized by dry heat. An alternative method is to prepare the 20-cm lengths of glass tubing with cotton-wool plugs in each end, wrap them in bundles of 8–10 in Kraft paper, sterilize in the hot-air oven and draw the capillaries in a flame just before they are required for use. These pipettes are useful for the sterile transfer of liquid in volumes that do not need to be measured accurately.

Capillary pipettes delivering measured drops. Small measured volumes are conveniently delivered with sterile capillary pipettes that have been prepared to give drops of a known volume. The pipettes are drawn from glass tubing as described above. When cool, the capillary is inserted into the appropriate hole of a Morse drill gauge and pressed through until it engages. For water drops of 0·020 ml the hole used is Morse 59 (i.e. 0·041 in diameter), for 0·025 ml Morse 55 (0·052 in), for 0·030 ml Morse 52 (0·063 in), for 0·035 ml Morse 47 (0·078 in) and for 0·040 ml Morse 43 (0·089 in). Exactly at its point of impaction in the hole, the capillary is scored with a glass-cutter (e.g. a vulcanite carborundum disk), and broken off squarely. The wide end of each pipette is then plugged with cotton-wool and the pipettes are packed in a large test-tube or a small tin and sterilized in the hot-air oven. In use, the liquid is drawn into the pipette by a teat. For accurate work, there should be a good volume of fluid in the pipette which should be held vertically, tip down, and the drops should be expelled at a constant rate of about 40 per minute, i.e. taking about $1\frac{1}{2}$ seconds for the gradual expulsion of one drop. The drop size may differ slightly in the case of liquids with different densities and surface tensions from that of water and the pipette should be calibrated directly for the particular liquid by measuring the volume of 100 drops. For further details consult Fildes (1931) or Miles and Misra (1938).

METHODS FOR MAKING SUBCULTURES

Since Petri dishes, tubes and bottles will be opened during inoculation of cultures and are therefore liable to contamination from the air, the bench should be free from dust and wiped with disinfectant at least before the start of each day's work and air currents should be reduced to a minimum by closing windows and doors and restricting the movement of people in the room. During inoculation, the culture medium should be uncovered for only a few seconds.

Formerly, when all tubes were fitted with cotton-wool plugs it was the practice to hold two or three tubes in the left hand and the plugs between the fingers of the right hand while inoculating from one tube to another. Push-on caps have now largely replaced plugs for tubes and are often either relatively loose or relatively tight because tubes vary by up to 1 mm in external diameter. For this reason it is unwise to attempt to manage more than one tube and its cap at a time. The same applies to bottles with screw caps because of the need for a screwing action to remove them.

In addition, when all tubes had cotton-wool plugs it was the practice to flame the mouths of all tubes before and after any manipulation, because the rims of tubes are not covered by plugs and are probably contaminated; in replacing the plug, organisms could be pushed down from the rim into the tube. The situation is quite different with metal caps and screw-caps. Accordingly, flaming of the mouths of tubes and bottles is not done as a routine, though the practice should be observed after any manipulation involving a container that has a cotton-wool plug.

CULTURE PROCEDURE

The following description applies to operators who are right-handed.

Place the lighted Bunsen burner and inoculating instruments to the right of the bench, and cultures and media to the back and the left. Plate cultures and uninoculated plates should be placed with the lid on the bench and the bottom containing the medium uppermost. The caps or plugs of tubes and bottles should be loosened for easy removal.

Media to be inoculated should be labelled at this stage, indicating the inoculum and the date, with a glass-marking pen or pencil or self-adhesive label. Labelling should be done on the bottoms of Petri dishes, on tubes and on bottles rather than on lids or caps which can be mistakenly placed on other cultures. Labels should be checked for accuracy while media are being seeded.

During inoculation the right hand holding the inoculating instrument charged with culture should be moved as little as possible and the left hand should bring the cultures and media to it.

Removal of Inoculum for Subculture

Subculture from a plate culture. Take the holder of the inoculating loop or wire in the first two fingers of the right hand (as in holding a pen) and flame it. Lift the plate culture with the left hand from its lid and hold it round the side with the thumb and middle finger. Cool the loop or wire by touching an uninoculated part of the medium and then pick the selected growth. Return the plate culture to its lid.

Subculture from a tube with a cotton-wool plug or a metal or plastic cap or a bottle with a screw cap. The inoculating instrument may be a loop or wire or, if the culture is in a liquid medium, a capillary pipette.

Hold the inoculating instrument in the right hand and flame it. Pick up the tube or bottle in the left hand and remove the cap or plug with the crooked third and fourth fingers of the right hand. If the culture is on a solid medium the loop or wire can be cooled by touching a portion of medium free from growth. If the culture is in a liquid medium it should not be touched with a hot loop, wire or capillary pipette because spluttering is particularly liable to form a contaminated aerosol. Remove the inoculum by scraping growth from the surface of solid medium or taking up a loopful or other aliquot of liquid medium with a cool inoculating instrument. Flame the mouth of the tube if it has a cotton-wool plug. Replace the cap or plug and return the tube or bottle to its place. After inoculation of the subculture check that the cap or plug has been replaced firmly.

Inoculation of Subculture

Seeding a plate. It is better to use a loop than a wire to seed a plate.

Lift the bottom of the Petri dish containing medium from its lid with the left hand and hold it round the side with the thumb and middle finger. In most cases the method of plating-out shown in Fig. 6.2 is employed. The inoculum is smeared thoroughly over area A to give a

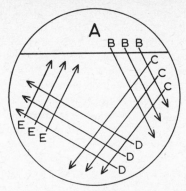

Fig. 6.2
The commonly adopted pattern of plating-out on solid medium. The area A is the well, and successive series of strokes B, C, D and E are made with the loop sterilized between each sequence.

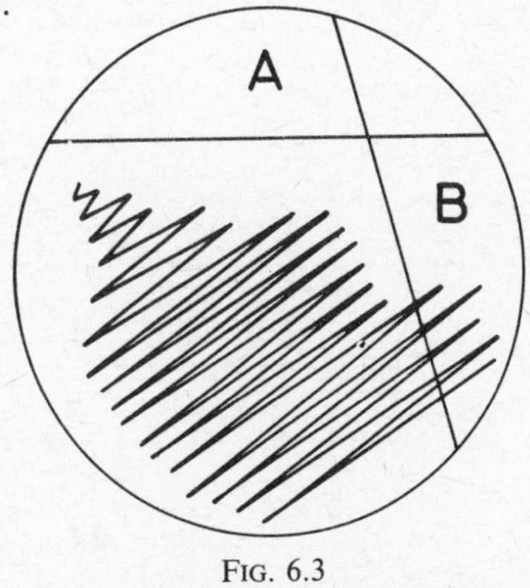

'well-inoculum' or 'well'. The loop is re-sterilized and then drawn from the well in two or three parallel lines on to the fresh surface of the medium (B, B, B); this process is repeated as shown, care being taken to sterilize and then cool the loop on uninoculated medium between each sequence. At each step the inoculum is derived from the most distal part of the immediately preceding strokes. Another quicker method of achieving a dilution of the inoculum that is high enough to yield separate colonies is to change to a 4-mm loop after spreading the well, sterilize it and use one side of the loop to spread an area B and the other side as a fresh sterile surface to make a succession of several strokes across the plate as shown in Fig. 6.3.

Fig. 6.3
An alternative plating procedure in which one edge of a larger loop is used to make a secondary well B. The other edge is then used to make a succession of strokes across the remaining unseeded area.

When the inoculum is small or the medium is selective it can be more heavily inoculated (Fig. 6.4). Several loopfuls of the specimen are used to spread the well (A); the loop is re-sterilized in a flame, recharged by rubbing it over area A and then used to seed the remainder of the plate by successive parallel strokes, B, C and D, drawn in the directions indicated in the diagram. When this method is used with small inocula or selective media, well separated colonies can be obtained from a heavy inoculation except, of course, in the well of the plate.

Subcultures from liquid media may be distributed with a spreader. This is made by bending a piece of glass rod of 3 mm diameter at a right angle in the blowpipe flame, the short limb used for spreading being 2 cm long. Spreaders may be sterilized in the hot-air oven, a number being packed in a metal tin with a 'press-on' lid loosely applied. Alternatively, a sterile capillary pipette held horizontally may be heated about 1 cm from its tip in the pilot flame of a Bunsen burner. As the glass softens, the end of the pipette bends at right angles and this forms a spreader. The inoculum is placed on the plate with an inoculating loop or capillary pipette and then, with a sterilized spreader, it is evenly distributed over the surface. If a large inoculum is used, incubation will result in a confluent growth called a 'lawn'. Media seeded in this way may be used for disk diffusion tests for assessing sensitivity to antibiotics and other chemotherapeutic agents or for phage typing.

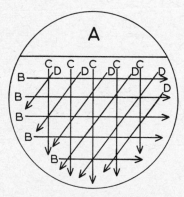

Fig. 6.4

A plating procedure used when the inoculum is scanty or when a highly selective medium is used (see text).

After the plate has been seeded, the bottom of the Petri dish is returned to its lid and the loop is flamed or the capillary pipette is discarded into a jar of disinfectant, care being taken to fill the pipette with the disinfectant. Plates are incubated in the inverted position with the lid underneath.

Seeding a tube fitted with a cotton-wool plug or a metal or plastic cap or a bottle with a screw cap. Pick up the tube or bottle with the left hand and remove the cap or plug with the crooked third and fourth fingers of the right hand. Slopes of solid media are seeded by lightly smearing the surface of the agar with the loop or wire in a transverse zig-zag pattern taking care not to wound the agar. Stab cultures in solid media are inoculated by plunging the wire into the centre of the medium and withdrawing it in the same line to avoid splitting of the medium. Liquid cultures are usually inoculated from a solid medium by inclining the tube or bottle at an angle of about 45° and depositing the inoculum on its wall above the surface of the liquid at its lower end. When the container is returned to the vertical position, the inoculum is below the surface of the liquid. Capillary pipettes or loops may be used for inoculation from liquid media.

After inoculation withdraw the loop, wire or pipette. Flame the mouth of the tube if it has a cotton-wool plug. Replace the cap or plug and return the tube or bottle to its place, at the same time flaming the loop or wire or discarding the pipette into disinfectant as described above. Check that the cap or plug has been replaced firmly.

Shake cultures are made by melting nutrient agar in a test tube, cooling it to 45°C and inoculating it while molten from a liquid medium with a drop from a capillary pipette or a wetted straight wire, depending on the desired size of inoculum. Withdraw the pipette or wire and flame the mouth of the tube if it has a cotton-wool plug. Replace the cap or plug and discard the pipette into disinfectant or flame the wire. Mix the contents of the tube by rotation between the palms of the hands before the agar solidifies.

Seeding several tubes and bottles of media from a single colony, as in the identification of enteric bacteria. It is best to use a wire to pick a single colony. The media are arranged in order for inoculation, firstly liquid media without carbohydrate, such as peptone water, then liquid media containing carbohydrate, then solid media for surface culture and lastly solid media for stab culture such as motility test medium. The wire charged with inoculum is lightly touched on the moist wall of each tilted liquid medium in turn, then streaked lightly on the solid media and plunged into the deep cultures, and then it is flamed.

Ørskov's method for studying the morphology of growing bacterial cells. This elegant method (Ørskov, 1923) allows the maintenance of living cultures under continuous observation so that the development of individual bacteria and also that of colonies can be studied.

Cubes of suitable size not exceeding 3–4 mm in thickness are cut out of an agar plate with a sterilized knife. They are transferred with the knife to a sterilized microscope slide. The agar is now inoculated with the organism by a fine stroke. With first a low-power objective the stroke is defined and then with a higher power an area is found where the bacteria lie sufficiently scattered. With a suitable lamp and objective and with the diaphragm closed down, young bacteria appear as strongly refractile and well-defined bodies. The area is then registered by means of the vernier scales on the mechanical stage. The slide is removed and placed in a Petri dish with a piece of moist filter paper in the bottom, and the dish is incubated at a suitable temperature. The selected area is then examined at intervals and the changing features observed. In this way the development of individual bacteria can be studied and also that of colonies at each stage. (An electrically heated microscope incubator allows a colony to be observed microscopically throughout its period of growth and this is very convenient for these and similar studies.)

Inoculation Hood or Cabinet

It is advisable, as far as possible, to carry out certain inoculation procedures under a hood, but the operator should clearly understand the operation of the particular system that he employs. Some systems are designed primarily to prevent contamination of the culture and

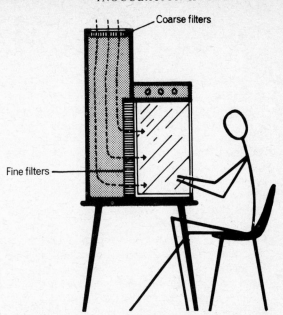

Coarse filters

Fine filters

Fig. 6.5

An inoculation cabinet in which a laminar flow of filtered air is delivered at the rear and passes forward over the handling area. Note that this system safeguards the work but must not be used for the manipulation of infective material as the airstream is directed towards the operator.

subculture media. For example, Fig. 6.5 illustrates a cabinet in which filtered air passes from the back panel to the front. This is useful for the manipulation of sterile media as in dispensing or plate-pouring procedures; it should be noted that this system blows virtually into the face of the operator and must not be used for the manipulation of potentially infective material.

A less expensive (and inevitably less effective) inoculation hood can be made as follows. A suitable size is 5 ft wide, 5 ft deep, and 7 ft 6 in high. The hood fits over the bench to form a completely enclosed chamber and access is provided via a sliding (not swing) door. All sides above the bench level consist of windows. Ventilation is secured by two holes in the roof; from the top of each is attached a vent pipe 3 in wide and 18 in long, and turned at right angles. The bench on which the hood is fitted should have a gas supply for the Bunser burner, and it is convenient to have a pipe from the roof 3 in in diameter with a funnel-shaped opening situated 24 in above the bench top, under which the Bunsen burner is placed so that the gas fumes are led directly away. The hood may be lighted by an electric lamp suspended from the roof.

The table under the hood is covered by a towel soaked in a disinfectant to destroy any organisms deposited in dust. The advantage of the hood depends on the relative absence of dust and air currents, which are likely to produce contamination of medium exposed in the process of inoculation. The inoculating hood may be used with advantage in the preparation of blood agar plates and other highly nutritive media and in conducting autopsies on animals under aseptic conditions.

A more simple inoculation box which is movable can be easily constructed as shown in the figure (Fig. 6.6). The frame is made of wood; it has a sloping glass window in front, and two apertures whereby the hands and arms can be inserted to carry out the necessary manipulation of the cultures. A convenient size is 3 ft wide, 2 ft deep and 3 ft high.

An effective inoculation hood or cabinet for the handling of *infective* material is designed so that air is pulled past the operator into the system and then discharged safely so that the immediate environment outside the cabinet is not contaminated. When work is done with dangerous pathogens, such as the tubercle bacillus, it is advisable that procedures are carried out in such a safety cabinet fitted with a ventilation system that does not allow contamination of the laboratory air and an ultraviolet lamp that can be used to disinfect the cabinet after the work is finished. A suitable cabinet has been described by Williams and Lidwell (1957). Convenient cabinets are available commercially, e.g. the 'Bassaire' cabinet supplied by John Bass Ltd., Crawley, Sussex. These safety cabinets are also quite suitable for carrying out dust-free inoculations and other procedures. For a discussion on the control of rate of air flow and the changing of filters in these cabinets see Kelsey *et al.* (1970).

The use of a laminar flow filtered airstream operating transversely in a cabinet offers many advantages. Laminar flow work cabinets provide maximal protection both to the worker and the work but, if they are recirculating systems, they demand a particularly high standard of maintenance (Akers *et al.*, 1969).

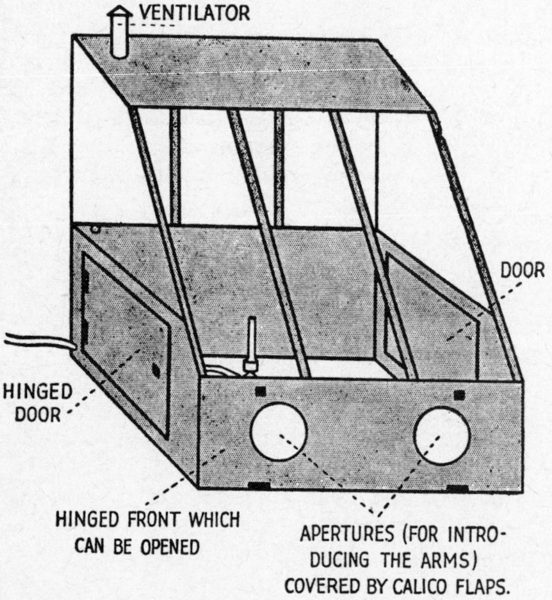

INCUBATION

Incubators

Students and others commencing work in a laboratory should familiarize themselves with the mechanism of the incubator, whereby any desired temperature may be constantly maintained. Incubators may be heated by electricity, gas or oil, according to the facilities of the laboratory.

All medical bacteriological laboratories have one or more incubators working at 37°C. This incubation temperature, which is the optimum for practically all pathogenic organisms of man, is that assumed when the temperature is not specified.

Some laboratories have a warm room kept at 37°C by gas or electricity in which large quantities of material can be incubated. The room has a regulating mechanism similar to that of the ordinary incubator to keep the temperature constant, and if electrically heated it should be fitted with a device to cut off the current for the room at the main switch if the temperature rises above 40°C.

FIG. 6.6
A simple inoculation box for manipulation of cultures.

Other temperatures for incubation are 30°C, used for cultivating leptospires and some bacteria, 25–28°C, used for many fungi, and 22°C ('cool incubator'), used for some fungi and for gelatin cultures (for viruses see Chaps 9 and 10).

In order to prevent drying of the medium when prolonged incubation is necessary, as in the cultivation of the tubercle bacillus, screw-capped bottles should be used instead of test-tubes.

ANAEROBIC INCUBATION

Obligate anaerobes are defined as organisms that will grow only in the absence of free oxygen. It has proved easier to culture them in the depths of liquid or solid media than on the surface of solid media and methods for preparing liquid semi-solid or deep media in tubes for the cultivation of anaerobes in the aerobic incubator are described in Chapter 5. For surface cultures, oxygen must be removed from the atmosphere above the culture either by using it for combustion or by replacing it with an inert gas.

The removal of oxygen by combustion is nearly always achieved by combining it with hydrogen to form water in the presence of a palladium catalyst. This method was originally used by McIntosh and Fildes (1916) to produce anaerobic conditions for plate cultures in tins or jars by coating asbestos wool with palladium and enclosing it in wire gauze to reduce the risk of explosion by conducting heat away on the Davy lamp principle. The capsules of catalyst had to be heated immediately before the jar was closed and depended on the heat of reaction to maintain the temperature necessary for their activity. The technique went through many refinements such as electrical heating of the palladiumized asbestos (Smillie, 1917; Brown, 1921), a modification that had the major disadvantage of requiring 20 to 40 minutes for complete combustion; the use of a pump to evacuate most of the air from the jar; and construction of more elaborate and more securely airtight jars. A full description of the operation of this type of jar is given by Cruickshank (1968). Concurrently, particularly in the U.S.A., a technique of repeated evacuation of jars and filling with an inert gas such as nitrogen

was used. This method tended to dehydrate cultures and it was modified for anaerobes that required prolonged incubation by using only one partial evacuation and catalysing the combustion of hydrogen with finely divided palladiumized asbestos in a flat porcelain dish uncovered by protective gauze and active at room temperature (Weiss and Spaulding, 1937). A significant advance was made when Wright (1943) increased the catalytic activity of palladium by presenting to the hydrogen and oxygen in the jar a large surface heavily impregnated with metallic palladium. Wright found that the palladium formed by the decomposition of 0·125 g (between 0·1 g and 0·15 g) palladium chloride coated on 0·15 g of finely teased-out asbestos and enclosed in copper gauze was spontaneously active at room temperature and suitable for a jar holding about 10 Petri dishes. This was a much heavier impregnation than had been used by McIntosh and Fildes (0·09 g palladium chloride on 0·15 g asbestos wool) and was used successfully at its minimum level by Hayward (1945) as a room-temperature catalyst. A full description of the operation of this type of jar is given by Cruickshank (1968).

A change from asbestos as the support was made when Heller (1954) advocated the use of 'Deoxo' pellets in which palladium is coated on alumina. This convenient form of the catalyst has now almost completely replaced palladiumized asbestos obtained commercially or prepared in the laboratory. 'Deoxo' pellets are available from Baker Platinum Ltd., London, and jars incorporating them as a room-temperature catalyst from Baird and Tatlock Ltd., Chadwell Heath, Essex, England.

The following technique is recommended (Collee, Rutter and Watt, 1971; Collee, Watt, Fowler and Brown, 1972) to provide anaerobiosis with an increased concentration of carbon dioxide in these jars (Fig. 6.7) as CO_2 enhances the growth of many clinically important anaerobes on solid media (Watt, 1973). The jar itself (8×5 in) should be made of metal with a lid that can be clamped down to make it airtight. Glass jars have been used in the past, but, as explosions occasionally occur, their use is not justified. The lid is furnished with two tubes and taps. One or

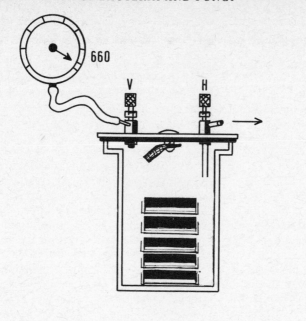

1. EVACUATE to - 660 mm Hg

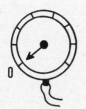

2. ADMIT 90 per cent. H_2 + 10 per cent. CO_2 mixture
    until gauge registers ZERO

3. CLOSE VALVES   V and H

LEAVE JAR AT ROOM TEMPERATURE FOR 10 MINUTES

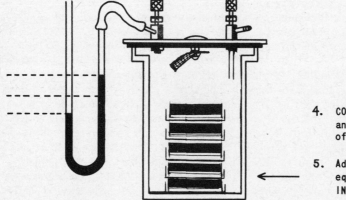

4. CONNECT VALVE V to manometer
    and confirm secondary vacuum
    of at least - 15 mm Hg

5. Admit H_2 : CO_2 mixture to
    equilibrate. Close valves.
    INCUBATE JAR.

FIG. 6.7   A standardized procedure for setting up an anaerobic jar fitted with a 'room-temperature' catalyst.

more capsules containing pellets of palladiumized alumina are suspended under the lid.

The most convenient source of hydrogen and carbon dioxide is cylinders of the compressed gases supplied commercially. The pressure in these cylinders is too great for them to be connected directly to the anaerobic jar and they should be fitted with reducing valves to deliver the gases at a constant pressure (e.g. 2–3 lb/in²) which can be predetermined or altered at will. Separate football bladders can be filled with the gases from the cylinders and used to deliver them to jars. Alternatively, a gas mixture of hydrogen 90 per cent and carbon dioxide 10 per cent can be held in one cylinder and delivered via one bladder. Tubes or Petri dishes with the medium uppermost and lid downwards are placed inside the jar. It is advisable to separate the lid about 1 mm from the rim of glass dishes by the insertion of a bent wire or fragment of blotting-paper or to make a few vertical cuts with a hot wire in the sides of plastic dishes, unless vented plates are used. Sealing of the lid to the bottom of an unvented Petri dish during evacuation of the jar by condensation moisture, interferes with removal of oxygen from inside the Petri dish. After putting the plates into the jar the lid is clamped on. Approximately $\frac{6}{7}$ of the air is evacuated (pressure reduced to 100 mmHg, i.e. 660 mm below atmospheric) and this is monitored on a vacuum gauge. The pump is disconnected and the gauge watched for a few seconds to check for leaks in the jar. The reduced pressure is brought up to 160 mmHg (600 below atmospheric) with carbon dioxide and then to 760 mmHg (i.e. atmospheric) or a slightly higher pressure with hydrogen from the rubber bladders, monitored on the vacuum gauge. The jar is then connected to a simple mercury manometer. Initially, the pressure in the jar is slightly above atmospheric, depending on the pressure of the gas supply via the hydrogen bladder, but if the catalyst is normally active, a decrease in pressure of at least 20 mm of mercury occurs within 10 min after the admission of hydrogen. This rapid development of an internal pressure change is important evidence that the palladium catalyst is active. More hydrogen is then introduced to equilibrate the pressure and the jar is incubated at 37°C.

Because a mercury manometer is used to detect pressure changes in the jar to indicate catalyst activity, wash bottles between the bladders and the jar are unnecessary.

The catalytic activity of the palladium may be seriously impaired by moisture which can be removed by heating the whole capsule in the outer part of a Bunsen flame. Moreover, inactive palladium sulphide may be formed from hydrogen sulphide evolved by cultures in the jar. When this happens, or if the catalyst becomes inactive for any cause other than moisture, it is best to discard the capsule. There is no precise information about the best relationship between the concentrations or amount of palladium on palladiumized alumina pellets and the volume of the jar. An awareness of this problem has always been apparent, from McIntosh and Fildes (1916) who said that a larger jar required more palladium to Collee et al. (1971) who used 3 capsules of palladiumized alumina pellets in each jar for their more exacting experiments.

An aerobic indicator is not necessary because the technique includes safeguards to ensure that the jar does not leak badly and that the catalyst capsule is active at room temperature.

Cultures on solid media for anaerobic incubation should be put in an anaerobic jar as soon as they are seeded. Many non-sporing anaerobes are readily killed by exposure to air and, even with clostridia, spores cannot be relied on to compensate for the toxicity of air to vegetative cells (Watt, 1972).

A more expensive but important alternative to this procedure, especially in laboratories where facilities and experience in anaerobic bacteriology are limited, is the 'Gaspak' system (Baltimore Biological Laboratories) devised by Brewer and Allgeier (1966). This is marketed by Becton, Dickinson, U.K. Ltd., York House, Empire Way, Wembley, Middlesex. Controlled trials have shown it to be satisfactory for the cultivation of a wide variety of anaerobes of clinical importance when it was used with the Baird and Tatlock anaerobic jar (Collee et al., 1972). Water is added to an aluminium foil packet containing pellets of sodium borohydride and cobalt chloride and of citric acid and sodium bicarbonate; the packet is immediately put in the jar and its lid is screwed on. The following reactions take place to supply hydrogen and carbon dioxide.

$$NaBH_4 + 2H_2O \longrightarrow NaBO_2 + 4H_2$$
$$CoCl_2 \text{ catalyst}$$

$$C_3H_5O(COOH)_3 + 3NaHCO_3 \rightarrow$$
$$C_3H_5O(COONa)_3 + 3CO_2 + 3H_2O$$

The complete 'Gaspak' system includes a special anaerobic jar. Palladiumized alumina in a safety screen to catalyze the combustion of hydrogen and removal of oxygen is attached under the lid of the jar which has no taps. The jar is made of transparent polycarbonate. No pumps and no cylinders of gas are required. A fresh foil pack of reagents is necessary each time the jar is set up. An anaerobic indicator, either traditional (Cruickshank, 1968) or modified (Brewer, Allgeier and McLaughlin, 1966) is necessary to check the activity of the palladium catalyst.

More meticulous anaerobic methods to prevent access of air to media during preparation, inoculation and incubation have been developed. One of these methods, the manipulation of all these procedures under oxygen-free gas, was pioneered in 1950 by Hungate (see Hungate, 1969), developed by Moore (1966) and has been applied to clinical specimens by McMinn and Crawford (1970). Surface colonies are grown in roll tubes in which a thin layer of agar coats the inside of the tube. The medium must be transparent for surface colonies to be visible, and this precludes the use of blood agar. In the other method, anaerobic cabinets have been used (e.g. Socransky, MacDonald and Sawyer, 1959; Drasar and Crowther, 1971), an ingenious one being a flexible plastic chamber kept in shape like a balloon by a slight excess in gas pressure over atmospheric pressure (Aranki et al., 1969). However, the benefit of these more complex methods over the more traditional procedure described here may be only marginal provided that specimens are not delayed in transit and are immediately put up in an anaerobic jar by a standardized procedure.

Culture in an Atmosphere with Added Carbon Dioxide

Some organisms, such as Brucella abortus, require extra carbon dioxide in the air in which they are grown and others, such as the pneumococcus and gonococcus, grow better in air containing 5–10 per cent carbon dioxide. An anaerobic jar can be used for the purpose, but this abuses the catalyst. The required amount of air is withdrawn with a pump and replaced with carbon dioxide from a cylinder or football bladder as described for anaerobic culture. Much simpler closed containers, such as a tin (8×10 in) with a press-on lid obtainable from A. Gallenkamp and Co., Ltd., London, or a screw-capped jar, are satisfactory because the concentration of carbon dioxide is not critical and carbon dioxide is heavier than air and is slow to leak out even if the container is not air-tight. Carbon dioxide can be generated inside the container by lighting a candle in it just before putting on the lid or by adding hydrochloric acid to a marble chip as described by Cruickshank (1968), but the more elegant procedure of adding relatively pure CO_2 gas to a proper container is preferable.

Whichever method is used, screw-caps on containers of liquid media such as blood cultures should be replaced by sterile cotton-wool plugs to allow entry of carbon dioxide.

ISOLATION OF PURE CULTURES

Most studies and tests of the physiological, serological and other characters of bacteria are valid only when made on a pure culture, i.e. the growth of a single strain free from mixture and contamination with other bacteria. For this reason, in the diagnostic examination of mixed infective material, an essential preliminary is the isolation of the pertinent organism in a pure culture. Several techniques are available:

1. *Plating out on a solid culture medium.* The solid medium most used is nutrient agar either plain or enriched and usually dispensed as plates. In order to ensure separation, i.e. growth of discrete colonies, the surface of the medium must be dry. The infective material is inoculated on the surface by one of the methods described above so that bacteria are ultimately

deposited singly. Where the bacteria are at a sufficient distance from each other (e.g. 1 cm) the whole progeny of each accumulates locally during growth to form a discrete mass, or colony, which is readily visible to the naked eye (e.g. 0·5–5 mm diameter). Each colony is presumed to be a pure culture, consisting exclusively of the descendants of a single cell; it may be picked with a sterile wire to prepare a pure subculture in a fresh medium.

In picking off single colonies, particularly when they are very close to one another, care must be taken that the point of the wire does not touch any of the neighbouring colonies. The culture should first be looked at through the medium held up to the light, by removing the dish from its lid and holding it round the side. The colonies selected should be indicated by marks on the bottom of the dish. To pick off the colony, first sit down with both elbows on the bench. Hold the plate vertically with the left hand, then grasp the holder of the sterilized wire, with the fingers quite close to the wire. Steady the right hand by placing the little finger on the left thumb in the way that artists support the hand when painting. The selected colony is then easily removed without touching the others. Return the plate to its lid, withdraw the right hand to the other end of the holder and inoculate the required medium in the manner previously described.

Plate culture microscope. Several makers produce low-power binocular magnifiers which are extremely useful for examining plate cultures of organisms; these have a long working distance so that a colony can also be picked off the plate while using the instrument. When dealing with bacteria forming small delicate colonies, or where the colonies of the desired organism are few in number, the low-power binocular is invaluable. A magnification of ten diameters is useful for general work, but with interchangeable eye-pieces and objectives, an instrument with magnifications from six to thirty diameters can be available.

Occasionally a mixed colony is formed from two bacteria that have been inoculated close together on the agar or that grow in association, e.g. aerobe and anaerobe. If there is any doubt as to whether a pure colony has been obtained for picking, the colony should be replated immediately on a fresh plate and a single colony picked from this second plating. A culture should not be assumed to be pure unless a sub-culture from a single colony has been plated, found to be pure and picked again from a single colony on the pure plate. The maintenance of pure cultures necessitates the use of sterilized media, containers and instruments and continuous covering against the deposition of dust-borne bacteria from the air.

2. *Use of selective, enrichment or indicator media.* Media such as tellurite media for the diphtheria bacillus, have been devised so that the majority of organisms likely to be associated with those for which the media are used will not grow, and the isolation of pure cultures is thus facilitated. The risk of contamination of single colonies from selective media is high because bacteria that do not grow may survive under colonies and grow in subcultures.

Enrichment cultures such as selenite broth for *Salmonella spp.* favour the multiplication of particular species as a step towards their isolation in pure culture.

Indicator media such as Willis and Hobbs' medium for *Clostridium spp.* contain ingredients that change in appearance with particular organisms and so assist in their isolation.

3. *Use of selective growth conditions.* The temperature and atmosphere chosen for a culture automatically preclude the growth of many bacteria. Incubation at 37°C, used for most medically-important bacteria, is too warm for some air contaminants which subsequently appear as colonies when plates are kept at room temperature. Strict anaerobes will not grow in air and most facultative anaerobes grow less vigorously under anaerobic than under aerobic conditions.

4. *Selective treatment of the specimen before culture.* Heating at 65°C for 30 min can be used to separate spores from vegetative bacilli but there is no guarantee that spores will germinate under subsequent cultural conditions (Collee, Rutter and Watt, 1971). Sputum for culture of tubercle bacilli is treated with a chemical, such as $1N$ NaOH or saturated trisodium phosphate, to kill accompanying bacteria.

5. *Animal inoculation.* Advantage is taken of the fact that laboratory animals are highly susceptible to certain organisms—for example,

the mouse to the pneumococcus. If a mixture of organisms containing the pneumococcus, e.g. sputum, is inoculated subcutaneously into a mouse, the animal dies of pneumococcal septicaemia in 12–48 h, and from the heart blood the organism can be obtained in pure culture. Similarly, the tubercle bacillus can be isolated from contaminating organisms by inoculation of an infected specimen into a guinea-pig. The tubercle bacillus is found in a pure state in the resulting lesions.

BLOOD CULTURE

In most bacterial infections of the blood in man the organisms are not numerous, and it is essential for their demonstration by blood culture that a relatively large amount of blood, e.g. 5–10 ml, should be used as the inoculum. When such a quantity of blood is added to a culture medium, its natural bactericidal or bacteriostatic action may readily interfere with the growth of any bacteria present and it is therefore essential that this effect should be annulled by diluting the blood with medium. Alternatively, the antibacterial effect may be prevented by some substance incorporated in the medium. While it is not strictly necessary that the blood should remain unclotted in the medium, it is better to add an anticoagulant because bacteria trapped in the fibrin clot may be unable to grow.

Requisites

1. A 10-ml sterile disposable plastic syringe is best but an 'all-glass' syringe (with a firmly fitting needle) sterilized in the hot-air oven as described in Chapter 3 is a good alternative.

If a syringe that will not withstand dry heat at 160°C is used it must be heated in boiling water for at least 15 min; the syringe must not come into contact with any antiseptic; it should not be removed from the sterilizing bath until it is immediately required, unless it is held in a rack within the sterilizer to facilitate drying; the parts should be taken out of the boiling water and fitted together with the aid of sterile forceps so that the needle, nozzle and piston are not touched by the fingers. Extraneous bacterial contamination of blood specimens is more frequent when the syringes are boiled

(10 per cent of specimens contaminated) than when they are sterilized in the hot-air oven (1 per cent contaminated). Syringes are liable to be contaminated with non-sporing bacteria while being assembled after their removal from the boiling water.

2. Gauze or cotton-wool, bandage, or rubber tourniquet, antiseptic (e.g. 2 per cent iodine or 0·5 per cent chlorhexidine in 70 per cent alcohol or plain 70 per cent alcohol), methylated spirit, collodion (sterile dissecting forceps, Bunsen burner or spirit lamp if blood culture bottle is not used).

3. *Culture media.* It is advisable to inoculate blood for culture into more than one medium, preferably three, the choice of media depending on the history of the patient. An anaerobic medium such as cooked-meat broth or broth containing a large strip of sheet iron almost as long as the column of liquid should be included routinely (Stokes, 1968). Anaerobic media are essential for the strict anaerobes such as *Clostridium*, *Bacteroides* and *Fusobacterium* species; they improve the growth of some aerobes such as streptococci and most other aerobes will grow in them. The best available broth should be used for at least one of the other media. Hartley's broth is recommended. The addition of 0·1 to 0·5 per cent glucose improves the growth of pneumococci and streptococci. One part of filtered Liquor trypsini Co. (Allen and Hanbury's) to 10 parts of medium neutralizes the antibacterial effect of blood. Broth supplemented with glucose and trypsin may be used for the isolation of pyogenic cocci. Acid formed from glucose fermentation tends to kill bacteria and the addition of glucose to all cultures is not recommended. In suspected cases of enteric fever the patient's blood may be diluted 1 in 10 in 0·5 per cent sodium taurocholate broth. Special procedures or culture media used for blood culture in the diagnosis of certain infections such as brucellosis and leptospirosis are described in the appropriate chapters.

Anticoagulants such as sodium citrate (0·2 per cent) or ammonium oxalate (1 per cent) may be added to media for blood culture but these are liable to be inhibitory. Liquoid (sodium polyanethol sulphonate) is recommended because its inhibitory effect is only slight and it also neutralizes the natural bactericidal action of blood, reducing the need for high dilution of blood in the medium. Saponin broth, in which blood does not clot and is promptly lysed, is sometimes favoured for the isolation of *viridans* streptococci which may be slightly sensitive to Liquoid. In patients on sulphonamide or penicillin therapy, *p*-aminobenzoic acid or pencillinase is added respectively (p. 114).

Castaneda's method of including an agar medium on one of the narrow sides of bottles of broth for blood culture is excellent because it allows a subculture to be made without opening the bottle.

For use, 5–10 ml patient's blood is mixed with the liquid medium and allowed to flow over the agar. The bottle is incubated in the upright position and the agar surface is examined daily for colonies, being re-seeded every 48 h from the blood broth by allowing it to flow gently over the agar by suitably tilting the bottle.

Broth for blood culture may be provided in flasks or tubes with cotton-wool plugs or rubber stoppers but it is preferably dispensed in a special blood-culture bottle and this is especially convenient when the patient is some distance from the laboratory.

Blood-culture bottle. This consists of a 3-oz (90 ml) round bottle or a 4-oz (120 ml) 'medical flat' bottle, with a screw-cap, similar to that used for storing nutrient agar in 50-ml amounts (Chap. 5). A hole is punched out of the cap and the rubber washer is re-inserted. In order to protect the surface of the cap and the exposed portion of the rubber washer from contamination before use, the cap and neck of the bottle are covered with a 'viskap'. This is a cellulose preparation which is slipped on moist and allowed to dry. In so doing the viskap shrinks, moulding itself tightly to the cap and neck of the bottle.

The apparatus is fitted up as follows. The bottles are supplied in a carton already washed, cleaned and capped, so that no further preparation is required. The rubber washer is removed, a $\frac{5}{16}$ in hole is punched out of the centre of the cap by means of a hollow punch, and the rubber washer re-inserted. Media are dispensed in 10–50 ml amounts and sterilized in the bottles. When the bottles are cool the viskap, No. 2 semi-opaque cut $1\frac{3}{8}$ in, is at once slipped on. Viskaps dry in a few hours. The broth can be stored without deterioration.

Media can be identified by colouring the top of the viskap with cellulose paint and putting either a coloured bead in the bottle or a small dab of paint on the shoulder of the bottle so that the medium is still identified when the viskap is removed. Coloured labels are preferable for large numbers of bottles.

Withdrawal of Blood

The media are taken to the patient's bedside and if they are in bottles the viskaps are removed. The blood is drawn by vein puncture: the skin of the patient's arm at the bend of the elbow is *thoroughly disinfected* by first washing with soap and water, then applying spirit and finally treating with the antiseptic spirit solution. Thorough disinfection is necessary to avoid contamination of the culture with skin organisms such as staphylococci. Several turns of a bandage are applied round the upper arm about the middle of the biceps to render the veins turgid, or a piece of rubber tubing is wound firmly, but not too tightly, once round the arm and clipped with pressure forceps to provide a convenient and easily released tourniquet for the purpose. The turgescence of the veins can be increased by the patient's alternately opening and clenching the hand. The needle of the syringe is inserted into a prominent vein and 5–10 ml of blood are drawn into the syringe. The tourniquet is then released. The needle is now withdrawn from the vein.

The patient should raise the arm after blood has been withdrawn and firm pressure should be applied to the site of the puncture to obviate haematoma formation. The puncture wound may be dressed with gauze or cotton-wool and collodion, but the operator must attend to the withdrawn blood without delay.

If the medium is in blood culture bottles, the needle of the syringe containing the withdrawn blood is immediately passed through each rubber washer to expel blood into each medium. Punctures in the washers seal themselves when the needle is withdrawn. It is advisable to wipe the exposed portions of the washers with a little spirit, but other chemical antiseptics should be avoided. At the laboratory, screw caps must be replaced by sterile cotton-wool plugs for bottles to be incubated in anaerobic jars or in carbon-dioxide.

If the medium is in flasks or tubes the needle is detached from the syringe by means of forceps so that the nozzle is not touched by the fingers. The flask of broth is unstoppered and the blood is added to the broth. The mouth of the flask is flamed and re-stoppered. The blood and broth are thoroughly mixed and sent to the laboratory for incubation.

Quantitative counts of bacteria in blood are sometimes useful in differentiating between bacteriaemia and septicaemia or for prognostic purposes. A simple procedure is to inoculate 1·0-ml amounts of blood into several tubes of melted agar and make pour plates either at the bedside or from unclotted blood in Liquoid in the laboratory.

'Clot' culture. When blood samples from a patient with suspected enteric fever have been submitted for the Widal test, it is useful as a routine to cultivate the clot after the serum has been removed (see below).

If it is known that the blood has been withdrawn with strict aseptic precautions, the clot may be placed in a wide tube (8 × 1 in), half-filled with broth, or in a wide-mouth screw-capped bottle (8-oz pot) containing 80 ml of broth. When there is any doubt as to the presence of contaminating organisms, and this is always a possibility when specimens of blood are sent to the laboratory from a distance, the clot should be transferred directly to a tube of sterile ox bile. After incubation overnight the bile culture is examined for enteric organisms in the usual manner.

A method of clot culture with streptokinase* has been recommended (Watson, 1955). Blood is taken from the vein in the usual way and 5-ml quantities are allowed to clot in sterile screw-capped Universal containers. The separated serum is removed and 15-ml of bile-salt streptokinase broth is added to each bottle. The streptokinase causes rapid clot lysis with release of bacteria trapped in the clot. The cultures are then incubated.

Examination of blood culture. Growth is most likely to occur on the surface of sedimented red cells where colonies may be visible or as a generalized turbidity. However, it is important to make subcultures to solid media as a routine; early growth sometimes produces no visible effect in the broth. Extreme care must be taken to avoid contamination when cultures are opened during subculture to test for growth. Subcultures should be made quickly so that blood cultures do not cool appreciably. It is suggested that the first subculture be made after incubation for 18–24 h and that subcultures every second day be continued for at least 3 weeks or until an isolation is made. The subcultures are incubated in air, anaerobically, or in carbon dioxide in the same way as the blood culture from which they were made. Castaneda's method has the great advantage that the blood broth is tilted over the agar to make a subculture without opening the bottle.

Disposal of Cultures

Cultures to be discarded should be killed by heat or antiseptics. If a non-disposable container is used, sterilization must be achieved before the container is cleaned for re-use.

Autoclaving is preferable and must be used for cultures of the tubercle bacillus and sporing organisms such as Cl. tetani and B. anthracis. The necessary exposure time depends on the depth and shape of the discard culture container, the presence of free water and the rate of heating of the autoclave chamber (Rubbo and Gardner, 1965; and see also Chapter 3 in this volume).

Disinfection with 3 per cent lysol or cresol in a large container can be used for non-sporing organisms; this involves the opening of tubes, bottles and plates. Caps of screw-capped bottles must be completely unscrewed, caps and plugs are removed from tubes and caps, plugs, tubes and bottles are then immersed in disinfectant. Glass Petri dish cultures are also similarly immersed in disinfectant. These operations carry an infective risk and a toxic hazard for laboratory staff; it is better practice to use the autoclave as a routine and to avoid

*Streptokinase is obtainable from Calbiochem, Ltd., 10 Wyndham Place, London W1H 1AS.

these risks and the uncertainty of chemical disinfection.

Plastic Petri dish cultures are conveniently disposed of by incineration if facilities are available. Otherwise they can be autoclaved and then handled as safe rubbish. Plastic Petri dish cultures must be autoclaved in a separate bin from glassware. In the autoclave the plastic melts and can be lifted out of the bin in a fused lump for incineration.

COLD STORAGE

It is essential to have some form of cold storage in the laboratory for the preservation of blood, serum, culture media, cultures, vaccines, etc.

Mechanical refrigeration is now universally used, and refrigerators are available in a large number of sizes from $1\frac{1}{2}$ cubic feet capacity to cold storage rooms of several thousand cubic feet. For the smaller laboratory one of the domestic refrigerators of 4–7 cubic feet capacity is suitable, while larger laboratories require a correspondingly larger instrument, or an insulated cold room with the refrigerating plant outside. Mechanical refrigerators can be obtained to work with electricity, gas or oil, and most of them have provision for making small quantities of ice. The temperature should be maintained between 4°–5°C (39°–41°F); it should never be so low as to cause freezing, as this may be detrimental to vaccines, bacterial suspensions, red cells and certain sera containing a preservative.

It should be noted that with the domestic type of refrigerator an accumulation of ice, due to freezing of water vapour, surrounds the freezing unit, and at intervals (about 10–14 days) it is necessary to 'de-frost' to remove this ice. The contents of the refrigerator are removed, the current (or gas) turned off and the doors opened. The melted water from the ice is caught in a suitable receptacle. When the ice is melted the interior of the refrigerator is wiped with a cloth, the contents replaced, and the refrigerating unit started again.

It is convenient also to have a refrigerator working at low temperatures for the preservation of sera, viruses, etc., and one of the commercial type of 'deep freeze' refrigerators working at −10° to −40°C is suitable for this purpose.

PRESERVATION OF CULTURES

Bacterial species vary greatly in the ability of their cultures to remain alive after the completion of growth (e.g. after twenty-four hours at 37°C). Some species such as *Neisseria gonorrhoeae* and *Streptobacillus moniliformis* are poorly viable and their cultures usually die out within a few days, whether kept at 37°C, at room temperature or at 4°–5°C; thus, they must be subcultivated every two to four days for maintenance in the laboratory. Other species are much hardier, especially sporing species which may remain viable for many years. There are also many non-sporing species (e.g. enterobacteriaceae) whose cultures, under suitable conditions, commonly remain viable for several months and often for as much as a few years. Their prolonged preservation requires the following: (1) that drying of the culture is prevented by hermetic sealing of the tube or bottle with a screw-cap and new rubber liner, or with a cotton-wool plug soaked in paraffin wax; (2) that the culture is stored in the dark, and either at room temperature or in a refrigerator at 4°–5°C, but not at 37°C; and (3) that the culture be grown on a suitable preservation medium or as a nutrient agar stab culture. Organisms of the enterobacteria group may be kept alive on egg saline medium (p. 143) for several years without subcultivation; they survive longer than on nutrient agar, and are less liable to vary to the 'rough' state. The culture is grown overnight at 37°C and the screw-cap of the bottle is firmly tightened before storing in a dark, cool cupboard. Survival is dependent on the culture not being allowed to dry out.

It is desirable that at least a moderate proportion of the cells in the culture should remain alive; if only a few survive, these may be exclusively resistant mutants, all cells of the original type being lost. Frequent subcultivation also tends to replace the original type by mutants and must therefore be avoided as far as possible. Specific recommendations for the short-term preservation of bacterial cultures have been made by Stokes (1962). Full discussions of media for the maintenance and preservation of bacteria (Lapage, Shelton and Mitchell, 1970) and of culture collections and the preservation of bacteria (Lapage *et al.*, 1970) have been published.

PRESERVATION OF CULTURES AND SERA BY FREEZE-DRYING *IN VACUO*

When dried and kept in the dry state under suitable conditions, bacterial cultures and virus suspensions may remain viable for several years, and antisera may be preserved without appreciable loss of antibody potency. If such materials are dried from the liquid state, a high salt concentration is produced in the later stages of drying, which causes denaturation of proteins, death of organisms and deterioration of serum. This is largely avoided by the 'freeze-drying', or 'lyophile' method, in which the culture or serum is dried rapidly *in vacuo* from the frozen state. The material is frozen by a suitable method and then dried by sublimation of the ice. The sublimation is effected by exposure to an atmosphere of very low pressure (e.g. 0·01 mmHg or less) which is dried by a chemical desiccant or refrigerated condenser. The dried material is preserved *in vacuo* or under an inert gas such as nitrogen in hermetically sealed ampoules which are stored in the dark, either at room temperature or, preferably, in a refrigerator at 4°–5°C. This is a convenient means of preserving stock strains of bacteria, guinea-pig complement serum and samples of antisera required for reference or standardization purposes. On a larger scale, it is used for preserving therapeutic antisera, human plasma, antibiotics and vaccines.

Freezing must be very rapid, with the temperature lowered to well below 0°C (e.g. to −20°C), since slow freezing would prolong exposure to the denaturing influence of the suspending salt solution as it was concentrated to its eutectic level by the formation of pure ice crystals. The liquid should be frozen in a shallow layer with a large surface available for evaporation. Two methods of freezing are available: (1) *prefreezing*, i.e. before the drying process is begun; and (2) *evaporative freezing*, effected during the first stage of the drying process.

Prefreezing is generally employed for large volumes. The liquid is frozen as a layer, or 'shell', lining the walls of the bottle, either by rotating the bottle while immersed nearly horizontally in a bath of ethyl alcohol and solid carbon dioxide, or of refrigerated coolant, or by spinning the bottle on its vertical axis in a current of refrigerated air.

Evaporative freezing is conveniently employed for the smaller quantities that generally suffice for laboratory purposes. The liquid is quickly frozen by the withdrawal of latent heat during its initial rapid evaporation when exposed to the vacuum applied for drying. Precautions must be taken against frothing and spilling during desolution of the atmospheric gases; the 'centrifugal' and 'degassing' methods have been developed for this purpose. **Greaves's centrifugal method of freeze-drying.** This is a most convenient method for preserving a number of cultures and it is described fully by Lapage *et al.* (1970). Frothing is prevented by centrifuging the liquid during the first stage of evacuation and drying, until freezing is complete. A suitable centrifugal freeze-dryer* consists of a glass bell-jar and metal chamber containing the centrifuge and trays of desiccant for the primary drying, a manifold for the secondary drying, a rotary oil-sealed pump capable of drawing a vacuum below 0·04 mmHg and a Pirani-type pressure gauge. The liquid cultures or suspensions are dried in special neutral soft glass tubes or ampoules with a stem bore of 6 mm. The procedure is as follows:

1. Place in each ampoule a small strip of Whatman No. 1 filter paper on which has been typed the number designating the culture to be introduced. Plug the ampoules with absorbent cotton-wool and sterilize lying horizontal at 20 lbs (125°C) in the autoclave for 25 min. With a sterile capillary pipette, put 0·25–0,5 ml of liquid culture into each small 'ampoule' (tube type) and up to 2·5 ml into each of the larger ampoules. Discard the original sterility plug into disinfectant and insert a fresh, *loose* plug of sterile, non-absorbent cotton-wool, pressing it wholly within the stem of the ampoule, or cap each ampoule with sterile surgical gauze folded over the top and stapled at both sides.

2. Prepare the chamber for primary drying by charging the metal desiccant trays with fresh phosphorus pentoxide to the extent of at

---

* Supplied by Edwards High Vacuum Ltd., Crawley, Sussex.

least 3 g (about 10 ml) of powder per ml of water to be absorbed. (*Note:* Phosphorus pentoxide is corrosive and care must be taken to avoid spilling it on the skin, clothing or freeze-dryer. After each use of the dryer, the expended desiccant must be washed from the trays with an excess of water, taking care to avoid the corrosive fumes evolved, and the trays are then thoroughly dried. The makers' instructions must be followed for cleaning the apparatus and removing spilt powder, which may interfere with the working of the centrifuge motor.)

3. *Primary Drying.* Place the ampoules in the nearly vertical holes of the constant speed centrifuge. Cover the centrifuge with the bell-jar and press this firmly into position on the sealing ring of the base plate. (The contact surfaces are previously cleaned with ether and lightly smeared with high-vacuum grease.*) While pressing down the jar, switch on first the centrifuge and then the rotary pump. Observe the fall of pressure on the gauge. When a low pressure of about 1 mmHg (1 Torr) has been achieved, in five to ten minutes, it can be assumed that the material is frozen as a thin layer on the inner wall of the ampoule. *Immediately switch off the centrifuge to avoid overheating.* Leave the rotary pump running for a period sufficient to complete the primary drying: about three hours for 0·25 ml volumes; six hours for 0·5 ml volumes and eight hours for 2·5 ml volumes. Then isolate the chamber, switch off the pump and leave the chamber evacuated until ready to remove the ampoules for the secondary drying. The ampoules must not be exposed to sunlight, nor, for more than a few hours, to weak daylight; if necessary, cover the apparatus to shield the ampoules from the light.

4. Open the chamber air-release valve, lift the bell-jar and remove the ampoules. Plug with sterile, non-absorbent wool if previously covered with gauze. Draw out the stem of the ampoule to form a thin capillary neck near the open end: first flame the opening and press the loose cotton-wool plug about $2\frac{1}{4}$ in (5·7 cm) down the stem. While rotating the ampoule, heat the stem in a small gas flame at about $1\frac{1}{4}$ in

(3·2 cm) from its open end, until the glass walls have softened and nearly doubled in thickness. Remove the ampoule from the flame and stretch it to form a capillary neck of about 2 mm external diameter and 1 mm bore. When cool, apply the open end to one of the rubber adaptors on the manifold used for the secondary drying; the manifold is placed so that the ampoules lie horizontally. Any adaptors not in use must be sealed by application of an empty ampoule.

5. *Secondary Drying.* Remove the expended desiccant from the trays and replace with fresh phosphorus pentoxide powder. Press the bell-jar into position, close the air-release valve and switch on the pump. Leave the pump running for a sufficient period to ensure complete drying, e.g. 6–18 h. Test the ampoules for vacuum tightness by briefly passing a high-frequency vacuum tester near the surface of the glass; a satisfactory vacuum is indicated by a blue-violet glow, failure of vacuum by long streaky discharges or absence of glow, and cracks in the glass by bright sparking. The Pirani gauge should show that a pressure as low as 0·05–0·01 mmHg is reached.

6. Seal the ampoules while they are attached to the manifold with the pump running: heat the capillary neck with a small gas flame; when the glass is melted, pull gently and allow the flame to sever the thin filament so formed, and hold the flame in position to seal the ends thoroughly. The Pirani gauge will show if a leak develops on the manifold side. When all the ampoules are sealed and set aside, open the air-release valve and switch off pump and Pirani gauge. After standing for half an hour, lay the ampoules on a metal surface and retest them for vacuum with the high-frequency tester; discard any not showing the blue-violet glow. Test the retained ampoules again on the following day.

Freeze-drying by the degassing method using a laboratory desiccator and high-vacuum pump. By this method, small volumes of culture may be freeze-dried with simple apparatus. From 0·25 ml to 2·5 ml of liquid culture is pipetted into a sterile glass tube or ampoule (stem bore 6 mm) which is then stoppered with a *loose*

* Edwards High Vacuum Ltd., supply Apiezon 'M' grease for glass joints and 'N' grease for glass-metal and glass-rubber joints.

cotton-wool plug. The ampoule is placed in a glass desiccator jar over phosphorus pentoxide and is supported in a sloping position so that its contents form a thin layer on one side. The rim of the desiccator jar is smeared with vacuum grease and the lid pressed firmly into position. A tap in the desiccator lid is connected with rubber pressure tubing through a drying column of calcium chloride to a high-vacuum pump (e.g. Hyvac pump), all joints being sealed with vacuum grease (footnote, p. 167). The desiccator tap should be a three-way tap which will allow air to be admitted independently to the desiccator or the pump.

Start the pump and exhaust the desiccator only until the liquid is seen to bubble slightly, and then maintain at this pressure for 20–30 min until the gentle degassing is complete. To do this, close the desiccator tap, admit air to the pump and switch off pump. If bubbling of the culture is marked, admit a very little air into the desiccator jar. When degassing is complete, reconnect the jar to the pump and rapidly exhaust it to high vacuum; the liquid in the ampoule is seen to freeze suddenly within a minute or so. Leave the pump running for about 1 h, then close the tap, switch off the pump and leave for 18–24 h in the dark for drying to continue in the evacuated jar. Finally remove the ampoule from the desiccator, press the cotton-wool plug about $2\frac{1}{4}$ in down the stem, heat the stem in a small gas flame at about $1\frac{1}{4}$ in from its open end and draw it there to form a capillary neck about 2 mm diameter. Attach the mouth of the ampoule stem to the rubber tubing leading to the vacuum pump and evacuate the ampoule to high vacuum for about one minute. Seal the ampoule by melting and severing the capillary neck in a small flame.

Cellophan method of freeze-drying (Rayner, 1943). Moderate quantities of agglutinating sera and guinea-pig complement serum may be preserved by this method. Disks of waterproof cellophan $2\frac{3}{4}$ in in diameter are placed over upturned lids of about 2 in diameter, e.g. the lids of 2-oz waxed cardboard (sputum) cartons. The disks are sterilized individually in Petri dishes in the hot-air oven and placed on the waxed cardboard lids by means of sterile forceps. The serum is pipetted in 1–5 ml amounts on to the cellophan disks. These are stacked in a desiccator over phosphorus pentoxide, and this is exhausted by means of a Hyvac pump. The serum rapidly freezes solid and dries in a short time, but is left overnight in the desiccator. The dried serum is detached quite easily by crumpling the cellophan, and is then placed in sterile $6 \times \frac{5}{8}$ in test-tubes. These are heated above the middle and constricted to a capillary neck about 2 mm in diameter. They are placed in the desiccator, which is again evacuated and left overnight. Finally, the tubes are connected individually to the Hyvac pump, evacuated to high vacuum and sealed by melting and severing the neck with a flame.

Suspending Media for Freeze-Drying of Bacteria
The survival of bacteria during freeze-drying is greatly influenced by the nature of the medium in which they are suspended. Nutrient broth containing 1 per cent of peptone and meat extract is a satisfactory medium for the most resistant organisms, e.g. *Strept. pyogenes* and *Staph. aureus*, and the moderately resistant, e.g. enterobacteria and brucellae. Broth cultures of these may be dried directly.

Special protective suspending media are necessary for the poorly resistant organisms such as *Neisseria gonorrhoeae*, *Vibrio cholerae* and *Haemophilus influenzae*. Organisms from a fresh stationary phase culture are suspended to a high density equivalent to Brown's opacity standard No. 4 (Chap. 14) in the sterile suspending medium just prior to freeze-drying. Various media have been advised, most of which contain sugar, peptone and a colloid (e.g. protein or dextran). Skimmed milk, containing lactose and protein, has been used with success. The media used at the National Collection of Type Cultures are 7·5 per cent glucose broth for the enterobacteria and 7·5 per cent glucose in horse serum sterilized by Seitz filtration for other organisms. Exceptionally fatty batches of serum are avoided.

Rehydration and Recovery of Freeze-Dried Bacteria
The provision of as rich a medium as possible and optimal growth conditions are recommended for revival after freeze-drying. It is

advisable to include a solid medium to detect aerial contamination which may occur during opening of ampoules. Organisms may take time to revive and frequently are not in optimum physiological condition, requiring several subcultures before fully regaining their characteristics.

REFERENCES AND FURTHER READING

AKERS, R. L., WALKER, R. J., SABEL, F. L. & McDADE, J. J. (1969) Development of a laminar air-flow biological cabinet. *American Industrial Hygiene Association Journal*, **30**, 177.

ARANKI, A., SYED, S. A., KENNEY, E. B. & FRETER, R. (1969) Isolation of anaerobic bacteria from human gingiva and mouse cecum by means of a simplified glove box procedure. *Applied Microbiology*, **17**, 568.

BREWER, J. H. & ALLGEIER, D. L. (1966) Safe self-contained carbon dioxide-hydrogen anaerobic system. *Applied Microbiology*, **14**, 985.

BREWER, J. H., ALLGEIER, D. L. & McLAUGHLIN, C. B. (1966) Improved anaerobic indicator. *Applied Microbiology*, **14**, 135.

BROWN, J. H. (1921) An improved anaerobe jar. *Journal of Experimental Medicine*, **33**, 677.

COLLEE, J. G., RUTTER, J. M. & WATT, B. (1971) The significantly viable particle: A study of the subculture of an exacting sporing anaerobe. *Journal of Medical Microbiology*, **4**, 271.

COLLEE, J. G., WATT, B., FOWLER, E. B. & BROWN, R. (1972) An evaluation of the Gaspak system in the culture of anaerobic bacteria. *Journal of Applied Bacteriology*, **35**, 71.

CRUICKSHANK, R. (1968) *Medical Microbiology*, 11th edn. (revised reprint). Edinburgh and London: Churchill Livingstone.

DARLOW, H. M. (1959) A device for flaming platinum loops. *Lancet*, **ii**, 651.

DRASAR, B. S. & CROWTHER, J. S. (1971) The cultivation of human intestinal bacteria. In *Isolation of Anaerobes. Society of Applied Bacteriology—Technical Series No. 5*, p. 93. Edited by D. A. Shapton and R. G. Board. London and New York: Academic Press.

FILDES, P. (1931) Measurement of small quantities of fluid. In *A system of bacteriology*, Vol. 9, p. 174. London: Medical Research Council.

GREAVES, R. I. N. (1944) Centrifugal vacuum freezing; application to the drying of biological material from the frozen state. *Nature, London*, **153**, 485.

HAYWARD, N. J. (1945) The examination of wounds for Clostridia. *Proceedings of the Association of Clinical Pathologists*, **1**, 5.

HELLER, C. L. (1954) A simple method for producing anaerobiosis. *Journal of Applied Bacteriology*, **17**, 202.

HUNGATE, R. E. (1969) A roll tube method for cultivation of strict anaerobes. In *Methods in Microbiology*, vol. 3B, p. 117. Edited by J. R. Norris and D. W. Ribbons. London: Academic Press.

KELSEY, J. C., LIDWELL, O. M., MARKS, J. & PARKER, M. T. (1970) *Precautions against tuberculous infection in the diagnostic laboratory*. London: Department of Health and Social Security.

LAPAGE, S. P., SHELTON, J. E. & MITCHELL, T. G. (1970) Media for the maintenance and preservation of bacteria. In *Methods in Microbiology*, vol. 3A, p. 1. Edited by J. R. Norris and D. W. Ribbons. London: Academic Press.

LAPAGE, S. P., SHELTON, J. E., MITCHELL, T. G. & MACKENZIE, A. R. (1970) Culture collections and the preservation of bacteria. In *Methods in Microbiology*, vol. 3A, p. 135. Edited by J. R. Norris and D. W. Ribbons. London: Academic Press.

McMINN, M. T. & CRAWFORD, J. J. (1970) Recovery of anaerobic microorganisms from clinical specimens in prereduced media versus recovery by routine clinical laboratory methods. *Applied Microbiology*, **19**, 207.

McINTOSH, J. & FILDES, P. (1916) A new apparatus for the isolation and cultivation of anaerobic microorganisms. *Lancet*, **i**, 768.

MARMION, B. P. & TONKIN, R. W. (1972) Control of hepatitis in dialysis units. *British Medical Bulletin*, **28**, 169.

MILES, A. A. & MIRSA, S. S. (1938) The estimation of the bactericidal power of the blood. *Journal of Hygiene*, **38**, 732.

MOORE, W. E. C. (1966) Techniques for routine culture of fastidious anaerobes. *International Journal of Systemic Bacteriology*, **16**, 178.

ØRSKOV, J. (1923) *Investigations into the Morphology of the Ray Fungi*. Copenhagen: Levin Munksgaard.

RAYNER, A. G. (1943) A simple method for the preservation of cultures and sera by drying. *Journal of Pathology and Bacteriology*, **55**, 373.

RUBBO, S. D. & GARDNER, J. F. (1965) *A Review of Sterilization and Disinfection*, p. 219. London: Lloyd-Luke.

SMILLIE, W. G. (1917) New anaerobic methods. *Journal of Experimental Medicine*, **26**, 59.

SOCRANSKY, S. S., MACDONALD, J. B. & SAWYER, S. (1959) The cultivation of *Treponema microdentium* as surface colonies. *Archives of Oral Biology*, **1**, 171.

STOKES, E. JOAN (1962) Short Term Preservation of Bacterial Cultures. Association of Clinical Pathologists, broadsheet No. 40 (new series).

STOKES, E. JOAN (1968) *Clinical Bacteriology*, 3rd edn., p. 26. London: Arnold.

WATSON, K. C. (1955) Isolation of *Salmonella typhi* from the bloodstream. *Journal of Laboratory and Clinical Medicine*, **46**, 128.

WATT, B. (1972) The recovery of clinically important anaerobes on solid media. *Journal of Medical Microbiology*, **5**, 211.

WATT, B. (1973) The influence of carbon dioxide on the growth of obligate and facultative anaerobes on solid media. *Journal of Medical Microbiology*. (In Press.)

WEISS, J. E. & SPAULDING, E. H. (1936–37) A simple method for obtaining effective anaerobiosis. *Journal of Laboratory and Clinical Medicine*, **22**, 726.

WILLIAMS, R. E. O. & LIDWELL, O. M. (1957) A protective cabinet for handling infective material in the laboratory. *Journal of Clinical Pathology*, **10**, 400.

WRIGHT, B. M. (1943) Improved catalyst for McIntosh and Fildes Anaerobic Jar. *Army Pathology Laboratory Service, Current Notes* No. 9, 8.

7. Tests for Identification of Bacteria

In this chapter a number of 'biochemical' tests and a few miscellaneous tests, used generally in the identification of microorganisms, are described. Tests used specifically for the identification of a particular organism are described elsewhere in the appropriate section dealing with that organism.

It should be realized that many of the tests described in this chapter are not 'all-or-none' tests; some distinguish between organisms that differ in the rate with which they carry out a particular reaction. It is therefore important to use a method of test that is suitably poised to differentiate the organisms under consideration. For many of the tests given here, a large number of variations have been developed in different laboratories. In these cases, it has been difficult to make a choice of a method and in some instances we have described more than one test for a given reaction. The results obtained with variations on a particular test may not be comparable and it is essential to bear this in mind. Moreover, there may be considerable variation in the commercially available preparations of the reagents used. For example, the tryptophane content of peptone varies considerably according to the mode of preparation and this markedly influences its value as a substrate in the indole test.

Unfortunately many routinely used tests are not yet standardized, but a start has been made by various organizations. For example, the International Committee on Bacteriological Nomenclature have published recommended biochemical methods for the group differentiation of the *Enterobacteriaceae* (Report, 1958) and much use has been made of these proposals in this chapter.

Diagnostic tables showing the biochemical reactions identifying many genera and species of pathogenic and saprophytic bacteria are given by Cowan and Steel (1965).

PREPARATION OF INOCULUM FOR TEST MEDIA

The validity of the identification of an unknown bacterial culture by its reactions in a range of biochemical tests depends absolutely on the use of a *pure* culture of the bacterium for inoculation of the test media. Single, well-separated colonies grown on a primary diagnostic plate that has been inoculated with material containing a mixture of bacterial species, e.g. sputum or faeces, are usually but not always pure. A small proportion of the colonies are likely to be contaminated with a minor admixture of bacteria of another kind, e.g. an anaerobic or other exacting species that does not grow well under the conditions of culture in the primary plate. If such a colony is accidentally picked and the test media are inoculated either directly from it or from an intermediate slope or broth subculture of it, the contaminating bacteria may grow out selectively in some of the media and give false results.

It is recommended, therefore, that the chosen colony should first be plated out on an unselective culture medium and that a well-isolated colony on the secondary plate should be used as the inoculum for the tests. This precaution is often omitted in medical diagnostic bacteriology, where speed in obtaining results is important. The results are then not fully reliable and if they are unexpected a freshly purified inoculum culture should be prepared and the tests be repeated.

If a larger number of test media have to be inoculated than can conveniently be done from a single colony, the colony should first be subcultured on an agar slope, or in a tube of broth, and this subculture should be used to inoculate the test media. The subculture can then be preserved for making confirmatory or other different tests on subsequent days. It is an unsound practice to use another, apparently similar colony from the primary plate to provide inocula for additional tests.

CONTROLS FOR TESTS

The sterility of each batch of test medium should be confirmed by incubating one or two uninoculated tubes of the batch along with the inoculated tests. If the uninoculated tubes show evidence of bacterial growth, the tests and the remainder of that batch of medium should be discarded.

Control tests are also made to confirm that the test media have been made up correctly and that they are used and observed under the proper conditions. One tube of each batch of test medium is inoculated with a stock culture of a bacterium known to give a positive reaction and another tube with a stock culture known to give a negative reaction. These positive and negative controls are incubated and examined along with the tests.

TESTS FOR METABOLISM OF CARBOHYDRATES AND RELATED COMPOUNDS

Bacteria differ widely in their ability to metabolize carbohydrates and related compounds. For purposes of identification these differences can be demonstrated by four varieties of test:

1. Test to distinguish between aerobic and anaerobic breakdown of a carbohydrate.

2. Tests to show the range of carbohydrates and related compounds that can be attacked.

3. Tests for specific breakdown products.

4. Tests to show ability to utilize a particular substrate.

Carbohydrates and related compounds may be altered when exposed to normal heat-sterilization temperatures. They may also be altered when heated in the presence of other ingredients of culture media, e.g. peptone, phosphate. For these reasons, it is recommended that the basal ingredients of test media should be heat-sterilized before the carbohydrate or related compound is added. A solution of the compound under test should be sterilized separately and the requisite amount subsequently added with aseptic precautions to the sterile basal medium.

Sterilization of solutions of test compounds by filtration is recommended. However, if heat is to be used, in general tyndallization (intermittent steaming) is less likely to alter the compound than autoclaving at 121°C. Some workers have strong reservations about the

reliability of tyndallization. Carbohydrates are particularly susceptible to heat in an alkaline environment and if a carbohydrate solution is to be sterilized by heat, the prior addition of one or two drops of phosphoric acid will ensure that the solution is not alkaline.

TEST TO DISTINGUISH BETWEEN AEROBIC AND ANAEROBIC BREAKDOWN OF A CARBOHYDRATE

This method (Hugh and Leifson, 1953) depends upon the use of a semi-solid tubed medium containing the carbohydrate together with a pH indicator. If acid is produced only at the surface of the medium, where conditions are aerobic, the attack on the sugar is oxidative. If acid is found throughout the tube, including the lower layers where conditions are anaerobic, the breakdown is fermentative.

Medium

Peptone	2·0 g
Sodium chloride, NaCl. . .	5·0 g
Dipotassium hydrogen phosphate, K_2HPO_4	0·3 g
Bromothymol blue (1 per cent aqueous solution) . . .	3 ml
Agar	3 g
Water	1 l

The pH is adjusted to 7·1 before adding the bromothymol blue and the medium is autoclaved in a flask at 121°C for 30 min. The carbohydrate to be added is sterilized separately and added to give a final concentration of 1 per cent. The medium is then tubed to a depth of about 4 cm.

Method. Duplicate tubes of medium are inoculated by stabbing, one tube is promptly covered with a layer of sterile melted petroleum jelly (yellow soft petroleum) to a depth of 5–10 mm and both are incubated for up to 30 days. Fermenting organisms (e.g. *Enterobacteriaceae*, *Aeromonas*, *Vibrio*) produce an acid reaction throughout the medium in the covered (anaerobic) as well as the open (aerobic) tube. Oxidizing organisms (e.g. *Pseudomonas*, *Loefflerella*) produce an acid reaction only in the open tube; this begins at the surface and gradually extends downwards, and may appear only after an alkaline reaction has been present for several days. Organisms that cannot break down the carbohydrate aerobically or anaerobically (e.g. *Alcaligenes faecalis*) produce an alkaline reaction in the open tube and no change in the covered tube.

It should be noted that this medium may also be used for recording gas production and motility.

TESTS TO SHOW THE RANGE OF CARBOHYDRATES AND RELATED COMPOUNDS THAT CAN BE ATTACKED

For practical purposes these tests are of two kinds. The majority are tests simply for the production of acid and gas or acid alone when a pure culture grows in the presence of the test compound. A negative reaction in these tests does not necessarily mean that the culture is unable to utilize the carbon compound. A minority of the tests are more complicated, the principal ones being those for tartrate and citrate fermentation in which breakdown of the substrate is confirmed by showing that it has been removed from the medium. These tests, in addition to fermentation of mucate, are used in the identification and fermentation typing of salmonellae. They are described in detail by Cruickshank (1968) and will not be repeated here.

Tests for Acid and Gas or Acid Alone: 'Fermentation Tests'

Constituents of Fermentation Test Media

1. A suitable *nutrient medium* as a base to allow the growth of the organism under test, free from substances that might yield acid products. The nature of this medium depends on the nutritional requirements of the organism. Peptone water, serum peptone water and serum agar are commonly used.

2. The *carbohydrate or related compound* under test. A large variety are used and they are often referred to loosely as 'sugars'.

Monosaccharides
Pentoses—Arabinose, xylose, rhamnose
Hexoses—Glucose, fructose, mannose, sorbose, galactose
Disaccharides
Sucrose, maltose, lactose, trehalose, cellobiose
Trisaccharide
Raffinose

Polysaccharides
Starch, inulin, dextrin, glycogen
Polyhydric alcohols
Glycerol, erythritol, adonitol, mannitol, dulcitol, sorbitol, inositol
Glycosides
Salicin, coniferin, aesculin
Organic acids
dextro—tartrate, *laevo*—tartrate, *meso*—tartrate, citrate, mucate, gluconate, malonate.

The test compounds in fermentation test media may be identified by a colour code (Chap. 5).

The test compound is usually added in the proportion of 0·5 per cent to peptone water or 1·0 per cent to serum bases. The majority can be prepared as 10 per cent aqueous solutions and sterilized, preferably by filtration. They can be kept conveniently in 10-oz screw-capped bottles fitted with a siphon and hooded pipette (Chap. 5). Rarer compounds may be stored in ½-oz bottles with a perforated cap and rubber washer, similar to the caps of blood culture bottles, and a sterile syringe can be used to withdraw solution from the bottle as required.

It is essential to prepare starch solution immediately before use because it undergoes gradual hydrolysis to glucose which is readily fermented by most medically-important bacteria and could give false reactions. Sufficient starch for about 24 bottles can be prepared by adding 5 ml sterile distilled water to 0·15 g soluble starch in a sterile Universal container, screwing on the cap and shaking vigorously. The bottle is placed in a pan of water, brought to the boil and boiled for about 5 min, shaking at intervals to ensure that all the starch is in solution and the contents are homogeneous. The solution is cooled and 0·15 ml is added to 3 ml nutrient medium, usually serum peptone water in bijou bottles (final concentration of starch, 0·15 per cent). The medium should be used within a few weeks after the starch is added.

3. A suitable *indicator* that will change colour only as a result of the formation of acids during the fermentation is required. A variety of indicators with a pK between pH 6 and 8 have been used:

Andrade's indicator is made by adding

1 N NaOH to a 0·5 per cent solution of acid fuchsin until the colour just becomes yellow. It is used at a final concentration of 0·005 per cent in the medium and it turns dark reddish pink at about pH 5·5. Andrade's indicator fades fairly rapidly when stored and should not be used unless the media can be utilized within a few months.

Bromocresol purple is made up as a 0·2 per cent solution. For use, 2·5 ml of this solution is added to each 100 ml medium to give a final concentration of 0·005 per cent. Bromocresol purple is yellow at pH 5·2 and violet-purple at pH 6·8. It is recommended instead of Andrade's indicator for media that are likely to be stored for several months.

Phenol red is made up as a 0·2 per cent solution as described on page 85, except that the phenol red is ten times as strong. For use, 5 ml of the 0·2 per cent solution is added to each 100 ml of medium giving a final concentration of 0·01 per cent. This indicator does not fade on storage and may be incorporated in bottled media that may not be used for some time. Phenol red is yellow at pH 6·8 and purple-pink at pH 8·4. It is used for serum media because it detects small changes in pH, characteristic of fermentation by nutritionally exacting bacteria.

Bromothymol blue is made up as a 0·2 per cent solution by dissolving 1 g in 25 ml 0·1 N NaOH mixed with 475 ml distilled water. For use, 1·25 ml of the 0·2 per cent solution is added to each 100 ml medium giving a final concentration of 0·0025 per cent. Bromothymol blue is yellow at pH 6·0 and blue at pH 7·6. It is an alternative to phenol red when the pH change is small and it is used in serum media, broth-based media and in media for organic acid fermentation tests.

4. A small inverted tube (*Durham tube*) completely filled with liquid and containing no air bubbles is usually included in each culture tube or bottle to detect gas (see below).

Preparation of Test Media

Peptone Water Fermentation Test Media

The commonest nutrient medium for fermentation tests is peptone water (p. 113).

Peptone water at pH 7·2 to 7·3   .   950 ml
Indicator solution (Andrade's 10
ml or bromocresol purple 25 ml)
Test compound, 10 per cent solution, sterile   .   .   .   .   50 ml

The nutrient medium is prepared and indicator is added. The complete medium cannot be handled in bulk because the process of heat sterilization is used to drive out the air from the Durham tubes which then fill with liquid as the medium cools and fermentation media cannot be heated after adding the test compound. Therefore the base and indicator must be dispensed, sterilized by autoclaving and cooled before the sterile solution of test compound is added aseptically to each individual tube or bottle.

Medium may be dispensed either in 5 ml amounts with 50×7 mm Durham tubes, in 125 or $150 \times 12·5$ mm test tubes with caps or cotton-wool plugs or in 3-ml amounts with 27×6 mm Durham tubes in bijou bottles. Medium in bottles can be stored and transported without risk of spilling or of alteration in concentration of ingredients. As a result of shaking during transit, air may enter the Durham tube, but it is easily removed by inverting the bottle, the amount of liquid being such that the open end of the tube is below the surface. When bottles have been seeded the caps should be loosely screwed on to allow access of air.

Broth fermentation media may be used instead of peptone water if a more nutritious base is needed.

Meat extract   .   .   .   .   5 g
Disodium   hydrogen   phosphate,
Na_2HPO_4 .   .   .   .   2 g
Water   .   .   .   .   950 ml
Indicator solution (bromothymol
blue)   .   .   .   .   12·5 ml
Test compound, 10 per cent solu-
tion, sterile   .   .   .   .   50 ml

Prepare, sterilize and dispense as for peptone water media.

Bitter medium has a special peptone base to distinguish only the reactions of strongly fermenting organisms. It is used with xylose for the 'fermentation typing' of organisms such as *S. typhimurium* and its preparation is described in Cruickshank (1968).

Serum Peptone Water Fermentation Media

These media are suitable for more exacting organisms such as *C. diphtheriae*.

Peptone water, pH 7·6 . .	800 ml
Serum	200 ml
Indicator solution (phenol red 50 ml or bromothymol blue 12·5 ml)	
Test compound . . .	10 g

Some samples of horse serum may contain saccharolytic enzymes and give fallacious results. Batches should be tested before use. Sheep or ox serum is preferable.

Serum media are best sterilized by filtration but if they are not acid they will not coagulate on heating and may be steamed for 20 min on three successive days.

Durham tubes are rarely required for serum media and alternative methods of preparation are therefore practicable. The complete medium can be prepared, sterilized by filtration and dispensed aseptically. Otherwise the nutrient medium and indicator can be prepared, dispensed and steamed for 20 min on three successive days, a sterile 10 per cent solution of the carbon compound being added to individual bottles or tubes with sterile precautions.

Hiss's serum water can replace serum peptone water. It consists of 25 per cent serum in distilled water.

Serum Agar Fermentation Media

These are recommended for organisms such as meningococci and gonococci that grow poorly in liquid media.

Basal medium

Peptone	20 g
Sodium chloride, NaCl .	5 g
Distilled water . . .	900 ml
Digest broth, pH 7·6 . .	100 ml
Agar	25 g
Phenol red solution, 0·2 per cent .	20 ml

Dissolve the peptone and salt in the water by steaming. Adjust to pH 8·4 by making just alkaline to phenolphthalein and steam for 30 min. Filter through a coarse filter paper. Adjust to pH 7·6. Add the broth and agar and steam at 100°C for 45 min or until the agar is dissolved. Filter through a hardened filter paper if necessary, bottle in 100-ml amounts

and add 2 ml phenol red to each bottle. Autoclave in 'free steam' for 1 h and then at 110°C for 5 min.

Complete medium

Basal medium . . .	100 ml
Sterile serum (guinea-pig or rabbit)	5 ml
Test compound, 10 per cent solution, sterile . . .	10 ml

Melt the basal medium, cool to 55°C, add the other ingredients with sterile precautions and dispense as slopes in sterile tubes or bijou bottles.

Solid Media in Plates for Strongly Fermenting Organisms

Plates of solid media containing carbohydrate may be used to test the fermentation of several pure cultures inoculated as streaks or spots, or to estimate the relative numbers of fermenting and non-fermenting organisms in a mixture plated on the medium. Eosin methylene blue agar or deoxycholate agar (Cruickshank, 1968) which gives better differentiation of crowded colonies, are recommended for this purpose. Deoxycholate agar is less inhibitory to *E. coli* than deoxycholate citrate agar because ferric ammonium citrate is omitted and the concentration of bile salt is halved. An even more suitable medium for *E. coli* substitutes dehydrocholic acid for deoxycholate.

Use of Test Media

Before inoculation, confirm the absence of bubbles of gas from Durham tubes in liquid media. Seed each medium with a speck of solid culture, or a drop or loopful of liquid culture, or a suspension of a solid culture in a sterile liquid. After incubation, examine the media for the presence of a colour change, indicating acid, and for gas formation in the Durham tube. Acid production in liquid serum media may cause coagulation of the serum.

Slopes of solid medium are seeded over the whole surface. The presence of a colour change after incubation indicates acid.

Fermentation reactions are commonly completed within a period of incubation of 24 h, or 48 h for slowly-growing species. The identification of many organisms is based on the results recorded at these times. However some quickly-growing organisms fail to ferment a given sugar in 24 h but will give 'late' fermentation if incubation is prolonged, up to 40 days. In such cases, tests should be inspected daily and the day on which fermentation first appears should be recorded.

TESTS FOR SPECIFIC BREAKDOWN PRODUCTS

Methyl Red Test

The methyl red test is employed to detect the production of sufficient acid during the fermentation of glucose and the maintenance of conditions such that the pH of an old culture is sustained below a value of about 4·5, as shown by a change in the colour of the methyl red indicator which is added at the end of the period of incubation.

Medium ('glucose phosphate peptone water')

Peptone	5 g
Dipotassium hydrogen phosphate, K_2HPO_4 . . .	5 g
Water	1 l
Glucose, 10 per cent solution, (sterilized separately) . .	50 ml

Dissolve the peptone and phosphate, adjust the pH to 7·6, filter, dispense in 5 ml amounts and sterilize at 121°C for 15 min. Sterilize the glucose solution by filtration and add 0·25 ml to each tube (final concentration 0·5 per cent).

Methyl red indicator solution

Methyl red . . .	0·1 g
Ethanol	300 ml
Distilled water	200 ml

Method. Inoculate the liquid medium lightly from a young agar slope culture and incubate at 37°C for 48 h. Add about five drops of the methyl red reagent (see above). Mix and read immediately. Positive tests are bright red and negative are yellow. If the results after 48 h are equivocal, the test should be repeated with cultures that have been incubated for 5 days. For some organisms, incubation at 30°C for 5 days is preferable to incubation at 37°C for 2 or 5 days.

Voges-Proskauer Test

Many bacteria ferment carbohydrates with the production of acetyl methyl carbinol (CH_3.

$CO.CHOH.CH_3$) or its reduction product 2, 3 butylene glycol ($CH_3.CHOH.CHOH.CH_3$). The substances can be tested for by a colorimetric reaction between diacetyl ($CH_3.CO.CO.CH_3$—formed during the test by oxidation of acetyl methyl carbinol or 2, 3 butylene glycol) and a guanidino group under alkaline conditions. This test is usually done in conjunction with the methyl red test since the production of acetyl methyl carbinol or butylene glycol usually results in insufficient acid accumulating during fermentation to give a methyl red positive reaction. An organism of the enterobacterial group is usually *either* methyl-red-positive and Voges-Proskauer-negative *or* methyl-red-negative and Voges-Proskauer-positive.

Medium. Glucose phosphate peptone water, as for the methyl red test.

Method 1 (O'Meara). Incubate at 37°C or 30°C for 48 h only. Add 0·5 ml of O'Meara reagent (40 g potassium hydroxide and 0·3 g creatine in 100 ml distilled water). Place tubes in a 37°C waterbath for 4 h. Aerate by shaking at intervals. A positive reaction is denoted by the development of an eosin-pink colour, usually in 2–5 min.

Method 2 (Barritt). Incubate at 37° or 30°C for 48 h. Add 1 ml of 40 per cent potassium hydroxide and 3 ml of a 5 per cent solution of α-naphthol in absolute ethanol. A positive reaction is indicated by the development of a pink colour in 2–5 min, becoming crimson in 30 min. The tube can be shaken at intervals to ensure maximum aeration. α-Naphthol is a carcinogen.

Stern's Glycerol Reaction

This reaction is used in the identification and fermentation typing of salmonellae. It depends on the ability of the organism to convert glycerol to an aldehyde that recolourizes fuchsin-sulphite. It is described in detail in Cruickshank (1968).

Gluconate Test

This is a test for the ability of an organism to oxidize gluconates to the 2 keto-gluconate which subsequently accumulates in the medium

(Shaw and Clarke, 1955; Carpenter, 1961). The basis of the test is the change from gluconate, a non-reducing compound when tested with a suitable reagent, to 2 keto-gluconate, which is a reducing compound when so tested.

Medium

Peptone	1·5 g
Yeastrel (Yeast extract) . .	1·0 g
Dipotassium hydrogen phosphate, K_2HPO_4 . . .	1·0 g
Potassium gluconate . . .	40·0 g
Distilled water	1 l

The pH, after solution, should be 7·0. Distribute in 10 ml quantities in screw-capped bottles and autoclave at 121°C for 15 min.

Method. Add 1 ml of the medium aseptically into a clean, sterile tube. Inoculate and incubate at 37°C for 48 h. Then add 1 ml of Benedict's reagent for reducing sugars, place the tube in a boiling water bath for 10 min and observe for the production of a coloured precipitate of cuprous oxide. Alternatively, add a 'Clintest reagent' tablet (Ames Co., Nuffield House, London W1) for the detection of reducing sugars.

Positive result = green to orange precipitate.
Negative result = the blue colour of the reagent is unchanged.

TESTS TO SHOW ABILITY TO UTILIZE A SPECIFIC SUBSTRATE

Bacteria that are capable of growing on a simple, chemically defined medium (i.e. *prototrophic* bacteria), can readily be tested for their ability to use a given compound as their sole source of carbon and energy. A defined medium such as that of Davis and Mingioli is prepared with the test compound substituted for the normal carbon and energy source (i.e. glucose and citrate in Davis and Mingioli's medium). The medium is usually made with agar and poured in plates. The organism is inoculated lightly in a streak or by plating out. After a suitable period of incubation the plate is examined and the appearance of bacterial growth indicates that the bacterium has been able to utilize the test compound.

Growth is often slower on a defined medium than on the ordinary peptone-containing media

and observations should be continued for up to 7 days during incubation at 37°C. Usually growth is well-developed at 2 days.

The inoculum for these tests should not be heavy and should not be made from a broth culture lest sufficient nutritive organic matter is carried over with the inoculum into the test medium to support a visible amount of growth. Preferably the bacterium is first grown for 18–24 h on an agar slope. A small amount of this growth is suspended in sterile saline solution to give a suspension of about $1–5 \times 10^8$ bacteria per ml and a small loopful of the suspension is used to inoculate the defined medium.

Bacteria that fail to grow on the simple defined medium when glucose and citrate are present as sources of carbon and energy generally do so because they require as additional nutrients one or more specific amino acids or vitamins; they are described as *auxotrophic*. Growth tests made on further defined media supplemented with single amino acids or vitamins, or different combinations of these, will enable the particular nutritional requirements of an auxotroph to be determined.

Citrate Utilization Test

This is a test for the ability of an organism to utilize citrate as the sole carbon and energy source for growth and an ammonium salt as the sole source of nitrogen. Koser's liquid citrate medium or Simmons' citrate agar may be used.

Koser's Medium (modified)

Sodium chloride, NaCl . .	5·0 g
Magnesium sulphate, $MgSO_4$.	0·2 g
Ammonium dihydrogen phosphate, $NH_4H_2PO_4$ . . .	1·0 g
Potassium dihydrogen phosphate, KH_2PO_4	1·0 g
Sodium citrate, $Na_3C_6H_5O_7.2H_2O$	5·0 g
Distilled water	1 l

The pH should be 6·8. The medium is dispensed and sterilized by autoclaving at 121°C for 15 min.

Simmons' Medium

Simmons' citrate medium is a modification of Koser's medium with agar and an indicator added.

Koser's medium . . . 1 l
Agar . . . . . 20 g
   Bromothymol blue,
   0·2 per cent (p. 173) . . 40 ml

Dispense, autoclave at 121°C for 15 min and allow to set as slopes.

Method. Inoculate from a saline suspension of the organism to be tested. Incubate for 96 h at 37°C.

The results are read as follows:
1. Koser's citrate medium:
   Positive = Turbidity, i.e. growth.
   Negative = No turbidity.

A positive test should be subcultured into a second tube to eliminate false positives due to an excessive initial inoculum.
2. Simmons' citrate medium:
   Positive = Blue colour and streak of growth.
   Negative = Original green colour and no growth.

Malonate Utilization Test

Note that utilization of malonate and deamination of phenylalanine can be combined in one test.

Medium
   Yeast extract . . . . 1·0 g
   Ammonium sulphate, $(NH_4)_2SO_4$ 2·0 g
   Dipotassium hydrogen phosphate, K_2HPO_4 . . . 0·6 g
   Potassium dihydrogen phosphate, KH_2PO_4. . . . 0·4 g
   Sodium chloride, NaCl . . 2·0 g
   Sodium malonate . . . 3·0 g
   Bromthymol blue . . . 0·025 g
   Distilled water. . . . 1 l

Adjust the pH to 7·4 if necessary. Sterilize by autoclaving at 121°C for 15 min.

Method. Inoculate from a young agar slope culture and incubate at 37°C for 48 h. Positive results are indicated by a change in colour of the indicator from green to blue due to the rise in pH consequent upon the utilization of sodium malonate.

TESTS FOR METABOLISM OF PROTEINS AND AMINO ACIDS

Proteolytic organisms digest proteins and consequently may liquefy gelatin or coagulated serum. Cultures in meat media cause blackening of the meat, decomposing it and reducing its volume with the formation of foul-smelling products. Some organisms decompose milk proteins. Whereas strongly proteolytic organisms may have all these properties, weakly proteolytic ones may only liquefy gelatin. Liquefaction of gelatin, being the commonest proteolytic property, is used routinely as an index of proteolytic activity but a positive result may take several days to develop.

GELATIN LIQUEFACTION

Nutrient Gelatin

For bacteriological use an edible grade of gelatin is preferred, since this is free from preservatives and inhibitory amounts of heavy metals. Gelatin will not by itself support the growth of many pathogens and it is added to a liquid nutrient medium to produce a firm gel called nutrient gelatin. The proportion of gelatin used varies, but 12 per cent is a suitable average.

It is important that the gelatin medium should not be exposed to a high temperature for longer than recommended, otherwise it may be partially hydrolyzed and will not solidify on cooling.

Medium
   Nutrient broth. . . . 1 l
   Gelatin . . . . . 120 g

Add the gelatin to the broth and allow it to stand at 4°C overnight. Warm to 45°C to dissolve the gelatin. Adjust to pH 8·4 and steam for 10 min. Cool quickly to 45°C and slowly add the beaten white of two eggs, or 10 g egg albumin dissolved in 50 ml water, or 50 ml serum; this helps to clear colloidal particles from the medium. Steam for 30 min, stirring occasionally. Filter through hardened filter paper. Adjust the pH to 7·6 and bottle in 12-ml amounts. Hold in the autoclave in free steam for 10 min followed by 115°C for 10 min. Remove from the autoclave as quickly as possible and keep at a low temperature.

The resulting medium is perfectly transparent when solid, and should be of firm consistency, yet not so stiff that it is split by the wire when inoculated.

Method. A stab culture is made using an

inoculum from an agar slope culture. Pathogenic bacteria are usually grown at 37°C and negative tests may be observed for as long as 30 days. Gelatin at the concentration used melts at about 24°C and is therefore liquid at 37°C. Liquefaction is tested for at intervals by removing the nutrient gelatin cultures from the incubator and holding them at 4°C for 30 min before reading the results.

Gelatin Agar

Gelatin breakdown can be demonstrated by incorporating it in a buffered nutrient agar, growing the culture and then flooding the medium with a reagent that differentially precipitates either gelatin or its breakdown products (Barer, 1946).

> *Medium*
> Nutrient agar . . . . 1 l
> Potassium dihydrogen phosphate,
> KH$_2$PO$_4$ . . . . 0·5 g
> Dipotassium hydrogen phosphate, K$_2$HPO$_4$ . . . 1·5 g
> Gelatin . . . . 4 g
> Glucose . . . . 0·05 g

Melt the agar and dissolve the phosphates, gelatin and glucose in it, taking care to ensure even distribution of the gelatin. Adjust the pH to 7·0. Sterilize in a flask at 121°C for 30 min. Pour plates.

> *Mercuric chloride solution*
> Mercuric chloride, HgCl$_2$ . . 15 g
> Hydrochloric acid, concentrated, HCl . . . . 20 ml
> Water . . . . 100 ml

Tannic acid solution. 1 per cent in water.
Method. Inoculate plates and incubate under appropriate conditions. Flood plates with either mercuric chloride which causes an opacity in the medium with clear zones around gelatin-liquefying colonies, slow to develop but not fading; or tannic acid which causes a relative opacity around gelatin-liquefying colonies, quick to develop but fading as the medium also becomes opaque.

Gelatin Charcoal Disks

The method of Kohn (1953) employing sterile disks or cubes of formaldehyde-denatured gelatin containing finely powdered charcoal is a very rapid and convenient test for proteolysis.

The sterile disk is picked from its bottle with a hot inoculating wire, to which it adheres, and is transferred into a newly inoculated or already grown culture in liquid medium. The culture is incubated with the disk for up to a week at 37°C. (The denatured gelatin does not melt at this temperature.) Liquefaction of the gelatin is shown by the settling of free carbon particles to the bottom of the medium and, later, by the complete disintegration of the disk.

If the disks are added to a culture that is already fully grown or to a dense suspension in peptone water of a young culture grown on agar, liquefaction may be observed after only a few hours' incubation at 37°C.

Lautrop (1956) has described a modification of the test for the demonstration of a special, calcium-dependent gelatinase present in certain organisms (e.g. *Salmonella abortus-bovis*, *S. schleissheim* and *S. texas*). Organisms grown at 22°C on agar are suspended to high density in 3–4 ml saline containing 0·01 M CaCl$_2$, a gelatin-charcoal disk is added and the test is incubated at 37°C for up to 3 days.

Digestion of Milk

Digestion of milk protein may be seen as a zone of clearing around colonies on milk agar. Results can be read in 24–48 h, less than the time usually necessary to see digestion of litmus milk.

> *Medium*
> Nutrient agar, sterile . . . 87·5 ml
> Skimmed milk, sterile . . 12·5 ml

Melt the agar, cool to 50°C, add the milk and pour plates.
Method. Inoculate, incubate and examine for zones of clearing.

Hydrogen Sulphide Production
(Combined with Gelatin Liquefaction)

Hydrogen sulphide can be produced at least in small amounts from sulphur-containing amino acids by a large number of bacteria. Methods showing hydrogen sulphide production by suspending strips of paper impregnated with lead acetate above cultures are of variable sensitivity and are of limited value. Precise tests must be poised at a definite level of sensitivity. The method described here is of a sensitivity suitable for group differentiation within the Enterobacteriaceae. Hydrogen sulphide is demonstrated by its ability to form black insoluble ferrous sulphide. The medium is solidified with gelatin and also indicates gelatin liquefaction.

Medium

Meat extract	7·5 g
Peptone	25 g
Sodium chloride, NaCl .	5 g
Gelatin	120 g
Distilled water . . .	1 l
Ferrous chloride, 10 per cent aqueous solution . . .	5 ml

Dissolve all the ingredients except ferrous chloride in water, adjust to pH 7·6, steam and filter. Heat in the autoclave in free steam for 10 min and then at 115°C for 10 min. Remove from the autoclave as quickly as possible and cool to about 55°C. Add the ferrous chloride solution, freshly prepared and sterilized by filtration. Tube the medium in narrow tubes and seal with corks impregnated with paraffin wax.

Method. Inoculate with a straight wire to a depth of 1 cm and incubate at 20°C for at least 7 days. Inspect daily for blackening due to production of hydrogen sulphide and for liquefaction of gelatin.

Indole Test

This test demonstrates the ability of certain bacteria to decompose the amino acid tryptophane to indole which accumulates in the medium. Indole is then tested for by a colourimetric reaction with *p*-dimethyl-aminobenzaldehyde.

Medium

Peptone (brand containing sufficient tryptophane) . .	20 g
Sodium chloride, NaCl .	5 g
Distilled water . . .	1 l

Adjust the pH to 7·4. Dispense and sterilize by autoclaving at 121°C for 15 min.

Kovac's Reagent

Amyl or isoamyl alcohol . .	150 ml
p-Dimethyl-aminobenzaldehyde .	10 g
Conc. hydrochloric acid, HCl .	50 ml

Dissolve the aldehyde in the alcohol and slowly add the acid. Prepare in small quantities and store in the refrigerator. Shake gently before use.

Method. Inoculate medium and incubate for 48 h at 37°C. Sometimes a period of 96 h at 37°C may be required for optimum accumulation of indole. Add 0·5 ml Kovac's reagent and shake gently. A red colour in the alcohol layer indicates a positive reaction.

Amino Acid Decarboxylase Tests

This test (Møller, 1955) is based on the ability of some bacteria to decarboxylate an amino acid to the corresponding amine with the liberation of carbon dioxide. The production of these decarboxylases is induced by a low pH and, as a result of their action, the pH rises to neutrality or above.

Medium

Peptone	5 g
Meat extract	5 g
Glucose	0·5 g
Pyridoxal	5 mg
Bromocresol purple (1 in 500 solution)	5 ml
Cresol red (1 in 500 solution) .	2·5 ml
Distilled water	1 l

Dissolve the solids in water and adjust the pH to 6·0 *before* the addition of the indicators. This is the basal medium and to it is added the amino acid whose decarboxylation is to be tested. Divide the basal medium into four portions and treat as follows:

1. Add 1 per cent L-lysine* hydrochloride.
2. Add 1 per cent L–ornithine* hydrochloride.
3. Add 1 per cent L-arginine* hydrochloride.
4. No additions (control).

Readjust the pH to 6·0 if necessary. Distribute 1 ml quantities in small tubes containing sterile liquid paraffin to provide a layer about 5 mm thick above the medium. Autoclave at 121°C for 15 min.

Method. Inoculate lightly through the paraffin layer with a straight wire. Incubate and read daily for four days.

* If the DL components are used, add 2 per cent of the amino acid.

The medium first becomes yellow due to acid production during glucose fermentation; later, if decarboxylation occurs, the medium becomes violet. The control should remain yellow.

Phenylalanine Deaminase Test

This test indicates the ability of an organism to deaminate phenylalanine with the production of phenylpyruvic acid which will react with ferric salts to give a green colour. Deamination of phenylalanine and utilization of malonate can be combined in one test.

Medium

Yeast extract . . .	3 g
DL-phenylalanine . .	2 g
(or L-phenylalanine . .	1 g)
Disodium hydrogen phosphate, Na_2HPO_4	1 g
Sodium chloride, NaCl .	5 g
Agar	12 g
Distilled water . . .	1 l

Adjust the pH to 7·4, distribute and sterilize by autoclaving at 121°C for 15 min. Allow to solidify in tubes as long slopes.
Method. Inoculate with a fairly heavy inoculum. Incubate for 4 h or, if desired, for up to 24 h at 37°C. Allow a few drops of a 10 per cent solution of ferric chloride to run down over the growth on the slope. If the test is positive, a green colour will develop in the fluid and in the slope.

TEST FOR METABOLISM OF FAT

Hydrolysis of Tributyrin

An emulsion of micro-droplets of the fat, tributyrin, in a solid medium makes it opaque. Lipolytic organisms remove the opacity by converting the fat to water-soluble butyric acid.

Medium

Peptone	5 g
Yeast extract . . .	3 g
Tributyrin (glyceryl tributyrate) .	10 g
Agar	20 g
Water	1 l

The medium is prepared so that the tributyrin forms a stable emulsion in the nutrient agar and the pH is adjusted to 7·5. For exacting orga-

nisms the medium may be enriched by addition of 5 per cent of Fildes' extract (Willis, 1960).
Method. Inoculate and incubate plates under appropriate conditions. Examine by transmitted light. Colonies of lipolytic organisms are surrounded by wide zones of clearing.

TESTS FOR ENZYMES

Catalase Test

This demonstrates the presence of catalase, an enzyme that catalyses the release of oxygen from hydrogen peroxide.

One ml of hydrogen peroxide solution, H_2O_2 (10 vol), is poured over a 24-h nutrient agar slope culture of the test organism and the tube is held in a slanting position.

Alternatively, a small amount of the culture to be tested is picked from a nutrient agar slope, using a clean sterile platinum loop or a clean, thin glass rod (a sealed capillary tube may be used for this purpose), and this is inserted intc hydrogen peroxide solution held in a small, clean tube. Enough material may be picked from a single colony to give a reaction by this method.

The production of gas bubbles from the surface of the solid culture material indicates a positive reaction. It occurs almost immediately. A false positive reaction may be obtained if the culture medium contains catalase (e.g. blood agar), or if an iron wire loop is used.

Oxidase Test

This test depends on the presence in bacteria of certain oxidases that will catalyse the transport of electrons between electron donors in the bacteria and a redox dye—tetramethyl-*p*-phenylene-diamine. The dye is reduced to a deep purple colour.

The test is used for screening species of *Neisseria*, *Alcaligenes*, *Aeromonas*, *Vibrio* and *Pseudomonas*, which give positive reactions (Steel, 1961) and for the exclusion of the Enterobacteriaceae, all species of which give negative reactions.
Plate method. Cultures are made on a suitable solid growth medium. A freshly prepared 1 per cent solution of tetramethyl-*p*-phenylene-dia-

mine dihydrochloride is poured on to the plate so as to cover the surface, and is then decanted. The colonies of oxidase-positive organisms rapidly develop a purple colour. If subcultures are required from the colonies, they should be made immediately; after 5 min exposure to the reagent it may not be possible to subculture them.

Dry filter paper method. Since the oxidase reagent is unstable and has to be freshly prepared for use, the following method is convenient. Strips of Whatman's No. 1 filter paper are soaked in a freshly prepared 1 per cent solution of tetramethyl-*p*-phenylene-diamine dihydrochloride. After draining for about 30 s the strips are freeze-dried and stored in a dark bottle tightly sealed with a screw cap. The papers have a light purple tint and will keep for several months in an airtight container at room temperature. For use, a strip is removed, laid in a Petri dish and moistened with distilled water. The colony to be tested is picked up with a platinum loop and smeared over the moist area. A positive reaction is indicated by an intense deep-purple hue, appearing within 5–10 s, a 'delayed positive' reaction by colouration in 10–60 s, and a negative reaction by absence of colouration or by colouration later than 60 s.

Wet filter paper method. A strip of filter paper is soaked with a little freshly made 1 per cent solution of the reagent and then at once used by rubbing a speck of culture on it with a platinum loop. The result is read as for the dry filter paper method.

Note that the reagent must be freshly made and the bacterial growth must be transferred to the test paper with a clean *platinum* loop or a clean glass rod, since traces of iron will catalyse the reaction and give false positive results. If the colony is small it may be necessary to pick up material from several similar colonies in order to have sufficient to give a strong reaction. When testing colonies from MacConkey's medium, a pink-violet colour is due to carry-over from the medium and is not a true oxidase reaction; the true reaction gives an intense purple hue. Dimethyl-*p*-phenylene-diamine oxalate, 1 per cent, may be used in place of the tetra-methyl-*p*-phenylene-diamine dihydrochloride in this paper-strip test.

Urease Test

Bacteria, particularly those growing naturally in an environment exposed to urine, may decompose urea by means of the enzyme urease:

$$NH_2 . CO . NH_2 + H_2O \longrightarrow 2NH_3 + CO_2$$

The occurrence of this enzyme can be tested for by growing the organism in the presence of urea and testing for alkali (NH_3) production by means of a suitable pH indicator. An alternative method is to test for the production of ammonia from urea by means of Nessler's reagent.

Medium 1 (Christensen's Medium)

Peptone	1 g
Sodium chloride, NaCl .	5 g
Dipotassium hydrogen phosphate, K_2HPO_4 . .	2 g
Phenol red (1 in 500 aqueous solution). . . .	6 ml
Agar	20 g
Distilled water . . .	1 l
Glucose, 10 per cent solution, sterile	10 ml
Urea, 20 per cent solution, sterile	100 ml

Sterilize the glucose and urea solutions by filtration. Prepare the basal medium without glucose or urea, adjust to pH 6·8–6·9 and sterilize by autoclaving in a flask at 121°C for 30 min. Cool to about 50°C, add the glucose and urea and tube the medium as deep slopes.

The medium may be used as a liquid by omitting the agar.

Method 1. Inoculate heavily over the entire slope surface and incubate at 37°C. Examine after 4 h and after overnight incubation, no tube being reported negative until after 4 days' incubation. Urease-positive cultures change the colour of the indicator to purple-pink.

Medium 2 (Elek's Test)

Urea	4 g
Potassium dihydrogen phosphate, KH_2PO_4, 0·2 M . .	50 ml
Sodium hydroxide, NaOH, 0·2 N	35 ml
Distilled water, ammonia-free .	115 ml

This substrate contains 2 per cent urea at pH 7·2. Sterilization of it is unnecessary. It can be stored in the refrigerator in a stoppered bottle with the stopper smeared with petroleum jelly. Freshly prepared substrate should be checked with a known urea-splitting organism, and for the test a negative control and an uninoculated blank must be included. The glassware must be scrupulously clean but not necessarily sterile.

Method 2. Emulsify sufficient of a 24-h culture of the organism to be tested, in 0·5 ml of the substrate in a $3 \times \frac{3}{8}$ in tube. The fluid should be distinctly opalescent. Place the tube in a water-bath at 37°C for 3 h. Remove the tube and add 0·1 ml of Nessler's reagent, and a similar amount to the negative control and blank tubes. Read the result 3 min after adding the Nessler's reagent. Both negative and control tubes must be absolutely colourless. A positive reaction is shown by a colour ranging from a pale but distinct yellow to a dark brown precipitate. The time of incubation is important and should be strictly adhered to.

When isolated colonies are to be examined, the volume of substrate is reduced to 0·3 ml and only one drop of Nessler's reagent used. Readings are taken 4–5 min after nesslerization.

Nitrate Reduction Test

This is a test for the presence of the enzyme nitrate reductase which causes the reduction of nitrate, in the presence of a suitable electron donor, to nitrite which can be tested for by an appropriate colourimetric reagent. Almost all enterobacteriaceae reduce nitrate.

Medium

Potassium nitrate, KNO_3 (nitrite-free) . . . . . 0·2 g
Peptone . . . . . 5·0 g
Distilled water . . . . 1 l

Tube in 5-ml amounts and autoclave at 121°C for 15 min.

Method. Inoculate and incubate for 96 h.

Test reagent

Solution A. Dissolve 8·0 g of sulphanilic acid in 1 l of 5 N acetic acid.
Solution B. Dissolve 5·0 g of α-naphthylamine in 1 l of 5 N acetic acid.

Immediately before use, mix equal volumes of solutions A and B to give the test reagent.

Add 0·1 ml of the test reagent to the test culture. A red colour developing within a few min indicates the presence of nitrite and hence the ability of the organism to reduce nitrate.

α-Naphthylamine is potentially carcinogenic.

Lecithinase Test

Some bacteria produce enzymes (lecithinases or phospholipases) that split lipoprotein complexes in human serum and hen egg-yolk and produce opalescence or turbidity when grown in media containing these substrates. When the reaction is produced with egg-yolk it is sometimes referred to as the lecithovitellin reaction. The reactions when the substrate is added to a liquid medium and when human serum is added to a solid medium are described here. The lecithinase test can also be done with egg-yolk in solid medium but it will be described under Combined Tests because lipase reactions can also be seen with this medium.

TUBE TEST (Hayward, 1941)

Medium

Nutrient broth, sterile . . 50 ml
Human serum, sterile . .
or   50 ml
Egg-yolk suspension, 10 per cent.

The egg-yolk suspension is prepared as described in Chapter 5 but is 10 per cent in saline instead of 50 per cent. A sterile egg-yolk broth is obtainable commercially (Oxoid, London).

Aliquots (0·3 to 1 ml) of medium are dispensed aseptically in sterile tubes. Aliquots of nutrient broth without human serum or egg-yolk are dispensed as controls.

Method. Test and control media are inoculated with a drop of liquid culture or a colony picked from a plate culture. A known lecithinase-producing organism may be inoculated into test and control media as a positive control. In some cases the test can be extended by inoculating an additional test medium and adding antitoxin to a specific lecithinase, e.g. *Cl. welchii* alpha antitoxin for the identification of *Cl. welchii* (Chap. 38). Some lecithinases are dependent on divalent cations and may be inhibited by sequestering agents or buffers containing calcium-binding salts.

The tubes are incubated under conditions suitable for growth of the species involved and examined for turbidity daily up to five days. A positive reaction usually develops within 24–48 h and is indicated by a pronounced turbidity with a yellowish curd on the surface of the test mixture, the lesser turbidity caused by growth being present in the control and antitoxin tubes. A modification of this method may be used for testing culture filtrates or centrifuged supernates for lecithinase activity using an incubation time of 1 h. Tests are more easily read after storage overnight at 4°C or centrifugation to deposit organisms at the bottom and raise the curd to the surface of the mixture in a positive test.

PLATE TEST (Hayward, 1943)

Medium
    Nutrient agar containing 3 per
    cent agar, sterile   .   .   . 100 ml
    Human serum, sterile   .   . 40 ml
Melt the agar, cool to 50°C, add the serum and pour plates. The medium may be enriched by the addition of 5 per cent Fildes' extract. A nutrient agar prepared with Evans' peptone stimulates lecithinase production by *Cl. welchii*.
Method Inoculate and incubate under conditions suitable for growth. Lecithinase-producing colonies are surrounded by zones of opalescence. In some cases an additional test can be included by spreading a few drops of antitoxin to a specific lecithinase over half the plate before it is inoculated. Opalescence should be inhibited around colonies on the antitoxin-treated half of the plate (Chap. 38).

Hyaluronidase Test

Hyaluronidase catalyses the hydrolysis of hyaluronic acid; it attacks the intercellular cement substances in tissues and acts as a 'spreading factor'. Hyaluronidase activity in bacterial culture filtrates can be demonstrated by a modification of the ACRA test (Burnet, 1948). A solution containing hyaluronic acid derived from synovial fluid is mixed with congo red. When a drop of this mixture falls into acid alcohol it produces a characteristic appearance. Progressive reduction of the amount of hyaluronic acid in the mixture, either by prior dilution or by enzymatic activity, leads to progressive changes in the pattern produced when a drop falls into acid alcohol. For an account of the procedure and details of factors influencing the test, the paper by Oakley and Warrack (1951) should be consulted.

Deoxyribonuclease Tests

The enzyme deoxyribonuclease attacks DNA present in the nuclei of leucocytes and influences their subsequent affinity for Romanowsky stains such as Jenner's. The enzyme also digests DNA present in tissues, e.g. horse spleen, and reduces the viscosity of solutions of semi-purified DNA extracts. The nucleic acid is precipitated by alcohol as a fibrous mass before but not after enzymatic decomposition. There are three tests for deoxyribonuclease activity and they are based on the above observations.

SLIDE TEST (Warrack, Bidwell and Oakley, 1951)

Substrate. Rabbits are bled into 1·6 per cent sodium oxalate, the leucocytes concentrated by centrifugation and resuspended in oxalated rabbit plasma, and trial films made. The concentration of leucocytes is adjusted to give 15–20 per $\frac{1}{12}$ in objective field. Films are made in a standard manner on slides $7·5 \times 1·2$ cm, dried in the air and fixed in methanol.

Test. The deoxyribonuclease activity of a culture filtrate is demonstrated as follows: A numbered slide bearing a fixed film is gently placed in each of a series of 4 ml volume doubling dilutions of the culture filtrate so that half of each film is submerged. After incubation in this position at 37°C for 18 h along with appropriate control tests, the slides are removed, rinsed with distilled water and stained with Jenner's stain. Each film is then examined microscopically, using the oil-immersion objective, and the half of each slide that was not immersed acts as a control for the number of intact leucocytes per field and for the efficiency of staining.

If the concentration of deoxyribonuclease is high, no stained leucocytes may be seen in the treated film. The first stage of action is reduction in nuclear staining of lymphocytes, progressing to production of unstained ('ghost') nuclei which are sharply demarcated from the surrounding faintly stained cytoplasm. Polymorphs are next affected and finally eosinophils are attacked.

OTHER TESTS FOR DEOXYRIBONUCLEASE.

A modification of the ACRA test of Burnet (1948) devised by Oakley and Warrack (1951), and the alcohol precipitation test (McCarty,

1949), may also be used to assess deoxyribonuclease activity.

COMBINED TESTS

Malonate Utilization and Phenylalanine Deaminase Test

This combines the two tests already described (Shaw and Clarke, 1955).

Medium

Ammonium sulphate, $(NH_4)_2SO_4$	2·0 g
Dipotassium hydrogen phosphate, K_2HPO_4 . . .	0·6 g
Potassium dihydrogen phosphate, KH_2PO_4	0·4 g
Sodium chloride, NaCl . .	2·0 g
Sodium malonate . . .	3·0 g
DL-phenylalanine . . .	2·0 g
Yeast extract	1·0 g
Distilled water	1 l

Steam for 5 min and filter through paper. Add 5 ml of a 0·5 per cent solution of bromothymol blue in absolute ethanol. Distribute in 10-ml quantities and autoclave at 121°C for 15 min.

Method. Distribute aseptically in 1 ml volumes in small sterile tubes. Inoculate, incubate overnight, and read results as follows:

1. Malonate utilization test.
Observe colour of medium.

> Blue = positive.
> Green = negative.

2. Phenylalanine deaminase test.

Having recorded the result of the malonate test, acidify with a few drops of 0·1 N HCl until the colour of the medium becomes yellow. Add a few drops of a 10 per cent aqueous solution of ferric chloride, shake and observe colour.

> Dark green = positive.
> Yellow-buff = negative.

Composite Media for Preliminary Identification of Enterobacteria

The following modification of Kohn's method (Gillies, 1956) is a reliable substitute for the conventional method of determining the biochemical identity of non-lactose-fermenting colonies prior to confirmation by serological typing.

Composite medium I

Beef extract	2 g
Proteose peptone No. 3 (Difco) .	15 g
Yeast extract . . .	2 g
Glucose	1 g
Mannitol	10 g
Agar	16 g
Indicator mixture . . .	26·5 ml
Distilled water . . .	1 l

Adjust pH to 7·2.

After autoclaving at 115°C for 15 min and cooling to 60°C, 50 ml of a 20 per cent urea solution sterilized by filtration are added and the medium is distributed aseptically in sterile test-tubes to a depth of 6·5 cm and allowed to solidify in a sloped position so as to provide a butt of 2·5 cm.

Indicator mixture. Three separate 0·2 per cent indicator solutions are made up.

Indicator	grams	0·05N NaOH	water
Bromothymol blue	0·20	6·4 ml	100 ml
Cresol red	0·20	10·6 ml	100 ml
Thymol blue	0·20	8·6 ml	100 ml

The final indicator is obtained by mixing the individual solutions in the following proportions:

Bromothymol blue . . .	12·5 ml
Cresol red	4 ml
Thymol blue	10 ml

Composite medium II

Agar	3 g
Bacto-peptone (Difco) . .	10 g
Tryptone (Difco) . . .	10 g
Sodium chloride, NaCl . .	5 g
Disodium hydrogen phosphate, $Na_2HPO_4.12H_2O$ . . .	0·25 g
Sucrose	10 g
Salicin	10 g
Bromothymol blue . . .	0·01 g
Sodium thiosulphate, $Na_2S_2O_3$. $5H_2O$	0·025 g
Distilled water	1 l

Adjust pH to 7·4.

The medium is distributed into cotton-wool-stoppered test-tubes in 8-ml amounts, autoclaved at 121°C for 15 min and allowed to set with the tubes in the vertical position.

Lead acetate papers. Strips (5 mm × 50 mm) of filter paper are impregnated with saturated lead acetate solution and dried in an oven at 70°C.

Indole test papers are similarly impregnated with the following solution:

p-dimethyl-aminobenzaldehyde . 5 g
Methanol   .   .   .   . 50 ml
o-phosphoric acid   .   .   . 10 ml

and are dried at 70°C for a minimum period.

Method

The two media are inoculated with a long straight wire charged from a colony of the organism to be identified; medium I is inoculated by both smearing the slant and then stabbing to the base of the butt; medium II is then inoculated by a single stab into its upper $\frac{1}{2}$ inch; finally, the two test papers are suspended above the latter medium and held by the cotton-wool stopper.

Results. In medium I the fermentation of glucose is indicated by the butt changing from deep green to yellow and that of mannitol by the development of a yellow slant. Urease production produces a deep blue colour throughout the medium. Gas production appears in varying degrees from a slight splitting along the wire track to disruption of the medium. In medium II, fermentation of sucrose or salicin or both changes the medium from light blue to yellow and accompanying gas production causes bubbles to form. Non-motile organisms grow only along the line of inoculation, whereas motile species show either a diffuse even growth spreading from the inoculum or more rarely localized outgrowths which are usually fan-shaped or occasionally nodular. H_2S production causes blackening of the lead acetate paper and the formation of indole gives a red colour in the yellow test paper.

Litmus Milk

Milk indicates both saccharolytic and proteolytic properties of bacteria by detecting whether they ferment lactose or digest casein. Lactose fermenters in litmus milk form acid and cause it to become pink. Large amounts of acid will precipitate the casein as a clot and if gas is formed during coagulation the clot will be disrupted by it ('stormy clot'). Proteolytic bacteria may decompose milk proteins to a transparent solution of soluble products. In litmus milk this shows as a change to a clear dark purple solution, usually taking several days and preceded by the formation of a soft, easily disintegrated clot.

Medium

Skimmed milk. Steam fresh milk for 20 min and allow it to stand for 24 h in order that the cream may separate. Siphon the milk off from the cream.

Litmus solution

Litmus granules   .   .   . 80 g
Ethanol, 40 per cent aqueous . 300 ml
                                 (approx.)
Hydrochloric acid, HCl 1N   . q.s.

Table 7.1   Identification patterns of organisms grown in the composite media of Gillies at 37°C for 18 h

| Organism | Results with Medium I | | | Results with Medium II | | | |
| | Fermentation of | | Production of Urease | Fermentation of Sucrose/Salicin | Motility | Production of | |
	Glucose	Mannitol				H_2S	Indole
Salmonella typhi	A	A	−	—	+	+	−
Other salmonellae	AG	A*	−	—	+	D	−
Shigella sonnei	A	A	−	—	−	−	−
Sh. flexneri	A	A	−	—	−	−	+
Sh. dysenteriae type 2	A	—	−	—	−	−	+
Proteus group	(—)	(—)	+	D	+	D	D

Key to Table: A = acid produced
                 AG = acid and gas produced
                  — = no reaction
               (—) = apparently no reaction
                  * = gas production not observable
                     from mannitol

− = negative
+ = positive
D = different results from
   different strains.

Grind up the granules, add to a flask containing 150 ml aqueous ethanol and boil for 1 min. Decant the solution, add remainder of the aqueous ethanol and boil for 1 min. Decant and combine the two solutions, making the volume up to 300 ml with 40 per cent aqueous ethanol. Add hydrochloric acid drop by drop, shaking continuously until the solution becomes purple. To test for the correct reaction, boil a tube of tap water and another of distilled water and add a drop of the solution to each. The tap water should be blue and the distilled water mauve.

Preparation of complete medium

Skimmed milk .	.	.	.	250 ml
Litmus solution	.	.	.	6·25 ml

Distribute in 5-ml amounts in tubes or screw-capped bottles. Steam for 20 min on three successive days.

The colour fades on storing and it is best to store the skimmed milk, steamed on three successive days, in bulk (e.g. 250 ml) and add the litmus immediately before distribution.

Egg-Yolk Agar

Egg-yolk indicates both lipase and lecithinase reactions of bacteria. On solid media containing egg-yolk, lipolysis is shown by the formation of a thin, iridescent 'pearly layer' overlying the colonies and a 'confined' opalescence in the medium underlying them, seen best when the colonies are scraped off. Copper sulphate can be used to form bright greenish-blue insoluble copper soaps with the fatty acids in both the pearly layer and the opalescence in the medium (Willis, 1960). Lecithinase is shown by wide zones of opalescence around colonies, more intense and larger than the zones caused by lipolysis. Neutralization by antitoxin may be possible (p. 119) (Chap. 37).

Medium

Nutrient agar, sterile.	.	.	85 ml
Egg-yolk suspension (p. 119)	.		15 ml

Melt the agar, cool to 55°C and add the egg-yolk. Pour plates.

The medium can be enriched with 5 per cent Fildes' extract. A sterile concentrated egg-yolk emulsion may be obtained from Oxoid, London.

Method. Inoculate, incubate and examine for wide zones of opalescence indicating lecithinase and for the iridescent layer indicating lipolysis. Flood the plate with a saturated aqueous solution of copper sulphate, stand for 20 min, drain off the excess solution and dry the plate for a short time in the incubator. The greenish-blue colour of copper soaps of fatty acids confirms lipolysis.

MISCELLANEOUS TESTS

Potassium Cyanide Test

This tests the ability of an organism to grow in the presence of cyanide (Rogers and Taylor, 1961).

Basal medium

Peptone .	.	.	.	3 g
Sodium chloride, $NaCl$	.	.	5 g
Potassium dihydrogen phosphate, KH_2PO_4.	.	.	.	0·23 g
Disodium hydrogen phosphate, $Na_2HPO_4.2H_2O$	.	.	5·64 g
Distilled water .	.	.	.	1 l

Adjust to pH 7·6 if necessary. Sterilize by autoclaving in a flask at 121°C for 30 min. Refrigerate the basal medium until totally chilled.

Cyanide solution

Potassium cyanide, KCN	.	.	0·5 g
Distilled water, sterile	.	.	100 ml

Preparation of complete medium

Basal medium .	.	.	1 l
Cyanide solution	.	.	15 ml

Add the cyanide to the cold medium. Distribute in 1-ml amounts in sterile bijou bottles, seal tightly without delay and store at 4°C. The medium will keep for 4 weeks under these conditions.

Method. Inoculate with one loopful from a 24 h nutrient broth culture and incubate at 37°C with the cap tightly screwed down to prevent air exchange. Observe after 24 h and 48 h for turbidity produced by growth.

After use the cyanide in the medium should be destroyed by adding ferrous sulphate and alkali before submitting the cultures for sterilization.

Niacin Test

This test is used in the differentiation of the mycobacteria. Tubercle bacilli of human type produce niacin (nicotinic acid) and this is detected with cyanogen bromide and aniline.

Reagents

Cyanogen Bromide. A 10 per cent aqueous solution is used. Cyanogen bromide liberates toxic fumes and should be prepared in a fume cupboard and stored in a dark-coloured, well-stoppered bottle in the refrigerator. It is made up once a fortnight.

Aniline. A 4 per cent (v/v) solution in 96 per cent ethanol is used. The aniline should be redistilled if coloured. The solution can be stored in the refrigerator for at least a month.

Method. Cultures of mycobacteria should be grown on slopes of a colourless medium, e.g. Dubos and Davis medium, incubated at 37°C. At intervals up to 10 weeks a slope is removed from the incubator and to it is added 1 ml of the cyanogen bromide solution, followed after five min by 1 ml of the aniline solution. The development of a yellow colour in the test fluid is regarded as positive. The yellow pigment of certain chromogenic strains does not diffuse from the colonies and so can be distinguished from a positive test. After the test has been read, a few ml of 10 per cent ammonia solution are added to the bottles to destroy the residual cyanogen bromide before submitting the cultures for sterilization.

Arylsulphatase Test

This test is particularly useful in distinguishing between *Myco. avium* (negative) and *Myco. intracellulare* (positive). *Myco. fortuitum* is very active on a concentration of 0·00025 M in 3 days.

Prepare a 6·25 per cent solution (0·1 M) of tripotassium phenolphthalein disulphate in water and sterilize by filtration. Add 1 ml to 100 ml Dubos and Davis liquid medium (see Chap. 5) to give a 0·001 M concentration. Inoculate a 5-ml volume of the above medium with a drop of a just-visible suspension of the culture. Incubate at 37°C for 2 weeks and then add, drop by drop, a solution (1·0 M) of sodium carbonate to detect the presence of

free phenolphthalein, which is demonstrated by the production of a pink colour.

Detection of Motility

In semi-solid agar media, motile bacteria 'swarm' and give a diffuse spreading growth that is easily recognized by the naked eye. Motility may thus be detected more easily than by the microscopical 'hanging drop' method.

The exact optimal concentration of agar depends on the particular brand used and must be determined by trial; usually it is about 0·4 per cent of Japanese agar or 0·2 per cent of New Zealand agar. This is dissolved in nutrient broth or peptone water. It is important that the final medium should be quite clear and transparent. Dispense 10-ml amounts in test-tubes and leave to set in the vertical position. Inoculate with a straight wire, making a single stab down the centre of the tube to about half the depth of the medium. Incubate under the conditions favouring motility. Examine at intervals, e.g. after 6 h and 1, 2 and 6 days when incubating at 37°C. Freshly-prepared medium containing 1 per cent glucose can be used for motility tests on anaerobes (see Chap. 5).

Non-motile bacteria generally give growths that are confined to the stab-line, have sharply defined margins and leave the surrounding

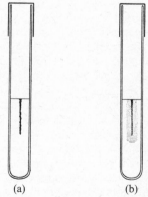

(a)   (b)

Fig. 7.1

Diagram showing growth of a non-motile organism (*a*) restricted to the stab line in semi-solid nutrient agar. The diffuse growth, or 'swarm', of a motile organism (*b*) extends as a zone of turbidity from the stab line.

medium clearly transparent. Motile bacteria typically give diffuse, hazy growths that spread throughout the medium rendering it slightly opaque. The outgrowth may reach the walls of the tube after a few hours and the foot of the tube after one or two days. It is best observed by contrast while there is still some transparent medium not yet invaded. With a non-motile strain that yields motile variants, a discrete line of growth is formed along the stab and diffuse outgrowths then fan out from one or two points. Sharply defined finger-like outgrowths may be given by some kinds of poorly motile bacteria, and also by some kinds of non-motile bacteria, apparently by their 'falling' through clefts in the medium; these doubtful cases may be resolved by use of the 'hanging drop' method.

Tests for Direct Bacterial Haemagglutinin

Adhesiveness for animal cells is commonly indicated by a tendency of certain bacteria to adhere to and bind together red blood cells and thus cause 'direct bacterial haemagglutination'. The bacterial haemagglutinin may be a fixed part of the bacterial surface (see *fimbriae*, Vol. I, Chap. 2) and this type of haemagglutinin is accordingly described as 'non-diffusible' or structural. A few bacterial species produce a soluble amorphous or 'diffusible haemagglutinin' which diffuses into the surrounding medium and, though reacting with red cells, cannot bind the bacteria to these or to other substrates.

TILE TEST FOR FIMBRIAL HAEMAGGLUTININ. Red cells separated from fresh citrated guinea-pig blood are washed twice in physiological saline and made up to a 3 per cent (v/v) suspension in fresh saline. A nutrient broth culture of the test organism is centrifuged to deposit the bacilli. After removal of the culture supernatant, the bacillary deposit is resuspended in the small amount of fluid remaining. A drop of the dense bacillary deposit is mixed with an equal drop of the red cell suspension in a depression on a white tile at 3–5°C, and the tile is then rocked gently for 5 min while it is warming to room temperature. In the case of most fimbriate organisms tests made at room temperature (15–20°C) without chilling the tile are entirely satisfactory. A few organisms, however, give haemagglutination at 3–5°C but not at higher temperatures.

The haemagglutination produced by fimbriate organisms is seen with the naked eye and usually develops as a coarse clumping within a few seconds. Weakly active cultures produce a fine granularity within 2–3 min. Very poorly haemagglutinating cultures may show positive reactions only if mixing is continued for up to 30 min.

Inhibition of Fimbrial Haemagglutination with Mannose. The incorporation of a small drop of a 2 per cent solution of D-mannose in the haemagglutination mixture (final mannose concentration 0·5 per cent) specifically inhibits fimbrial haemagglutination (see Duguid and Gillies, 1957).

TUBE TEST FOR SOLUBLE HAEMAGGLUTININ. To doubling dilutions of the test culture supernatant in physiological saline (0·5-ml volumes), 0·5-ml aliquots of a 1 per cent (v/v) red cell suspension in saline are added. The tubes are shaken and allowed to stand at room temperature for 1–2 h. The red cells settle into a characteristic pattern at the foot of each tube and this is conveniently viewed in a mirror. In the absence of haemagglutinin, the red cells form a dense central button. In the presence of soluble haemagglutinin, the red cells fall in a reticulum and this covers the base of the tube. The patterns are very similar to those described by Salk (1944) for myxovirus haemagglutination.

REFERENCES

BARER, G. (1946) The rapid detection of gelatin-liquefying organisms. *Monthly Bulletin of the Ministry of Health Laboratory Service,* **5,** 28.

BURNET, F. M. (1948) The mucinase of *V. cholerae. Australian Journal of Experimental Biology and Medical Science,* **26,** 71.

CARPENTER, K. P. (1961) The relationship of the Enterobacterium A 12 (Sachs) to *Shigella boydii* 14. *Journal of General Microbiology,* **26,** 535.

COWAN, S. T. & STEEL, K. J. (1965) *Manual for the Identification of Medical Bacteria.* London: Cambridge University Press.

CRUICKSHANK, R. (1968) *Medical Microbiology,* 11th edn. (revised reprint). Edinburgh: Churchill Livingstone.

DUGUID, J. P. & GILLIES, R. R. (1957) Fimbriae and adhesive properties in dysentery bacilli. *Journal of Pathology and Bacteriology,* **74,** 397.

GILLIES, R. R. (1956) An evaluation of two composite media for preliminary identification of shigella and salmonella. *Journal of Clinical Pathology,* **9,** 368.

HAYWARD, N. J. (1941) Rapid identification of *Cl. welchii* by the Nagler reaction. *British Medical Journal,* 1, 811.

HAYWARD, N. J. (1943) The rapid identification of *Cl. welchii* by Nagler tests in plate cultures. *Journal of Pathology and Bacteriology,* 55, 285.

HUGH, R. & LEIFSON, E. (1953) The taxonomic significance of fermentative versus oxidative metabolism of carbohydrates by various Gram negative bacteria. *Journal of Bacteriology,* 66, 24.

KOHN, J. (1953) A preliminary report of a new gelatin liquefaction method. *Journal of Clinical Pathology,* 6, 249.

LAUTROP, H. (1956) *Acta pathologica et microbiologica scandinavica,* 39, 370.

McCARTY, M. (1949) The inhibition of streptococcal desoxyribonuclease by rabbit and human antisera. *Journal of Experimental Medicine,* 90, 543.

MØLLER, V. (1955) Simplified tests for some amino acid decarboxylases and for the arginine dihydrolase system. *Acta pathologica et microbiologica scandinavica,* 36, 158.

OAKLEY, C. L. & WARRACK, G. H. (1951) The ACRA test as a means of estimating hyaluronidase, deoxyribonuc-lease and their antibodies. *Journal of Pathology and Bacteriology,* 63, 45.

REPORT (1958) Recommended methods for group differentiation with the enterobacteriaceae. *International Bulletin of Bacteriological Nomenclature and Taxonomy,* 8, 53.

ROGERS, K. B. & TAYLOR, J. (1961) Laboratory diagnosis of gastro-enteritis due to *Escherichia coli. Bulletin of the World Health Organization,* 24, 59.

SALK, J. E. (1944) A simplified procedure for titrating hemagglutinating capacity of influenza-virus and the corresponding antibody. *Journal of Immunology,* 49, 87.

SHAW, C. & CLARKE, P. H. (1955) Biochemical classification of *Proteus* and Providence cultures. *Journal of General Microbiology,* 13, 155.

STEEL, K. J. (1961) The oxidase reaction as a taxonomic tool. *Journal of General Microbiology,* 25, 297.

WARRACK, G. H., BIDWELL, E. & OAKLEY, C. L. (1951) The beta-toxin (deoxyribonuclease) of *Cl. septicum. Journal of Pathology and Bacteriology,* 63, 293.

WILLIS, A. T. (1960) The lipolytic activity of some clostridia. *Journal of Pathology and Bacteriology,* 80, 379.

8. Tests for Sensitivity to Antimicrobial Agents

Antimicrobial agents and their activities have been described in Volume I, Chapters 6 and 56. They include the disinfectants and the antimicrobial drugs (i.e. chemotherapeutic agents and antibiotics). The clinical bacteriologist is nowadays required to spend much time assessing the range of sensitivity of pathogenic bacteria isolated from patients to different antimicrobial drugs. He may also be required to assay the antimicrobial content of serum and other body fluids from patients receiving drug therapy and to test the effectiveness of disinfectants under specified conditions. Guidance in the use of these substances is part of his province and he is often expected to discuss disinfection and antibiotic policies with clinicians and to give advice on codes of practice and their implementation.

Testing of Disinfectants

Many different disinfectant compounds are in use, some with a wide range of activity and others more specific in their effects. A knowledge of the properties of the individual compounds is necessary for the proper testing of their activity and such information is usually readily obtained from the manufacturers.

A number of variables affect the activity of all disinfectants and these must be considered when interpreting the results of laboratory tests and their application in practice. The most important factors are the following:

Concentration. In general, the higher the concentration of the disinfectant the greater its killing activity. The careful preparation of fresh in-use solutions at the correct dilution is especially important in the case of compounds, such as those of the phenolic group, the activity of which falls off rapidly with dilution (i.e. which have a high concentration coefficient).

Time and temperature. The number of organisms killed increases with the length of time they are in contact with the disinfectant and a certain minimum time, usually not less than 10 minutes, is normally required for proper disinfection. Speed of killing increases with an increase in temperature, the upper limit of the increase depending on the heat stability of the disinfectant used.

Inactivating agents. The activity of all disinfectants is reduced by organic matter and this inactivation occurs particularly in the presence of the proteins in such body fluids as faeces, blood and pus. Soap, incompatible detergents, hard water and materials such as plastic or cork also inactivate certain disinfectants. Some disinfectants, such as hypochlorite, are unstable and may be readily inactivated by exposure to organic materials and metal surfaces. It is thus essential that, when practicable, the objects to be disinfected should be made as clean as possible.

Number of organisms. The larger the number of organisms to be killed the greater will be the time required for disinfection. Spores are highly resistant to destruction by most disinfectants.

Principles of Different Tests

The tests generally used are carried out under conditions quite different from those found in practice and the simulation of natural conditions is extremely difficult due to the influence of many variables, such as the presence of organic matter and the different types, numbers and location of the organisms at the sites to be disinfected. A wide range of tests is available, each of which is appropriate for a different purpose, and their particular applications must be appreciated when interpreting the results. The tests most commonly used are as follows:

1. The minimum inhibitory concentration (MIC) test measures the lowest concentration of the disinfectant that will inhibit the growth of a known strain of bacterium, e.g. *Salmonella typhi*, in nutrient medium.

2. The Rideal-Walker test compares the bactericidal activity of the disinfectant with that of phenol, i.e. it measures the phenol coefficient of the disinfectant under standard conditions (British Standards specification 541).

3. The Chick-Martin and Garrod tests also determine the phenol coefficient of the disinfectant but are more rigorous than the Rideal-Walker in that a standard amount of organic matter is incorporated in the test mixture (British Standards specification 808).

4. Tests for disinfecting action on surfaces.

5. The capacity use-dilution test measures the effect of repeated challenge by the addition of fresh bacteria on the antibacterial effectiveness of the disinfectant.

6. The stability test measures the stability and long-term effectiveness of diluted disinfectant in clean and dirty situations; it supplements the capacity use-dilution test.

7. The in-use test determines whether living bacteria are present in samples of liquid disinfectants taken from utensils and containers, such as hospital buckets and laboratory discard jars. This simple test is the only test for disinfectants that need be done in hospitals, where it has many obvious applications (Kelsey and Maurer, 1972).

All these tests have a common principle. After the indicator bacteria have been exposed to contact with the disinfectant, their viability is tested by subculture on medium prepared without disinfectant. Some disinfectant, however, is carried over in the inoculum of the test mixture into the subculture and its subsequent static or cidal action on bacteria that have survived in the test mixture is a common cause of overestimation of the disinfectant's activity. It is important, therefore, that the disinfectant carried over into the subculture should be neutralized either by its being diluted to a subinhibitory concentration in the subculture medium or by the addition to the medium of a substance that inactivates it. Simple 1 in 10 dilution in broth is sufficient to neutralize phenols and alcohols, but is inadequate for the neutralization of many disinfectants with lower concentration coefficients. Chlorine compounds, iodine and iodophors can be neutralized by the addition of 0·5 per cent sodium thiosulphate to the subculture medium, chlorhexidine by 2 per cent Lubrol W with 0·5 per cent lecithin, quaternary ammonium compounds by 3 per cent Lubrol W with 2 per cent lecithin, and formaldehyde and glutaraldehyde by 1 per cent sodium bisulphite.

Minimum Inhibitory Concentration (MIC) Test

Plate test. Prepare suspensions of different indicator bacteria from young (e.g. overnight) cultures on solid medium by adding the bacteria to sterile distilled water until it appears faintly turbid. Incorporate different known concentrations of the disinfectant under test in plates of nutrient agar and inoculate streaks of the different bacterial suspensions on the surface of each plate. Incubate the plates for 48 h at 37°C. The lowest concentration of disinfectant that entirely prevents the growth of an indicator bacterium on the plate is the minimum inhibitory concentration of the disinfectant for that particular bacterium.

Tube test. Incorporate different known concentrations of the disinfectant in tubes of broth or serum (sterile ox serum previously heated at 56°C) and inoculate a standard volume of a suspension of indicator bacteria into each tube. Incubate the tubes for 48 h at 37°C and then examine them with the naked eye for turbidity. The lowest concentration of disinfectant that prevents the development of turbidity is the MIC. To confirm the naked-eye reading and to demonstrate cidal as well as static effects, streak-inoculate a loopful of each mixture on to an agar plate. The subculture from the tube containing the MIC will form no more than a few colonies derived from inoculated bacteria that have survived exposure to the disinfectant. Subcultures from tubes containing less than the MIC will give heavy growths and subcultures from tubes containing cidal concentrations, e.g. the minimum cidal concentration (MCC), will give no growth.

Rideal-Walker Test

The bactericidal potency of disinfectants is most frequently assessed by measuring the rate of kill of a selected range of bacteria under specified conditions. Most methods employ phenol as a standard reference so that a *phenol coefficient* is frequently cited for disinfectants. This coefficient expresses the bactericidal power of a particular disinfectant as compared with that of pure phenol. The principal methods are those of the Rideal-Walker, Chick-Martin, Garrod and United States (FDA) tests. These tests are mostly used for comparing disinfectants composed of phenolic coal-tar derivatives that are water-soluble or water-miscible. They are of no use for comparing the merits of different classes of compounds, e.g. for comparing coal-tar derivatives with quaternary ammonium compounds. The Rideal-Walker test is described below. For full details of the technique see *Technique for Determining the Rideal-Walker Coefficient of Disinfectants*, British Standards Specification, No. 541 (1934) with amendments dated 1943 and 1961; obtainable from British Standards Institution, 28 Victoria Street, London SW1.

Materials

1. Standard loop of 28 SWG wire, 4 mm internal diameter, bent almost at a right angle to the wire, so that in the subsequent manipulations the plane of the loop is horizontal.

2. Culture of *Salmonella typhi*. It is important to use a standard culture. A suitable culture may be obtained from the National Collection of Type Cultures, Central Public Health Laboratories, Colindale Avenue, London, if the purpose for which the culture is required is stated. Make three successive subcultures in a standard broth at intervals of 24 h and use the third 24-h culture as the inoculum for the test.

Method

1. Determine the minimum inhibitory concentration (MIC) of the disinfectant under test for the standard strain of *S. typhi* and make up a series of five graded concentrations in distilled water, the lowest being slightly greater than the MIC. Dispense 5 ml volumes of the different concentrations into stoppered sterile test-tubes.

2. Make up 100 ml of a 5 per cent stock solution of pure phenol in sterile distilled water, and from it prepare the following dilutions of phenol: 1 in 95, 1 in 100, 1 in 105, 1 in 110 and 1 in 115. Dispense 5 ml volumes of the different concentrations into stoppered sterile test-tubes. To each of the tubes containing 5 ml volumes of the solutions of the disinfectant under test, add with a sterile pipette 0·2 ml of the 24-h broth culture of *S. typhi* and shake the mixtures. Before and during the test, keep the tubes in a water-bath at 18°C.

4. At intervals of 2·5 min up to 10 min remove a large loopful from each mixture with the standard wire loop and transfer to tubes of 5 ml standard broth. (If the bacterial suspension in (3) is added to the tubes of disinfectant solutions in succession at definite intervals, e.g. 30 sec, the loop-transfers from each tube of disinfectant into standard broth can be accurately timed after 2·5, 5, 7·5 and 10 min.)

Table 8.1

Disinfectant	Dilution of disinfectant	Growth of *S. typhi* after exposure to disinfectant for test period (min)			
		2·5	5	7·5	10
Disinfectant under test	1 in 400	−	−	−	−
	1 in 500	−	−	−	−
	1 in 600	+	−	−	−
	1 in 700	+	+	−	−
	1 in 800	+	+	+	+
Phenol	1 in 95	+	−	−	−
	1 in 100	+	+	−	−
	1 in 105	+	+	+	−
	1 in 110	+	+	+	−
	1 in 115	+	+	+	+

Phenol coefficient of disinfectant under test $= \dfrac{700}{100} = 7 \cdot 0$.

5 and 6. Carry out with the phenol solutions the same procedure as in (3) and (4).

7. Incubate the broth tubes for 48 h and then note the tubes in which the development of turbidity indicates the occurrence of growth.

8. Calculate the *phenol coefficient* by dividing the figures indicating the dilution of the disinfectant that shows bacterial growth after exposure for 2·5 and 5 min, but no growth after longer exposure, by the figure indicating the dilution of phenol that shows growth after exposure for 2·5 and 5 min but no growth after longer exposure (see Table 8.1).

CHICK-MARTIN AND GARROD TESTS

The Rideal-Walker test, just described, compares the action of the test disinfectant with that of phenol on *S. typhi* in distilled water. It does not necessarily give a measure of the activity of the disinfectant under practical conditions where much organic matter is usually present. The Chick-Martin test simulates natural conditions more closely than the Rideal-Walker in that it tests the disinfectant in the presence of organic material. For the purpose of the test the organic material is the quantity of solid matter present when heat-sterilized liquid faeces containing 10 per cent of solids is mixed with twice its volume of disinfectant. The use of faeces in this test is open to several objections and Garrod has devised a modification of the Chick-Martin test with yeast instead of faeces. The yeast is suspended in distilled water to a concentration equivalent to 5 g dry yeast per 100 ml and for the test 48 ml is added to 2 ml of *S. typhi* broth culture. To 2·5 ml portions of this mixture is added 2·5 ml of separate parallel dilutions, varying by 10 per cent, of the disinfectant and phenol. The phenol coefficient of the disinfectant under test is calculated by dividing the mean of the highest concentration of phenol producing sterility with the corresponding mean for the disinfectant. Thus, if there were no growth with 2·0 per cent phenol, but growth with 1·8 per cent, the mean would be 1·9. Similarly, if there were no growth with 0·457 per cent of the disinfectant, but growth with 0·411 per cent, the mean would be 0·434. The result then would be expressed in the following form:

$$\text{Phenol coefficient of disinfectant} = \frac{1\cdot 9}{0\cdot 434} = 4\cdot 4.$$

OTHER TESTS OF DISINFECTANTS

Tests for Surface Disinfection

The rapidly expanding use of disinfectants and antiseptics for removing microorganisms from surfaces has focused attention on tests of the ability of the disinfectant to kill microorganisms on the surfaces of objects. Recent techniques utilize glass cylinders (Mallman and Hanes, 1945) and squares of test material such as steel, linoleum or tile (Stedman, Kravitz and Bell, 1954). The original papers should be consulted for details.

Capacity Use-Dilution Test

This test (Kelsey and Sykes, 1969) measures the effect of repeated bacterial challenge upon the bactericidal efficiency of the disinfectant. It is carried out by adding successive volumes of a suspension of a suitable test bacterium at standard time intervals to the disinfectant diluted in a standard hard water solution. After each addition of the organism, portions of the mixture are removed and cultured for survivors.

Stability Test

This test (Maurer, 1969) is used to supplement the information obtained from the capacity use-dilution test. It is designed to check the stability and long-term effectiveness of disinfectants in their recommended dilutions.

In-Use Test

Take samples of disinfectant from any place or container in which it is being used, such as floor-mop buckets, cleansing buckets, laboratory discard jars, disinfectant solutions in which instruments, crockery, bedpans, etc., have been rinsed, and closed containers of diluted disinfectants ready for use. Determine the numbers of living bacteria, if any, in these in-use samples by making cultures.

Transfer 1 ml of the disinfectant sample to 9 ml of quarter-strength Ringer's solution or, in the case of a non-phenolic disinfectant, to 9 ml of an isotonic solution that inactivates it, e.g. nutrient broth containing 0·5 per cent sodium thiosulphate for hypochlorites and iodophors. With a '50-dropper' pipette, immediately transfer 10 small drops (about 0·02 ml) of the decimal dilution on to separate areas of the surface of each of two dried agar plates. Incubate for 72 h one plate at 37°C and the other at room temperature. Examine the plates and score the growth from each drop. Growth from more than 5 out of 10 drops on either plate indicates failure of disinfection. Such a result corresponds to approximately 1000 living organisms per ml in the sample of disinfectant. Regard the result as satisfactory if only an occasional sample drop shows growth.

The method and use of this test in the control of hospital disinfection programmes is described by Kelsey and Maurer (1972) who give further references and advise that it is *the only test for disinfectants that need be done in hospitals*.

ANTIBIOTIC SENSITIVITY TESTS AND ASSAYS

A wide range of techniques is available which correspond to those used in other forms of microbiological assay. The principle of these tests is similar, namely the preparation of a concentration gradient of the antibiotic in a nutrient medium and the observation of whether or not growth takes place when the medium is seeded with the indicator bacterium and incubated. The concentration gradient may be continuously varied, as in agar diffusion tests, or discontinuously varied as in a series of tubes of liquid medium or plates of agar medium (see Fig. 8.1). In tests to determine the *sensitivity* of a newly isolated bacterium, known amounts of antibiotic are added to the medium. In *assays*, or *titrations* of antibiotics, e.g. in body fluids, a bacterium of known sensitivity to the antibiotic is used as an indicator.

These tests are artificial laboratory models and often do not closely simulate conditions in the tissues of the host during treatment. As long as this limitation is realized, and the method of testing is carefully controlled, the results are of great value. Many variables are involved in sensitivity and assays tests, such as the size of the inoculum, the nature of the culture medium, the presence of inhibitors, the concentration of agar in the medium, the thickness of the medium in the plate, the conditions and time of incubation, and the composition of antibiotic disks. The effect of these variables has been fully investigated and the findings used in recommendations for standardization of techniques and the use of quality control (Bauer *et al.*, 1966; Anderson, 1970; Ericsson and Sherris, 1971; Garrod, Lambert and O'Grady, 1973, pp. 491–508). Whatever method is used, the number of variables should be kept to a minimum and consultation should be

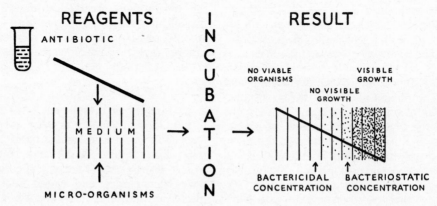

FIG. 8.1

Principles of antibiotic sensitivity tests and microbiological assays (Gould, J. C. (1960). *British Medical Bulletin*, **16**, 29)

maintained between the microbiologist and the clinician about the interpretation of the results obtained in the laboratory.

In a conventional disk-diffusion or tube-dilution test on primary cultures of clinical specimens, the results will be available only after 24 h, and those of tests on pure sub-cultures only after 36–48 h or longer. In some cases, it may be important to report the sensitivity of an organism more rapidly and this can be done by the use of special techniques, e.g. tests involving turbidometric readings, which are applicable only to pure cultures and are not always reliable. Speed in obtaining results is probably more important in the assay of antibiotics in body fluids than in testing the sensitivities of bacterial isolates as the main indication for assays relates to the toxicity of antibiotics such as the aminoglycosides.

Techniques for testing the sensitivities of fresh bacterial isolates to a range of potentially therapeutic antibiotics are described below and techniques for assaying antibiotics in the blood or other body fluid of a patient under therapy are described towards the end of this chapter.

SENSITIVITY TESTS FOR CLINICAL USE

Large numbers of isolates of bacteria from patients are examined in the clinical laboratory in order to determine which antibiotics are likely to be effective in curing the infections. The tests are, therefore, done in such a way as to show whether the isolate is sensitive to a concentration of the antibiotic likely to be produced in the infected tissues during treatment of the patient by the methods and dosage rates employed by the physicians. The concentration of a drug in the tissues varies considerably from patient to patient and from time to time in the same patient, so that for most clinical purposes it is pointless to employ laborious methods to measure accurately the minimum inhibitory and cidal concentrations (MIC and MCC) of the drug for the isolate. It is sufficient to use a simple, empirically-based test which distinguishes isolates as 'sensitive' or 'resistant' in fair concordance with the probable outcome of therapy.

In a survey made in 1970, Castle and Elstub (1971) found that 99 per cent of laboratories in Britain used the *disk-diffusion test*. In this test, small absorbent paper disks or tablets impregnated with known amounts of antibiotics are placed on an agar culture plate that has been seeded uniformly with bacteria of the isolate to be tested. After incubation, the size of the zones of inhibition of growth produced by the antibiotics diffusing from the disks into the surrounding agar is observed. The critical decisions to be made in the laboratory which affect the clinical validity of the disk test are those fixing the amount of antibiotic to be contained in each disk and the size of the zone to be read as the boundary between 'sensitivity' and 'resistance'. It is generally considered that for infections in most parts of the body a bacterium may be considered 'sensitive' to an antibiotic if the antibiotic's MIC for it is not more than one-quarter to one-half the average concentration of antibiotic maintained in the blood of a patient receiving ordinary dosage (for many antibiotic schedules this is in the range $0 \cdot 1$–$1 \cdot 0$ μg per ml). The MIC of an antibiotic for a fresh bacterial isolate can be estimated from the diameter of the zone of inhibition of growth around a disk by reference to 'standard graphs' (regression lines). These relate the zone diameter to the antibiotic content of the disk for a standard organism for which the MIC is known (Gould and Bowie, 1952; Ericsson, 1960). Most laboratories, however, use a simpler, empirical method for determining the conditions of sensitivity readings, by comparing the zone of inhibition of the test isolate with that of a standard organism known to be sensitive to therapy at ordinary rates of dosage.

Oral and parenteral administrations generally produce much higher (e.g. ×10 to ×100) concentrations of antibiotics in the urine than in the blood and tissues. For the treatment, therefore, of urinary tract infections in which there is no significant invasion of tissues, a bacterium may be considered 'sensitive' to an antibiotic whose MIC for it is up to 10 or more times as great as that acceptable for the treatment of other kinds of infections. This difference is taken into account by the use of disks containing, for example, 10 times larger amounts of antibiotic in tests of isolates from urine than in those of isolates from other parts of the body.

Other tests based on antibiotic diffusion gradients are controlled and interpreted in much the same way as the disk tests. In the *cup test* solutions of different antibiotics or of different concentrations of the same antibiotic are placed in circular holes cut with a cork-borer in a uniformly seeded culture plate. In the *ditch test* an antibiotic dissolved in nutrient agar is poured into and allowed to set in a rectangular ditch formed by cutting a strip of agar from a plate; a number of bacterial isolates as well as a standard organism as control are then inoculated in streaks crossing the ditch at right angles.

There are only a few clinical circumstances that require a fairly precise measurement of the MIC and MCC of an antibiotic for the patient's infecting organism, e.g. the need accurately to control the therapy of subacute bacterial endocarditis (Garrod, Lambert and O'Grady, 1973, p. 318). In these cases the MIC and MCC are measured in serial dilution tests in tubes or plates. Serial dilution tests with different concentrations of antibiotic in each of a set of tubes or plates are also used for sensitivity tests of organisms such as the tubercle bacillus and *Actinomyces israelii* which grow so slowly that tests based on diffusion gradients are unreliable.

DISK-DIFFUSION TESTS OF SENSITIVITY TO ANTIBIOTICS

The disk-diffusion method provides a simple and reliable test specially applicable in routine clinical bacteriology. It consists of impregnating small disks of a standard filter paper with given amounts of a chosen range of antibiotics. These are placed on plates of culture medium previously spread uniformly with an inoculum of the bacterial isolate to be tested. After incubation, the degree of sensitivity is determined by measuring the easily visible areas of inhibition of growth produced by the diffusion of the antibiotic from the disks into the surrounding medium (Gould and Bowie, 1952).

The width of the zones of inhibition of growth depends upon variables that influence the diffusion of the antibiotic, such as the pH, depth, hydration and concentration of the agar

medium, as well as on the type of nutrients in the medium, the numbers and rate of growth of the inoculated bacteria, and the conditions of incubation. Because, however, the majority of pathogens encountered in the clinical laboratory grow at similar rates and the experimental conditions can be standardized, diffusion tests can give results of a high standard of reproducibility as well as a reasonable degree of accuracy. Replicate tests and control tests are easily set up and several different antibiotics can be tested against the same bacterial isolate on a single plate. Suggestions for the standardization of variables and for a uniform method of performing the disk test have been made by Garrod and Waterworth (1971) and Stokes and Waterworth (1972) and form the basis of the following recommendations.

Primary-culture and Pure-subculture Tests

Sensitivity disk-diffusion tests done on primary cultures from clinical specimens have the advantage that their results are generally available as early as the day following the receipt of the specimen. When the specimen contains a mixture of bacteria they may also be helpful, either by showing which antibiotic is effective against all the potentially pathogenic strains present, or by facilitating the separation and identification of strains through the production of selective zones. Swabs well soaked in pus and specimens of urine showing bacteria by microscopy are suitable for primary-culture tests, but throat swabs, faeces and vaginal swabs are not. The main disadvantage of primary-culture tests is that the number of bacteria in the inoculum cannot be standardized and sometimes is so small that results cannot be read or properly assessed; a further test must then be done on a pure subculture of the suspected pathogen.

Pure-subculture tests are done with inocula of bacteria taken from one or more colonies in a primary culture of the clinical specimen. Their results, therefore, are not available until at least two days after the receipt of the specimen. Their main advantage is that the inoculum can be standardized at the optimum density for the test.

Preparation of Disks

It is most convenient to use dry antibiotic disks prepared and supplied commercially. The disks are usually about 6 mm in diameter and consist of absorbent paper impregnated with antibiotic. Some brands consist of a vehicle, binding agent and antibiotic compressed into a tablet (Sleigh, 1958). They are marked with letters to show which antibiotic they contain. When large numbers of isolates from the same type of clinical specimen have to be tested against a standard set of antibiotics, time and labour are saved by the use of multi-disks or rings which carry several different disks at an appropriate spacing and may be applied to the culture plate in a single action. Three-quarters of the laboratories in Britain surveyed by Castle and Elstub (1971) used mainly such multi-disks or rings. It is recommended they should not contain more than six drugs because zones may not be distinct when larger numbers of drugs are tested on an 8·5 cm plate.

Commercially prepared disks may not always contain the correct amount of antibiotic and if they are used, it is recommended that they should be compared in control tests with fresh disks of known potency prepared in the laboratory (see Greenberg et al., 1957). Methods for preparing wet disks with a reliable content of antibiotic (Gould and Bowie, 1952) and for their colour coding with dyes to indicate which antibiotics they contain (Bowie and Gould, 1952) are described in the Appendix to this chapter.

Dry disks can be stored at −20°C for at least a year without loss of potency and for a shorter period at 4°C. The manufacturer's expiry date should be observed. Wet disks retain their potency for several months at 4°C.

Drug Content of Disks

A choice has to be made between disks with 'high' contents of antibiotics and disks with 'low' contents. High-content disks give wide zones of inhibition (e.g. 30–50 mm diameter) with organisms sensitive to the therapeutic concentrations of antibiotics commonly produced in the blood and tissues, and narrower zones (e.g. 15–30 mm) with organisms resistant to such concentrations though sensitive to the higher concentrations therapeutically attainable in the urine. Low-content disks give moderate-sized zones (e.g. 20–40 mm) with organisms sensitive to the commonly produced blood concentrations and narrower zones (e.g. 10–20 mm) or no inhibition at all with organisms resistant to the blood concentration though perhaps sensitive to urine concentrations.

High-content disks are often used with a view to estimating the degree of sensitivity of organisms over a wide range and to detect the lower degrees of sensitivity in bacteria that would be susceptible to therapy in the urinary tract. Their use, however, carries the disadvantages that in multi-disk tests the very large zones obtained with sensitive organisms may merge and be difficult to measure and that the bacteriologist may be reluctant to report as 'resistant' the strains that show the substantial zones of inhibition (e.g. 20 mm) indicative of resistance to the usual therapeutic concentrations of antibiotic.

It is probably better to use low-content disks for tests on bacteria from infections of parts of the body other than the urinary tract and a separate high-content set of disks for bacteria from urine. A suitable range of contents, which is based mainly on the recommendations of Garrod and Waterworth (1971) and Stokes and Waterworth (1972), is shown in Table 8.2.

Choice of Drugs for Disk Test

When large numbers of sensitivity tests have to be done on isolates from clinical specimens, it is convenient to restrict the routine 'first-line' tests to the number of antibiotics that can be accommodated on a single culture plate. Preferably not more than six disks should be tested on a plate and certainly not more than eight. Different appropriate first-line sets of six or eight drugs, e.g. on multi-disks, may be chosen for use with the different types of clinical specimen, e.g. exudates, sputum, urines, or, in the case of tests on pure subcultures, for different groups of bacteria, e.g. staphylococci, other Gram-positive bacteria, and coliform bacilli. The set of drugs chosen should reflect the frequency of usage of the different drugs by the clinicians served and the common

Table 8.2   Suitable drug contents (μg) for sensitivity-test disks

Drug	Bacteria from sites other than urine	Bacteria from urine
Ampicillin	2	30
Carbenicillin*	100	100
Cephaloridine	5	30
Chloramphenicol	10	30
Clindamycin	2	...
Colistin*	50	50
Erythromycin	10	...
Fucidin	10	...
Gentamicin	10	30
Kanamycin	10	30
Lincomycin	2	...
Methicillin	10	...
Nalidixic acid	...	30
Neomycin	10	...
Nitrofurantoin	...	200
Novobiocin	5	...
Penicillin (benzyl-)	1	30
Polymyxin B*	30	30
Streptomycin	10	30
Sulphonamide (Sulphafurazol)	100	500
Tetracycline	10	30
Trimethoprim	1·25	1·25
Trimethoprim/sulphamethoxazole†	1·25/23·5	1·25/23·5

*For *Pseudomonas aeruginosa* only.
†Cotrimoxazole.
Other disks: for sensitivity tests on yeasts, nystatin 100 μg; for identification of *Streptococcus pyogenes*, bacitracin 2·5 units; for diagnosis of clostridia, neomycin 100 μg; for identification of pneumococcus, optochin 5 μg.

sensitivity patterns of the local endemic pathogens. In special cases requiring tests against other drugs, a second plate may be put up with a supplementary set of drugs. Examples of suitable first-line sets of drugs for different purposes are as follows.

1. *For cultures from specimens other than urine* (e.g. blood, exudates, pus, sputum, swabs from wounds and mucosae): ampicillin cotrimoxazole, erythromycin, penicillin (benzyl), tetracyline and gentamicin (or cephaloridine or streptomycin).

2. *For cultures from urine:* high-content disks of ampicillin, cotrimoxazole, nalidixic acid, nitrofurantoin, sulphonamide and kanamycin (or cephaloridine or tetracycline).

3. *For staphylococcus:* erythromycin, fucidin, penicillin (benzyl), tetracycline, lincomycin (or clindamycin), cotrimoxazole (or gentamicin or novobiocin) and, separately by special method, methicillin.

4. *For other cocci and Gram-positive bacteria:* ampicillin, cephaloridine, cotrimoxazole, erythromycin, penicillin (benzyl) and tetracycline.

5. *For most Gram-negative bacilli:* ampicillin, cephaloridine, cotrimoxazole (or sulphonamide), streptomycin (or kanamycin) and tetracycline; for *Salmonella typhi* include chloramphenicol.

6. *For Haemophilus:* ampicillin, cephaloridine, chloramphenicol, cotrimoxazole, sulphonamide and tetracycline.

7. *For Pseudomonas aeruginosa:* carbenicillin, colistin (or polymyxin B) and gentamicin.

8. *For clostridia and anaerobic Gram-negative bacilli:* ampicillin, clindamycin, fucidin, penicillin (benzyl) and tetracycline.

Culture Medium

A nutrient agar medium should be used which is as free as possible from substances inhibitory to the action of the antibiotics, e.g. inhibitors of sulphonamides and tetracycline. Suitable 'sensitivity test agars' are available from commercial suppliers. The pH should be 7·2–7·5. Glucose and reducing substances such as thioglycollate should not be added. Blood should be added when testing *Streptococcus pyogenes* or pneumococcus, heated ('chocolated') blood when testing haemophilus, and lysed horse blood (Harper and Cawston, 1945) when testing sulphonamides and trimethoprim. A volume of about 20 ml should be poured in 8·5 cm diameter petri dishes with flat bottoms lying on a horizontal surface to give a uniform layer of agar 3–4 mm deep.

Harper and Cawston's (1945) lysed blood agar for sulphonamide tests is prepared from a base consisting of Evans peptone 20 g, sodium chloride 2·5 g, sodium glycerophosphate 2·0 g, Davis New Zealand agar 10 g and water 1 litre. Dissolve the ingredients in the water. Add 11 ml N-Na_2CO_3 per litre. Adjust to pH 7·2–7·4. Bottle in 100 ml amounts and autoclave at 121° for 15 min. Melt the medium and add 6 per cent of oxalated horse blood which has been freshly lysed by the addition of 2 ml of a 10 per cent solution of saponin to each 100 ml blood. Mix thoroughly, pour plates and store for 12 h before use.

Test Procedure

Dry the culture plate in the incubator with the lid ajar until its surface is free from visible moisture. Inoculate the bacteria to be tested by one of the procedures described below and, if inoculation is by flooding, dry the plate again for up to 30 min. Without further delay, apply the chosen antibiotic disks at adequate spacing (2 cm or more apart) to the surface of the plate with sterile fine-pointed forceps and press gently to ensure full contact with the medium and moistening of the disk. At once transfer to the incubator and incubate for the minimum time needed for normal growth, usually for 18–24 h at 37°C.

Inoculum

The method used for inoculation of the bacteria to be tested should aim at producing a uniform, nearly confluent lawn of growth covering the whole surface of the plate on which the disks are to be placed. The zones of inhibition are smaller the greater the number of bacteria inoculated and it is, therefore, best to adjust the density of the inoculum so that the growth appears as numerous small, nearly confluent colonies and not as a continuous film. Such adjustment is difficult in primary-culture tests but can be done reasonably well in tests on pure subcultures.

For *tests on primary cultures*, rub a swab well soaked in pus over the whole or half of a culture plate to give a heavy, uniform inoculum; if only half the plate is thus seeded, stroke out the inoculum on the other half to yield separate colonies. Inoculate urine by placing a 5 mm flat loopful of uncentrifuged, well mixed urine on the plate and spread evenly with a dry sterile swab. Place disks on the uniformly seeded area of the plate, spacing them so that their centres are at least 2 cm apart.

For *tests on pure subcultures*, use one of the following methods:
Inoculation by flooding. Suspend bacteria from the culture to be tested in sterile isotonic saline solution to a concentration of 10^5–10^6 bacteria per ml. Do this by adding to 5 ml saline a small loopful (about 0·01 ml) of an overnight broth culture (about 10^9 bacteria/ml) or a suspension of a few colonies in broth at a similar density. With a sterile Pasteur pipette transfer about 2 ml of the dilute suspension to the plate, tip the plate in different directions to wet the whole of its surface, remove all the excess fluid with the pipette, dry the plate inverted and with its lid ajar in the incubator for up to 30 min or on the bench for one hour and finally apply the disks.
Inoculation by spreading. Place on the plate a loopful of an overnight broth culture or a broth suspension of colonies at similar density and spread it evenly over the whole plate or test area with a sterile bent glass rod or a dry sterile cotton-wool swab of the throat-swab type.

Control Cultures

Because the results of disk-diffusion tests vary with a number of experimental conditions that are difficult to standardize, it is necessary to evaluate them by comparison with those of a control test with a standard organism of known sensitivity. The Oxford strain of *Staphylococcus aureus* (National Collection of Type Cultures No. 6571) is a suitable control for tests of bacteria from most kinds of infections (except those of the urinary tract) against most kinds of antibiotics (except polymyxin). For controlling tests of bacteria from urine for sensitivity to the high concentrations of antibiotics that may be achieved in urine, an 'antibiotic-sensitive' strain of *Escherichia coli*, such as NCTC10418, is recommended. The *Esch. coli* strain can be used as a control for tests with polymyxin. Tests of *Pseudomonas aeruginosa* should be controlled by a test with a 'sensitive' strain of the same species (e.g. NCTC10662) because zone sizes are smaller than those with *Esch. coli*.

Control on same plate as test. The most satisfactory way to use the control culture is to grow it alongside the test culture on the same plate and compare the zones of inhibition produced in the two cultures by the same disk (Stokes, 1960). Inoculate the clinical specimen or a pure subculture in a broad band across the middle of the culture plate and inoculate the control culture on the sectors on either side of this band, carefully leaving an unseeded strip not more than 5 mm wide between the test and control areas. When a clinical specimen is inoculated as the test, make the control inoculum from an overnight broth culture diluted 1 in 100 in fresh broth; this dilution gives an inoculum similar in density to that of many clinical specimens. After inoculation, apply up to four disks, two on each of the unseeded strips between the test and control inocula.

Control on separate plate from test. Although not excessively laborious, the method just described is sufficiently exacting to be almost impracticable for routine use in laboratories with a large daily receipt of specimens and an ungenerous level of staffing. In such laboratories the easier procedure of inoculating the test bacterium over the whole surface of the culture plate and applying a multi-disk is usually adopted. When this is done, one plate in each batch of tests with a given set of disks should be inoculated with the standard bacterium to serve as a control for the batch and the zone sizes produced on the bacteria under test should be compared with those produced on the standard bacterium. This procedure does not control variations between the amounts of an antibiotic in different disks or variations between the conditions in the different culture plates in the batch poured for the tests. It does, however, control certain other variables and the repeated daily observation of the sizes of the zones produced with the standard bacterium indicates the probable limits of variability in the test.

Reading and Interpretation of Results

Measure the diameters of the zones of inhibition of growth (including the 6 mm diameter of the disk itself) by the use of calipers or by viewing the plate against a ruler or ruled screen. Compare the zones produced by each drug on the test bacteria with that produced on the standard bacterium. It is recommended that when a strain shows a zone smaller than that of the control bacterium and a confluence of its growth shows that the inoculum has been too dense, the test should be repeated.

Report the strain under test as *sensitive* (i.e. probably susceptible to clinical therapy at ordinary dosage rates) if the diameter of its zone of inhibition by a drug is greater than, equal to, or not more than 4 mm less than that on the control culture.

Report the strain as *moderately sensitive* if its zone diameter is at least 12 mm but is reduced by over 4 mm as compared with the control (see Fig. 8.2).

Report the strain as *resistant* (i.e. unlikely to respond even to high-dosage therapy) if it shows no zone of inhibition of growth or if the diameter of its zone is not more than 10 mm (i.e. 2 mm on each side of a 6 mm disk).

It is important that criteria such as these should be clearly defined for the bacteriologists and technicians reading and reporting tests in a clinical laboratory, and that it should not be left to each worker arbitrarily to determine his own criteria for reporting sensitivity or resistance. The procedure of measuring zones need not be very laborious. When a bacteriologist is reading large numbers of tests, he should be able, after measuring the zones in the control culture, to read most of the test cultures at sight. It is very disturbing that only 100 out of

330 British hospital laboratories surveyed by Castle and Elstub (1971) controlled their reading of sensitivity tests by comparison with a standard organism.

Penicillinase-producing staphylococci may show large inhibition zones when tested against a penicillin or ampicillin disk, but show a sharp, heaped-up edge consisting of full-sized colonies which contrasts markedly with the smooth tapering edge seen in control tests with the penicillin-sensitive control culture. Regardless of zone size they should be reported as 'resistant' to penicillin and ampicillin.

Because the use of cotrimoxazole (sulphamethoxazole + trimethoprim) to treat patients infected with bacteria that are highly resistant to sulphonamide may lead to the development of resistance to trimethoprim, it may be wise not to report strains as being cotrimoxazole-sensitive unless they also show some degree of sensitivity to sulphonamide alone. Trimethoprim diffuses rapidly and produce very wide zones in sensitive strains.

Tests with Penicillin-resistant Penicillins and Cephalosporins

The resistance of staphylococci to methicillin, cloxacillin, flucloxacillin, cephaloridine and other cephalosporins cannot be tested by the disk methods described above, but should be assessed in a separate test with a 10 μg methicillin disk on a plate incubated at 30°C (Hewitt, Coe and Parker, 1969) or on medium containing 5 per cent NaCl at 37°C. Only methicillin should be used. If methicillin-resistance is demonstrated, the strain will also be resistant to cloxacillin, flucloxacillin and the cephalosporins.

Determination of MIC by Disk Method

The MIC of any antibiotic for a bacterial isolate can be estimated from a measurement of the zone of inhibition in the disk test by reference to a standard graph, or regression line, previously prepared, which relates the MIC to the zone diameter for a standard organism of a known degree of sensitivity (Gould and Bowie, 1952). The validity of the method depends on very careful standardiza-

tion of the conditions of the tests and an effective method has been defined by Ericsson and Sherris (1971). The principle of the construction and use of a standard graph may be explained as follows.

Disks containing different amounts of the antibiotic are tested under carefully standardized conditions against a standard organism of known sensitivity, e.g. the Oxford (Heatley) strain of *Staph. aureus* (NCTC6571). The organism is grown for 18 h in broth, diluted to approximately 10^8 bacterial cells per ml and inoculated on to nutrient agar plates by flooding. The open plates are dried, the disks are applied and the plates are incubated overnight at 37°C. For each antibiotic the diameters of the circular areas of inhibition are plotted against the logarithms of the amounts of antibiotic in the disk and the resultant graph is approximately a straight line.

When a fresh bacterial isolate is later tested under the same conditions, the concentration of antibiotic required for the inhibition of its growth (MIC) may be calculated from the measurement of the diameter of the zone of inhibition by reference to the standard graph. The sensitivity of the standard bacterium (*Staph. aureus* strain NCTC6571) is known (e.g. MIC penicillin = 0·03 units per ml, i.e. 0·018 μg per ml). Therefore, the calculation of the degree of sensitivity of the new isolate under test is as follows:

$$\text{MIC of bacterium under test} = \frac{\begin{array}{c}\text{Amount of antibiotic} \\ \text{per disk required to} \\ \text{inhibit the bacterium} \\ \text{under test at a given} \\ \text{size of zone}\end{array}}{\begin{array}{c}\text{Amount of antibiotic} \\ \text{per disk required to} \\ \text{inhibit the standard} \\ \text{bacterium at the} \\ \text{same size of zone}\end{array}} \times \begin{array}{c}\text{MIC of} \\ \text{standard} \\ \text{bacterium}\end{array}$$

For routine tests, disks contain the same amount of any given antibiotic. The amount required to inhibit the standard bacterium is constant, and the amount required to inhibit the bacterium under test is obtained from the standard graph as in the following example for penicillin. Suppose the diameter of the zone of

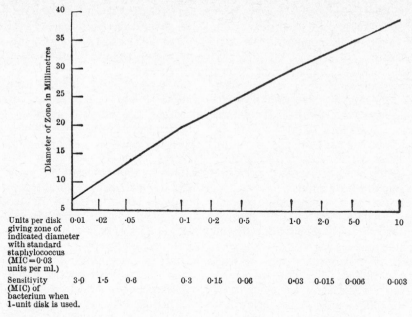

Fig. 8.2

Graph relating the diameter of the zone of inhibition of the standard strain of *Staph. aureus* to the number of units of benzylpenicillin in the disk in a disk-diffusion sensitivity test.

inhibition of the bacterium under test produced by a disk containing 1 unit of penicillin is 13 mm. The graph for penicillin indicates that a disk containing 0·05 units penicillin inhibits the standard bacterium to 13 mm. Therefore the MIC of penicillin for the bacterium under test is $\frac{1}{0·05} \times 0·03 = 0·06$ units per ml.

Replica Plate Test for Cidal Action

A zone of inhibition of growth may be produced around an antibiotic disk irrespective of whether the antibiotic is bactericidal or only bacteriostatic. The replica plate method of Elek and Hilson (1954) demonstrates whether or not bacteria have survived in this zone.

Prepare a 'stamp' from a cylindrical, flat-ended block of wood 3 cm in length and slightly less in diameter than a Petri dish by attaching to one end with latex adhesive a piece of close-piled velvet about 2·5 mm thick; face the pile away from the wood and trim its edges to the block. Autoclave the stamps and store in pairs, velvet faces in contact. Use repeatedly until velvet becomes matted.

Press the velvet face of a sterilized stamp evenly and without lateral movement on to the growth on the incubated disk-sensitivity plate. Lift the stamp and press it firmly on a fresh (replica) plate without antibiotic. After removal of the stamp, incubate the replica plate and examine it for growth within the areas corresponding to the inhibition zones on the disk-sensitivity plate. About 1 per cent of the bacteria are transferred from plate to plate and it can be seen whether these had been killed or merely inhibited on the sensitivity plate.

SERIAL DILUTION TESTS OF ANTIBIOTIC SENSITIVITY

Tube Dilution Test for MIC

Prepare in broth, or other suitable liquid medium, a solution of antibiotic at a known concentration, e.g. 20 μg/ml, at least twice the highest concentration likely to be found in the tissues. Make in parallel two series of doubling dilutions of this solution in broth in sterile stoppered test-tubes, extending down to a concentration of antibiotic half that inhibiting the most sensitive member of the species being tested. Add to each series a tube of medium without antibiotic. Inoculate the bacterial isolate under test into one series and a standard organism, e.g. the Oxford strain of *Staph. aureus*, into the other by adding to each tube one drop of an overnight broth culture diluted to such an extent that after inoculation the text mixture will contain about 10^6 bacteria per ml. With each group of tests include tubes of uninoculated medium with and without antibiotic to act as controls of the sterility and clarity of the media. Incubate the tests for 18–24 h at 37°C and examine for turbidity due to bacterial growth. Read the tube with the highest dilution of antibiotic showing no visible turbidity as the one containing the minimum inhibitory concentration (MIC) of the antibiotic for the bacterial isolate tested. The value for the new bacterial isolate should be accepted as valid only if that for the standard organism is given correctly, e.g. 0·03 units (0·018 μg) of penicillin per ml for the Oxford staphylococcus.

Tube Dilution Test for MCC

The tube dilution test just described may readily be modified so that it measures the minimum cidal concentration (MCC) as well as the minimum inhibitory concentration (MIC) of an antibiotic for an isolate. Before incubating each series of seeded tubes, remove a large loopful, e.g. 0·02 ml, from the tube without antibiotic and spread it uniformly over quarter of a plate of agar free from antibiotic. After incubation of the tubes, similarly spread a loopful from each tube not showing growth over a different sector of a plate. Where available, use an inactivator of the antibiotic, e.g. penicillinase, in the plating medium. Incubate the plate cultures for 24 h. Read the tube culture containing the highest dilution of antibiotic that yields no growth in the plate subculture as the one containing the MCC of the antibiotic for the bacterial isolate tested. Compare the plate subcultures yielding growth with that seeded from the antibiotic-free tube cultures before incubation to determine whether there was some bactericidal action or only bacteriostasis.

Plate or Slope Dilution Test for MIC

Tests on plates or slopes of solid medium are used for organisms such as haemophili, meningococci, Gram-negative anaerobes and tubercle bacilli which grow poorly or slowly in liquid media. Pour a series of plates or slopes of a suitable solid medium containing different concentrations of the antibiotic and spread or streak-inoculate on each a loopful of a suspension of the culture under test diluted to a standard density, e.g. 10^6 bacteria per ml. On a separate area on each plate or on parallel slope cultures inoculate a standard organism. When incubation has to be prolonged, as for tubercle bacilli, use slopes in screw-capped bottles. Read the MIC as the lowest concentration entirely preventing growth.

TESTS FOR COMBINED DRUG ACTION

There are three main reasons why a physician may treat a patient with more than one antibiotic at the same time.

1. Treatment with two drugs with different modes of action to both of which the infecting bacterium is originally sensitive prevents the outgrowth of mutant bacteria resistant to either drug, e.g. in the dual or triple drug therapy of tuberculosis. The success of this method may be predicted from the demonstration that a culture from the patient is sensitive to each drug by itself and it is not dependent on the two drugs having a 'synergistic' or mutually enhancing action.

2. Two drugs may be given because the identity or sensitivity of the infecting bacterium is still unknown, e.g. kanamycin and polymyxin for Gram-negative bacteriaemic shock.

3. Two drugs may be given together because they are synergistic in their bactericidal action, being strongly cidal in combination though not completely cidal when used separately. Synergistic cidal effect is required mainly in the treatment of subacute infective endocarditis in which a complete bactericidal effect is essential for cure because any surviving bacteria in the vegetations are protected from the natural body defence mechanisms. Certain combinations of drugs are known to be likely to show synergy, e.g. (a) penicillin or cephaloridine with strepto-mycin, kanamycin or vancomycin for strepto-

cocci, (b) methicillin, cloxacillin or cephaloridine with streptomycin, kanamycin or vancomycin for penicillinase-producing staphylococci, and (c) ampicillin, carbenicillin, cephaloridine or polymyxin with streptomycin, kanamycin or gentamicin for Gram-negative bacilli. Other combinations are known to be ineffective; the penicillin group of drugs are antagonized by bacteriostatic drugs such as chloramphenicol and tetracycline. The culture from the patient may be tested for sensitivity to the cidal action of suitable pairs of drugs by the *cellophane transfer method* of Chabbert and Waterworth (1965) or the *half-chess-board test in liquid media* described by Garrod, Lambert and O'Grady (1973, p. 512).

Half-Chess-Board Test for Synergistic Bactericidal Action

Perform bactericidal tests in tubes of broth containing each antibiotic at a single concentration attainable in the blood during conventional therapy, e.g. 10 μg per ml, both separately and in all possible combinations in different tubes. For streptococci from subacute bacterial endocarditis, penicillin, streptomycin, cephalosporin, erythromycin and kanamycin might be tested. Inoculate a drop of a diluted culture of the bacterial isolate under test into each tube with antibiotic and a control tube without antibiotic to give a final density of about 10^6 bacteria per ml. Inoculate plate subcultures before and after incubation as described for the tube dilution test for MCC and examine for a combination of drugs giving a greater bactericidal effect than given by any one drug by itself.

SENSITIVITY TESTS OF MYCOBACTERIUM TUBERCULOSIS

Several antimicrobial drugs such as streptomycin, para-aminosalicylic acid (PAS) and isonicotinic acid hydrazide (isoniazid) have a beneficial effect in cases of tuberculosis if the organism is sensitive to the drug. Unfortunately, drug-resistant mutant bacilli may grow out selectively during treatment with a single drug, so that it is customary to administer two or more drugs simultaneously. It is essential that strains isolated from the patient before and at intervals during treatment should be tested for their sensitivity to the various antituberculous drugs to guide the physician in making necessary changes to his choice of drugs for therapy. The criteria for interpreting resistance from the tests to be described have been determined by closely correlating the results of sensitivity tests with clinical findings.

Danger to Laboratory Personnel

Aerosols of suspensions of cultures of tubercle bacilli are notorious for their ability to infect laboratory workers. Great care should be taken to avoid spilling or splashing the infected fluids and by gentle procedures to minimize the formation of aerosols. It is essential, moreover, that all procedures of inoculation and preparing inocula, especially the shaking of culture suspensions, should be done in a safety cabinet of approved design.

Sensitivity to Streptomycin

Strains of tubercle bacilli are tested for sensitivity to streptomycin in cultures on Löwenstein-Jensen medium. Dihydrostreptomycin is used because of its stability on heating. The concentrations of streptomycin tested are 1 μg per ml rising by two-fold increments to 64 μg per ml. These are the actual concentrations in the medium before it is inspissated. A control bottle of medium without the drug is included. The medium containing streptomycin is dispensed in 1·25 ml amounts into 6-ml screw-capped bottles, inspissated for 60 min at 85°C to produce a firm medium and stored in the refrigerator at 4°C; it may be kept for at least one month without loss of potency.

To prepare the inoculum, sterilize screw-capped 6-ml bottles containing 0·1 ml water and six 5-mm glass beads. Make a suspension of the culture to be tested by shaking a loopful of the growth in the 0·1 ml water on a mechanical shaker for a few minutes and dilute to a standard suspension. With a wire loop of 2·5 mm internal diameter and 22 SWG diameter streak a loopful of the suspension up the centre of the control slope and each antibiotic-containing slope. This inoculum will consist of about 10^4–10^5 bacterial aggregates per slope.

In each batch of tests include a control test using the standard drug-sensitive strain of *Myco. tuberculosis* H37 Rv. Read after 28 days incubation at 37°C.

The end-point is the lowest concentration of the antibiotic that inhibits growth (MIC). Growth is considered to be inhibited if fewer than 20 colonies appear on the slope. The result is expressed as a *resistance ratio* by comparison with the control culture as follows:

$$\text{Resistance ratio} = \frac{\begin{array}{c}\text{Lowest concentration of the}\\ \text{antibiotic that inhibits the}\\ \text{patient's strain of } Myco.\\ tuberculosis\end{array}}{\begin{array}{c}\text{Lowest concentration of the}\\ \text{antibiotic that inhibits the}\\ \text{standard drug-sensitive strain}\\ \text{H37 Rv.}\end{array}}$$

For example, if the patient's strain is inhibited by 16 μg per ml and the standard, drug-sensitive strain by 4 μg per ml, then the resistance ratio is $\frac{16}{4} = 4$.

Strains are considered to be resistant to streptomycin if the resistance ratio is 8 or more. A ratio of 4 is suggestive of resistance, but not conclusive. In such a case, other cultures of the patient's strain should be tested and the previous chemotherapy considered.

Sensitivity to Para-aminosalicylic Acid (PAS)

Sensitivity tests to PAS are performed in the same way as for streptomycin but with concentrations of PAS ranging in two-fold steps from 0·25 to 16 μg per ml. Sodium PAS is used because it is more stable and more soluble than PAS itself. Strains are considered resistant to PAS if the resistance ratio is 8 or more. A ratio of 4 is suggestive, but not conclusive. In such a case, other cultures of the patient's strain should be tested and the previous chemotherapy considered.

Sensitivity to Isoniazid

The following method is that recommended by the Medical Research Council (1953). The medium, method of inoculation and period of incubation are the same as for testing streptomycin sensitivity and the concentrations of isoniazid in the media are 0·2, 1·0, 5·0 and 50 μg per ml. The end-point is the lowest concentration inhibiting growth to 20 colonies or less. Strains are resistant to isoniazid if growth occurs on 1 μg per ml or more. Growth on 0·2 μg per ml is suggestive of resistance, but is not conclusive. In such a case other cultures of the patient's strain should be tested and previous chemotherapy considered.

Alternatively, a closer range of isoniazid concentrations, from 0·25 to 0·8 μg per ml, may be used and the results reported as the resistance ratio. A ratio of 4 indicates resistance.

For alternative methods for estimating the sensitivity of *Myco. tuberculosis* to these drugs see Canetti *et al.* (1963).

Sensitivity tests for other antituberculous drugs. Tests with viomycin, cycloserine and oxytetracycline may be done in a manner similar to that for streptomycin.

ASSAYS OF ANTIBIOTICS IN THE BLOOD AND OTHER BODY FLUIDS

An estimate of the amount of an antibiotic in the blood of a patient receiving treatment may be required to ensure that the dosage being given is adequate for a curative effect or that it is not so high as to cause accumulation of toxic antibiotics in excessive amounts. The methods employed, tube-dilution and diffusion tests, are similar to those used to determine the sensitivity of bacteria. For assay, however, a stock bacterium of known sensitivity is used as the inoculum and the unknown factor to be measured is the inhibitory content of the fluid. Collect two samples of the blood or fluid from the patient at fixed times in relation to a dose of antibiotic, e.g. immediately before a dose and one hour after it. Note whether any antibiotics are being given apart from that for which the test is to be made. If the fluid is likely to be contaminated with microorganisms, remove these by filtration. Withdraw blood by venepuncture and separate the serum; if necessary, centrifuge the serum to free it from suspended red cells. Carry out the test as soon as possible after the specimen has been collected.

Prepare dilutions of the serum or body fluid in broth and inoculate a standard organism of known sensitivity, such as the Oxford strain of *Staph. aureus*, which is sensitive to the concentrations of antibiotics easily attained in the tissues. Garrod, Lambert and O'Grady (1973, p. 519) give a list of organisms suitable for assays of the different antibiotics. Include a control tube containing the medium alone. Incubate the tubes for 18–24 h and examine them to find the tube with the highest dilution of body fluid that has no turbidity.

Set up a parallel control test with a fresh sample of the same body fluid known not to contain any bacterial agent but to which a known amount of the agent being assayed is added. By comparing the dilutions that inhibit the growth of the standard organism estimate the concentration of antibiotic in the body fluid. In doing this, take account of any bacteriostatic action in the fluid under test; e.g. if the specimen of body fluid inhibits growth at a dilution of 1 in 60 and the control fluid containing 5 μg antibiotic per ml does so at a dilution of 1 in 120, the specimen contains $\dfrac{60}{120} \times 5 = 2.5$ μg antibiotic per ml.

Estimation of one antibiotic in the presence of another. When the patient is receiving two antibiotics, estimation of the level of one in the presence of the other can be carried out in one of two ways: (a) by using as test organism a strain that is resistant to the unwanted antibiotic and which has a low MIC (e.g. less than 1 μg per ml) to the antibiotic being tested; or (b) if the unwanted antibiotic is a penicillin or cephalosporin, by destroying it by the addition of β-lactamase (Waterworth, 1973).

Estimation of streptomycin in serum and cerebrospinal fluid. The method recommended by the Medical Research Council Subcommittee (Medical Research Council Subcommittee Report, 1948) can be used when a rapid clinical assay is required. When a more precise determination is required, the method of Mitchison and Spicer (1949) may be used.

There are many detailed techniques, both chemical and biological, for assaying individual antibiotics, and for these appropriate textbooks should be consulted (e.g. Kavanagh, 1963).

APPENDIX

Preparation of Wet Disks for Antibiotic-sensitivity Tests (See Table 8.3)

Method. Punch disks 6·25 mm in diameter from No. 1 Whatman filter paper, dispense batches of 100 in screw-capped bottles and sterilize by dry heat at 140°C for 60 min. Prepare solutions of antibiotics so that 1 ml contains 100 times the amount of antibiotic required in the disk. Add 1 ml solution to each bottle of 100 disks and, as the whole of this volume will be absorbed, assume that each disk will contain approximately 0·01 ml. Store the disks in the wet conditions. They will retain their moisture and potency for at least three months if kept in screw-capped bottles with the caps screwed on tightly.

Antibiotic content of disks. Disks containing the following amounts of antibiotics and other chemotherapeutic agents are used in routine tests:

Ampicillin	10 and 100 μg
Bacitracin	10 units (diagnostic for *Strept. pyogenes* 2·5 units)
Carbencillin	10 μg
Chloramphenicol	25 μg
Clindamycin	10 μg
Colistin or polymyxin	1000 units
Cycloserine	100 μg
Erythromycin	10 μg
Fusidic acid	10 μg
Gentamicin	10 μg
Kanamycin	10 and 100 μg
Methicillin	10 μg
Neomycin	10 μg (diagnostic for clostridia 100 μg)
Nitrofurantoin	100 μg
Nystatin	100 μg
Penicillin (benzyl-)	1, 10 and 100 units
Streptomycin	10 and 100 μg
Sulphonamide	250 and 500 μg
Tetracycline	10 and 25 μg

The disks containing the different antibiotics may be identified by typed or printed letters on them or by colour applied to plain paper or paper on which black spots or lines have been stencilled. Colouring is done with 'cotton' dyes which are fast to the paper and do not interfere with the activity of the antimicrobial agents or exert any antibacterial activity themselves in

Table 8.3

Antimicrobial drug	Dye	Colour of disk
Ampicillin	red diluted 1 in 10	pink
Bacitracin	2:2:1 mixture of scarlet:orange:blue	brown
Benzyl-penicillin	red	red
Chloramphenicol	3:1 mixture of yellow:blue	green
Colistin	blue diluted 1 in 10	pale blue with spots
Cycloserine	1:4 mixture of orange:yellow	orange
Erythromycin	1:1:8 mixture of orange:blue:red	puce
Fusidic acid	none	white with spots
Gentamicin	red diluted 1 in 10	pink with spots
Kanamycin	scarlet	scarlet with spots
Methicillin	turquoise	turquoise
Neomycin	1:9 mixture of blue:yellow	light green
Nitrofurantoin	yellow	yellow with spots
Polymyxin	1:5 blue:red	purple with spots
Streptomycin	none	white
Sulphonamide	blue	blue
Tetracycline	1:1 mixture of orange:scarlet	terra-cotta

the concentrations recommended (Bowie and Gould, 1952). A useful range of such dyes and a scheme for coding antibiotics with them is shown below.

'Chlorazol' sky blue ICI FF 200   blue
'Diphenyl'   pink BK Ciba-Geigy   red
'Durazol'   fast orange ICI R 150   orange
'Durazol'   scarlet ICI 4B, 150   scarlet
'Durazol'   turquoise blue ICI FBF   turquoise
'Durazol'   yellow ICI GR 200   yellow

Prepare a stock solution of 25 mg dye per ml in distilled water and autoclave. This solution will keep indefinitely. Before use, dilute the stock solution to 5 mg dye per ml in sterile water. Except in the case of streptomycin, polymyxin, bacitracin and sulphonamides, make a solution of the antibacterial drug at twice the required final concentration by adding sterile water to a commercial preparation of the drug, e.g. benzyl-penicillin 200 units per ml (for 1 unit disks), 2000 units per ml (for 10 unit disks). Mix equal parts of the antibacterial solution and dye solution and add 1 ml of the mixture to a bottle containing 100 disks (2 ml to 200 disks and *pro rata*).

Streptomycin, Polymyxin, Bacitracin and Sulphonamide Disks. These drugs precipitate the dyes in solution, and although the precipitation does not interfere with the activity of the drug, the colouring of the disks is unsatisfactory. For streptomycin, use uncoloured disks. For polymyxin and bacitracin, first colour the disks with the dye, then dry and impregnate with the drug. Make up the solutions of these drugs as follows: streptomycin 1000 μg per ml, polymyxin 10000 units per ml, and bacitracin 1000 units per ml. Add 1 ml solution to each bottle of 100 disks. Dye disks for sulphonamide blue and then impregnate with a solution of the sodium salt of the sulphonamide at 12·5 mg per ml.

REFERENCES AND FURTHER READING

ANDERSON, T. G. (1970) Testing of susceptibility to antimicrobial agents and assay of antimicrobial agents in body fluids. *Manual of Clinical Microbiology*, edited by J. E. Blair, E. H. Lenette & J. P. Truant, pp. 299–310. Bethesda, Maryland: American Society for Microbiology.

BAUER, A. W., KIRBY, W. M. M., SHERRIS, J. C. & TURCK, M. (1966) Antibiotic susceptibility testing by a standardized single disk method. *American Journal of Clinical Pathology*, **45**, 493.

BOWIE, J. H. & GOULD, J. C. (1952) Colouring agents for use in disc-antibiotic sensitivity tests. *Journal of Clinical Pathology*, **5**, 356.

CANETTI, G., FROMAN, S., GROSSET, J., HAUDOROY, P., LANDEROVÁ, M., MAHLER, H. T., MEISSNER, G., MITCHISON, D. A. & SULA, L. (1963) Mycobacteria: laboratory methods for testing drug sensitivity and resistance. *Bulletin of the World Health Organization*, **29**, 565.

CASTLE, A. R. & ELSTUB, J. (1971) Antibiotic sensitivity testing: a survey undertaken in September 1970 in the United Kingdom. *Journal of Clinical Pathology*, **24**, 773.

CHABBERT, Y. A. & WATERWORTH, PAMELA M. (1965) Studies on the 'carry-over' of antibiotics using the cellophane transfer technique. *Journal of Clinical Pathology*, **18**, 314.

ELEK, S. D. & HILSON, G. R. F. (1954) Combined agar diffusion and replica plating techniques in the study of antibacterial substances. *Journal of Clinical Pathology*, **7**, 37.

ERICSSON, H. (1960) Rational use of antibiotics in hospital: studies on laboratory methods and discussion of the biological basis for their clinical application. *Scandinavian Journal of Clinical Laboratory Investigation*, **12**, Supplement 50.

ERICSSON, H. M. & SHERRIS, J. C. (1971) Antibiotic sensitivity testing: report of an international collaborative study. *Acta pathologica microbiologica Scandinavica B*, Supplement 217.

GARROD, L. P., LAMBERT, H. P. & O'GRADY, F. (1973) *Antibiotic and Chemotherapy*, 4th edition. Edinburgh: Churchill Livingstone.

GARROD, L. P. & WATERWORTH, PAMELA M. (1971) A study of antibiotic sensitivity testing with proposals for simple uniform methods. *Journal of Clinical Pathology*, **24**, 779.

GOULD, J. C. & BOWIE, J. H. (1952) The determination of bacterial sensitivity to antibiotics. *Edinburgh Medical Journal*, **59**, 178.

GREENBERG, L., FITZPATRICK, K. M. & BRANCH, A. (1957) The status of the antibiotic disc in Canada. *Canadian Medical Journal*, **76**, 194.

HARPER, G. J. & CAWSTON, W. C. (1945) The *in vitro* determination of the sulphonamide sensitivity of bacteria. *Journal of Pathology and Bacteriology*, **57**, 59.

HEWITT, J. H., COE, A. W. & PARKER, M. T. (1969) The detection of methicillin resistance in *Staphylococcus aureus*. *Journal of Medical Microbiology*, **2**, 443.

KAVANAGH, F. (1963) *Analytical Microbiology*. New York and London: Academic Press.

KELSEY, J. C. & MAURER, ISOBEL M. (1972) *The use of chemical disinfectants in hospitals*. Public Health Laboratory Service Monograph Series No. 2. London: H.M. Stationery Office.

KELSEY, J. C. & SYKES, G. (1969) A new test for the assessment of disinfectants with particular reference to their use in hospitals. *Pharmaceutical Journal*, **202**, 607.

MALLMAN, W. L. & HANES, M. (1945) The use-dilution method of testing disinfectants. *Journal of Bacteriology*, **49**, 526.

MAURER, I. M. (1969) A test for stability and long term effectiveness in disinfectants. *Pharmaceutical Journal*, **203**, 529.

MEDICAL RESEARCH COUNCIL REPORT (1953) Laboratory techniques for the determination of sensitivity of tubercle bacilli to isoniazid, streptomycin and PAS (MRC isoniazid Trial: Report No. 3). *Lancet*, **2**, 213.

MEDICAL RESEARCH COUNCIL SUBCOMMITTEE REPORT (1948) Specific laboratory tests in streptomycin therapy of tuberculosis. *Lancet*, **2**, 862.

MITCHISON, D. A. & SPICER, C. C. (1949) A method of estimating streptomycin in serum and other body fluids by diffusion through agar enclosed in glass tubes. *Journal of General Microbiology*, **3**, 184.

SLEIGH, J. D. (1958) Difficulties encountered in reporting penicillin sensitivity of staphylococci. *Scottish Medical Journal*, **3**, 454.

STEDMAN, R. L., KRAVITZ, E. & BELL, H. (1954) Studies on the efficiencies of disinfectants for use on inanimate objects. *Applied Microbiology*, **2**, 199 and 322.

STOKES, E. JOAN (1960) *Clinical Bacteriology*, p. 163. London: Arnold.

STOKES, E. JOAN & WATERWORTH, PAMELA M. (1972) Antibiotic sensitivity tests by diffusion methods. *Association of Clinical Pathologists*, Broadsheet 55.

WATERWORTH, PAMELA M. (1973) An enzyme preparation inactivating all penicillins and cephalosporins. *Journal of Clinical Pathology*, **26**, 596.

9. Cell, Tissue and Organ Culture

Over the last decade methods have evolved that have made the establishment and maintenance of eukaryotic cells *in vitro* much easier. It is possible to produce a monolayer of cells by enzymatic treatment, e.g. trypsinization of almost any normal tissue. These 'primary' cell cultures closely resemble their cells of origin. They can be removed from the supporting surface and seeded to a number of fresh containers giving secondary cultures which are commonly used in attempting to grow viruses. These cultures will continue to divide for a limited number of generations but eventually die out. Early preparations of these cultures may be stored at low temperatures when the cells remain viable and form a reserve of cells for the laboratory. This is frequently done with cells derived from foetal embryo lungs because it is often impossible to use the whole yield of cells at the time of trypsinization or if cells of identical passage are required.

Other cell cultures, mainly those derived from carcinomatous tissue, e.g. HeLa cells, will go on dividing *ad infinitum;* are useful for the growth of many viruses and they can be stored at low temperatures giving a reserve of cells should the laboratory stock become contaminated or fail for other reasons.

Small pieces of organized tissue can also be employed either secured in a matrix or simply adhering to the supporting surface. When the tissue is in a matrix of, say, clotted plasma or agar, the cells grow out from the piece of tissue to form a sheet. This is a useful method for the growth of epidermal cells. When the piece of tissue is merely adhering to the surface, the purpose is not to produce outgrowths but to study the effect of the virus on organized tissue or as they are now called 'organ cultures'.

All these cell cultures require nutrition generally supplied in the form of a defined medium with a serum supplement to which is added certain antibiotics. The buffering of the medium depends to some extent on the carbon dioxide and a tendency to acidity produced during cellular respiration; this is partly balanced by the addition of sodium bicarbonate to the medium but there is usually some phosphate buffer also present. Recently the introduction of the Zwitterionic buffer N-2-hydroxyethylpiperazine-N^1-3-ethanesulphonic acid, HEPES, (Good *et al.*, 1966) has simplified the growth of tissue cultures since it overrides all other buffers present and it allows incubation of the cell culture in an open system, i.e. a Petri dish, without the need for an atmosphere of carbon dioxide to maintain the appropriate proportion of carbon dioxide in the gaseous phase.

This chapter is not a complete account of cell culture techniques, but attempts to set out the methods in general use in a diagnostic virology laboratory. For further information on specific techniques, texts such as Paul (1970) and Willmer (1965) should be consulted.

Apparatus

Glassware. Pyrex or neutral glass test-tubes, flasks and bottles may be employed. Soda glass may also be used provided the containers have first been treated with 2 per cent HCl to remove excess soda. The glassware must be scrupulously clean (washing procedure is described in Chapter 4).

Disposable plastic containers are now widely used in virology and there are many grades. If primary cells are being established 'Falcon' grade plastic may be required, but established cell cultures will grow readily on routine grade plastic such as that supplied by 'Nunclon'. (Supplier: J. A. Jobling.)

Stoppers and rubber tubing. These should be either of white rubber such as that supplied by ESCO or of silicone. Silicone has the advantage that it is non-toxic and does not become sticky on repeated sterilization but it is expensive and contracts at a different rate to glass so the stoppers are liable to fall out of the test-tubes at low temperatures. Black or red rubber stoppers should be avoided due to their toxicity.

Filters. Sintered glass filters should be cleaned after use by treatment with strong acid. Concentrated sulphuric acid to which crystals of sodium nitrate and sodium chlorate have been added is allowed to seep through the filter. Afterwards the filter must be rinsed thoroughly with a large volume of distilled water.

Seitz filter pads are made from asbestos which is alkaline. To remove the alkalinity and also loose asbestos fibres, 200 ml Hanks' BSS (see below) is passed through the sterile filter before use.

Millipore filters may also be used (see Chap. 3). They have the advantages of being used under positive pressure which reduces some of the risk of contamination of the final product and of not being alkaline. There is a range of porosities. The disadvantage of such filters is that they easily become clogged so that a range of filters of decreasing porosities needs to be used. These filters may be sterilized by autoclaving but care must be taken not to exceed 121°C.

Instruments. These should be clean and sterile. Prepacked disposable sterile scalpel blades are very useful because they do not have any coating of grease and so are not toxic to cells.

Roller drum apparatus. After monolayer cell cultures have been established in test tubes, it is convenient to place them in a rotating drum. The drum consists of sheet metal or plastic such as Perspex, pierced with holes of the appropriate size to hold the culture tubes and mounted on a horizontal shaft. The drum is tilted at an angle of five degrees in order to prevent the medium touching the stoppers of the tubes; it is rotated at 12–20 revolutions per hour by an electric motor fitted with a reduction gear.

'Burler' apparatus. It is often useful to grow cells in 2-litre Winchester bottles so a similar device to that described above is used. The main difference is that the bottles are held horizontal, either fitted into a perspex holder or laid on the drive spindles. A speed of 12 revolutions per hour will allow some cell cultures to adhere to the whole of the glass surface, but when dealing with epitheloid cells, e.g. HEp-2, the revolutions should be reduced to five per hour until the cells have attached to the glass. The bottles can then be rotated at the faster rate.

Carbon dioxide incubator. These incubators can be purchased commercially or an ordinary, water-jacketed incubator may be adapted by passing rubber tubing through the thermometer hole. This tubing should be connected to either a cylinder or 5 per cent CO_2 in air or to a flow meter mixing device, to produce 5 per cent CO_2 in air from a CO_2 cylinder and compressed air. It should lead through a filter and a water reservoir in the incubator to ensure that the atmosphere is kept humid.

Inverted microscope. Such a microscope (Leitz) is very useful for examining cells in Roux bottles and 2-litre Winchester bottles. It is also essential for the examination of cells growing in Petri dishes and microtitre plates.

Media should be prepared from glass distilled water and analytically pure reagents.

Hanks' Balanced Salt Solution (BSS)

Stock Solution A

1. NaCl . . 160 g
   KCl . . 8 g
   $MgSO_4.7H_2O$. 2 g
   $MgCl_2.6H_2O$. 2 g
   Distilled water . 800 ml
2. $CaCl_2$ . . 2·8 g
   Distilled water . 100 ml

Mix these two solutions slowly and make up volume to 1000 ml with distilled water. Add 2 ml chloroform—store at 4°C.

Stock solution B

$Na_2HPO_4.12H_2O$ . . . 3·04 g
KH_2PO_4 . . . . 1·2 g
Glucose . . . . 20 g
Distilled water . . . 800 ml

When chemicals have dissolved add 100 ml of 0·4 per cent phenol red in NaOH. Make up volume to 1000 ml with distilled water. Add 2 ml chloroform and store at 4°C.

For use

Stock solution A . . . 100 ml
Stock solution B . . . 100 ml
Distilled water . . . . 800 ml

Dispense in 100-ml amounts. Sterilize by autoclaving at 15 lb (121°C) for 20 min. Store at 4°C.

Dulbecco's Phosphate Buffered Saline (PBS) Solution 'A'

NaCl	. . . .	8 g
KCl	. . . .	0·2 g
Na_2HPO_4	. . .	1·15 g
KH_2PO_4 .	. . .	0·2 g
Distilled water .	. . .	1000 ml
1 per cent aqueous phenol red	.	1 or 2 drops

(or until solution is pale pink)

Distribute in 100-ml amounts and autoclave for 20 min at 115°C. Store at 4°C.

Dulbecco's PBS Solution 'B'

$CaCl_2$	. . . .	2·0 g
$MgCl_2.6H_2O$.	. .	2·0 g
Distilled water .	. .	100 ml

Dispense in 2·5-ml amounts in bijoux, sterilize for 20 min at 121°C. Store at 4°C.

Add 0·5 ml solution B to 100 ml Dulbecco solution A to make the complete salt solution.

Phenol Red 1 per cent

Dissolve 10 g phenol red in 325 ml N/10 NaOH
Make up to 1000 ml with distilled water
Distribute in 20-ml amounts
Autoclave for 15 min at 121°C.

Sodium Bicarbonate Solution 1·4, 4·4 and 8·0 per cent

$NaHCO_3$	. .	14 g or 44 g or 80 g
Water	. .	1000 ml

Dissolve $NaHCO_3$ in distilled water. Add a few drops 1 per cent phenol red and pass CO_2 through the solution until colour is pale pink.

Distribute in 1-oz bottles with as little air space as possible and screw caps on tightly. Autoclave for 20 min at 115°C. Store at 4°C.

Earle's Solution

As in Hanks' solution the calcium salt should be dissolved separately and added slowly.

NaCl	. . . . .	6·80 g
KCl	. . . . .	0·40 g
$CaCl_2$	. . . . .	0·20 g
$MgSO_4.7H_2O$.	. .	0·10 g
$NaH_2PO_4.H_2O$	. .	0·125 g
Glucose .	. . . .	1·00 g
Phenol red solution .	. .	12·5 ml
$NaHCO_3$	. . .	2·20 g
Water to make .	. . .	1000 ml

Earle's solution contains greater amounts of sodium bicarbonate than Hanks' solution; it is useful when cultures produce much acid or have a large cell population. When used for cultures with small numbers of cells they may lose their CO_2 and become alkaline; such cultures need to be 'gassed' with 5–10 per cent CO_2 in air when set up and after the medium is changed.

Serum

Calf serum is commonly used in media for cell culture. It may be purchased commercially as either foetal or 'new born'. The foetal calf serum obtained before suckling is sometimes necessary for the establishment of primary cell cultures, but in many instances serum from calves of less than one week old is quite satisfactory. Some laboratories process serum obtained from the slaughterhouse as follows:

1. Collect the whole calf blood in plastic containers.

2. Allow to clot.

3. Aspirate the serum—possibly with some free red blood cells.

4. Centrifuge for 45 min at 1500 rev/min to remove the red cells.

5. Filter five litres serum through a Whatman Gamma-12 'in-line' filter using unsterile filter tubes in the following order:
(a) Grade 20, (b) Grade 12, (c) Grade 03.

6. Filter serum through the following unsterile membrane filters:
(a) porosity 0·45 μm and (b) 0·22 μm.

7. Filter serum through sterile membrane filter of porosity 0·22 μm. Collect in a sterile aspirator.

8. Dispense aseptically in convenient volumes and store at −20°C.

9. Test for sterility at 37°C, 28°C and room temperature by adding 10 ml serum to 50 ml glucose broth. The cultures should be observed for at least one week.

In some cases human serum can be used but here it should be realized that the serum may contain Hepatitis B antigen or antibodies to the

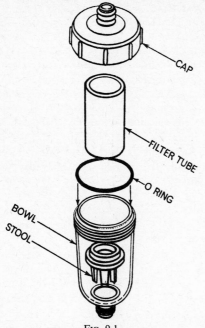

CAP

FILTER TUBE

O RING

BOWL

STOOL

FIG. 9.1
Whatman Gammo-12 in-line filter.

virus under study. Bovine serum may contain antibodies to parainfluenza or enteroviruses.

All sera should be checked for sterility, and also for possible toxicity to the tissue culture cells before issue for use. In some instances serum should be inactivated by heating for 30 min at 56°C.

Hepes

HEPES buffer may be incorporated in most cell culture media at a concentration of 10–40 mM depending on the medium (Shipman, 1969). As the buffer equilibrates with air, it is independent of cellular metabolism and is apparently non-toxic to many cell types and viruses. It gives a much more uniform medium for the growth of cells and the pH of passaged material does not become alkaline on repeated sampling. The incorporation of this buffer in media for petri dish cultures removes the necessity for incubation in an atmosphere of 5 per cent carbon dioxide.

Antibiotics

Nearly all the culture media in general use contain antibiotics to control chance contamination during the handling of cell cultures.

For this purpose, stock solutions of penicillin and streptomycin are held in small amounts at $-20°C$ and are added to the media immediately before use. A solution of 10^6 units of benzyl penicillin and 1 g of streptomycin is made in 10 ml distilled water. Final concentrations of 100 units of benzyl penicillin and 100 μg of streptomycin per ml of the medium are sufficient for the purpose and are not toxic to the cells. Fungal contamination may be held in check by mycostatin (nystatin Squibb) added to give a concentration of 20–50 μg per ml but this antibiotic is unstable at 37°C and after 24 h its influence is lost. Tylosin or sodium aurothio-malate (myocrysin) may be added to the medium in an attempt to control mycoplasma infection (Cross, Goodman and Shaw, 1967).

Trypsin

Difco Trypsin 1:250 .	.	.	10 g
Distilled water .	.	.	1000 ml

Leave for 2–3 h at 37°C to dissolve. Seitz filter. Distribute in 10-ml amounts using aseptic technique. Store at $-20°C$.

TEST FOR STERILITY. Pipette aseptically 0·1 ml from each 10-ml amount into 5 ml glucose broth. Incubate for 7 days at 37°C.

TEST FOR THE ACTIVITY OF TRYPSIN—I. It is necessary to check from time to time the activity of the trypsin used in solutions to disaggregate the cells of tissues such as monkey kidney. This can be carried out by preparing a series of about 10 doubling dilutions from 1 in 10 onwards of the trypsin solution in Hanks' balanced salt solution. One drop of each dilution is placed on a strip of X-ray film together with one drop of Hanks' solution as a control. The strip is then placed on moist blotting-paper in a Petri dish, covered and incubated for thirty minutes at 37°C. The strip is removed and allowed to cool to room temperature or cold water run over the reverse side (no film) until the gelatin has set firmly. Now flood the whole film gently with cold water. Wherever trypsin was present the gelatin will have been digested to water-soluble products and a punched-out hole will appear in the film. The control area (Hanks' solution) is not dissolved at all.

TEST FOR THE ACTIVITY OF TRYPSIN—II. Again prepare a series of doubling dilutions of the trypsin solution in Hanks' solution in 5-ml amounts. To each dilution, and a control tube containing Hanks' solution only, add a charcoal gelatin disc (Oxoid). Incubate for 90 min at 37°C. Examine every 30 min for trypsin activity, i.e. charcoal particles in suspension.

Methocel (Methyl Cellulose) (5 per cent)

1. Put 500 ml distilled water in refrigerator at 4°C.
2. Heat 500 ml distilled water to 90°C and add the methocel to wet it.
3. Cool this mixture in a bucket of ice and then add the 500 ml of chilled water.
4. Dispense in 50-ml amounts in 100-ml bottles.
5. Autoclave for 20 min at 121°C.
6. Store at 4°C.

For use, 0·75 per cent w/v of this methocel is incorporated in the overlay.

Formol Saline

Formalin (40 per cent)	.	.	500 ml
NaCl	. . .	.	25 g
Na₂SO₄	. . .	.	75 g
Demineralized water	.	.	4500 ml

Formalin (40 per cent) . . 500 ml
NaCl . . . . 25 g
Na_2SO_4 . . . . 75 g
Demineralized water . . 4500 ml

Agar for Plaques

Difco agar (Nobel) . . . 2·4 g
Water . . . . . 100 ml
Sterilize for 15 min at 121°C in 20-ml amounts.

For use, prepare equal volumes of double strength growth medium and place in a 45°C water bath. Melt the agar and cool to 45°C in water bath. Mix quickly and pipette on to monolayers of cells.

Versene

Sequestric acid, disodium salt
(BDH) . . . . . 10 g
Distilled water . . . 1000 ml
Distribute in 1·5-ml amounts in bijou bottles. Autoclave for 20 min at 121°C.

For use, add 1·25 ml of the stock versene to 100 ml of Dulbecco 'A' and store at 4°C.

Glycerol

Glycerol should be sterilized in containers with aluminium foil (not rubber) tops in the hot air oven for 1 h at 160°C. It is then incorporated in media in 10 per cent v/v amounts.

Nutrient Media

Many defined nutrient media have been devised incorporating amino acids, vitamins, enzymes, accessory growth factors, glucose and inorganic salts in varying proportions. They are used without supplementation to maintain established cultures for periods of three or four days when cell multiplication is not required. With serum or tissue extracts added they are used to promote the active growth of cells.

Eagle's medium is widely used and the stock medium may be obtained at ten times strength commercially (Wellcome Reagents Ltd.).

Eagle's Medium

Eagle's (MEM) × 10 . . . 8 ml
Calf serum . . . . 10 ml
Tryptone phosphate broth (Oxoid) 10 ml
Sodium bicarbonate 1·4 per cent . 3 ml
Penicillin and streptomycin . 0·1 ml
Distilled water to . . . 100 ml

The medium may also be made in the laboratory according to the 1959 modification (see below).

Eagle's Medium—1959 Modification (based on Eagle, 1959)

Solution No. 1
L-Arginine HCl . . . 10·5 g
L-Histidine HCl . . . 3·1 g
L-Lysine mono. HCl . . 5·8 g
L-Leucine (with Isoleucine) . 5·2 g
L-Isoleucine . . . 5·2 g
L-Methionine . . . 1·5 g
L-*p*-phenylalanine . . 3·2 g
L-Threonine . . . 4·8 g
L-Tryptophan . . . 1·0 g
L-Valine . . . . 4·6 g
Hanks' BSS . . . 1000 ml

Solution No. 2
L-Tyrosine . . . . 0·2 g
L-Cystine . . . . 2·4 g

Mix tyrosine and cystine in 100 ml distilled water. Add conc. HCl until clear then add distilled water to make 1 litre.

Solution No. 3

Choline	0·1 g
Nicotinamide	0·1 g
Pathothenic acid (calcium salt) .	0·1 g
Pyridoxal	0·1 g
Aneurine HCl	0·1 g
Riboflavin	0·01 g
i-Inositol	0·2 g
Hanks' BSS . . .	1000 ml

Solution No. 4

Folic acid . . . . 0·1 g/l

Dissolve folic acid in a few ml of N/10 NaOH—make up to 1 litre with Hanks' salt solution.

Solution No. 5

Glucose 100 g/l in Hanks' salt solution

Solution No. 6

L-Glutamine 29·2 g/l in distilled water

Solution No. 7

Sodium pyruvate 11·006 g/l in Hanks' salt solution

Solution No. 8

L-Alanine	0·891 g
L-Asparagine	1·321 g
L-Aspartic acid . . .	1·331 g
L-Glutamic acid . . .	1·471 g
L-Proline	1·311 g
L-Serine	1·051 g
Glycine	0·751 g
Hanks' BSS . . .	1000 ml

All solutions are sterilized by filtration through a 5/3 sintered glass filter. Dispensed aseptically in 11-ml amounts and stored at −20°C.

Earle's Salt Solution (1959 Modification)

NaCl	6·8 g
KCl	0·4 g
CaCl$_2$	0·2 g
MgCl$_2$.6H$_2$O . . .	0·2 g
NaH$_2$PO$_4$.2H$_2$O . .	0·15 g
0·4 per cent phenol red . .	3 ml
Distilled water to . . .	1000 ml

Dispense in 80-ml amounts. Sterilize for 20 min at 115°C. Store at 4°C.

1. *Working Stock Solution* (*WSS*)

The 8 solutions numbered 1 to 8 are pooled in equal amounts, i.e. 10 ml of each, and stored at 4°C not more than one week.

2. *Complete Medium*

	Growth
Earle's salt solution . . .	70 ml
Working stock solution . .	8 ml
Tryptose phosphate broth (Oxoid)	10 ml
Calf serum—heated . . .	2 ml
Penicillin—streptomycin . .	0·1 ml
8 per cent NaHCO$_3$ . . .	1 ml

For details of other defined media, such as Parker 199, the reader is referred to Paul (1970).

Preparation of Cell Cultures from Fresh Tissue

Cell cultures can be prepared from both foetal and adult tissue and from both normal and malignant material. For primary cell cultures human amnion or normal monkey kidney (Plate 9.1) provide good sources of cells. Foetal material such as lung or kidney also gives a good yield of cells and is useful for the growth of certain viruses. Some tissues may not disaggregate with trypsin and in that case collaginase treatment may be effective (Freshney, 1972).

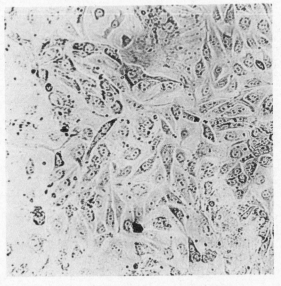

PLATE 9.1
Monolayer of normal monkey kidney cells

Preparation of Human Amnion Tissue Cultures
(Duncan and Bell, 1961)

It is essential that any placenta that is to be used for tissue culture is not brought into contact with disinfectant. A placenta from a Caesarian section is preferable. The placenta should be placed in a sterile beaker, covered and transported to the laboratory *without chilling*.

1. Suspend the placenta by the umbilical cord and free the amniotic membrane using scalpel, scissors and forceps.
2. Place the membrane in 100 ml Hanks' BSS with antibiotics.
3. Spread out the membrane in a large Petri dish and remove the mucus and blood clots by gentle scraping with the edge of a sterile microscope slide.
4. Wash three times in Hanks' BSS with antibiotics.
5. Put pieces of the membrane in a flask with 200 ml 0·25 per cent trypsin in Hanks' BSS and antibiotics and trypsinize for 30 min at 37°C either shaking every five minutes or preferably using a magnetic stirrer.
6. Change the trypsin and leave 4–4½ h at 37°C shaking every 30 min.
7. Filter through sterile gauze and wash filter with 100 ml Hanks' BSS with antibiotics.
8. Spin filtrate for 10 min at 1000 rev/min.
9. Discard supernatant.
10. Resuspend in 20 ml of propagating medium without serum.
11. Estimate the number of viable cells and dilute to give $3·5 \times 10^5$ cells/ml.
12. Inoculate Roux bottles with 100 ml of cells and leave 3–4 days undisturbed.
13. Change medium.
    Trypsin can be diluted in Dulbecco's solution instead of Hanks' BSS because the pH is less likely to become alkaline.

Method for Foetal Lung Fibroblasts

The lungs should be removed under aseptic conditions and sent to the laboratory with the least possible delay in a sterile container.
Method
1. Using sterile scalpel blades chop the lung into small pieces.
2. Wash twice in Hanks' BSS containing antibiotics.

3. Suspend the fragments in 50–100 ml 0·25 per cent trypsin in Hanks' BSS.
4. Place in a shaking water bath for 30 min at 37°C, or shake regularly and then pipette the suspension vigorously. If an even suspension does not result, return to the water bath for a further 10–15 min.
5. Add 3 ml calf serum to each 30 ml of suspension to stop the action of the trypsin and spin for 5 min at 1000 rev/min.
6. Resuspend the cells in Eagle's growth medium containing 10 per cent foetal calf serum.
7. Count the cells.
8. Dilute the suspension to contain 10^5 cells/ml and dispense in bottles.

CULTIVATION OF CELL STRAINS

Cell strains grow uniformly as sheets on the surface of glass. Often it is important to be able to examine the cells during their growth and for this purpose they are manipulated so that a layer one cell thick 'monolayer' is formed on the side of test-tubes. This can be viewed with $\frac{2}{3}$ in objective of the microscope. For other purposes cells may be cultivated on the flat surfaces of Carrel flasks or Petri dishes; when required in greater numbers they are propagated on the sides of ordinary flat prescription bottles, Pyrex baby bottles (4–8 oz), Roux bottles, or in rolling 2-litre Winchester bottles.

The Removal of Cells from Glass

This can be achieved either by the use of the chelating agent 'versene' or enzymatically by trypsin.

1. *Versene*. To suspend the cells remove the growth medium and wash the surface of the cell sheet with an equal volume of balanced salt solution (Ca and Mg free), e.g. Dulbecco 'A' warmed to 37°C. Replace the salt solution with one-tenth the volume of the versene solution and incubate the culture for 10–15 min at 37°C. As soon as the cells have left the glass disperse them by gentle pipetting. The cells in this suspension are then counted in a haemocytometer and diluted to give a concentration of the order of 100 000 per ml. With delicate or slow-growing cells, concentrations

as high as 500 000 per ml may be required for seeding.

2. *Proteolytic enzymes* may be used to release cells from the surface of the glass. A stock solution of 1 per cent trypsin (Difco 'Trypsin 1:250') in water is kept at $-30°C$. Before use the trypsin is diluted in Dulbecco 'A' and the pH adjusted to 8·0 with 4·4 per cent sodium bicarbonate. The final concentration of the trypsin should be 0·1 per cent. The culture medium is removed from the monolayers which are then washed with an equal volume of Dulbecco 'A'. One-tenth of the volume of 0·1 per cent trypsin is added to the monolayer, when the cells develop a ground glass appearance, the trypsin is decanted and the container placed at 37°C for a few minutes. When the cells detach from the glass they should be resuspended in 10 ml medium, counted and inoculated to fresh containers.

A mixture of trypsin (0·1 per cent) and versene (0·02 per cent) is useful for fibroblastic cultures.

The density of the cells inoculated into a vessel will depend on the type of cell, the size of the vessel and the approximate date when the cells will be needed for use. Each laboratory will have to study the behaviour of its cell cultures, but as a general guide it has been found that 50 000 HEp2 or HeLa cells are sufficient to establish a monolayer in a test-tube containing 1 ml of medium, and 8×10^6 similar cells in a Roux bottle with 100 ml medium should give a confluent monolayer in about 5 days.

The medium used for growth of the cells varies with the cell strains but the following is one of those in common use:

Eagle's medium with the addition of 5–10 per cent calf serum.

For maintenance of cell cultures the calf serum content may be reduced to 2 per cent and the buffering power increased by the inclusion of more sodium bicarbonate. If the cells are to be incubated in an open system, i.e. in Petri dishes, they must be placed in a humid atmosphere containing 5 per cent CO_2 in air to compensate for the loss of CO_2 by diffusion or HEPES buffer should be added to the medium. In the routine maintenance of cell strains it is convenient to handle them at 3–5 day intervals but the cells should be removed from the glass when the cell sheet is confluent. It is often convenient to hold suspensions of tissue culture cells at 4°C in growth medium. From such stocks it is possible to inoculate tubes, Petri dishes or larger vessels as the need arises successfully up to one week from the time of trypsinization.

Tissue and Organ Culture

Instead of disaggregating organs and tissues enzymatically it is sometimes better to use small pieces of organized tissue. These may be taken at biopsy or at hysterotomy. The tissues to be used should be excised aseptically, placed in a sterile container and sent to the laboratory as quickly as possible. On arrival, the tissue is cut into small 1 mm^3 pieces and depending on the ultimate aim, incubated in growth medium. In some instances, e.g. human skin biopsies, the small fragment of tissue is anchored to the vessel and then the cells, on division, spread out and migrate from the tissue. Such cells may be removed by trypsin and used to produce monolayer cultures. On the other hand, it is sometimes useful to be able to study the growth of a virus in a piece of the original tissue. Here the 'explant' is anchored in its place but the migration of dividing cells is discouraged by omission of serum from the growth medium. This technique has been employed with ferret trachea and by this method it has been possible to isolate previously undetected viruses (Tyrrell and Bynoe, 1965).

To anchor the small pieces of tissue to the culture vessel, it may be sufficient to place the tissue on the roughened surface of a plastic Petri dish but with glass sometimes it is necessary to employ either clotted plasma or 0·5 per cent agar (Paul, 1970). The method of choice depends on the final use of the cells. Sometimes it is better to allow the cells to attach to, say, vilene on the top of a stainless steel raft. This has the advantage that the tissue, when ready for examination at the end of the experiment, can be removed complete with vilene and treated to produce histological sections for either the light or the electron microscope.

Preservation of tissue culture cells at low temperatures. Tissue culture cells suspended in suitable media may be frozen slowly to $-70°C$ or $-190°C$. At these temperatures the cells remain viable and can be taken out as the need arises. When the cells are to be reintroduced into glass vessels they should be thawed quickly and placed in medium warmed to 37°C. There are two methods for the preservation of cells: (1) by the inclusion of glycerol in the medium and (2) by the use of dimethyl sulfoxide (DMSO).

The cells, which should be in a logarithmic stage of growth, are removed from the glass, counted and either resuspended at a concentration of $2–8 \times 10^6$ per ml in growth medium which incorporates 10 per cent sterile glycerol or in growth medium to which is added 10 per cent DMSO. The suspensions are then put in ampoules in 2 ml amounts, sealed and cooled slowly. This may be achieved by placing the ampoules in an expanded polystyrene box in a refrigerator at $-60°C$ or by using a special holder which fits in the mouth of the liquid nitrogen container. When the cells have cooled down they are quickly transferred to the liquid nitrogen container. To recover the cells, thaw in water at 37°C taking precautions to avoid a leaking ampoule exploding, then either introduce the cells into at least 25 ml of warm (37°C) medium, or the cells can be spun out of the preserving medium before resuspension in fresh growth medium. Once the cells adhere to the vessel (possibly after overnight incubation) the medium should be changed.

At regular intervals during passage and before cells are stored at low temperatures they should be examined for the presence of *Mycoplasma spp.* and only cells free of *Mycoplasma spp. should be stored*; if contaminated they should be rejected. This may be carried out as follows:

Isolation of Mycoplasmas from Tissue Cultures

1. Inoculate cell suspension as follows:
    (a) On 2 plates of PPLO agar.
    (b) In one bottle of PPLO sloppy agar.
2. (a) Incubate one plate in a closed humidified container (such as a plastic lunch box) under aerobic conditions, at 37°C, and the other plate under anaerobic conditions with the addition of 10 per cent CO_2, at 37°C.
    (b) Incubate the sloppy agar cultures at 37°C and subculture two drops to each of two PPLO agar plates at 3, 7 and 14 days. Incubate one plate aerobically and one plate anaerobically with 10 per cent CO_2 at 37°C.
3. All plates are examined microscopically after 3, 7, 10 and 14 days' incubation before discarding as negative.
4. Plates with mycoplasma colonies or suspect mycoplasma colonies are removed for further investigation as follows:
    (a) Stain a sample of colonies or suspect colonies by Dienes' stain.
    (b) If 'Dienes stain positive' cut out a block of agar and incubate the block into PPLO broth (Vol. II, Chap. 43). Incubate for 3–4 days aerobically or anaerobically with 10 per cent CO_2 at 37°C, and use the broth culture to inoculate plates (0·1 ml per plate for the growth inhibition test).
5. Colonies from 'positive' plates may also be transferred to microscope slides and stained by the indirect method for immunofluorescence microscopy to identify the mycoplasma species.
6. Cell suspensions may be used to prepare 'flying coverslip' cultures which may be examined by immunofluorescence microscopy with antisera to those mycoplasmas commonly found as cell contaminants (e.g. *M. orale*, *M. hyrhinis*, *M. arginini* etc. (Chaps 11 and 43).

Other Contaminants of Tissue Culture Cells

Tissue culture can be contaminated with viruses, e.g. parvoviruses (Hallauer, Kronaver and Siegl, 1971) or with other tissue culture cells. It has been claimed that a considerable proportion of established cell cultures of human origin are in reality HeLa cells which have contaminated the 'primary' culture. It is, therefore, important to be able to examine cells and determine their species or in some instances subspecies. This may be done by:
1. Chromosome counting.
2. Mixed haemagglutination test (Coombs *et al.*, 1961).

3. Analysis of isoenzyme pattern (Gartler, 1967).

4. Immunofluoresence (Simpson and Stulberg, 1963).

5. Cytotoxicity test (Greene, Coriell and Charney, 1964).

REFERENCES AND FURTHER READING

BUSBY, D. W. G., HOUSE, W. & MACDONALD, J. R. (1964) *Virological Techniques*. London: Churchill.

COOMBS, R. R. A., DANIEL, M. R., GURNER, B. W. & KELAS, A. (1961) Recognition of the species of origin of cells in culture by mixed agglutination. 1. Use of antisera to red cells. *Immunology*, **4**, 55.

CROSS, G. F., GOODMAN, M. R. & SHAW, E. J. (1967) Detection and treatment of contaminating mycoplasmas in cell culture. *Australian Journal of Experimental Biology and Medical Science*, **45**, 201.

DUNCAN, I. B. R. & BELL, E. J. (1961) Human amnion tissue culture in the routine virus laboratory. *British Medical Journal*, **ii**, 863.

EAGLE, H. (1959) Amino acid metabolism in mammalian cell cultures. *Science*, **130**, 432.

FOGH, J. (1973) *Contamination in tissue culture*. New York: Academic Press.

FRESHNEY, R. I. (1972) Tumour cells disaggregated in collagenase. *Lancet*, **ii**, 488.

GARTLER, S. M. (1967) Genetic markers as tracers in tissue cultures. *NCI Monograph*, **26**, 167.

GOOD, N. E., WINGET, G. D., WINDER, W., CONNOLLY, T. N., IZAWA, S. & SINGH, R. M. M. (1966) Hydrogen ion buffers for virological research. *Biochemistry*, **5**, 467.

GREENE, A. E., CORIELL, L. L. & CHARNEY, J. (1964) A rapid cytotoxic antibody test to determine species of cell cultures. *Journal of the National Cancer Institute*, **32**, 779.

HALLAUER, G., KRONAUER, G. & SIEGL, G. (1971) Parvoviruses as contaminants of permanent human cell lines. *Archiv für die gesamte Virusforschung*, **35**, 80.

PAUL, J. (1970) *Cell and Tissue Culture*, 4th edn. Edinburgh: Livingstone.

SCHMIDT, N. J. (1969) Tissue culture methods and procedures in diagnostic virology. In *Diagnostic Procedures for Viral and Rickettsial Infections*, 4th edn. Edited by E. H. Lenette and N. J. Schmidt. American Public Health Association.

SHIPMAN, C. JR. (1969) Evaluation of 4−(2-hydroxyethyl) −1-piperazine-ethanesulphonic acid (HEPES) as a tissue culture buffer. *Proceedings of the Society for Experimental Biology and Medicine*, **130**, 305.

SIMPSON, W. F. & STULBERG, C. S. (1963) Species identification of animal cell strains by immunofluorescence. *Nature (London)*, **199**, 616.

TYRRELL, D. A. J. & BYNOE, M. L. (1965) Cultivation of a novel type of common-cold virus in organ cultures. *British Medical Journal*, **i**, 1467.

WILLMER, E. N. (1965) *Cells and Tissues in Culture. Methods, Biology and Physiology 1 & 2*. New York: Academic Press.

10. Isolation and Identification of Viruses

Specimens taken from patients in the acute phases of viral diseases may be highly infectious to the laboratory worker. Special care is needed in handling them and manipulations are best carried out in a safety cabinet that can subsequently be disinfected by ultra-violet light. The whole subject of safety in laboratory work is dealt with in Volume II, Chapter 16.

Most viruses recovered from infected patients are isolated and identified in a tissue culture system. When a specimen is received in the laboratory it may require to be treated with antibiotics to remove contaminating bacteria before it can be inoculated into appropriate tissue culture systems depending on the provisional clinical diagnosis, e.g. to attempt to grow an adenovirus, HEp2 or HeLa cells will suffice but monkey kidney cells are superior for the growth of the enteroviruses.

Transport and Treatment of Specimens

SPECIMENS. These should be collected as soon after the onset of the illness as possible and sent to the laboratory in the appropriate manner.

Scrapings from conjunctival lesions or from localized skin infections can be sent on microscope slides *unfixed*. Vesicle fluid may be collected in capillary tubes, sealed and sent in any suitable containers. Blood for serum should be collected in a dry, sterile tube; it should be allowed to clot and should *not be frozen* before sending to the laboratory. If the blood specimen is from a suspected case of serum hepatitis, the container should be wrapped in a polythene bag. It is then placed in a second polythene bag together with the request form and the whole package clearly marked 'Hepatitis'.

Throat swabs, throat washings, rectal swabs, mouth swabs, corneal scrapings or conjunctival scrapings may be placed in 2 ml of Hanks' BSS containing protein (1 per cent BSA or gelatin) and antibiotics, frozen and sent to the laboratory as swiftly as possible. Leibovitz (1969) charcoal virus transport medium (CVTM) may

also be used. If there is any possibility that a chlamydia might be involved, antibiotics should be omitted from the transport medium. Faecal specimens, urine and CSF should be kept cold but should not be placed in transport medium.

For transport the specimens may be packed in solid carbon dioxide in a thermos jar or packed in a polythene bag and then surrounded by ice and salt in a second polythene bag and the whole package placed in an insulated box.

If respiratory syncytial virus infection is suspected the specimen should not be chilled because the virus is sensitive to low temperatures. The best method to attempt to isolate respiratory syncytial virus is to have the tissue culture monolayers available near the bedside and to inoculate the throat swab material on the spot.

TREATMENT OF SPECIMENS. Throat swabs, vesicle swabs and rectal swabs should be placed in a bijou containing 2–3 ml of a transport medium, e.g. Hanks' BSS with 1 per cent BSA and antibiotics (1000 units of benzyl penicillin and 5000 μg streptomycin per ml). The specimen should be left on the bench for about 3 h to allow the antibiotics to act on the logarithmic phase of the contaminating bacteria. The specimen may then be inoculated into tissue cultures.

FAECES. A 10 per cent suspension is made in Hanks' BSS containing protein and antibiotics. After standing on the bench for 3 h, centrifuge at 2500 rev/min for 15 min. The supernate is collected and used as the inoculum. CSF is usually inoculated directly to the cell system, but sometimes it must be added to larger cell sheets in increased volumes of medium so as to dilute out the virus antibody present in the CSF.

Inoculation of Cell Cultures

The inoculum (0·2 ml) may either be introduced into the medium or it can be added to the cell sheet, allowed to adsorb for 2 h, the cell sheet washed and fresh medium added. This latter method has the advantage that any toxic material in the sample is removed from the tissue culture cells. Duplicate cultures are usually inoculated with every specimen and the tubes incubated either rolling or stationary. The cells are examined at two-day intervals for the appearance of CPE. The medium is changed regularly (every 3–4 days) to ensure that the pH does not become too acid. This tendency can also be counteracted by lowering the serum and increasing the sodium bicarbonate content of the medium (maintenance medium). It should be possible to maintain infected tissue culture monolayers for 14–28 days depending on the type of cell.

If a CPE develops in any of the cell monolayers the tubes are frozen at −30°C or −70°C or are subjected to ultrasonication in a bath, unless respiratory syncytial, cytomegalo or varicella zoster viruses are thought to be present (see below). Either of these methods will lyse the infected cells and release the virus. The suspension can then be introduced (0·2 ml) to fresh culture tubes. If the CPE was not caused by a virus but was a toxic effect, usually no CPE can be seen on the second passage due to dilution; but if the CPE was due to a virus the CPE may develop faster than on the first passage. From the source of the specimen, clinical diagnosis and the type of CPE which develops it is possible to make an educated guess as to which virus is present (see Table 10.1).

The identity of the virus is confirmed by neutralization with specific antiserum. In the mouth swab—herpes simplex virus example—this is a relatively simple matter since there are only two closely related serotypes of herpes simplex virus.

Neutralization Test

1. Titrate the virus in cell cultures.
2. Dilute the virus suspension to contain about 100 TCID50/0·1 ml.
3. Mix an equal volume of the diluted virus suspension with diluent—*virus control*.
4. Mix an equal volume of the virus suspension with a suitably diluted antiserum—*test*.
5. Allow these two mixtures to react at 4°C for 1 h. (Herpes is a heat labile virus.)
6. Inoculate two tubes with 0·2 ml of the respective mixtures.
7. Examine the cells daily for the production of CPE in the virus control.
8. When the virus control tubes are showing complete CPE, examine the test cell sheets. If they show no or very little CPE, the virus has been neutralized and identified.

Sometimes the virus breaks through in the test system; this may be due to too much virus being present or to the antiserum losing its potency, e.g. perhaps due to repeated freezing and thawing.

There are more than 30 human serotypes of adenovirus so it is convenient to make pools of neutralizing antisera, e.g. each containing antisera to three different adenoviruses. The new virus isolate is tested against each of the pools and if it is neutralized then subsequent mixing of the virus with each component of the pool identifies the virus.

Enteroviruses are even more complicated than the adenoviruses since the CPE may be caused by any one of the three polioviruses, two of the coxsackie A and six of the coxsackie B viruses or 34 echoviruses. Pools of antisera to polioviruses 1, 2 and 3, and to the coxsackie viruses can be applied as above and if neutralization is effected by either pool the test is

Table 10.1

Specimen	CPE	Possible virus
Throat swab	Ballooning of cells Clustering of cells	Adenovirus
Throat swab	Syncytia	Parainfluenza, RSV, measles
Faecal specimen	Pyknotic cells Cell lysis	Enterovirus
Mouth swab	Rounding of cells	Herpes simplex virus

completed using the single type specific antisera. In the case of the echoviruses a slightly different system is used. Antibody to 25 common types of virus is made up into ten pools, viz.:

	(f)	(g)	(h)	(i)	(j)
(a)	1	2	3	4	5
(b)	6	7	8	9	10
(c)	11	12	13	14	15
(d)	16	17	18	19	20
(e)	21	22	23	24	25

(a) contains antibody to virus 1–5 and (f) to 1, 6, 11, 16 and 21. These numbers are convenient but in practice the antisera to the 25 most common of the 34 serotypes should be used. The virus isolate is mixed with each of the 10 pools, allowed time to react, and tested for residual infectivity. If pools (c) and (h) neutralized the effect of the virus then the probable identity of the virus would be type 13. This could then be confirmed by neutralizing the virus with antiserum specific to echovirus type 13.

Before performing a neutralization test it is sometimes useful to carry out a complement fixation test using the virus isolate as the antigen, e.g. the adenoviruses share the same complement-fixing antigen so a positive reaction would confirm that the isolate was an adenovirus.

1. Freeze and thaw the virus isolate and a control uninoculated culture.

2. Heat for 30 min at 56°C.

3. Prepare two-fold dilutions of both the virus and the control culture in complement fixation buffer.

4. Using the above preparation as antigen carry out a complement fixation test.

Adenoviruses may also be grouped by haemagglutination of monkey or rat erythrocytes (Vol. I, Chapter 42 and Vol. II, Chapter 11).

In a few cases it is unwise to freeze infected cells because the virus loses its infectivity on release from the cells. The respiratory syncytial, cytomegalo and varicella zoster viruses fall into this category and infected cells should be passed to fresh monolayers. As the virus is poorly released from cells, neutralization tests cannot be used to identify these viruses. Fluorescent antibody tests (Vol. II, Chapter 11) can be used or in the case of cytomegalovirus, inclusions may be demonstrated in the cells following staining with Giemsa's stain.

If a CPE does not develop in the inoculated cell culture it should be passed 'blind' to fresh tissue culture cells in the same manner as above. The tubes are again examined for 14–28 days and in some cases a cytopathic effect may develop during the second passage. Such virus isolates are dealt with as above. If, however, no CPE develops it cannot be assumed that no virus is present, especially if influenza or parainfluenza virus infection is suspected. In monkey kidney cells no CPE develops, but the surface of the infected cells may be so altered that red blood cells of a suitable species will adhere to the infected cells. This is known as *haemadsorption* and is useful for the detection of the ortho- and paramyxoviruses. The identity of the virus can be determined by haemadsorption inhibition or fluorescent antibody tests.

Method for Haemadsorption

1. Remove the medium from one control and one infected cell sheet.

2. Wash the cell sheets twice with 1 ml of Dulbecco's phosphate buffered saline (PBS).

3. Add 1·0 ml 0·5 per cent guinea-pig or human group 'O' cells.

4. Allow to adsorb for 1 h at 4°C.

5. Wash twice with PBS.

6. Examine for the adsorption of red blood cells to the infected cells. There should be no adsorption to the control cells. If red cells have adsorbed to the infected cells the identity of the virus responsible can be determined either by fluorescent antibody or by inhibition of haemadsorption.

Inhibition of Haemadsorption

1. Remove the medium from two uninfected and one infected cell sheet.

2. Wash twice with PBS.

3. Add specific antiserum to one of the infected cell sheets and PBS to the other and to the control cell sheet.

4. Allow to react for 1 h at 37°C.

5. Wash twice with PBS.

6. Continue as from step 3 of the haem-adsorption test.

If haemadsorption is found on the untreated infected cell sheet but not on either the control or the serum treated cell sheet then the haem-adsorption has been inhibited and the virus identified.

Rubella virus does not produce a CPE in all types of cell, but it can be detected because it can interfere with the growth of a challenge virus, e.g. echovirus 11. Interference, however, is not the easiest way in which to detect rubella virus and it is much better to employ cells which do develop a CPE, e.g. RK 13 cells.

If no CPE develops and no haemadsorption is found after two passages in tissue culture cells, it is usually concluded that none of the viruses that would normally grow under the conditions employed was present in the specimen.

Inoculation of Fertile Eggs and Animals

Inoculation of fertile eggs. Throat washings from patients with suspected influenza can be inoculated into fertile eggs as influenza virus can be grown on primary inoculation in 10–12-day-old eggs following the introduction of 0·05–0·2 ml into the amniotic cavity. The presence of virus is noted when the amniotic fluid, harvested 72 h later, is spot-checked for haemagglutination. The harvested amniotic fluid is passed in further eggs either blind or to increase the yield of virus. From the agglutination obtained it is possible to predict the group of influenza virus present (Table 10.2). The group can be confirmed by determination of the complement-fixing antigen from the chorio-allantoic membrane or amniotic fluid and the specific type of virus from the inhibition of haemagglutination.

Smears from macules submitted to the laboratory on slides may be washed off with saline and used as the inoculum in suspected cases of smallpox. Vesicle fluid or swabs in transport medium from such cases or from suspected cases of herpes may all be inoculated to the chorioallantoic membrane of 10–12-day-old fertile eggs. The inoculum is 0·2 ml and the eggs are incubated for 72 h following inoculation. If a virus is present pocks may develop and from their appearance some idea of the type of virus is obtained (Table 10.3).

As with all the other methods of growing viruses, blind passage is carried out if no pocks grow at the first passage and the identity of the virus is confirmed by neutralization of the isolate with the specific antiserum. To distinguish between variola major and variola minor the eggs should be incubated at 38·5°C and at 37·5°C. Variola major will grow at both temperatures whereas variola minor will only produce pocks at the lower temperature.

Strains of herpes simplex virus can be divided into two types: type 2 strains produce

Table 10.2

	4°C		22°C	
	Guinea-pig	Fowl	Guinea-pig	Fowl
Influenza A	+	−	+	−
Influenza B	+	+	+	+
Influenza C	+	+	−	−

Table 10.3

Pock	Virus
Small, white, discrete	Smallpox, herpes
Creamy, larger, necrotic	Vaccinia
Haemorrhagic, necrotic	Cowpox

pocks greater than 1 mm in diameter when the eggs are incubated for 7 days after infection, whereas type 1 strains produce only minute pocks which do not increase in size after the third day of incubation.

Inoculation of animals. Specimens from patients suffering from a clinical condition thought to be caused by the enterovirus are first inoculated into tissue cultures, but if these prove negative the specimen should be inoculated into suckling mice as the coxsackie A viruses are difficult to grow in tissue culture. Mice less than 48 h old are used and 0·02 ml of the specimen is injected intracerebrally and subcutaneously (see Vol. II, Chapter 15). The mice are examined daily for 14 days for the paralysis of the hind limbs. Any developing paralysis are (a) killed and sections stained by haematoxylin and eosin are examined histologically for the presence of muscular changes (Vol. I, Chapter 45), and (b) passed to further suckling mice to increase the yield of virus. Identification of the specific type of virus is determined by neutralization, i.e. the prevention of paralysis of suckling mice by type specific antisera and also by the patient's own convalescent serum.

Direct Demonstration of Virus or Virus Antigens

In the *electron microscope* it is possible to visualize virus particles provided that they are present in sufficient quantity. This technique can be used for vesicle fluid from cases of suspected smallpox, chickenpox or herpes; for warts or molluscum bodies or for lysates of cell cultures which have developed a CPE.

Method

1. Prepare copper grids with a collodion/carbon membrane (Vol. II, page 27).
2. Tease out the wart or molluscum body in distilled water.
3. Transfer the vesicle fluid, cell lysate or aqueous suspension from step 2 to the grid.
4. Allow to dry.
5. Irradiate with ultraviolet light for 30 min at 10 cm.
6. Wash with water to remove any crystalline deposit.
7. Apply a drop of phosphotungstic acid for 30 sec (see Vol. II, page 29).
8. Blot off excess stain.

9. Dry for 30 min in a desiccator over calcium chloride before examining in the electron microscope.

Light microscopy

Conjunctival smears, urine deposits, smears from suspected cases of smallpox or chickenpox or infected cell cultures can be stained by Giemsa's method and examined in the light microscope for the presence of inclusions or giant cells. Acridine orange staining of cell cultures can be useful in some instances and if the specific antisera are available, fluorescent antibody staining will allow identification of the virus (Vol. II, Chapter 11).

Gel Diffusion

Some viruses or their antigens can be identified by the gel diffusion technique with specific antisera. This test is employed in suspected cases of smallpox, serum hepatitis, etc.

Reagents for variola diagnosis

1. 1·0 per cent agarose (Noble).
2. Hyperimmune antivaccinial antiserum (rabbit).
3. Non-immune rabbit serum.
4. Known vaccinial antigen.
5. Unknown material.

Method

1. Prepare a slide coated with agar.
2. Punch holes (see Plate 10.1).
3. Place antiserum in centre well S+.
4. Place known antigen in 2 left-hand wells A+.
5. Place unknown antigen in 2 top wells AT.
6. Place non-immune serum in 2 right-hand wells S−.
7. Incubate for half-an-hour at 37°C in a moist atmosphere.
8. Examine for lines of identity.
9. If necessary, reincubate.

Hepatitis virus B antigen may be detected by a number of methods:

(a) Complement fixation (Purcell *et al.,* 1969).
(b) Haemagglutination (Vyas and Shulman, 1970).
(c) Radioimmuno-assay (Hollinger, Vordam and Dreesman, 1971), (Ling and Overby, 1972).

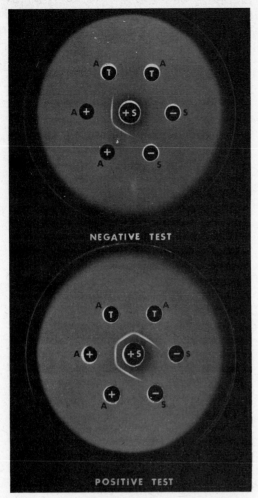

PLATE 10.1

The Agar-gel Precipitation Test

+S Centre wells: Positive rabbit antivaccinial serum.

TA Top wells: Test antigen made from material taken from the skin lesions of a case of smallpox.

+A Left: Positive antigen prepared from the crusts of a known case of smallpox.

−S Right: Normal rabbit serum from an animal known to be devoid of antibodies to variola.

Above A negative test. There is no precipitation between the test antigen (TA) and the positive serum (+S). The only lines of precipitation are between the positive serum and the positive control antigen (+A).

Below. A positive test. The lines of precipitation between the positive serum (+S) and the test antigen (TA) join the lines between the positive control antigen (+A) and the positive serum (+S).

(From Swain and Dodds (1967) *Clinical Virology*. Edinburgh: Livingstone.)

(d) Counter immune electroosmophoresis (CIEOP) (Prince and Burke, 1970).

This latter test will be described in detail as it is the most commonly used test.

Materials

Kodak projection slides ($3\frac{1}{4} \times 3\frac{1}{4}$)

Sterilin 10 cm square plastic petri dishes

Levelling table

Template and cutter

Electrophoresis chamber (Shandon)

Power pack (Shandon)

Chromedia 81 glass fibre paper (Whatman GF 81)

0·025 M veronal buffer pH 8·6

0·9 per cent agarose in 0·025 M veronal buffer pH 8·6

1·0 per cent tannic acid

Lyphogel (Gelman Instrument Co., supplied by Hawksley & Sons Ltd., 12 Peter Road, Lancing, Sussex)

Antiserum

Control antigen and unknown specimens.

The template has 2 mm holes in double rows 3 mm apart. The double rows are separated from the adjacent double rows by 5 mm. There are 35 pairs of holes on the template.

Method

1. Clean the projection slide with alcohol and cover with a thin layer of agar (6 ml per slide).

2. Dry quickly by heat, e.g. place on top of a boiling sterilizer. The agar will form a skin to accept a second layer of agar and keep it in place. Also it will stop the reagents running under the agar.

3. Place coated slide in the Sterilin petri dish on a levelling table.

4. Pour 25 ml 0·9 per cent agarose over the slide and leave till set.

5. Cut the slide away from the surrounding excess agar.

6. Cut the holes. It is convenient to have the cutter connected to a water pump to suck out the agar.

7. Place the antiserum in the well which will be nearer the anode of each of the pairs of wells to be used.

8. Pre-run in the electrophoresis chamber for 5 min at 30 milliamps per slide.

9. Refill these wells with antiserum.

10. Place the specimens in the adjacent

(cathode) wells and include a known positive antigen control.

11. Return the slide to the electrophoresis chamber with the antiserum wells at the anode. Electrophoresis for at least an hour at a constant current of 30 milliamps per slide.

12. Provided the positive control has produced a line, the slide is examined for precipitin lines. These may be enhanced as follows.

13. Leave the slide overnight in saline.

14. Wash with distilled water.

15. Flood the slide with 1 per cent tannic acid for 10 min and examine immediately.

16. If a line is produced with an unknown specimen it must be examined for the foundation of line of identity with the precipitate of a known positive reaction. This can be done by gel diffusion or by CIEOP (Das et al., 1971).

The sensitivity of the CIEOP test can be increased by concentration of the specimen with Lyphogel (a polyacrylamide gel).

1·48 g of Lyphogel is added to 10 ml of specimen and left 5 h at room temperature. The volume is then reduced to 2 ml. The concentrated specimen is then tested as above, neat, and at a 1 in 2 dilution for the presence of antigen. This latter dilution is required as high titred antigen may produce a prozone at times 5 concentration.

Antibody to hepatitis B antigen can also be detected by CIEOP. In this case the specimen is placed in the anode well and a known positive antigen in the cathode well. If a precipitin line develops it can be checked for specificity by performing the line of identity test including a known positive antibody. (This test is not particularly sensitive for the detection of antibody.)

Growth of Stock Viruses

To grow stocks of virus it is best to choose if possible, a system where a CPE develops as it is much easier to judge when to harvest the virus. As an example, to produce a stock of herpes simplex virus, the following procedure may be performed with baby hamster kidney cells (BHK cells) in Eagle's medium with 10 per cent calf serum.

1. Inoculate 0·2 ml of a suspension of seed herpes simplex virus into a test-tube monolayer.

2. When the CPE is complete, harvest the culture.

3. Lyse cells to release virus either by freezing and thawing or by ultrasonication.

4. Propagate a monolayer of 4×10^6 cells in 10 ml medium.

5. Decant the medium.

6. Inoculate the 1 ml from 3 into the monolayer and allow the virus to adsorb to the cells for 4 h at 35°C.

7. Replace medium.

8. Incubate overnight at 35°C after which all cells should show CPE.

9. Remove cells from glass with gentle pipetting or glass beads.

10. Repeat step 3.

11. Propagate 60×10^6 cells as a monolayer in a Roux bottle with 100 ml medium. Repeat steps 5 to 8 using 5 ml as inoculum.

12. After overnight incubation all the cells should show CPE.

13. Remove 10 ml of medium.

14. Decant rest of medium.

15. Resuspend infected cells in the 10 ml of medium.

16. Treat as step 3.

17. Propagate 200×10^6 cells as a monolayer in a 2 litre Winchester bottle with 200 ml medium. Repeat steps 5 and 6 using the 10 ml from 16 as the inoculum.

18. Allow the bottle to roll for 4 h to adsorb the virus.

19. Incubate overnight with or without the remainder of the medium.

20. Harvest the infected cells into 10–15 ml of medium.

21. Treat as step 3.

22. Titrate the virus suspension (see page 220).

23. If the titre of the virus is high enough store in small amounts at −70°C.

The resulting suspension of herpes simplex virus type 1 should have an infectivity of at least 10^8 pfu/ml and if kept in small amounts should retain its titre over a long period. Repeated freezing and thawing of virus stocks leads to loss of titre. Similar procedures may be adopted with most other viruses, but with varicella zoster, cytomegalo and respiratory syncytial virus, the infected cells should *not* be lysed or frozen. The above procedure may be stopped at any stage when sufficient virus has been produced; to act, say, as an antigen in a neutralization test.

Quantitation of Viruses

The infectivity of a suspension of an animal virus may be estimated in one of two ways, (a) quantal response and (b) focal response.

1. QUANTAL RESPONSE. This is an all or nothing response and may be measured in animals, fertile eggs or tissue culture monolayers. In the first two cases death or life are taken as the two parameters. Similarly, if a tissue culture is more than two-thirds destroyed it is scored as dead and less than that as alive or according to the convention of the laboratory. In order to make the quantal test an accurate one it is necessary to have a very large number of observations on each dilution of virus. This is not always possible so Reed and Muench (1938) proposed a method which would increase the number of observations. The premise is that any subject killed with a dilution of, say, 10^{-4}, would likewise be killed by inoculation with all more concentrated suspensions. From this it is possible to calculate a cumulative number dead (see Chapter 14). The virus infectivity is expressed as LD50 or TCID50, EID50, and in tissue cultures it is usual to employ 100 TCID50 in neutralization tests.

2. FOCAL RESPONSE. In this method viruses are allowed to infect monolayers of cells and the medium is such that released virus cannot spread; thus foci of infection or *plaques* are formed. After a suitable incubation period the plaques may be counted and the infectivity can be expressed as plaque-forming units per ml (pfu/ml). To contain the viruses in the neighbourhood of the first cell infected the following substances may be added to the medium: (a) antiserum to the virus—this will prevent spread of released virus through the medium so only closely adjacent cells will be infected; (b) agar—this is useful for small viruses such as polioviruses (Vol. II, Chapter 9). This method has the disadvantage that if the overlay is too hot, it will kill the cells and if too cool, cannot be pipetted; (c) methocel—is incorporated in the medium at a final concentration of 0·75 per cent. This overlay is much easier to handle but is only sufficiently viscid to inhibit the diffusion of large viruses such as the herpes and pox viruses.

Production of plaques. This can be done using either preformed monolayers or by infecting cells in suspension.

Preformed Monolayers

Method

1. Seed 5 cm Petri dishes with sufficient cells in 10 ml of medium to give a monolayer. Incubate in a carbon dioxide incubator or in medium containing herpes buffer.

2. Prepare dilutions of the virus in a suitable medium (1·0 per cent skim milk is useful), changing pipettes for each transfer. It is convenient to use 9 ml of diluent and 1 ml of inoculum for ten-fold dilutions.

3. Drain the medium from the Petri dishes.

4. Introduce 0·2 ml of the diluted virus suspension or suspending medium on to the monolayer.

5. Incubate for 1–4 h at 37°C depending on the virus.

6. Remove any unadsorbed virus.

7. Cover with an overlay containing serum or agar.

8. Incubate in the carbon dioxide incubator or in medium containing HEPES buffer for the required time.

9. To stain the plates overlaid with medium containing antiserum, drain off the medium and cover the cells for 5 min with formol methyl violet. Drain off stain and count plaques.

The cells under agar should be fixed for 2 h at least with formol saline (Vol. II, Chapter 9). The agar can then be shelled out and staining carried out as above. In some cases it is necessary to add DEAE to the agar overlay as agar contains substances which are inhibitory to some viruses.

Cells in Suspension (Russell, 1962)

Method

1. Prepare the required number of bijou bottles containing, e.g. $2·5 \times 10^6$ BHK cells in 1·8 ml of medium for a 5 cm Petri dish.

2. Prepare dilutions of virus.

3. Introduce 0·2 ml of virus suspension or suspending fluid into the bijou and shake for 20 min at room temperature.

4. Place 6 ml of methocel overlay medium in each 5 cm Petri dish.

5. Transfer the content of one bijou to each Petri dish.

6. Incubate as above and stain as in step 8 above.

Standardization of a Virus Suspension by a Particle Count

It is sometimes necessary to perform a total count of all the particles present in a suspension when preparing an antigen for gel diffusion. This can be done in the electron microscope using a suspension of polystyrene latex spheres as a comparison. (Polystyrene latex obtainable from Dow Chemical Company, Midland, Michigan, U.S.A., in sizes ranging from 90 nm to 1170 nm.)

Method

1. Accurately measure out 1 ml of a suspension of latex spheres of required diameter.

2. Heat to constant weight (M).

3. Using the specific gravity (d) of latex calculate the volume of latex ($V_1 = M/d$).

4. Using the radius (r) of the latex spheres calculate the volume of one sphere ($V_2 = 4/3 \pi r^3$).

5. Determine the number of spheres present in 1 ml of latex (V_1/V_2).

6. Mix equal quantities of the latex and virus suspensions.

7. Place a drop on a prepared copper grid and stain as *p*.

8. Count the relative numbers of latex particles and viruses in about 20 fields and by proportion calculate the concentration of the virus suspension.

Growth of Animal Viruses and Chlamydiae in Fertile Hens Eggs

The eggs should have white shells and should, if possible, come from a disease-free flock: the hens should not have been fed on a diet containing antibiotics (such eggs are useless for the growth of chlamydiae). After laying, the eggs should be kept for not more than one week at 4°C to 20°C before being set. A commercial egg incubator at 39°C is suitable for incubation. After about seven days they are examined to check for viability which is judged by the movement of the embryo and the clarity of the blood vessels. Candle the eggs in a dark room by placing over the opening of an illuminated box.

Four routes of inoculation are in common use (Table 10.4).

In all cases the eggs are candled, the air sac outlined with pencil and for the first two routes a cross is marked on the shell over the area where the chorio-allantois is best developed, avoiding any blood vessel.

Chorio-allantois

1. Using a dental drill fitted with a carborundum disc cut a slit 2–3 mm long in the air sac. This should pierce the shell membrane.

2. Carefully drill a square with 5 mm sides around the marked area taking care not to pierce the shell membrane.

3. Gently lever the shell from the shell membrane with a blunt dissecting needle.

4. Place a drop of sterile saline on the exposed shell membrane.

5. Carefully draw a dissecting needle across the exposed shell membrane through the saline drop at right angles to the fibres.

6. Apply negative pressure to the slit over the air sac with a rubber bulb. This will allow the

Table 10.4

	Sites	Organism	Age of embryo
1.	Chorio-allantois	Pox and herpes group	10–12 days
2.	Amniotic sac	Fresh isolates of orthomyco- and paramyxoviruses	7–12 days
3.	Allantoic sac	Egg adapted orthomyxoviruses	10–12 days
4.	Yolk sac	Chlamydiae and rickettsiae	6–7 days

saline drop to enter and separate the chorio-allantois from the shell membrane and to form a false air sac.

7. Introduce 0·2 ml inoculum through the shell membrane.

8. Rock the egg to distribute the inoculum evenly over the chorio-allantois.

9. Seal with clear adhesive tape.

10. Incubate for the required time at the appropriate temperature in a humid atmosphere (Vol. I, Chapter 40).

11. Chill for at least 2 h at 4°C. This will kill the embryo and reduce haemorrhage.

12. Place the egg in a suitable holder on cellulose wadding which can be discarded. Put on a pair of gloves.

13. With sharp pointed scissors and starting from the slit over the air sac cut right round the egg in its longest diameter. Discard the holder, embryo, and lower hemisected shell in a polythene bag.

14. Remove the inoculated area of the chorio-allantois from the hemisected shell with forceps.

15. Float in sterile saline in a Petri dish.

16. Examine for the presence of pocks against a dark background. The chorio-allantoic membrane may be used for the production of antigen by grinding in a tissue grinder and resuspension in sterile saline.

Amniotic Sac

1. Candle egg and mark boundary of natural air sac.

2. Drill round egg just inside the boundary of the air sac.

3. Remove the cap thus created.

4. Clarify the underlying shell membrane—chorio-allantoic membrane—by painting with sterile liquid paraffin on a cotton swab.

5. With a fine pair of forceps (iris forceps) penetrate the clarified membrane and pick up a fold of the amnion and insert the needle into it so as to gently prod the embryo and then expel the inoculum. (A small bubble of air may be expelled with the inoculum to check the correct position of the needle in the amniotic cavity.)

6. The air sac is then covered with wide adhesive tape and may be incubated, air sac upwards, in a commercial egg rack.

7. To harvest, chill and remove allantoic fluid with Pasteur pipette with side hole (see below) and then harvest amniotic fluid; the sac may be washed out with saline if the yield of amniotic fluid is low.

8. The fluids may be checked for viral haemagglutinins at an approximate dilution of 1/10; note that strong concentrations of amniotic fluid (1/1 to 1/3) may give false positive haemagglutination.

Allantoic Sac

1. Drill a 2–3 mm slit in the air sac piercing the shell membrane.

2. Make a depression in the shell over the marked area using a 'burr' and taking care not to damage the shell membrane.

3. Inoculate 0·2 ml of suspension through this area. The syringe should penetrate about 2 mm into the egg.

4. Cover the depression with a molten mixture of equal quantities of vaseline and paraffin wax.

5. Incubate in a humid atmosphere for the required time at the appropriate temperature.

6. Chill the egg for at least 2 h at 4°C.

7. Pierce the egg through the wax vaseline mixture with a warmed probe or forceps.

8. Aspirate the allantoic fluid using a Pasteur pipette with a hole in the side.

(To make such a pipette, pull a Pasteur pipette of fairly wide bore—about 2 mm. Seal the end. When the pipette is cool, attach a rubber teat and hold the pipette beside a pilot light about $\frac{1}{2}$ in from the sealed end. The glass will melt and due to the pressure applied on the bulb a hole will be produced.)

The allantoic sac inoculation route can be used for the production of the V or S antigens of the ortho- and paramyxovirus groups.

The V antigen is prepared from the harvested fluid.

1. Inoculate allantoic cavities of 10–12-day-old embryos with 0·1 ml of a virus suspension diluted 10^{-3} to avoid autointerference.

2. Incubate 40–44 h at 35°C.

3. Chill 1 h at 4°C.

4. Harvest allantoic fluid.

5. Test for haemagglutination. If the titre is 1280 or greater the antigen is ready for use and may be stored with the addition of 0·08

per cent sodium azide at $-30°C$. If the titre is not sufficiently high then the virus should be passed at least once more in eggs.

The S antigen is prepared from the chorio-allantois of the infected eggs.

1. By passage of the virus in the allantoic cavity, prepare a virus stock which on dilution to 10^{-4} will ensure a good response, i.e. a haemagglutination titre of 256 on inoculation of an egg.

2. Inoculate a batch of 11–13-day-old eggs with 0·1 ml of the above diluted stock.

3. Incubate 48 h at 35°C.

4. Harvest the allantoic fluid, without chilling.

5. Test for the presence of haemagglutination.

6. If the haemagglutination titre is 64 or greater harvest the chorio-allantoic membrane by first tipping out the embryo and then pulling the chorioallantois from the shell membrane and then dissecting it free.

7. Wash the membranes in 0·08 per cent azide saline to remove any blood or yolk.

8. Dry between filter papers.

9. Weigh.

10. Suspend in 5–10 ml azide saline.

11. Freeze and thaw three times.

12. Make a mixture to 40 per cent w/v in azide saline.

13. Homogenize.

14. Spin lightly to remove coarse debris.

15. Add a few drops of chloroform.

16. Leave overnight at 4°C.

17. Spin in an angle head centrifuge for 1 h at 1500 g.

18. Store, preferably as freeze dried material, for 1 month at $-30°C$.

Yolk Sac Inoculation

1. Drill a 2–3 mm slit in the air sac piercing the shell membrane.

2. Place the egg in a holder, air sac uppermost, at an angle of 15° to the vertical.

3. Using a 3 cm 12–14 gauge needle introduce 0·2 ml of the inoculum by inserting the needle vertically through the slit right up to the hilt.

4. Seal the hole with nail varnish.

5. Incubate at 35°C in a humid atmosphere.

6. Candle the eggs daily; discard any eggs which die in the first 48 h after inoculation, but examine any which die later.

7. Live eggs should be chilled before harvesting.

8. Remove the shell over the air sac, peel off the shell membrane and slit the exposed chorioallantois with sharp scissors.

9. Tip out the embryo and yolk sac into a sterile Petri dish.

10. Dissect yolk sac and prepare smears from the stalk which has been wiped free of yolk.

11. Fix the smear and stain by modified Brucella, Castaneda, Giminez or Machiavello's methods (Vol. II, Chapter 3).

12. Place yolk sac in PBS in a bijou and store at $-70°$.

Concentration and Purification of Virus Preparations

To obtain high titre virus a number of steps may be taken. If the virus is mainly cell associated, the infected cells may be harvested in a small volume of medium, artificially lysed and the cellular debris removed by centrifugation for 15 min at 2000 g. If the virus is released into the medium then both the medium and the cells should be harvested. After lysis of the cells and clarification of the fluid by a similar centrifugation as above the volume can be reduced by either (1) placing dialysis tubing containing polyethylene glycol in the virus suspension, Kohn (1959) or (2) by ultracentrifugation of the suspension—the time and speed required depending upon the virus. The pellet can then be resuspended in a small volume of medium. This latter method can be deleterious to the virus and also resuspension of the pellet is difficult so a sucrose cushion is often placed in the bottom of the tube. The concentration of the sucrose should be sufficient to exclude the virus which will then collect in a band on top of the sucrose.

The reduction, by polyethylene glycol, of the volume of fluid in a virus suspension will result in a concentration of both virus and cellular material and in the ultracentrifuge the virus will be contaminated with cellular material which co-sediments with it. The virus can be separated from the contaminating cellular material in a number of ways;

    (a) by adsorption to and elution from red blood cells (Laver, 1969),

    (b) by exclusion chromatography (Philipson, 1967),

    (c) by centrifugation in a sucrose rate-zonal or a caesium chloride equilibrium gradient (Laver, 1969; Crawford, 1969),

    (d) by adsorption and elution from calcium phosphate (Burness, 1969).

ACTION TO BE TAKEN WITH SPECIMENS AND POSSIBLE VIRUS ISOLATES

Adenovirus

Clinical syndromes. Febrile pharyngitis, respiratory disease and pneumonia in young children, conjunctivitis, mesenteric adenitis.
Specimens. Throat swab, eye swab, rectal swab or faeces, biopsy material.
Suggested tissue culture. HeLa or HEp2.
CPE. Clustering of cells and cytoplasmic strands.
Identification:

    (a) Use the virus isolate suspension as a complement-fixing antigen.

    (b) Haemagglutination of monkey and rat cells.

    (c) Neutralization by type-specific antiserum.

Arbovirus

Staff handling arboviruses should be protected by immunization where available.
Clinical syndromes. Fever, encephalitis in areas where insect-borne disease is common and haemorrhagic fever.
Specimens. Blood serum, blood clot, cerebrospinal fluid, insect vectors.
Culture system. Intracerebral inoculation of weanling mice. Egg yolk sac. Care should be taken when dealing with inoculated mice since the excreta may contain large amounts of virus. Special caging can be useful (Lennette and Schmidt, 1969).
Identification. Neutralization and haemadsorption inhibition tests.

Cytomegalovirus

Clinical syndromes. Cytomegalic inclusion disease. Post transfusion mononucleosis.

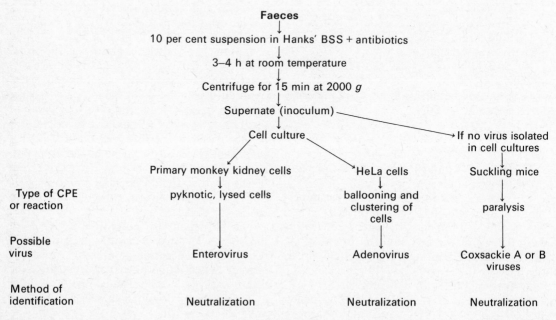

FIG. 10.1

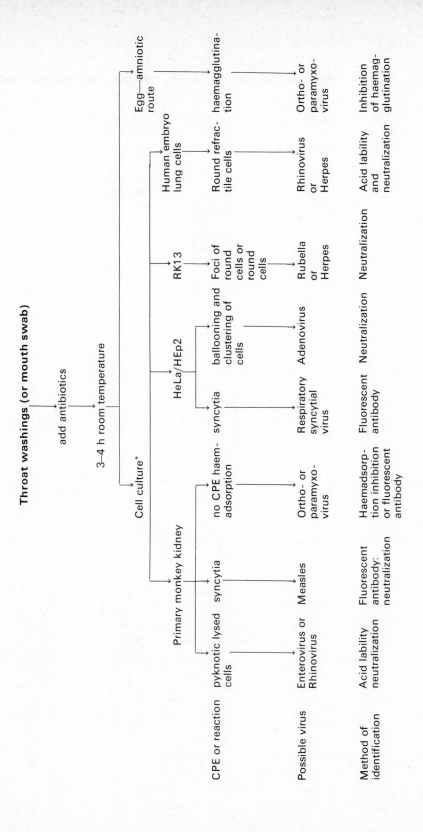

Throat washings (or mouth swab)

add antibiotics

3–4 h room temperature

Cell culture*

	Primary monkey kidney		HeLa/HEp2		RK13	Human embryo lung cells	Egg—amniotic route
CPE or reaction	pyknotic lysed cells	syncytia	no CPE haem-adsorption	syncytia	ballooning and clustering of cells	Foci of round cells or round cells	Round refractile cells	haemagglutination
Possible virus	Enterovirus or Rhinovirus	Measles	Ortho- or paramyxo-virus	Respiratory syncytial virus	Adenovirus	Rubella or Herpes	Rhinovirus or Herpes	Ortho- or paramyxo-virus
Method of identification	Acid lability neutralization	Fluorescent antibody: neutralization	Haemadsorption inhibition or fluorescent antibody	Fluorescent antibody	Neutralization	Neutralization	Acid lability and neutralization	Inhibition of haemagglutination

Fig. 10.2

*According to clinical information to decide on appropriate culture system.

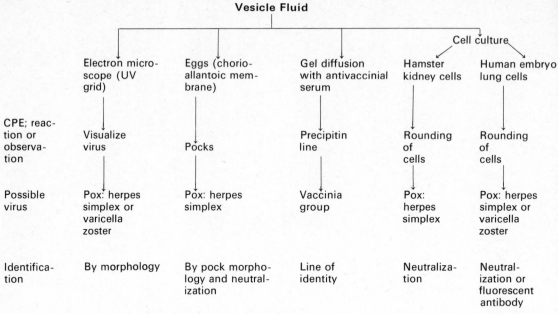

Fig. 10.3

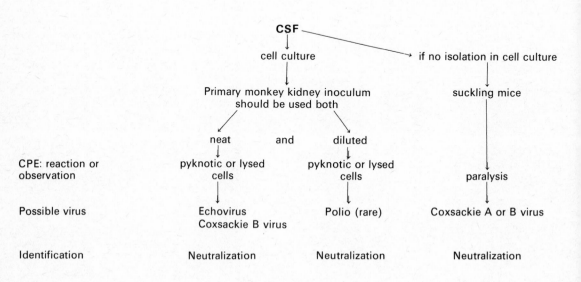

Fig. 10.4

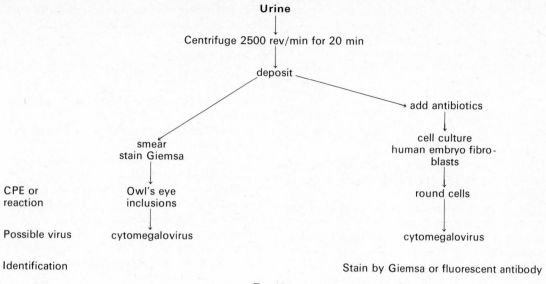

FIG. 10.5

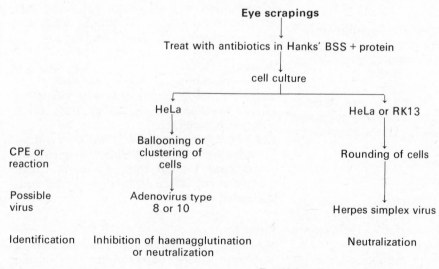

FIG. 10.6

Specimens. Urine, saliva, tears, liver biopsy. These specimens should *not* be frozen.

Suggested tissue culture. Human embryo fibroblast cells (e.g. lung cells).

Identification. Stain the infected cells and look for large intra-nuclear 'owl eye' inclusions.

Enterovirus

Staff should be protected by poliovirus immunization.

Clinical syndromes. Aseptic meningitis, paralysis, exanthemata, pericarditis, myocarditis, pleurodynia, gastroenteritis.

Specimens. Faeces or rectal swabs, throat swab, cerebrospinal fluid.

Suggested tissue culture. Primary monkey kidney cells.

CPE. Round, dense, pyknotic cells.

Identification. Neutralization for polio, coxsackie A and B, or echo virus.

If no virus is isolated in tissue culture the specimen should be inoculated intracerebrally or intraperitoneally into suckling mice to attempt to isolate coxsackie A or B viruses (Vol II, Chapter 15).

The wild and vaccine strains of polio may be distinguished by various special tests, e.g. the rct 40 test or dextran test.

Hepatitis

Clinical syndromes. Infectious hepatitis virus A (short incubation). Serum hepatitis virus B (long incubation). Specimens. Clotted blood, Liver biopsy and necropsy materials.

Cultural methods are not yet available.

Identification of virus B antigen is by counter-immune electrophoresis complement-fixation and radio immuno-assay. Haemagglutination methods are also in use.

Herpes Simplex Virus

Clinical syndromes. Stomatitis, dendriform ulcers, whitlows, herpes labialis, herpes genetalis, one form of Kaposi's varicelliform dermatitis, encephalitis.

Specimens. Swabs from mouth, eye, vesicle fluids, vulva, urethra or cervix uteri, CSF.

Suggested tissue cultures. Human amnion, W1–38, human embryo lung or BHK.

CPE. Rounding of cells or syncytial formation. Identification is by neutralization tests.

Orthomyxoviruses

Clinical syndromes. Influenzal illnesses.

Specimens. Throat washings, throat swabs from young children, lung tissue taken at necropsy.

Suggested tissue culture. Primary or secondary monkey kidney cells.

Detection is by haemadsorption or haemagglutin. CPE is not usual.

Identification. Complement-fixation or fluorescent antibody tests give the group: haemadsorption inhibition indicates the type.

The specimen may be inoculated into the amniotic cavity of 12 day-old chick embryos and is detected by haemagglutination. Strain specific identification is by inhibition by specific antisera of haemagglutination.

Paramyxoviruses

Measles

Specimens. Throat washings, urine, cerebrospinal fluid or necropsy materials.

Suggested tissue cultures. Human embryonic kidney, human amnion, monkey kidney cells.

CPE. Syncytia or stellate cells (in epitheloid cells).

Identification is by staining inclusions with acridine orange (Vol II, Chapter 2) or neutralization or haemagglutination inhibition.

Mumps

Specimens. Saliva or cerebrospinal fluid.

Suggested tissue culture. Monkey kidney or HeLa. Amniotic inoculation of 8-day chick embryos is preferable.

CPE. Cytolytic effects and haemadsorption.

Identification. Haemagglutination inhibition, complement fixation with egg fluids, haemadsorption in infected monolayers and neutralization.

Poxvirus

Staff handling material from potential cases of smallpox should be protected by regular vaccination.

Specimens. Scrapings from macules, papules, vesicle fluid and crusts. (Vol I, Chap. 40)

Laboratory diagnosis. (a) Electronmicroscopical examination to search for pox viruses of typical morphology, (b) gel diffusion to establish lines of identity with known positive antigen and known antibody, (c) inoculation of 0·2 ml to chorio-allantoic membrane of 10 to 12 day-old chick embryo. Incubate 72 h and examine membranes for the production of pocks. Identify by the appearance of the pocks and the presence of poxvirus virions by electronmicroscopy and in stained films of crushed lesions.

Variola major may be distinguished from variola minor by incubation of inoculated eggs at 37·5°C at which temperature variola minor will not grow.

Rabies virus

This virus and specimens from suspected cases of rabies should only be handled in licenced laboratories.
Clinical syndromes. Hydrophobia and fatal encephalitis, following a bite from a dog or any other mammal (see Vol I, Chap. 48).
Specimens. Nerve tissue from autopsy—animal or human, or saliva from dog, or saliva from the patient. Great care should be taken when handling such specimens as the virus can infect man via the conjunctiva or abrasions of the skin. Gloves should be worn and the face and eyes should be protected by a suitable plastic face shield. When it is necessary to inoculate animals, they should be handled with forceps (Lennette and Schmidt, 1968).
Treatment of specimens. Inoculate mice intra-cerebrally and look for flaccid paralysis.
Identification. Histological staining of tissue smears or sections for Negri bodies by specific labelled fluorescent antibody for rabies virus, or by conventional histological methods.

Respiratory syncytial virus

Clinical syndromes. Bronchiolitis and less severe illnesses and the common cold.
Specimens. Throat swab or sputum (*do not chill*).
Suggested tissue cultures. Bristol HeLa cells: HEp2 cells inoculated at bedside.
CPE. Syncytia formation. Identification. Complement fixation or fluorescent antibody.

Rhinovirus

Clinical syndrome. Common cold.
Specimens. Nasal washings, nasopharyngeal swabs or throat washings.
Suggested tissue cultures. Organ cultures of human embryonic trachea, primary human embryonic kidney cells or for a few strains, secondary monkey kidney cells. Incubate at 33°C. Rotate.
CPE. Rounding and shrivelling of cells.
Identification. These viruses may be distinguished from enteroviruses by lability at low pH. At pH 3 the virus is almost completely destroyed in 3–4 h at room temperature.

Varicella-zoster virus

Clinical syndromes. Chickenpox, shingles, encephalitis.
Specimens. Vesicle fluid (or cerebrospinal fluid).
Suggested tissue culture. Human amnion or embryonic lung cells. Do *not* freeze infected cells.
CPE. Rounding of cells following the aggregated spirals of cells.
Identification. Fluorescent antibody or complement fixation tests.

REFERENCES

BURNESS, A. T. H. (1969) Purification and separation of encephalomyocarditis virus variants by chromatography on calcium phosphate. In *Fundamental Techniques in Virology*, edited by K. Habel and N. P. Salzman. New York: Academic Press.
CRAWFORD, L. V. (1969) Purification of polyoma virus. In *Fundamental Techniques in Virology*, edited by K. Habel and N. P. Salzman. New York: Academic Press.
DAS, P. C., HOPKINS, R., CASH, J. D. & CUMMING, R. A. (1971) Rapid identification of hepatitis associated antigen and antibody by counter-immunoelectrophoresis. *British Journal of Haematology*, **21**, 673.
HOLLINGER, F. B., VORDAM, V. & DREESMAN, G. R. (1971) Assay of Australia antigen and antibody employing double-antibody and solid-phase radioimmunoassay techniques and comparison with the passive haemagglutination methods. *Journal of Immunology*, **107**, 1099.
KOHN, J. (1959) A simple method for the concentration of fluids containing protein. *Nature, London*, **183**, 1055.
KORITZ, R. L., KLAHS, D. R., RITMAN, S., DAMUS, K. & GITNICK, G. L. (1973) Post transfusion hepatitis in recipients of blood screened by newer assays. *Lancet*, **ii**, 694–696.
LAVER, W. G. (1969) Purification of influenza virus. In *Fundamental Techniques in Virology*, edited by K. Habel and N. P. Salzman. New York: Academic Press.

LEIBOVITZ, A. (1969) A transport medium for diagnostic virology. *Proceedings of the Society for Experimental Biology and Medicine,* **131,** 127.

LING, C. M. & OVERBY, L. R. (1972) Prevalence of hepatitis B antigen as revealed by direct radioimmune assay with ^{125}I-antibody. *Journal of Immunology,* **109,** 834.

PHILIPSON, L. (1967) Chromatography and membrane separation. In *Methods in Virology,* Vol. 2, edited by K. Maramorosch and H. Koprowski. New York: Academic Press.

PRINCE, A. M. & BURKE, K. (1970) Serum hepatitis antigen (SH): rapid detection by high voltage immuno-electrophoresis. *Science,* **169,** 593.

PURCELL, R. H., HOLLAND, P. V., WALSH, J. H., WONG, D. C., MORROW, A. G. & CHANOCK, R. M. (1969) A complement-fixation test for measuring Australia antigen and antibody. *Journal of Infectious Diseases,* **120,** 383.

REED, L. J. & MEUNCH, H. (1938) A simple method for estimating fifty per cent endpoints. *Journal of Hygiene,* **27,** 493.

REESINK, H. W., DUIMEL, W. J. & BRUMMELHUIS, H. G. J. (1973) Evaluation of a new haemagglutination technique for the demonstration of hepatitis-B antigen. *Lancet,* **ii,** 1351–1353.

RUSSELL, W. C. (1962) A sensitive and precise plaque assay for herpes virus. *Nature, London,* **195,** 1028.

VYAS, G. N. & SHULMAN, N. R. (1970) Haemagglutination assay for antigen and antibody association with viral hepatitis. *Science,* **170,** 332.

FURTHER READING

BEVERIDGE, W. I. B. & BURNET, F. M. (1946) The cultivation of viruses and rickettsiae in the chick embryo. *Special Report Series of the Medical Research Council (London),* No. 256.

BUSBY, D. W. G., HOUSE, W. & MacDONALD, J. R. (1964) *Virological Technique,* London: Churchill.

CRAMER, R. (1964) Purification of animal viruses. In *Techniques in Experimental Virology,* edited by R. J. C. Harris. New York: Academic Press.

GRIST, N. R., ROSS, C. A. C. & BELL, E. J. (1974) *Diagnostic Methods in Clinical Virology,* 2nd edition. Oxford: Blackwell.

LENETTE, E. H. & SCHMIDT, N. J. (1969) *Diagnostic Procedures for Viral and Rickettsial Infections,* 4th edition. New York: American Public Health Association Inc.

11. Immunological and Serological Methods in Microbial Infections

The Interaction of Antibody with Antigen

An antibody, as has been pointed out, is an immunoglobulin molecule secreted into the tissue fluids from lymphoid cells which have been exposed to a foreign substance—an antigen. An antigen may be potentially harmful, such as a bacterium or virus, or it may be a harmless bland substance such as foreign serum protein. The antibody can combine only with antigen which is identical or nearly identical with the inducing antigen and not with unrelated antigens. When molecules of antibody and antigen are brought together in solution, they interact with each other by the formation of a link between an antigen-binding site on the immunoglobulin molecule—part of the Fab fragment—and the particular chemical groupings which make up what is termed the antigenic determinant of the antigen molecule. The molecules are held together by non-covalent intermolecular forces which are effective only when the antigen-binding site and the antigenic determinant group are able to make close contact. The better the fit the closer the contact and the stronger the antigen-antibody bond, these factors determining what is often called the affinity of the antibody molecule; antibodies of varying combining quality exist and the overall tendency to combine with antigen is the average ability of the antibodies to combine with antigen or the average intrinsic association constant. This can be calculated experimentally by application of the concepts of chemical equilibria to antigen-antibody interactions. Studies of this type have shown that the affinity of antibodies increases as immunization proceeds and that the dose of antigen can influence the quality of antibody.

The methods used for the detection of antigen-antibody reactions in the laboratory fall into two functional groups: first, procedures designed to elucidate the cytodynamics of antibody formation which involve the study of the behaviour of single cells or small populations of cells; the second group, which is the subject of the present discussion, concerns the detection and quantitation of *secreted antibody* circulating in the blood or present in the tissue fluids.

The methods used here range in their application from highly specialized studies of the physico-chemical aspects of antigen-antibody interaction to widely used procedures designed to aid in the diagnosis of disease.

Primary Interaction and Secondary Effects

In practical terms, the union of antibody with antigen can be detected at two different levels. The first level is that following *primary union* of the two reactants and usually requires that one or other reactant is labelled with a suitable marker such as a fluorescent dye or a radioactive isotope. A simple example of this is the microscopic localization in a tissue of a particular microorganism utilizing an antiserum prepared against the microorganism and labelled with a dye that fluoresces under UV light.

The second level at which antigen-antibody combination can be detected depends on the development, after primary union, of certain changes in the physical state of the complex, resulting in precipitation or agglutination of the components or, alternatively, in the activation of non-antibody components such as serum complement or histamine from mast cells. Reactions of this type occurring subsequent to primary union are termed *secondary phenomena*. This discussion is concerned with the principles of a few of these secondary phenomena which are in common use.

Secondary Effects: Interpretation and Applications

Before considering these reactions individually, it is important to be aware of the difficulties in interpreting results of such tests. The initiation and development of the secondary phenomena constitute a complicated series of events involving many variables such as the type of antibody taking part, the relative proportions of antibody and antigen, characteristics of the antigen molecule, presence of electrolytes, inhibitory substances and unstable components.

Despite these formidable difficulties, the widely and long used secondary phenomena such as precipitation, agglutination and complement fixation have an important role to play as aids in the diagnosis of disease and in the identification of microorganisms.

The secondary phenomena, as already indicated, can bring about several readily observable changes when carried out *in vitro* and these are used in tests to demonstrate the presence of antibody in the sera of patients suffering from infectious disease, or producing an antibody response to cell antigens as might, for example, occur after incompatible blood transfusion, tissue grafting or in autoimmune states.

Reactions of this type can also be used to identify antigens in the tissues or body fluids and, for example, would be utilized for blood grouping, tissue typing or the identification of microorganisms.

Among the most important of these reactions are *precipitation*, which occurs between antibody and antigen molecules in soluble form; *agglutination*, in which the antibodies directed against surface antigens of particulate materials such as microorganisms or erythrocytes link them together in large clumps or aggregates; and *complement fixation* in which antibody molecules, after reaction with antigen, activate the complex blood components which make up serum complement.

In addition to these widely used serological tests, a number of other effects of antigen-antibody interaction are of medical importance. These include neutralization tests used for example in virus identification, immobilization tests with bacteria and protozoa and skin tests for the reaginic antibody characteristic of anaphylactic states.

Quantitative Tests: Dilutions and Titres

In diagnostic serology it is often necessary to determine the *amount* of a specific antibody in the patient's blood serum in order to distinguish between the presence of a large amount of antibody produced in response to a current infection and that of a small amount of 'natural' or cross-reacting antibody unrelated to the patient's illness. In routine tests it is impracticable to isolate the specific antibody and measure its mass. Instead, the amount of the antibody is estimated by determining the greatest degree to which the serum may be diluted without losing the power to give an observable primary reaction or secondary effect in a mixture with the specific antigen. Different dilutions of the serum are tested in mixtures with a constant amount of antigen and the *greatest reacting dilution* is taken as the measure, or *titre*, of the concentration of antibody in the undiluted serum.

Dilutions may be expressed in one of two ways: (1) they may be expressed in terms of the way in which they are made, e.g. a dilution of '1 in 8' is a dilution made by mixing one volume of serum with seven volumes of diluent (usually physiological saline); (2) alternatively, they may be expressed as the factor by which the dilution of the reagent (antibody) is increased, e.g. a dilution of '8' represents an eight-fold increase in dilution.

It is incorrect to express dilutions as fractions, e.g. $\frac{1}{8}$, because the higher dilutions are then represented by the smaller values. In a dilution of 1 in 8, it is the concentration, not the dilution of the reagent that is reduced to $\frac{1}{8}$. It is, moreover, inadvisable to express dilutions in the form '1:8', as this is the notation generally used to express a ratio; its use for a dilution might be taken to indicate either the ratio between the volume of the serum and that of the diluent or the ratio of the volume of the serum to that of the final mixture of serum with diluent.

Titres should be expressed by the *integers* representing the greatest reacting dilutions, e.g. if the greatest reacting dilution of the serum is 8, the titre is 8. The term 'reciprocal titre' is commonly used in an incorrect sense based on the mistaken use of a fraction to express the end-point dilution; it should therefore be avoided. Where the end-point dilution is 1 in 8, it is the titre, not the reciprocal titre, that is 8.

Titres cited by bacteriologists normally indicate the dilution of the serum in the reaction mixture after all the other reagents have been added, e.g. bacterial suspension and saline diluent. Most titres cited by virologists indicate either the dilution of the serum in the primary reaction mixture with virus or haemagglutinin, or the initial dilution of the serum without adjustment for the further dilution with the added reactants; in the latter case the value is meaningful only in the context of knowledge of the volumes of the reactants added to each mixture.

PRECIPITATION

Optimal Proportions

As a result of the interaction of antibody and antigen molecules in solution, complexes of the two types of molecule will form and precipitation may occur depending on the relative concentration of the two reactants. If a series of tubes is set up (Fig. 11.1), each containing a constant amount of antiserum, and decreasing amounts of antigen are added to the tubes in the row, a haziness will start to appear in the tubes gradually increasing to visible aggregates or precipitates. The amount of precipitation will be seen to increase along the row, reaching

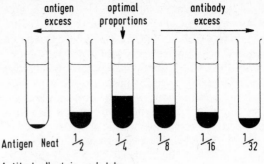

Antigen Neat $\frac{1}{2}$ $\frac{1}{4}$ $\frac{1}{8}$ $\frac{1}{16}$ $\frac{1}{32}$

Antibody Neat in each tube.

FIG. 11.1

a maximum and then falling off with the lower antigen concentration. The tubes where most precipitate appears contain the *optimal proportions* of antigen and antibody for precipitation and the proportions are constant for all dilutions of the same reagents. The composition of the precipitate varies with the original proportions of the antibody and antigen; if antigen is in excess the precipitate will contain relatively more of this component and similarly more antibody if it is present in excess. As can be seen from Figure 11.2, on the antigen excess side of optimal proportions less precipitate appears and this is due to the inability of the antigen-antibody complexes formed to link up

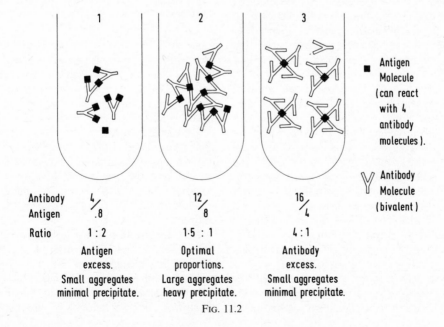

	1	2	3
Antibody	4	12	16
Antigen	.8	8	4
Ratio	1 : 2	1.5 : 1	4 : 1
	Antigen excess.	Optimal proportions.	Antibody excess.
	Small aggregates minimal precipitate.	Large aggregates heavy precipitate.	Small aggregates minimal precipitate.

■ Antigen Molecule (can react with 4 antibody molecules).

Y Antibody Molecule (bivalent)

FIG. 11.2

to other complexes and so make a large aggregate or lattice which will appear as a visible precipitate (tube 1, Fig. 11.2). Large aggregates of antibody and antigen can form best under conditions of optimal proportions where the antibody and antigen proportions are such that after initial combination of the molecules, free antigen-binding sites and antigen determinant groups remain, enabling the complexes to link up into a large lattice formation (as in tube 2 of Fig. 11.2). In antibody excess all the free determinants of the antigen molecule are soon taken up with antibody, so that very little linking can take place between the complexes (as in tube 3 of Fig. 11.2).

Applications

The precipitin test can be carried out in a quantitative manner by estimating the protein content of the precipitate at optimal proportions. The qualitative test is much more widely used and is of considerable value in detecting and identifying antigens, having applications in the typing of streptococci or pneumococci. This is done by layering an extract of the organism over antiserum. After a short while, a ring of precipitate forms at the interface (this is called the ring test). The technique is also used in forensic studies and in detecting adulteration of foodstuffs. A modification of the test in which precipitation is allowed to occur in *agar gel* is very widely used for detecting the presence of antibody in serum or antigen in unknown preparations, and is valuable for showing the identity of different antigen preparations (Fig. 11.3). A concentration gradient forms in the gel, the concentration of a substance decreasing as the molecules diffuse away from the well in which they were placed. Precipitin bands form in the gel in the position where the antigen and antibody molecules reach optimal proportions after diffusion. When a large number of different antigens are present in a solution, it is difficult to separate the precipitin bands for each of the antigen-antibody reactions by the simple gel-diffusion method just described. In such a situation, a variation of this method can be used to identify the individual components. This modification is particularly valuable in

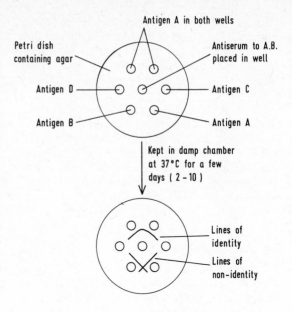

FIG. 11.3

Immunodiffusion or gel diffusion test. Wells are cut in a layer of agar in a Petri dish. Antiserum and antigen solutions are placed opposite each other in the wells and after allowing a few days for diffusion to take place precipitin bands will form where antibody and antigen meet in suitable proportions (optimal proportions). No reactions take place with antigens C and D as the antiserum in the central well contains antibodies only for antigens A and B. Lines of identity as formed between the two A wells enable the technique to be used for identifying unknown antigens.

analysing a multicomponent system such as serum. The individual components of serum are first separated by electrophoresis in agar gel and an antiserum, prepared against the serum, is allowed to diffuse towards the separated components, resulting in the formation of precipitin bands. This method, known as immunoelectrophoresis, is particularly valuable for showing the presence of abnormal globulin constituents in the serum of patients with myelomatosis and other serum protein abnormalities.

A microimmunodiffusion test with wells cut in a layer of agar on a microscope slide is a convenient modification of the Petri dish method. This procedure has come into wide use for the detection in human serum of the *Australia antigen* which is associated with serum hepatitis. The routine screening of blood products by a modification of this technique using specific antisera prepared in animals has become an important laboratory test in the prevention of serum hepatitis outbreaks.

IMMUNODIFFUSION

Double diffusion carried out in tubes 5 cm × 2 cm in which the antigen and antibody diffuse towards each other in a layer of agar is the basis of the Oakley and Fulthorpe (1953) and Preer (1956) techniques. The antigen and antibody solutions may be introduced in liquid form particularly when the concentration of either is low and dilution is not desirable. More conveniently the antigen and antibody can be mixed with agar. The three layers of the system then consist of antigen and antibody mixed with agar separated by a layer of agar. The concentration of the agar used is commonly 0·6 per cent. The precipitin bands form in the middle layer and with strong antisera may be seen within a few hours. Dilution of the antisera or antigen causes displacement of the band towards the antiserum-agar or antigen-agar interface respectively. This type of immunodiffusion technique in tubes has the distinction of being the most sensitive type of precipitin test available with respect to the quantities of reactants required for the formation of visible precipitates. Quantities of reactants too small

to form visible precipitates if they were simply mixed together are concentrated in a very narrow zone and can thus form an observable precipitate (Crowle, 1961). The number of precipitin bands observed in the agar tubes does not necessarily indicate the total number of systems present as some of the bands in complex mixtures may be hidden by others and would only be identified by procedures of high resolving power such as immunoelectrophoresis.

Immunodiffusion has been extensively used in microbiology for the identification of different types and strains of bacteria and viruses.

The smallpox virus can be detected in the exudate from the skin lesions and poliomyelitis virus can be typed (Grasset, Bonifas and Pongratz, 1958). Fungi can be identified by immunodiffusion and a diagnostic test has been developed for histoplasmosis (Heiner, 1958).

Double Diffusion in Plates

Sufficient 1 per cent agar in 0·85 per cent NaCl or 0·2 M phosphate buffer pH 7·2 containing 0·1 per cent sodium azide is poured into a small, flat-bottomed Petri dish to give a perfectly level surface (about 10 ml). When this has solidified, wells are cut in the agar with a cork borer in positions determined by a pattern drawn on a piece of paper which is placed under the Petri dish. More conveniently

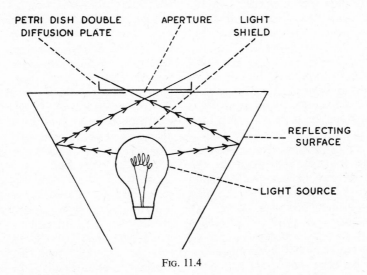

FIG. 11.4

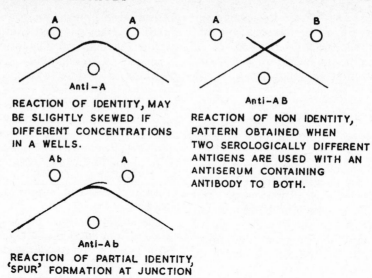

FIG. 11.5

Commonly observed patterns found in double diffusion plates where two antigen solutions are compared using antiserum as the analytic agent.

wells are cut with a gel cutter with, for example, a central well surrounded by six satellite wells (Shandon Scientific Company). A very large number of different sizes and shapes and arrangements of wells have been used in this technique, the circular central well with equidistant satellite wells is perhaps the most popular. After the wells have been filled, using separate clean Pasteur pipettes, with the antigen and antiserum solutions, e.g. the antiserum in the central well and the antigens in the peripheral wells, the plate is covered and placed in a damp chamber (e.g. a plastic lunch box with a piece of wet filter paper in the base). Diffusion is allowed to occur in the cold (4°C) overnight or longer if necessary. Incubation at 37°C may be used and gives more rapid but less clear cut results; however, certain labile antigens may be denatured at this temperature. The plate is examined by means of incident light using a simple arrangement consisting of a 60 watt electric light bulb with the top covered with a metal light shield, light being reflected into the gel plate from below through an aperture in the light box as shown in the diagram (Fig. 11.4). The types of precipitin bands commonly observed are shown in Figure 11.5. They take the form essentially of one of three different patterns: (1) the reaction of

identity where the lines are continuous from one well to the next; (2) the reaction of non-identity where the lines cross each other; and (3) the reaction of partial identity which is similar to (1) except for spur formation at the junction of the precipitin bands.

IMMUNOELECTROPHORESIS

Immunoelectrophoresis can be used for the identification of myeloma proteins for increase in globulin, and the changes in such diseases as virus hepatitis, cirrhosis and the reticuloses are distinct enough to suggest the appropriate diagnosis. Techniques have been developed for the simple quantitation of γ globulin in patients being treated by passive transfer of this protein (Gell, 1957). The use of immunoelectrophoresis in analysis of human pathological sera has been reviewed by Scheiffarth and Goetz (1960) and Crowle (1961) (Fig. 11.6).

A glass slide is coated with 1 per cent agar about 1 mm thick made up in either veronal buffer pH 8·6 (diethylbarbituric acid 1·38 g sodium veronal 8·76 g, calcium lactate 0·38 g, distilled water, 1 litre) or 0·02 M phosphate buffer pH 7·2. The former is the buffer commonly used in paper electrophoresis and is available commercially; the latter, however,

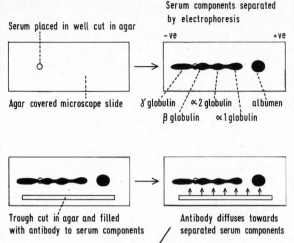

Serum placed in well cut in agar

Agar covered microscope slide

Serum components separated by electrophoresis

−ve   +ve

γ globulin   α2 globulin   albumen
β globulin   α1globulin

Trough cut in agar and filled with antibody to serum components

Antibody diffuses towards separated serum components

IgG   IgA IgM   Alb

Precipitin bands form where antibody and antigen (i.e. serum components) meet at optimal proportions. Approximately 30 components can be detected in human serum in this way. The position of the main immunoglobulins is shown.

FIG. 11.6
Immunoelectrophoresis. The antigen, for example, serum, is placed in a small well cut in a layer of agar on a microscope slide. A direct current is applied and differential migration of the serum components takes place. (They are not normally visible in the agar and will show up only if suitably stained.) After electrophoresis for an hour or so, a trough is cut longitudinally in the agar and an antiserum against the electrophoresed antigen is placed in the trough. The two components diffuse towards each other and precipitin bands form. These can be shown up more clearly by staining with a protein stain. This is a very powerful analytic technique and can show up about 30 different components in human serum compared with 4 or 5 by electrophoresis.

gives better resolution of the precipitin bands and has a more suitable pH for immunodiffusion. A pattern is made in the agar with a cutter which can be constructed by forcing two large gauge hypodermic needles (1–2 mm internal diameter) with their points sawn off through the centre area of a large cork stopper 4 cm in diameter about 7 mm apart. Between the needles are placed the two halves of a razor blade inserted into the cork so that they are parallel and separated from each other by 1 mm. The cutter is lowered onto the agar on a slide to cut the required pattern and the agar plugs are removed from the wells cut with the needles (a fine Pasteur pipette on a water pump is suitable). The agar between the two parallel cuts made by the razor blades is left *in situ* until after electrophoresis. The prepared slide is used as a bridge between the two compartments of the electrophoresis apparatus, and is connected to the buffer at each end by means of filter paper wicks. It is important that the wicks are kept damp as they tend to heat up and dry due to the passage of the current. Electrophoresis of the antigen (placed in the peripheral wells) is carried out using about 50 volts requiring approximately 2·5 ma per slide for a period (45 min–4 h) sufficient to give adequate separation of the different components of the antigen. Following this the band of agar in the trough between the two razor blade slits is removed and the antiserum run into the trough. The slide is then placed in a humid atmosphere at 4°C or 37°C to allow the development of the precipitin reaction. The preparation is examined at intervals using the viewing box depicted in Figure 11.4. Any precipitin bands formed can be recorded by drawing the pattern obtained on a piece of paper or the preparation can be photographed. Staining of the bands with a protein stain improves the clarity of the patterns and may even show up precipitin bands which cannot be seen in the unstained preparation. Such stained preparations can conveniently be dried and kept for reference. A suitable procedure for staining and drying is as follows:

1. The unprecipitated protein is washed out of the agar by immersion of the slide for 24 h in the buffer used to make up the agar solution.

2. The slide is then washed for 15 min in 1 per cent acetic acid to remove excess salts.

3. Staining is carried out with a protein stain such as naphthalene black made up to a 1 per cent solution in a solvent containing glacial acetic acid 1 ml, distilled water 49 ml, and methylated spirit 50 ml. Staining should be carried out for about 30 min with this stain.

4. Excess stain is washed out with the solvent to give a preparation with dark blue precipitin bands on a clear background.

5. The preparation is finally soaked in 1 per cent acetic acid containing 1 per cent glycerol for 15 min and dried at 37°C in an incubator.

AGGLUTINATION

In this reaction the antigen is part of the surface of some particulate material such as a red cell, bacterium or perhaps an inorganic particle (e.g. polystyrene latex) which has been coated with antigen. Antibody added to a suspension of such particles combines with the surface antigens and links them together to form clearly visible aggregates or agglutinates (Fig. 11.7). In its simplest form an agglutination test is set up in round-bottomed test-tubes or perspex plates with round-bottomed wells and doubling dilutions of the antiserum are made up in the tubes (neat, 1 in 2, 1 in 4, etc.). The particulate antigen is then added and after incubation at 37°C agglutination is seen in the bottom of the tubes. The last tube showing clearly visible agglutination is the end point of the test. The dilution of the antiserum at the end point, e.g. 256, is known as the *titre* of the antiserum and is a measure of the number of antibody units per unit volume of serum, e.g. if the end point occurs at a 256 dilution of the antiserum and if the test has been carried out in 1 ml volumes, the titre of the serum is 256 units per ml of serum. One practical difficulty of importance in agglutination tests is the occasional inhibition of agglutination in the first tubes of an anti-serum dilution series, agglutination occurring only in those tubes containing more dilute antiserum. This is known as the *prozone phenomenon* and is probably, in part, due to the stabilizing effects of high protein concentration on the particles, the protein coating the particles, increasing their net charge and so bringing about increased electrostatic repulsion between individual particles, thus opposing the efforts of the antibody molecules to link the particles together. However, once the protein concentration is reduced by dilution the antibody molecules can then exert their aggregating effect and bring about agglutination. The agglutination reaction has been shown to require the presence of electrolytes in the suspending medium and is usually performed for this reason at physiological salt concentration.

Applications

Blood specimens for agglutination tests are taken by vein puncture, so as to obtain a satisfactory amount of serum for the complete test. At least 5 ml of blood should be obtained, and the blood immediately transferred from the syringe to a dry stoppered sterile tube or screw-capped bottle and allowed to clot. When the serum has separated, it is pipetted off into a sterile tube.

One of the classical applications of the agglutination test in diagnostic bacteriology is the Widal test used for the demonstration of antibodies to salmonellae in serum specimens taken from suspected enteric fever cases (see Chap. 29). Agglutination is the basic technique used in blood grouping, the A, B or O group of the red cells under test being determined by agglutination with a specific antiserum—an anti-A serum, for example, will agglutinate A cells but not B or O cells. Red cells and inert particles such as polystyrene latex can be coated with various antigens and suitably coated particles are used in a variety of diagnostic tests such as thyroid antibody tests using

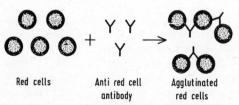

FIG. 11.7
Agglutination reaction. The IgM molecule with at least five antigen-binding sites is particularly effective in bringing about agglutination.

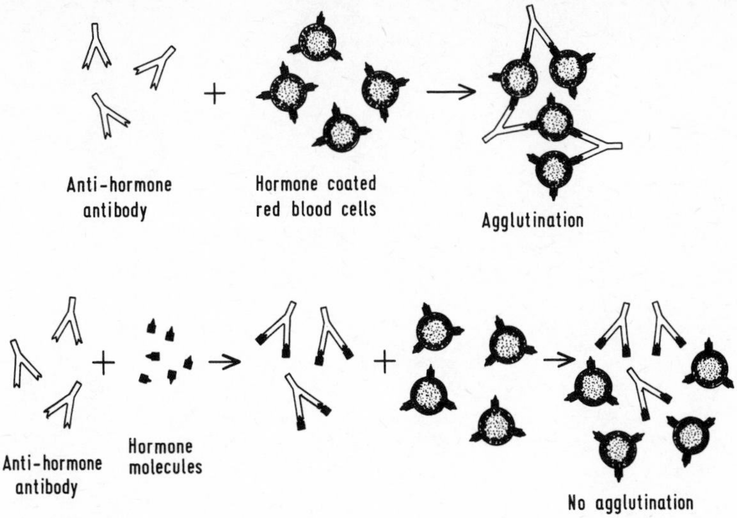

FIG. 11.8

Principle of hormone assay by agglutination inhibition. Red cells coated with hormone are agglutinable by antihormone antibody. The addition to the antiserum of a test sample containing free hormone will block the antigen-binding sites and prevent agglutination. The test can be carried out quantitatively by comparing the activity of a known standard hormone preparation with the test sample.

thyroglobulin-coated cells or latex particles. Hormone-coated red cells or inert particles are used in many hormone assay procedures which are based on the inhibition of the antibody-induced agglutination of the hormone-coated particles by hormone added in the sample under test (Fig. 11.8). Tests of this type are in wide use in pregnancy diagnosis.

Certain viruses, e.g. the orthomyxo and paramyxo viruses causing influenza and mumps, have the property of bringing about agglutination of red cells (haemagglutination). Inhibition of haemagglutination by antibody in patients' serum is a widely-used diagnostic procedure. The presence of antibody in the patient's serum is thus detected by its ability to link with virus particles and prevent them from bringing about agglutination of the red cells (Fig. 11.9).

IgM antibodies capable of agglutinating human red cells (including those of the individual producing the antibody) between 0 and 4°C are sometimes found in certain human diseases including primary atypical pneumonia, malaria, trypanosomiasis and acquired haemolytic anaemia.

The presence of antibody globulin on a red cell may not result in direct agglutination of the cells, for example in some Rh-negative mothers

with Rh-positive infants or in acquired haemolytic anaemia. It is, however, possible to show that the red cells are coated with antibody by using an antiglobulin serum (produced in the rabbit by injecting human globulin) which will bring about agglutination of the cells. This is the basis of the Coombs test which is a very widely used serological procedure (Fig. 11.10).

SLIDE AGGLUTINATION

This method is useful where only small quantities of culture are available, as in the identification of the whooping-cough bacillus, or where agglutination is carried out with undiluted serum, e.g. in typing pneumococci or typing streptococci by Griffith's method, and it is necessary to use as small a quantity as possible. The method may be applied likewise for identifying organisms of the *Salmonella* and dysentery groups. Slide agglutination is only practicable when the clumping of organisms occurs within a minute or so; it is not suitable where the mixture of organisms and serum has to be incubated.

The procedure can be carried out quite readily on an ordinary slide, but where a

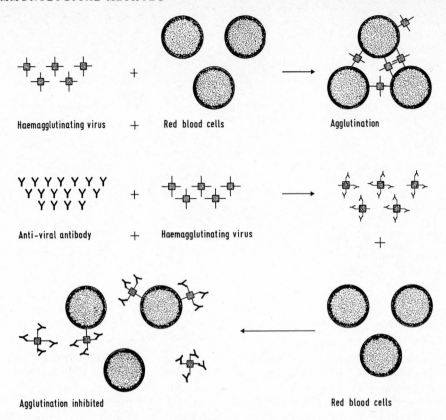

Haemagglutinating virus   +   Red blood cells   →   Agglutination

Anti-viral antibody   +   Haemagglutinating virus

Agglutination inhibited   Red blood cells

FIG. 11.9

Virus haemagglutination inhibition test. Red cell agglutination is brought about by a variety of viruses (see text). This can be inhibited by mixing the virus with anti-viral antibody as shown in the diagram. The test can be quantitated by comparison of serial dilutions of virus alone and virus-antibody mixture (Clarke and Casals, 1958).

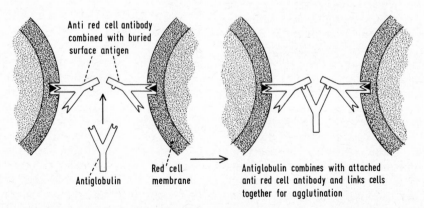

Anti red cell antibody combined with buried surface antigen

Antiglobulin

Red cell membrane

Antiglobulin combines with attached anti red cell antibody and links cells together for agglutination

FIG. 11.10

Coombs antiglobulin test. The red cell antibody, probably because it is directed against an antigen situated deep in the cell wall, cannot link two red cells together for agglutination. The addition of an antiglobulin serum brings about agglutination by linking two attached immunoglobulins to one another.

number of agglutination tests have to be made it is more convenient to use a piece of $\frac{1}{4}$-in polished plate glass about 6 in × 2 in. A long horizontal line is ruled with a grease pencil through the middle of the glass from end to end and then a number of lines are ruled at $\frac{1}{2}$-in intervals at right angles to this line, thereby dividing the glass into a series of divisions.

A drop of saline is placed in one of the divisions and a small amount of culture from a solid medium emulsified in it by means of an inoculating loop. It is then examined through a hand-lens (8 or 10×), or the low-power microscope, to ascertain that the suspension is even and that the bacteria are well separated and not in visible clumps. With a small loop, $1\frac{1}{2}$ mm diameter, made from thin platinum wire take up a drop of the serum and place it on the slide just beside the bacterial suspension. Mix the serum and bacterial suspension and examine with the hand lens, or place on the stage of the microscope. Agglutination when it occurs is rapid and the clumps can be seen with the naked eye, but the use of some form of magnification is an advantage. For control purposes, two drops of saline can be placed in adjacent divisions and bacterial culture emulsified in both, one only being mixed with the serum. With streptococci a broth culture is used, and methods for obtaining suitable suspensions for the agglutination test are described in Chapter 19. Two drops of suspension are placed on the side and a small loopful of the serum mixed with one of them and examined as described above.

While the slide agglutination test is rapid and convenient, its limitations must be realized. In order to obtain rapid agglutination the serum is used undiluted or in low dilutions. In consequence, it may contain normal agglutinins which give non-specific agglutination with organisms other than that against which the serum was prepared. Thus, with regard to the *Salmonella* group particularly, slide agglutination with its high concentration of agglutinins may show low-titre reactions with organisms outside the group, e.g. '*paracolon bacilli*' which may also have somewhat similar biochemical reactions. It is important therefore to confirm the slide test by quantitative tests in tubes, particularly when any doubt arises or where

precise results from agglutination tests are desired.

AGGLUTININ-ABSORPTION TESTS

Agglutinins, like other antibodies, combine firmly with their homologous antigens, and by treating an agglutinating antiserum with the homologous bacteria and then separating the organisms by centrifuging, it is found that the agglutinin has been 'absorbed' or removed by the organisms from the serum.

In certain cases, to prove the serological identity of an unknown strain with a particular species, it may be necessary to show not only that it is agglutinated by a specific antiserum to approximately its titre but also that it can absorb from the serum the agglutinins for the known organism. This becomes necessary owing to the fact that, on immunizing an animal with a particular bacterium, 'group antibodies' for allied organisms are developed, and in some cases these may act in relatively high titre. 'Absorption' with a heterologous strain would remove only the group agglutinins without affecting the specific agglutinin. These effects are exemplified in the *Salmonella* and *Brucella* groups. The general method of carrying out such absorption tests is to mix a dense suspension of the organism—e.g. 24 hours' growth on a 4-in plate of nutrient agar, suspended in 1 ml saline and killed at 60°C (30 min) —with an equal volume of a suitable dilution of the serum, e.g. 64 times the concentration of the known titre. (The bacterial growth must have been thoroughly washed with normal salt solution, i.e. by mixing with several volumes of saline, centrifuging and repeating the process 2—3 times). Thus, if the titre is 1600, the dilution used would be 1 in 25. The mixture is incubated for three to four h at 37°C and the serum is then separated from the bacteria in a high-speed centrifuge. (In some cases for complete absorption the process may require to be repeated with a similar fresh quantity of bacteria.) The dilution of the serum would now be approximately double the original dilution— in the example taken (see above) 1 in 50. From the treated serum a series of doubling dilutions is prepared as in direct agglutination tests, so that, when an equal volume of bacterial suspension is added, the series will reach to the known titre of the serum. In the example taken above, the following series of dilutions would be tested:

1 in 50   1 in 100   1 in 200   1 in 400   1 in 800,

and after the addition of bacterial suspension these would become:

1 in 100   1 in 200   1 in 400   1 in 800   1 in 1600

A control tube is also included, containing suspension but no serum, and the general technique is that employed in direct agglutination tests.

Thus, the identity or non-identity of an unknown culture (X) with a known (A) may be investigated by agglutinin-absorption as follows:

1. Absorb, as above, antiserum to A with a dense suspension of organism $X = X$-absorbed serum.

2. Test the agglutinating power of X-absorbed serum for A and X.

(A control test would show that the antiserum to A after absorption with A agglutinates neither organism.)

Results

(*a*) The absorbed serum agglutinates neither A nor X. This indicates that the organisms are identical, because X has absorbed agglutinins for A; to establish this conclusion completely an antiserum to X after absorption with A should agglutinate neither organism.

(*b*) The absorbed serum fails to agglutinate X, but still agglutinates A. This shows that the organisms are not identical, because X has not absorbed the agglutinins for A, though it has removed the heterologous agglutinins.

Some Common Diagnostic Applications of Agglutination Tests

The agglutination test already referred to for the sero-diagnosis of salmonella infections is known as the Widal test. It is usual to test dilutions of the patient's serum against standard suspensions of somatic (O) antigen and flagellar (H) antigen of each organism likely to be encountered in the patient's environment.

The test usually becomes positive with both suspensions, a week after the onset of the illness but may be weakly positive with one of the antigens even earlier. The titre in an acute infection rises to a maximum by the end of the third week. Complications in interpretation of the results may arise in patients who have been immunized with typhoid-paratyphoid vaccine (TAB). A rising titre may be of some help in diagnosing an infection; furthermore some months after immunization the titre of O agglutinins tends to fall off leaving only H agglutinins. Normal sera sometimes have low titres of agglutinins for salmonella organisms and this varies in populations in different parts of the world. Again the importance of a rising titre becomes a significant factor.

Another widely used agglutination test is the Paul-Bunnell reaction. This is used for the diagnosis of infectious mononucleosis in which agglutinins develop for sheep erythrocytes. Normal serum may agglutinate sheep cells in low dilutions and a titre of 128 is taken as suggestive and 256 as positive for the test. In some individuals who have received horse serum as a therapeutic agent (e.g. antitetanus serum) agglutinins develop for sheep cells because of the presence in the horse serum of an antigen very widespread in nature, known as the Forssman antigen. This antigen is present in the red cells of sheep and the cells of a number of other species, including the guinea-pig. The usual way of differentiating the two types of antibody is to mix the serum with minced guinea-pig tissue (usually kidney). This treatment will absorb out the anti-Forssman antibody leaving the anti-sheep cell antibody unaffected. Ox red cells which contain both the Forssman antigen and an antigen similar to that on sheep cells, which reacts with the Paul-Bunnell antibody, will absorb out both types of antibody.

An agglutination test is widely used for the the diagnosis of rheumatoid arthritis; the sera of 70–80 per cent of patients with this disease contain an IgM antibody which is able to combine with the IgG globulin from various species. Detection of the antibody depends on the agglutination of sheep red cells or inert particles (polystyrene latex) coated with IgG globulin. Sheep red cells for example may be coated with specific rabbit antibody and will then be agglutinated by the IgM antibody in the rheumatoid patient's serum. The antibody is known as rheumatoid factor. Occasional low titres (less than 16 are found in normal sera, 2–5 per cent) and the test is not entirely specific for rheumatoid arthritis.

THE PAUL-BUNNELL REACTION

During and after an attack of infectious mononucleosis there is present in the serum a non-specific agglutinin that is of diagnostic significance. These Paul-Bunnell antibodies agglutinate the red blood cells of sheep, horses and oxen, but not of men. They are known to be IgM globulins.

SLIDE SCREENING TEST. Fresh horse blood is used and the erythrocytes are washed five times in the centrifuge; 25 ml of the packed cells are then suspended in 175 ml of iso-osmotic phosphate buffer pH 7·2 and formalized by the technique described by Dacie and Lewis (1968). The cells are then made up in a 25–50 per cent suspension which can be stored for up to six months at 4°C. For use, this suspension is diluted to 4 per cent in saline. Formalized cells of this type can be purchased commercially.

The test is carried out by placing one drop of patient's serum on a glass slide with one drop of the horse red blood cell suspension. After thorough mixing and rotation, naked-eye agglutination is looked for after two minutes with oblique illumination. Positive and negative control sera as well as saline must be included in these tests. A kit containing all the necessary reagents and full instructions is conveniently supplied for 'the Monospot' slide test for infectious mononucleosis by Ortho-Diagnostic through Stayne Laboratories.

THE FULL TEST. Heat the serum at 55°C for 20 min. Make a series of doubling dilutions of the serum with saline in 0·5 ml amounts in 3-in $\times \frac{1}{2}$-in tubes, ranging from 1 in 16 to 1 in 1024. A control tube containing only saline is included. Add to each tube 0·5 ml of a 1 per cent suspension of sheep red corpuscles in saline, washed as for the Wassermann test. Shake the tubes thoroughly and incubate at 37°C for 4 h. Note which tubes show agglutination of the red cells, and state the titre of the reaction in terms of the final dilution of the serum: 1st tube, 1 in 32; 2nd, 1 in 64; etc. Normal serum may agglutinate in low dilutions. A suggestive titre is 128. Repeated tests may reveal a rising titre. A significant titre is 256.

If a second reading of results is made after the tubes have stood overnight at room temperature or in the refrigerator, they should be replaced in the incubator at 37°C for 1 or 2 h. This avoids fallacious results from 'cold agglutination' which is reversible at 37°C and, so far as is known, is not associated with infectious mononucleosis.

It should be noted that the reaction is negative in tuberculosis, leukaemia and Hodgkin's disease.

In persons who have recently received an injection of a therapeutic serum (from the horse), an apparently similar heterophile antibody (Forssman's antibody) may be present in considerable amount in the blood, since horse serum contains the appropriate heterophile antigen and stimulates the production of an antibody for sheep red cells. However, the type of antibody present in infectious mononucleosis differs in certain respects from the Forssman antibody, and also from that found in normal serum, and this difference can be determined by agglutinin-absorption tests as shown in Table 11.1.

Table 11.1

Antibody	Treated with emulsion of guinea-pig kidney	Treated with ox red cells
Normal serum	Absorbed	Not absorbed
After serum therapy	Absorbed	Absorbed
Infective mononucleosis	Not absorbed	Absorbed

It may be found, however, that the antibody present after serum therapy is not absorbed by ox red cells and only partially absorbed by guinea-pig kidney tissue, i.e. more closely resembles the antibody in normal serum.

PAUL-BUNNELL TEST WITH DIFFERENTIAL ABSORPTION. The following method, a modification of Barrett's (1941) technique, may be adopted for determining these absorption effects.

Reagents

1. *Patient's serum* 1·0 ml is required. Heat the serum in a water-bath at 56°C for 30 min.

2. *Physiological saline* (0·9 per cent NaCl).

3. 20 *per cent guinea-pig kidney emulsion in saline*. Take several fresh guinea-pig kidneys and, after removing any fat, cut into small pieces with scissors. Wash several times with saline to remove all the blood, and mash the tissue into a fine pulp in a blender for 2 min. Autoclave for 20 min at 121°C and blend once again to obtain a fine suspension. Next deposit the kidney fragments by centrifugation and wash in two changes of saline. The deposit is now resuspended to about four times its volume in 0·5 per cent phenol saline. Next estimate the concentration of kidney tissue in the suspension by centrifugation in a haematocrit tube. Then add sufficient phenol saline to give a 1 in 6 suspension. The absorbing power of the antigen must be tested against known positive and negative sera. This reagent is used without further dilution and is stable for about a year at 4°C.

4. 20 *per cent ox red cell suspension in saline*. Make a 20 per cent suspension of washed ox cells in saline and treat in exactly the same way as the 20 per cent guinea-pig kidney emulsion described above. This antigen keeps well at 4°C.

5. 2 *per cent suspension of sheep red cells*. Wash the sheep cells in saline and make a 2 per cent suspension in saline. The cells should be more than one day and less than seven days old. Formalinized sheep cells preferably not more than seven days old may be used.

The Test

Use 3-in $\times \frac{3}{8}$-in test-tubes.

In three separate test-tubes, (a), (b) and (c) place:

(a) 1·0 ml saline.

(b) 1·25 ml* of guinea-pig kidney emulsion.

(c) 1·25 ml* of ox cell suspension.

To each tube add 0·25 ml of heated serum. Allow to stand for two hours or overnight at 4°C, and then centrifuge tubes (b) and (c).

Set up a rack containing three rows of 10 tubes. Into the last 9 of each row put 0·25 ml saline. Into the first two tubes of the front row place 0·25 ml of the diluted serum (a). From the mixture in the second tube carry over 0·25 ml to the third tube, and continue doubling dilutions to the end of the row. Repeat this process using the supernatant fluid from (b) and (c) in the middle and back rows respectively.

To every tube add 0·1 ml of the 2 per cent suspension of sheep cells and mix thoroughly by shaking.

The final serum dilutions are 1 in 7, 1 in 14, 1 in 28, 1 in 56, etc.

The test is read, after the tubes have stood for 24 h at room temperature, by removing the tubes from the rack and attempting to resuspend the cells by flicking the tubes with the finger. The end-point is the highest dilution of serum in which the cells cannot be evenly suspended. The end-point can be made more clear-cut if the tubes are centrifuged for 2 min before resuspension of the cells is attempted.

A preliminary report can be made after the test has been set up for an hour, if the tubes are centrifuged before making the reading, but a final report should be postponed until the following day.

A typical report in a case of glandular fever would be:

Heterophile agglutinin for sheep cells present in dilutions up to 1 in 448. The agglutinin is completely absorbed by ox cell suspension, but unaffected by guinea-pig kidney emulsion.

With the absorption technique, as detailed above, even a titre of 28 in rows (a) and (b) is significant.

---

* The extra quantity of material in these tubes is because 1·25 ml of a 20 per cent emulsion or suspension contains only 1·0 ml of fluid.

STREPTOCOCCUS MG AGGLUTINATION TEST

Reagents

1. *Patient's serum.* 1·0 ml is required. Two samples of serum should be tested: the first taken during the acute phase of the illness and the second after an interval of 12–18 days.

Note. The sera must not be inactivated at 56°C as this lowers the titre.

2. *Streptococcus 'MG' Suspension.* Remove the growth from a 48 h digest broth culture of the organism by centrifugation and wash it three times with sterile saline. Kill the suspension by heating in a water-bath at 100°C for 30 min. After one further washing with saline make the suspension up to a standard density (Brown's opacity tube No. 5, see Chap. 13) and add merthiolate 1 in 10 000 as a preservative.

3. *Standard positive rabbit antiserum.*

4. *Physiological saline.*

The test. Use $3 \times \frac{1}{2}$ in tubes: Set up a rack containing 7 tubes. In the first tube place 0·8 ml saline and 0·5 ml in the remaining tubes. Add 0·2 ml serum to the first tube, mix thoroughly and transfer 0·5 ml of the mixture to the second tube and continue preparing doubling dilutions to the end of the row. Include a control tube containing 0·5 ml saline only. To each tube add 0·5 ml Streptococcus MG suspension. Final serum dilutions are 1 in 10, 1 in 20, 1 in 40, 1 in 80, 1 in 160, 1 in 320, and 1 in 640.

With each batch of tests a titration of the positive rabbit serum should be included.

The tubes are incubated overnight in the water-bath at 37°C.

A rising titre between acute and convalescent sera (at least four-fold) is regarded as significant. A titre of 20 or over is regarded by some workers as suggestive.

Sera should not be screened by using a single low dilution tube method as a *prozone* is frequently observed.

'COLD AGGLUTINATION' REACTION

It has been shown that in cases of primary atypical pneumonia the serum may agglutinate at low temperatures human erythrocytes of the blood group O. This reaction is absent in other types of pneumonia, other infections of the respiratory passages and normal individuals,

and has been suggested as a means of confirming a diagnosis of atypical pneumonia. The reaction, however, tends to be late in its appearance during the illness. The test can be carried out quantitatively by preparing a series of nine doubling dilutions of serum from 1 in 8 to 1 in 2048 and adding to each an equal volume of 0·2 per cent suspension of washed group O human red cells. The mixtures are placed in a refrigerator at 0°–4°C overnight after which readings of agglutination are made by shaking the tubes and observing clumped cells with the naked eye. As the agglutinin is readily absorbed by erythrocytes at low temperature, the serum should be separated from the blood specimen at a temperature above 20°C. A titre of 32 or 64 (in terms of the final dilution of serum after addition of red cells) may be considered significant, but much higher titres have been recorded.

A high proportion of the cases of primary atypical pneumonia (85–90 per cent) that have positive cold agglutination reactions are associated with infection with *Mycoplasma pneumoniae*, see Vol. I, Chapter 52.

COATED-PARTICLE AGGLUTINATION REACTIONS

The inert particles of polystyrene latex, collodion and bentonite, and red cells both treated with tannic acid and untreated, can be coated with a variety of protein antigens and also in the case of untreated red cells, with polysaccharide antigens. They can then be used for the detection of antibody as shown by the agglutination of the coated particles. The haemagglutination tests are the most sensitive and can detect as little as $0·003 \mu g$ of antibody measured as antibody nitrogen, which is about 10 times more sensitive than the most sensitive gel diffusion techniques.

The value of these tests has increased considerably with the development of techniques for storing antigen-coated red cell preparations. A large batch of cells can be coated with antigen and a standardized preparation is then available for use for some months afterwards. Of the various methods available probably the most useful is that described by Csizmas (1960) in which the cells are formalinized by placing a dialysis bag of formalin into a beaker of carefully washed cells. After recovery from the formalin, the cells can be stored in the refrigerator and after tanning and coating with the antigen, they may be stored at $-20°C$. These techniques have the advantage that in common with other agglutination reactions they can be used as antibody titration methods. A large variety of antigens can be adsorbed on to cells or particles, and even two different antigens have been applied to the same red cells (Lecocq and Linz, 1962) or latex particles (Singer et al., 1961). The methods are simple to use and once a particular test is standardized reproducible results can be obtained.

Tanned Red Cell Agglutination Tests

The surfaces of red blood cells are altered and the cells rendered much more agglutinable by treatment with tannic acid. This enables cells coated with various antigens—proteins and viruses—to be agglutinated by specific antibody. The method here described employs thyroglobulin but this could be replaced by any one of a large number of antigens. (For detailed consideration of the application of the test to the detection of thyroglobulin autoantibodies see Fulthorpe et al., 1961.)

Reagents

1. Phosphate buffered saline 0.15 M KH_2PO_4, 0.15 M Na_2HPO_4 mixed in suitable proportions (see Chap. 4) to give the pH required— e.g. pH 7.2 for the thyroglobulin antibody test. One volume of this buffer is added to 9 volumes of 0.85 per cent NaCl.

2. Tannic acid solution, 1 in 20 000 made up fresh before use (12.5 mg of analytical grade tannic acid dissolved in 250 ml of the buffer).

3. Defibrinated sheep blood not more than 1–2 days old.

4. Antigen at a concentration of 2 mg/ml in the buffered saline e.g. human, thyroglobulin prepared by the method of Derrien, Michel and Roche (1948).

5. 0.85 per cent NaCl.

6. Rabbit or horse serum which has been inactivated for 30 min at $56°C$ and absorbed for 10 min at room temperature with washed sheep red blood cells (approx. 0.1 ml of packed cells to 10 ml of serum).

Method

1. Wash about 20 ml of the sheep blood three times (twice with 0.85 per cent NaCl and once with the phosphate buffered saline) in a one-ounce universal container. Centrifuge finally at 750 g for 15 min to pack the cells.

2. Pipette 0.6 ml of the packed cells into each of two universal containers and add 10 ml of buffered saline to each bottle to resuspend the cells.

3. Add 10 ml of the 1 in 20 000 tannic acid solution to each container, shake and incubate for 15 min at $37°C$.

4. Centrifuge the bottles at 750 g for 5 min and discard the supernatant, resuspend cells in each container in 20 ml of buffer, centrifuge for a similar period and discard the supernatant.

5. Lay one container of cells aside; this will be used as the source of uncoated cells for absorbing the heterophile agglutinins in the sera to be tested, and for various controls.

6. Resuspend the cells in the other container in 10 ml of buffer and then add 10 ml of buffer containing the antigen to be coated on to the cells. Incubate for 30 min at $37°C$ shaking occasionally.

7. Centrifuge the coated cells for 5 min at 750 g and remove the supernatant.

8. Wash these cells and the cells set aside (5) three times with the buffered saline made up to contain 1 per cent normal rabbit or horse serum (previously inactivated and absorbed), centrifuge for 5 min at 750 g, on each occasion and discard the supernatant. (Make sure each bottle is correctly labelled.)

9. Finally make up both batches of cells, i.e. the coated and the uncoated, to 50 ml with the buffer to which has been added the 1 per cent serum as in (8).

The test

1. Inactivate the test sera for 30 min at $56°C$ (not necessary for formalinized cells, see above).

2. Add 0.1 ml of inactivated serum to 0.9 ml of the uncoated cell preparation, leave on bench for 15 min and centrifuge for 5 min at 750 g to recover the serum—which is now diluted 1 in 10.

3. Make 8 or more doubling or trebling dilutions of the serum in the buffered saline in 0.1 ml volumes using a WHO plate. Add 0.1 ml of the 1 per cent coated cells to each well and to

a control well containing 0·1 ml of buffer only. Set up controls using uncoated cells with and without serum.

Read first for agglutination after 2 h on the bench (20°C) and after leaving overnight at 4°C. The end point is taken as the last cup showing a smooth mat of agglutinated cells with a crenated rim. Doubtful results appear as a smaller circle of cells having a dark outer rim and a negative result shows as a closely packed button of cells. The controls should always be negative.

Formalinization of Red Cells (prior to tanning and coating)

Mammalian or avian red blood cells can conveniently be preserved by the method of Csizmas (1960). The treated cells are morphologically identical to normal red cells and withstand treatment with water or freezing and thawing. They may even be freeze dried without damage. They retain most of the surface properties of fresh red cells and can be tanned and coated with antigens or agglutinated by viruses.

Method

1. Fresh (sheep) blood is washed five times with 0·85 per cent saline and the cells packed after the final wash (for 15 min at 750 g). (It is important to avoid any lysis).

2. 25 ml of packed cells are resuspended to 200 ml in phosphate buffered saline pH 7·2 and placed in a 500 ml conical flask.

3. 50 ml of formalin (40 per cent formaldehyde) is introduced into a length of dialysis tubing and tied off so that the tubing is only $\frac{2}{3}$ full, but air is excluded, i.e. the knot is tied in the tubing which has not been distended with air one third of the total length of the tubing above the top of the formalin.

4. The two-thirds filled dialysis tube is submerged in the cell suspension in the conical flask, stoppered, and the whole *gently* agitated for 3–4 h at room temperature (20°C). Gross foaming should be avoided (a Matburn blood cell suspension mixer with a wire mesh glassware crate attached is a suitable arrangement).

5. After 3–4 h the swollen dialysis sac is punctured, the formalin allowed to mix directly with the cells and the empty sac removed. Gentle mixing is continued overnight.

6. At the end of this period the dark brown cell suspension is carefully decanted from the flask into centrifuge bottles, leaving the surface scum of froth and damaged cells behind (the cells may be filtered through gauze to achieve this). The cells are then washed 5 times with 0·9 per cent saline to remove the formalin (for 10 min at 750 g). Gentle stirring of the deposit with a glass rod helps to ensure adequate resuspension at each wash.

7. The cells are finally made up to a 25 or a 50 per cent suspension in 0·85 per cent saline and stored at 4°C or at −20°C to be made up to a 1 per cent suspension before use.

The supernatant from the first wash after formalinization is normally very dark.

LATEX FIXATION TEST FOR RHEUMATOID FACTOR

The following is a simplification of the method of Singer and Plotz (1956).

Reagents

1. Polystyrene latex uniform sized particles 0·81 μm in diameter (Difco Bacto-latex). Add 20 ml of distilled water to 2 ml of the latex suspension and filter through Whatman 40 filter paper (the suspension will keep for months at 4°C).

2. Borate buffer pH 8·2 (see page 89).

3. Stock gamma-globulin solution—0·5 per cent in borate buffer. To 0·1 g of lyophilised human fraction II gamma-globulin add borate buffer in small increments, mixing well until 20 ml has been added and the gamma-globulin completely dissolved. This preparation will keep for several weeks at 4°C.

The Test. (Bywaters and Scott, 1960).

1. Add 1 ml of the borate buffer to a series of $3 \times \frac{1}{2}$ tubes, include one tube for each test serum and one for a positive control and another for a control with buffer only.

2. Inactivate the sera for 30 min at 56°C and add 0·05 ml of serum to each tube (i.e. a dilution of 1 in 21 of the serum).

3. To each serum dilution and to the controls add 1 ml of a mixture containing 1 per cent

stock latex and 5 per cent stock gamma globulin in borate buffer (for 10 ml add 0·1 ml of stock latex and 0·5 ml of stock gamma-globulin to 9·5 ml of buffer).

4. Shake the tubes carefully and incubate in a 56°C water bath for 2 h.

5. Prior to reading the tests centrifuge for 3 min at 1000 g.

Readings

Opaque suspension, no deposit, −ve.

Opaque suspension, minimal deposit, ± doubtful.

Partially cleared suspension, granular deposit, +.

Clear or almost clear supernatant, granular deposit, + +.

A reading of + or + + is regarded as positive, ± is of doubtful significance.

HAEMAGGLUTINATION AND HAEMAGGLUTINATION INHIBITION TEST

Apparatus (Sever, 1962)

1. Permanent lucite 'U' or 'V' plates or disposable (Rigid Styrene) 'U' or 'V' plates.
2. Microtitre droppers 0·025 ml.
3. Microtitre diluters 0·025 ml.

Reagents

1. Complement fixation test diluent is suitable for influenza as it contains Ca^{2+} and Mg^{2+} ions.
2. Viral antigen.
3. Serum heated to 56°C for 30 min and suitably treated to remove non-specific inhibitors (see below).
4. Red cells of the optimum species and concentration.

Titration of Virus

1. Place one drop of buffer in each of, say, 10 wells of the microtitre plate and in one more well to act as a cell control.
2. Place one drop of virus in first well giving a 1 in 2 dilution and using a micro-diluter prepare doubling dilutions of the virus discarding the last 0·025 ml.
3. Add one drop of red cells to each well including the cell control.

4. Incubate at the appropriate temperature till the control cells have settled to a discrete button.

5. Read the titre of the virus as the highest dilution that gives haemagglutination (1 HAU).

Haemagglutination Inhibition Test (Table 11.2)

1. Place one drop of buffer in the second and each of the remaining, say, 10 wells for the serum dilutions and to the control wells.
2. Place one drop of serum dilution in 1st and 2nd well and in serum control well.
3. Make doubling dilutions of the serum using a microdiluter.
4. Add one drop 4 HAU virus to each of the test wells and to one of the antigen control wells. Add 2, 1 and $\frac{1}{2}$ HAU to the other three antigen control wells.
5. Incubate to allow serum and virus to interact for 1 h at room temperature.
6. Add one volume of red cells to each well, the test, and the serum and the four antigen controls, as well as the cell control.
7. Incubate as when titrating the virus.
8. Read the result, when the cell and serum controls are discrete buttons and the virus controls show a diminishing amount of haemagglutination. The limiting dilution of antibody is that which causes *complete* inhibition of haemagglutination and is the titre of the serum.

Removal of Non-Specific Inhibitors from Serum

Heat. By holding the sera at 56°C for 30 min the Chu inhibitors are destroyed.

Receptor Destroying Enzyme (RDE) obtainable from Wellcome Reagents Ltd. removes the Francis' inhibitor or mucoid inhibitor. Mix 4 parts of RDE with 1 part serum. Incubate overnight at 37°C and follow by incubation for 1 h at 56°C to destroy any remaining RDE. The serum has been diluted 1 in 5. This method depends on the potency of the RDE so if it was not purchased commercially, it needs to be standardized by titration against normal rabbit serum.

Trypsin and periodate will also remove the Francis' inhibitor or mucoid inhibitors.

Reagents: Trypsin 1:250 dissolved in M/10

Table 11.2 Conditions for the Haemagglutination Inhibition Test

Virus	Optimal type of red cell and concentration	pH	Temperature of incubation	Time of incubation (for reaction of virus and serum)	Diluent	Treatment of serum to remove non-specific inhibitors
Adenovirus	Monkey, rat 0·75% stabilized with rabbit serum	7·2	37°C	1 h	Saline	Kaolin and red cells
Arbovirus	Goose 0·3%	5·7–7·4	4°C	Overnight	Borate saline solution pH8–9, according to virus strain	Kaolin pH9 and red cells
Enteroviruses	Human 'O'	5·8 or 7·4	4°C or 37°C		PBS	Kaolin. Animal sera have to be absorbed with red cells
Influenza A (in O phase)	Human 'O' Guinea pig 0·5%	7·2	22°C	30 min–1 h	PBS	
(in D phase)	Fowl 0·5%	7·2	22°C	30 min–1 h	PBS	Heat, RDE or trypsin/periodate
Influenza B	Human 'O' Guinea pig Fowl	7·2	22°C	30 min–1 h	PBS	
Influenza C	Human 'O' Guinea pig Fowl	7·2	0–4°C	30 min–1 h	PBS	
Measles	Monkey 0·5%	7·2	37°C	30 min–1 h	PBS	Heat. Absorb with monkey red cells overnight at 4°C
Mumps and NDV	Chicken Human 'O' Guinea pig. 1·0%	7·2	4°C or 22°C	30 min–1 h	PBS	As influenza A
Reovirus	Human 'O' Day-old chick cells 0·25%	7·2 / 7·3	22°C / RT	1 h / 1 h	Saline / DGV	Kaolin / Kaolin
Rubella	Pigeon 0·25%	6·2	RT	1 h	HSAG	Heparin $MnCl_2$

phosphate buffer pH 8·2 at a concentration of 4 μg/ml. This solution should be clear and requires prolonged shaking; M/90 potassium periodate.

1. Mix 1 vol serum and 1 vol trypsin.

2. Place immediately for 30 min in 56°C water-bath.

3. Cool to room temperature.

4. Add 3 volumes of M/90 potassium periodate.

5. Incubate for at least 15 min.

6. Add 3 vol of 1 per cent glycerol-saline solution. This gives a 1 in 8 dilution of the serum.

Kaolin for removal of non-specific inhibitors for rubella.

Reagents: Physiological saline, 25 per cent acid washed Kaolin.

1. Make a 1 in 5 dilution of serum in saline.

2. Add an equal volume of washed Kaolin; the serum is now diluted 1 in 10.

3. Allow to stand 20 min at room temperature.

4. Deposit the Kaolin by centrifugation.

Red blood cells of the appropriate species.

Reagent: Packed erythrocytes.

1. Add 0·1 ml packed cells to 1·0 ml 1 in 10 dilution of serum.

2. Incubate for 1 h at 4°C.

3. Remove the red cells by centrifugation at 4°C.

4. Test the serum for residual agglutinins at 37°C.

5. If any remain repeat steps 1 to 4.

Heparin MnCl$_2$ for absorbing non-specific inhibitors for the rubella virus.

Reagents: Sodium Heparin—5000 iu/ml; MnCl$_2$4H$_2$O—prepare 1 molar MnCl$_2$ stock solution.

1. Sterilize M MnCl$_2$4H$_2$O solution by filtration through a millipore membrane, 0·22 μm pore size.

2. Add equal parts heparin and 1·0 M MnCl$_2$.

3. Store at 4°C (can be used for up to two weeks).

4. Add to 0·3 ml HSAG diluent, 0·2 ml serum.

5. Add 0·2 ml of Heparin-MnCl$_2$ and mix gently.

6. Hold for 15 min at 4°C.

7. Add 0·4 ml of 50 per cent red cells and shake gently to mix.

8. Add 0·7 ml HSAG diluent to tube and mix gently.

9. Centrifuge for 20 min at 4°C at 900 g.

10. Recover supernate—final dilution of serum is 1 in 8.

HSAG Diluent

A. HEPES saline ($\times$ 5 concentrated solution)

HEPES	29·8 g
NaCl	40·95 g
CaCl$_2$2H$_2$O	0·74 g
Distilled water to	1000 ml

Dissolve in approximately 900 ml distilled water. Adjust the pH to 6·5 by adding 1N NaOH. Add distilled water to 1000 ml. Sterilize by filtration through a 0·22 μm membrane and store at 4°C in convenient amounts.

B. Bovine Serum Albumin ($\times$ 2 concentrated solution)

Bovine albumin powder	20 g
Distilled water to	1000 ml

Dissolve albumin; sterilize and store as above.

C. Gelatin ($\times$ 10 concentrated solution)

Gelatin	0·025 g
Distilled water to	1000 ml

Dissolve gelatin and sterilize by autoclaving for 15 min at 121°C. Store at 4°C in convenient amounts.

To make 1000 ml of complete HSAG diluent combine:

200 ml of solution A
500 ml of solution B
100 ml of solution C
200 ml of sterile distilled water.

At 25°C the pH of the HSAG diluent should be 6·2. Store at 4°C for up to 2 months if kept sterile.

Dextrose-Gelatin-Veronal Buffer (DGV)

As used in the rubella haemagglutination inhibition test.

Veronal (barbitone, diethylbarbituric acid)	0·58 g
Gelatin	0·60 g

Dissolve veronal and gelatin in 125 ml RP water by gentle heating.

Sodium veronal (sod. barbitone,		
sod. barbiturate)	. . .	0·38 g
Calcium chloride (anhydrous)	.	0·02 g
Magnesium sulphate .	. .	0·12 g
Sodium chloride	. . .	8·5 g
Dextrose .	. . .	10·0 g
RP water .	. . .	875 ml

Combine with veronal/gelatin. Sterilize by autoclaving at 115°C for 10 min (pH 7·3).

COMPLEMENT FIXATION

The fact that antibody, once it combines with antigen, is able to activate the complement system is used as a way of showing the presence of a particular antibody in a serum, e.g. the Wassermann antibody in syphilis (Price, 1949; 1950a,b) or in the identification of viral antigens.

The complement system consists of a group of at least nine serum factors of globulin nature present in the serum of normal individuals. The complement of most species will react with antibody derived from other species and guinea-pig serum is a common laboratory source of complement—some of the components of complement are heat labile and are destroyed by heating at 56°C for 20–30 minutes. The individual components of the complement system are taken up by the antigen-antibody complex in a particular order and destruction of the heat-labile components which are taken up early prevents the remaining components from taking part.

For most antigens the reaction of the complement system with the antigen-antibody complex causes in itself no visible effect and it is necessary to use an indicator system consisting of sheep red cells coated with anti-sheep red cell antibody. Complement has the ability to lyse the antibody-coated cells, probably by virtue of the esterase activity of one of the components acting on the red cell membrane. In a test the antibody, complement and antigen are first mixed together and after a period of incubation the indicator system, antibody-coated sheep cells, is added. The complement

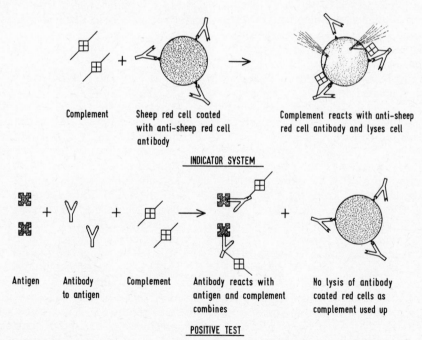

Complement   Sheep red cell coated   Complement reacts with anti-sheep
with anti-sheep red cell   red cell antibody and lyses cell
antibody

INDICATOR SYSTEM

Antigen   Antibody   Complement   Antibody reacts with   No lysis of antibody
to antigen   antigen and complement   coated red cells as
combines   complement used up

POSITIVE TEST

FIG. 11.11

Complement-fixation test. The indicator system (sheep red cells coated with antibody to sheep red cells) is normally lysed in the presence of complement (fresh guinea-pig serum)—top. If another antibody-antigen system is first mixed with the complement it will no longer be available to lyse the indicator system—bottom.

will, however, have been taken up during the incubation stage by the original antibody-antigen complex and will not be available to lyse the red cells. Thus, a positive complement fixation test is indicated by absence of lysis of the red cells whilst a negative test, with unused complement, is shown by lysis of the red cells (Fig. 11.11).

Reagents

Complement fixation test diluent (see veronal—NaCl diluent, Chap. 4) obtainable in tablet form from Oxoid.

Complement

Fresh or specially preserved guinea-pig serum is used. It contains an active haemolytic complement for the red corpuscles of the ox or sheep sensitized with the homologous haemolytic antibody. When fresh serum is used, the blood is obtained 12 to 18 h before the test by severing the large vessels of the neck over a 6-in funnel, from which the blood is collected in a measuring cylinder; it is allowed to co-agulate and stand overnight in the refrigerator. The complement in serum too recently withdrawn is apt to be excessively 'fixable', and in consequence is unsuitable for the Wassermann test.

If possible the pooled serum of several guinea-pigs should be used.

It should be noted that complement is unstable and deteriorates on keeping at ordinary temperatures. It is advisable throughout the experiment to keep the guinea-pig serum on ice. If storage at $-30°C$ is available the fresh serum may be divided into small portions and kept frozen for a few weeks.

It is now a general practice to use specially preserved serum pooled from a number of animals and it is recommended that it should be absorbed with packed sheep erythrocytes (0·1 ml cells/ml guinea-pig serum for 30 min at 4°C).

Preservation of complement. For the preservation of complement two principles have been applied: (1) rapid drying of the serum from the frozen state *in vacuo* ('freeze-drying') and the reconstitution of the serum when required by dissolving the dried material in the appropriate amount of distilled water; this is exemplified by *Rayner's method* for the preservation of bacterial cultures and serum (Rayner, 1943); and this technique is also recommended for complement-serum, particularly when the complement may not be used for some time; (2) addition to the liquid serum of sodium chloride or other salts in hypertonic concentration; this is exemplified by *Richardson's method* and the *sodium acetate boric acid method*. Preservation of the complement-serum in the liquid state constitutes a simple and convenient procedure. It is available commercially (Wellcome Reagents Ltd.). It may be obtained either in liquid form which will keep for a few months at 4°C or in the freeze dried state. Once the freeze-dried reagent is reconstituted it should be stored at 4°C and used within one week.

Richardson's Method. Preservation of liquid complement-serum in hypertonic salt solution is effective provided the pH is adjusted to 6–6·4. A convenient method, employing borate-buffer-sorbitol for control of pH, is described here (Richardson, 1941).

Two stock solutions, which keep indefinitely, are used:

(*a*) Boric acid (H_3BO_3) 0·93 g, borax ($Na_2B_4O_7$, $10H_2O$) 2·29 g, and sorbitol ($C_6H_{14}O_6$, $\frac{1}{2}H_2O$) 11·74 g are dissolved in and made up to 100 ml with saturated NaCl solution. The *resulting* molar concentrations are: 0·27 M boric acid, 0·12 M sodium borate, 0·6 M sorbitol in saturated sodium chloride.

(*b*) Borax 0·57 g and sodium azide (NaN_3) 0·81 g are dissolved and made up to 100 ml with saturated NaCl solution. The *resulting* molar concentrations are: 0·03 M boric acid, 0·03 M sodium borate, 0·125 M sodium azide in saturated sodium chloride.

To preserve complement-serum, mix 8 parts of serum with 1 part of solution *b*, followed by 1 part of solution *a*. This treated serum keeps very well even at room temperature. At 0°–3°C, loss of titre is not noticeable until after six to nine months. The mixture contains 0·03 M boric acid, 0·015 M sodium borate, 0·06 M sorbitol, and 0·0125 M sodium azide.

For use as 1 in 10 complement, 1 part of preserved serum is diluted with 7 parts of distilled water. Any further dilution from this 1 in 10 mixture is made with saline. Diluted serum should not be kept more than an hour or two. According to Richardson, no case of faulty behaviour in the Wassermann reaction attributable to preserved serum has come to notice.

Preservation by Sodium Acetate. A very simple and most convenient method of preserving complement is to add to the serum an equal volume of a solution of 12 per cent sodium acetate and 4 per cent boric acid in distilled water (Sonnenschein, 1930). The serum is kept in sterile screw-capped bottles at approximately 4°C. The full haemolytic activity of the serum and the fixability of the complement in the Wassermann reaction are maintained for about six months. It should be noted in using this preserved complement that it represents a 1 in 2 dilution of the original serum.

It should be noted that traces of zinc reduce the haemolytic activity of complement. Since Analar preparations of sodium chloride do not at present limit the presence of zinc, it is a wise precaution to check the diluents and solutions used in preparing complement. Traces of zinc are detected by turbidity on the addition of a freshly prepared solution of 0·1 per cent sodium di-ethyl-dithiocarbamate (Wilkinson, 1950).

Patient's Serum

A specimen of blood is obtained by vein puncture as for blood culture. The blood is then placed in a sterile stoppered test-tube or screw-capped bottle and allowed to coagulate. It is advisable to obtain about 5 ml of blood. The serum is pipetted off after separation and heated in a water-bath at 56°C for 30 min. Heating *eliminates the fallacy of non-specific fixation effects which may occur with normal unheated sera* plus *the antigen*; it also deprives the serum of its complementary property.

Viral Antigens at their Optimal Concentration

These may be bought commercially or made in the laboratory. See Lenette and Schmidt, (1969).

Sheep Red Blood Cells (Oxoid)

Either defibrinated or in Alsever's solution. Wash in saline at least three times, till supernate is colourless. Resuspend the red cells in saline and estimate the concentration of red cells in a haematocrit tube by centrifuging at 3000 rev/min for 20 min.

Rabbit or Horse Anti-sheep Cell Serum (Wellcome Reagents Ltd.)

This should have a high haemolytic titre but a low haemagglutinating titre. It is often referred to as 'Immune Body' or IB (Darter, 1953).

Applications

The classical complement fixation test is the Wassermann reaction used in the diagnosis of syphilis in which the test system consists of cardiolipin antigen mixed with dilutions of the patient's serum in the presence of guinea-pig complement (see Chap. 39). After the antigen

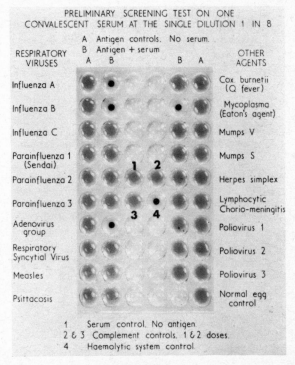

PLATE 11.1
Preliminary screening in complement fixation reactions. (From Swain and Dodds, 1967.)

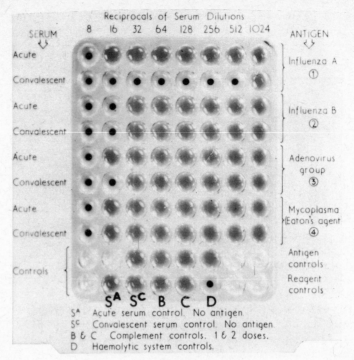

Reciprocals of Serum Dilutions

SA   Acute serum control. No antigen.
SC   Convalescent serum control. No antigen.
B & C   Complement controls. 1 & 2 doses.
D   Haemolytic system controls.

PLATE 11.2
The full complement fixation reaction as carried out after
screening. (From Swain and Dodds, 1967.)

and patient's serum have had time to react and take up the limited amount of complement available in the system, the indicator system is added to show whether or not there is free complement. Controls are included to ensure that none of the reagents are anti-complementary (able to take up complement non-specifically as might, for example, occur with contaminated serum) and positive and negative control sera are tested in parallel. Complement fixation tests are used on occasion for detecting viruses in tissue cultures that have been inoculated with specimens of blood or tissue fluids from humans with probable virus infections.

COMPLEMENT FIXATION TEST FOR THE DETECTION OF VIRAL ANTIBODIES

The method described is based on that of Bradstreet and Taylor (1962) but has been modified for use in microtitre plates. All the serum titres quoted here and elsewhere in this chapter are those in normal virological use, i.e.

they are initial dilutions before the addition of the test system.

Apparatus

1. Cooke microtitre disposable 'U' plates (rigid styrene) or permanent lucite 'U' plates (Flow Labs.). These plates have 12 × 8 wells.

2. Permanent or disposable 0·025 ml pipettes (Flow Labs.) with filters.

3. Microdiluters 0·025 ml (Flow Labs.).

4. Go-no-Go sheets to test volume delivered by pipettes and microdiluters (Flow Labs.).

5. Automatic syringe (1 ml to deliver 0·1 ml) (Turner and Co.).

6. 1 ml rubber teat.

Titration of complement and anti-sheep cell haemolytic serum

1. Prepare dilutions of the complement in 20 per cent steps as follows. If Richardson's preserved complement is being employed it should be prepared by adding 7 volumes of distilled water to 1 volume of complement. This will give a dilution equivalent to that of 1 in 10 which can subsequently be diluted with

Table 11.3

Tube	1	2	3	4	5	6	7	8	9
Complement	0·1	—	—	—	—	—	—	—	—
Distilled water	0·7	—	—	—	—	—	—	—	—
Buffer	1·6	0·5	0·5	0·5	0·5	0·5	0·5	0·5	0·5
		2 ml	2 ml	2 ml	2 ml	2 ml	2 ml	2 ml	2 ml
Resulting dilution	1 in 30	1 in 38	1 in 47	1 in 59	1 in 73	1 in 92	1 in 114	in 143	1 in 179

buffer. When using the Microtitre plates only a very small volume of the complement dilutions is required. The quantities suggested are shown in Table 11.3.

2. Using the micropipette put two drops (0·05 ml) of buffer in each of 70 wells (10 × 7) of a microtitre plate. These two drops replace the antibody and antigen in the actual test.

3. Beginning with row ten, add one drop of buffer to each of the seven wells, then one drop of the 1 in 179 complement to each of the seven wells of row nine and so on till all the wells contain a total of three drops.

4. Cover the plate and incubate overnight at 4°C to mimic the actual test because the virus-antibody reaction requires 18 h to reach completion.

5. Prepare 1 ml amounts of doubling dilutions of the anti-sheep cell serum from 1 in 25 to 1 in 800 (7 tubes). Add an equal volume of 4 per cent sheep red cells to these dilutions of serum and to 1 ml buffer. This serves as a control to ensure that the cells do not lyse in the absence of the haemolytic antiserum. Place for 10 min at 37°C and incubate at 4°C overnight.

6. On the following day incubate the disposable tray and sensitized red cells for 30 min at 37°C.

7. Beginning with the tube without any haemolytic antiserum add one drop of the cells to each well of row seven. Continue to add the sensitized red cells row by row finishing with the mixture containing the 1 in 25 haemolytic antiserum.

8. Tap plate gently to keep cells in suspension and incubate for 30 min at 37°C. The plate should be shaken at 10 min intervals.

9. Place at 4°C to allow unlysed cells to settle. The plate is read according to the degree of haemolysis.

$$0 = 100 \text{ per cent}$$
$$1 = 75 \text{ per cent}$$
$$2 = 50 \text{ per cent}$$
$$3 = 25 \text{ per cent}$$
$$4 = 0 \text{ per cent}$$

The optimal sensitizing concentration (OSC) of the haemolytic serum is that dilution which gives most haemolysis with the highest dilution of complement. In the example shown in Table 11.4 it would be 1 in 100. The haemolytic dose of complement (HD50) is that dose of comple-

Table 11.4

Row	1	2	3	4	5 '	6	7	8	9	10	Dilution of Immune Body
1	0	0	0	2	4	4	4	4	4	4	25
2	0	0	0	0	0	1	3	4	4	4	50
3	0	0	0	0	0	0	1	2	4	4	100
4	0	0	0	0	1	2	4	4	4	4	200
5	0	0	0	4	2	4	4	4	4	4	400
6	1	3	4	4	4	4	4	4	4	4	800
7	4	4	4	4	4	4	4	4	4	4	0
Dilution of Complement 1 in	30	38	47	59	73	92	114	143	179	0	

Table 11.5

	Antiserum dilutions								Antigen C
	8	16	32	64	128	256	512	1024	
Antigen dilutions 2	4	4	4	3	0	0	0	0	0
4	4	4	4	4	2	0	0	0	0
8	4	4	4	4	3	0	0	0	0
16	4	4	4	4	3	0	0	0	0
32	4	4	2	0	0	0	0	0	0
64	2	0	0	0	0	0	0	0	0
sc	0	0	0	0	0	0	0	0	
cc	4	0	1	2					

ment at which lysis of 50 per cent of the cells occurs in the presence of the OSC of haemolytic serum. In the above example the HD50 would be 1 in 143.

In most cases it is advisable to titrate the complement in the presence of the antigen and if this is so, one volume of the buffer is replaced by one volume of antigen, before the overnight incubation at 4°C.

The complement fixation test—full checkerboard

1. Prepare doubling dilutions of the inactivated serum from 1 in 8 to 1 in 1024 (8 wells) or desired level. This may be done either in tubes before subsequent transfer of the serum dilutions to the plate or in the plate itself by the use of the microdiluters. For this latter method one drop of buffer is added to 56 wells (8 × 7) beginning with the second vertical row; one drop of serum diluted to 1 in 8 is added to all the wells of the first and second vertical rows. The loops are then placed, one in each of the wells of the second row, rotated and transferred

to the wells of the third row with 0·025 ml. This is continued until the eighth row is reached when the remaining 0·025 ml is discarded. The 9th well contains buffer only and will serve later as the antigen control (Takatsy, 1955).

2. Add one drop of 3HD50 complement to all the wells of the test.
Controls:
   one well with three drops of buffer and no complement—(cell control).
   three wells with two drops of buffer and one drop of 3, 2 and 1 HD50 complement.

3. Prepare six doubling dilutions of antigen in test tubes remembering to change pipettes at each dilution to avoid carry over of antigen. Beginning with the bottom row add one drop buffer to all the wells of that row (serum control) and continue up the concentrations of antigen allowing one row per dilution.

4. Incubate overnight at 4°C.

5. Prepare and sensitize the haemolytic system using OSC of IB.

Table 11.6

	Antiserum dilutions								Antigen C
	8	16	32	64	128	256	512	1024	
Antigen dilutions 2	4	4	4	4	4	4	3	1	0
4	4	4	2	0	0	0	0	0	0
8	4	3	0	0	0	0	0	0	0
16	0	0	0	0	0	0	0	0	0
32	0	0	0	0	0	0	0	0	0
64	0	0	0	0	0	0	0	0	0
sc	0	0	0	0	0	0	0	0	
cc	4	0	1	2					

6. Next day place both plate and haemolytic system for 30 min at 37°C.

7. Add one drop of haemolytic system to all wells; incubate as for complement titration.

8. Read the test (Table 11.5).

This is the more normal reaction and from this it can be seen that the titre of the serum is 128 and the optimal dilution of the antigen is 16 (Table 11.6).

This can occur with sera from young children or in a convalescent serum following a primary infection. Here the limiting dilution of the serum is 512 and the optimal dilution of the antigen is 2. This shows that in some cases it is wise either to carry out a full checkerboard titration or to include a more concentrated antigen as was suggested by a PHLS report.

In the diagnostic laboratory it is often convenient to fix the sensitizing dose of horse or rabbit anti-sheep cell serum and then to titrate the complement in the presence of each antigen at its optimal dilution. This will give the HD50 of complement for each antigen. A screening test can then be performed on the inactivated unknown serum at dilutions of 1 in 8 and 1 in 32. Any serum which fixes complement in the presence of an antigen (provided the controls are satisfactory) should be titrated out to establish the end point dilution of the antibody for that antigen.

The following viral and other antigens may be incorporated in a screening test:

1. Serum from patients with respiratory tract infection. Influenza A, influenza B, influenza C, sendai, adenovirus, respiratory syncytial virus, measles, *Mycoplasma pneumoniae*, *Coxiella burnetii* and Psittacosis.

2. In encephalitis and meningitis, mumps S and V, herpes, measles.

3. Endocarditis—*Coxiella burnetii*.

If any serum should be anticomplementary, i.e. fixes complement in the absence of antigen, it should be treated by adding fresh guinea-pig serum (4 vols patient's serum to one volume guinea-pig serum) and incubating overnight at 4°C. After heating for 30 min at 37°C dilute with buffer to give a 1 in 8 dilution and inactivate any free complement by heating for 30 min at 56°C.

Antigen-antibody Reactions using Fluorescent Labels

The precise localization of tissue antigens or the antigens of infecting organisms in the body, of

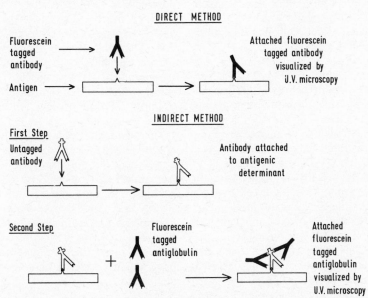

FIG. 11.12

Fluorescent antibody technique—direct and indirect methods. The indirect method can be seen to be more sensitive as two or more fluorescein-tagged antiglobulin molecules can be attached to each immunoglobulin molecule bound to its antigen.

anti-tissue antibody and of antigen-antibody complexes was achieved by the introduction of the use of fluorochrome-labelled proteins by Coons and Kaplan in 1950. The adsorption of ultra-violet light between 290 and 495 nm by fluorescein and its emission of longer wave-length green light (525 nm) is used to visualize protein labelled with this dye. The technique is more sensitive than precipitation or com-plement fixation techniques, and fluorescent protein tracers can be detected at a concen-tration of the order of 1 μg protein per ml body fluid.

Applications. Some of the uses to which the technique has been put include the localization of the origin of a variety of serum protein components, for example immunoglobulin pro-duction by plasma cells and other lymphoid cells. The demonstration and localization in the tissues of antibody globulin in a variety of auto-immune conditions has been shown, in-cluding an anti-nuclear antibody in the serum of patients with systemic lupus erythematosus and thyroid auto-antibodies in the sera of patients with Hashimoto's thyroiditis. In the diagnostic field most human pathogens can be demonstrated by immunofluorescence and a tentative diagnosis may be made much sooner than by cultivation; the fluorescent method at present can be used to supplement rather than replace conventional methods.

There are two main procedures in use, the direct and indirect methods (Fig. 11.12). The *direct method* consists of bringing fluorescein-tagged antibodies into contact with antigens fixed on a slide (e.g. in the form of a tissue section or a smear of an organism), allowing them to react, washing off excess antibody and examining under the UV light microscope. The site of union of the labelled antibody with its antigen can be seen by the apple-green fluores-cent areas on the slide. The *indirect method* can be used both for detecting specific antibodies in sera or other body fluids and also for identi-fying antigens. This method differs from the direct method in the use of a non-labelled antiserum which is layered on first, in the same way as described above. Whether or not this antiserum has reacted with the material on the slide is shown by means of a fluorescein-tagged *antiglobulin serum* specific for the

globulin of the serum applied first. Such an antiglobulin serum can be used to detect antibody globulin in sera to a variety of different antigens which gives it a considerable advan-tage over the direct test; it is also more sen-sitive.

Conjugation of Antiserum with Fluorescein Isothiocyanate

Prior to conjugation it is necessary to separate the globulin fraction from the antiserum and this is conveniently carried out by 50 per cent saturation with ammonium sulphate as follows:

1. Equal volumes, e.g. 10 ml of antiserum and saturated ammonium sulphate are chilled separately in universal containers until ice crystals start to form in the antiserum, and then mixed by pouring the ammonium sulphate (all at once) into the antiserum. The mixture is then shaken well and left for 2 h in the cold at 4°C.

2. The precipitated globulin is separated from the supernatant albumin by centri-fugation at 3000 g in a refrigerated centrifuge at 4°C.

3. The supernatant is removed and the pre-cipitate dissolved in a small volume of distilled water, *just sufficient* to dissolve the globulin completely. The globulin solution is then dialysed overnight against 0·85 per cent NaCl at 4°C to remove the ammonium sulphate.

4. The total protein of the dialysed globulin is then estimated by a convenient method, e.g. the quantitative Biuret method. Provided only a small volume of distilled water was used in the previous step the protein concentration should be 20–30 mg/ml.

Conjugation. Proteins contain several differ-ent chemical groups which can be used for the attachment of fluorochromes. These include the free amino and carboxyl groups at the ends of each protein chain and free amino groups in the lysine side chains. The optimal quantity of fluorescein has been estimated by Coons and Kaplan (1950) as 0·05 mg/mg of protein. Above this level no further conjugation takes place and progressively larger amounts of protein are denatured.

Conjugation with Fluorescein Isothiocyanate.

1. The globulin fraction prepared as in-dicated above is diluted to 10 mg of protein

per ml with 0·5 M carbonate-bicarbonate buffer pH 9·2 (made up fresh before use) so that the final mixture contains 10 per cent buffer.

2. The solution is chilled to 4°C and 0·05 mg of fluorescein isothiocyanate (British Drug Houses) per mg. of protein is added. During the addition of the fluorochrome and for the next 18 h the mixture should be stirred continuously, e.g. with a magnetic stirrer, and kept at 4°C.

4. Following conjugation excess fluorescein is dialysed away against phosphate buffered saline (physiological 0·85 per cent NaCl buffered with 0·01 M phosphate) in the cold, changing the buffer frequently until the dialysate contains no further dye.

5. The conjugate is finally centrifuged for 45 min at 3000 g at 4°C to remove any precipitated denatured protein.

Conjugation with Lissamine Rhodamine B (RB200). The fluorochrome is used as the sulphonyl chloride prepared by grinding 0·5 g of RB200 with 1 g of PCl_5 in a mortar (using a fume cupboard). After mixing, 5 ml of acetone is added with stirring for a few minutes and the mixture filtered. This solution should be used within 48 h of preparation. The conjugation process is similar to that for fluorescein isothiocyanate except that 0·2 ml of the solution is used for every 100 mg of protein and after mixing with the globulin stirring need only be continued for 30 min.

Storage of conjugates. Conjugates may be stored at 4°C with the addition of preservative, e.g. merthiolate 1/10 000; alternatively they may be stored at −20°C or freeze dried. Prior to use non-specific fluorescence will require to be absorbed out from the conjugate.

FLUORESCENT ANTIBODY TECHNIQUE FOR ESTIMATION OF VIRAL ANTIBODY

This test may be applied to detect membrane fluorescence (using unfixed cells) or as a less well-defined fluorescence (using fixed cells).

Membrane Fluorescence

Apparatus

1. Plastic test-tubes 3 in × ½ in.
2. Microscope slides less than 1 mm thick. These slides should be cleaned by placing in chromic acid for at least a day. They are then rinsed in running water overnight and stored in alcohol.
3. No. 1 coverslips.
4. Fluorescent microscope.

Reagents

1. Known positive, negative and unknown sera all absorbed with uninfected tissue culture cells. To each serum add 10^8 uninfected cells for each 1 ml of undiluted serum. Mix at 4°C for 1 h or at 37°C for 1 h followed by 4°C overnight. Remove the cells by centrifugation at 4000 rev/min for 15 min and subsequent millipore filtration.
2. Fluorescent antiserum at optimal dilution and absorbed as above.
3. Monolayers of uninfected tissue culture cells.
4. Virus of known infectivity.
5. Trypsin to remove the infected cells.
6. Foetal calf serum to quench the action of the trypsin.
7. Tris buffer saline.
8. Alcohol.
9. Glycerol mountant. (Nairn, 1969.)

Method (Smith *et al.,* 1972).

1. Infect the monolayer of cells with virus at a multiplicity of 1–2 p.f.u./cell.
2. Incubate, e.g. 20 h for herpes simplex virus.
3. Wash the cells with Tris buffer saline.
4. Remove the cells with trypsin.
5. Resuspend the cells in 10 ml Tris buffer saline containing 10 per cent foetal calf serum.
6. Centrifuge the cells at 1000 rev/min for 5 min (all subsequent centrifugations are at this speed and for this time).
7. Count the cells.
8. Adjust the concentration to 1×10^6/ml.
9. Dispense in 1 ml amounts in plastic tubes.
10. Wash twice in Tris buffer saline.
11. To different tubes add 0·1 ml (a) buffer, (b) known positive, (c) known negative and (d) unknown serum.
12. Incubate at 37°C for ½ h.
13. Wash three times with Tris buffer saline.
14. Add 0·1 ml fluorescent antiserum to all tubes.
15. Incubate at 37°C for ½ h.
16. Wash three times with Tris buffer saline.
17. Put a small drop from each tube on a clean slide.

18. Allow to dry in air.

19. Fix in alcohol.

20. Mount in glycerol mountant and examine.

Results

The infected cells treated with negative serum or buffer should show no fluorescence. Fluorescence of cells treated with buffer indicates that the fluorescent antiserum has been insufficiently absorbed with uninfected cells. The cells treated with known positive serum should show good membrane fluorescence. If these three controls are acceptable the unknown serum can be titrated to find the limiting dilution of the antibody.

Fixed Cells

These can be used either for the titration of Epstein–Barr virus antibody with cells grown in a suspension, or for the titration of other viral antibodies using cells which are growing on coverslips.

Reagents

1. Infected tissue culture cells.

2. Acetone (A.R.).

3. Known positive, negative and unknown sera, adsorbed usually with liver powder or cell powder.

4. Fluorescent labelled antiserum at optimal dilution and adsorbed as above.

5. Phosphate buffer saline pH 7.6.

6. Mounting fluid.

7. Clean slides.

Method

1. Fix the dried smears from suspension cultures or coverslips in acetone for 10 min.

2. Apply the known positive, known negative, unknown serum and buffer to different smears or coverslips.

3. Incubate in a humid atmosphere for 30 min at 37°C.

4. Wash in buffer with agitation. (Four changes of buffer in 20 min.)

5. Blot dry.

6. Apply the fluorescent antiserum.

7. Incubate, as in 3.

8. Wash as in 4.

9. Blot dry.

10. Mount in glycerol mountant.

11. Examine.

Results. The buffer and the known negative serum should give no fluorescence. Known positive serum should show fluorescence. If these controls are in order the test can be read. The limiting dilution of the antiviral antibody can also be determined using this method.

TITRATION OF VIRAL NEUTRALIZING ANTIBODY

Neutralizing antibodies are capable of forming a complex with their homologous virus by attaching to the capsid or envelope. This renders the virus incapable of expressing itself in the indicator system. The antibody does not, however, destroy the virus as, apparently unaltered, infective virus can be detected after dissociation of the virus-serum complexes by dilution or alteration of the pH of the reaction mixture. The formation of the virus-serum complex is time-, temperature- and concentration-dependent and the sensitivity of the reaction will be governed by the indicator system.

When carrying out neutralization tests it is necessary to include a virus-diluent control which is treated in exactly the same manner as the virus-serum mixture since some viruses are thermolabile and their titre may fall during the reaction. The interaction of the virus control with the indicator system is used as the baseline for the determination of the limiting dilution of antibody.

The titration of neutralizing antibody can be applied to any virus, provided there is a method for the titration of the residual virus. This indicator system may be animals, eggs or cell cultures but here only cell cultures will be considered. In such a system the viral activity may be measured as a focal, quantal or metabolic response.

Quantal Method

Reagents

1. Serum heated for 30 min, at 56°C.

2. The diluent used can be either 1 per cent skim milk or growth medium.

3. Virus at the required challenge dose, e.g. 100 TCID50/unit volume.

Test

1. Prepare two-fold dilutions of the serum.

2. Add an equal volume of the challenge dose of virus.

3. Incubate for 1 h at 4°C for a heat labile virus or at room temperature for other viruses.

4. Controls: (i) Serum+diluent; (ii) Virus+diluent. Both incubated as above.

5. Inoculate replicate test systems with aliquots of virus-serum mixtures: serum control: antigen control and diluent (to act as cell control). When the CPE is complete in the virus control, the amount of CPE should be recorded in each of the tests and the antibody level is expressed as the highest dilution of serum at which the virus is fully inhibited.

This test is used to estimate the amount of antibody to each of the 6 Coxsackie B viruses and other enteroviruses since they are antigenically distinct.

Focal Method, e.g. plaque reduction test.

The reagents are as above but the challenge dose usually contains 100 p.f.u.

The reduction in the number of plaques gives a measure of the neutralizing power of the serum. Plaque reduction of 50–90 per cent is usually taken as the limiting dilution.

Metabolic Inhibition Test

This is a useful colorimetric test to determine the limiting dilution of antibody to the enteroviruses. It is based on the fact that cells that are respiring normally produce acid and change the colour of the medium (containing phenol red indicator) from orange red to yellow. If the virus is a cytotoxic virus it inhibits the respiration of the cells resulting in a rise in pH indicated by a dark red colour. Neutralisation of the virus with specific antiserum will allow the cells to continue to respire normally and the medium will develop a yellow colour.

Reagents

1. Sterile Cooke microtitre disposable 'U' (rigid styrene) plates. (These plates may be sterilized in the laboratory by exposure to U.V. light at a distance of 10 cm for two hours).

2. Suspension of HEp–2 cells at a concentration of 5×10^5/ml.

3. Medium containing high glucose content.

4. Pipettes.

5. Microdiluters.

6. Covers or sellotape.

7. Virus suspension.

8. Sera heated to 56°C for 30 min.

Method: Titration of the virus

1. Prepare eight tenfold dilutions of the virus in medium.

2. Add two volumes of medium to all wells serving as cell controls and one volume to all other wells (10×8).

3. Add one volume of cells to all the wells.

4. Beginning with the most dilute virus suspension add one volume to, say, 10 wells; continue till all the dilutions have been added.

5. Seal the plate.

6. Incubate at 37°C for six days.

7. Remove plate from incubator.

8. Remove seal and allow any CO_2 to escape.

9. Reseal plate.

10. Reincubate plate overnight at 37°C.

11. Read result (shown in Table 11.7).

Table 11.7

	Virus dilutions								Cell control
10^1	10^2	10^3	10^4	10^5	10^6	10^7	10^8	0
R	R	R	R	R	Y	Y	Y	Y
R	R	R	R	R	Y	Y	Y	Y
R	R	R	R	Y	R	Y	Y	Y
R	R	R	R	R	Y	Y	Y	Y
R	R	R	R	Y	Y	Y	Y	Y
R	R	R	R	Y	R	Y	Y	Y
R	R	R	R	R	R	Y	Y	Y
R	R	R	R	R	Y	Y	Y	Y
R	R	R	R	R	R	Y	Y	Y
R	R	R	R	Y	Y	Y	Y	Y

R = red
Y = yellow

Table 11.8

	Serum dilutions							Antigen C	Cell control
	8	16	32	64	128	256	512		
SC	Y	Y	Y	Y	Y	Y	Y	R	Y
Test	Y	Y	Y	Y	Y	R	R		

R = red
Y = yellow

The titre of the virus suspension/unit volume can be calculated using the formula of Reed and Muench (page 315). Here the result would be $10^{5.5}$/unit volume.

Method: Test

1. Prepare doubling dilutions of serum in the microplates using microdiluters (see CFT).

2. Add unit volumes of virus suspension containing 100 TCID50.

3. Set up serum control in which medium replaces virus.

4. Set up virus control in which medium replaces serum.

5. Cover and incubate one hour at room temperature.

6. Remove cover and add one volume of cells to all wells and to cell control which contains two volumes of media in lieu of both serum and virus.

7. Seal and continue as from 6 in titration above (see Table 11.8).

Results. The cell controls should be yellow. The serum controls should be yellow. The virus controls should be red. Here the serum has a limiting dilution of 1 in 128.

SEPARATION AND ASSAY OF IMMUNOGLOBULINS

It is often important to be able to distinguish the various classes of immunoglobulin in a serum, e.g. to detect a recent infection with rubella virus. This can be done either by separation of the classes on a sucrose density gradient and subsequent assay of their amount and activity or by direct examination of the serum by gel diffusion or immunofluorescence using specific anti-immunoglobulins.

Sucrose Density Gradient

Apparatus

1. High speed centrifuge, e.g. Spinco with a swing-out head.

2. Plastic liners for the centrifuge buckets.

3. Holder for the plastic liners.

4. Vibration-free refrigerator.

5. 1 ml syringe with a needle bent at right angles, bevel down, or a rubber stopper to fit the plastic liners. This stopper should have a piece of rubber tubing controlled by a jubilee clip attached to it by a piece of glass tubing.

6. A gradient maker or pipettes.

Reagents

1. PBS pH 7·2.

2. Serum.

3. A series of sucrose solutions in PBS. 40, 30, 20 and 10 per cent are convenient, or 40 and 10 per cent if a gradient maker is available.

Method

1. Place the plastic liners in the holder.

2. Prepare the gradients in the plastic liners either using a gradient maker or by means of a pipette. For the 5 ml liners, the following schedule is appropriate if a pipette is being used. Place 1·22 ml 40 per cent sucrose in the bottom of the liner. 1·12 ml of 30 per cent is then run slowly down the inside of the liner taking care to preserve the interface. Repeat this using 1·12 ml of the 20 and 10 per cent sucrose.

3. Place the gradients in a vibration-free refrigerator at 4°C and allow to equilibrate overnight.

4. Dilute the serum 1 in 2 in PBS.

5. Centrifuge at 750 g for 10 min.

6. Carefully layer 0·5 ml diluted serum on the surface of the gradient again taking care to preserve the interface.

7. With a bacteriological stab wire bent at right angles, carefully mix the serum with the top of the gradient. (This is to prevent globule formation when spinning commences.)

8. Place the plastic liners in the buckets of a precooled centrifuge head ensuring that the head is balanced.

9. Centrifuge at 134,000 g for 16 h under refrigeration and without the brake.

10. When the centrifuge has stopped, remove the liner and place it carefully in a clamp.

11. Remove the fractions either from the top using the 1 ml syringe and abstracting 0·5 ml aliquots or place the rubber stopper in the plastic liner; close the rubber tubing by means of the jubilee clip; pierce the bottom of the tube with a needle and collect the drops. As the solution is expelled from the liner, it is necessary to release the jubilee clip gradually. This second method allows smaller fractions to be collected but sometimes the fractions are not so clean as the sucrose tends to 'tail' in the liners.

The fractions can now be examined for their immunoglobulin class by gel diffusion or by estimation of the amount of specific antibody present in each fraction. This is carried out using one of the standard techniques, e.g. haemagglutination inhibition, complement-fixation or neutralization. It must be remembered, however, that the presence of the sucrose tends to make the fractions anticomplementary, so if this test is being used, the fractions must be dialysed against PBS before examination. The sucrose does not appear to interfere with haemagglutination inhibition or neutralization tests.

Gel Diffusion

This can be applied to the fractions from the sucrose density gradient to establish their immunoglobulin class or to the whole serum.

Instead of placing antibody and antigen in separate wells and allowing them to diffuse towards each other, the antibody can be incorporated in the agar and the antigen placed in wells. This technique is known as *single radial immunodiffusion* and depends upon diffusion of antigen from the well until a point is reached where the concentration is optimal for precipitation to occur. Close to the antigen well the concentration of antigen will be high and although the antigen will combine with antibody in the agar, the complexes will be unable to form the large lattice structure necessary for precipitation to take place (Fig. 11.2) and will thus remain as soluble complexes. The precipitin band that forms at optimal proportions of antigen and antibody will show up as a ring around the antigen well. The distance the ring forms from the antigen well will be dependent on the concentration of the antigen in the well. In practice, the diameter of the ring is measured around a well containing an unknown concentration of antigen and this is compared with the diameter of the rings formed with known con-

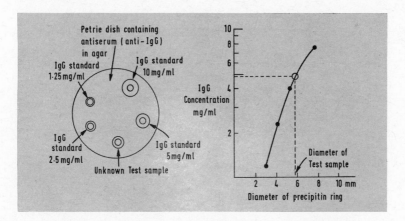

FIG. 11.13
Diagram of single radial immunodiffusion plate with antiserum incorporated in agar and antigen dilutions and test sample in wells. Reference Graph drawn using 3 concentrations of antigen standard showing the diameter of precipitin ring obtained with each concentration (●). Diameter of unknown sample (○) when plotted enables determination of its antigen concentration.

centrations of the antigen, thus enabling the estimation of the concentration of antigen in the unknown preparation. This technique is widely used to estimate the quantity of the various immunoglobulin classes in human serum samples. An antiserum to a particular immunoglobulin class (e.g. IgG) is incorporated in the agar and the test serum sample is placed in a well. The diameter of the precipition band that forms after incubation is then compared to the diameter obtained with standard IgG preparations of known concentration. The diameters of the rings with the standard IgG preparations (e.g. 3 or 4 dilutions of a known concentration) can be plotted graphically against the concentration of IgG and the diameter obtained with the unknown sample can be read off against concentration on this reference graph (Fig. 11.13).

Immunofluorescence

As specific anti IgG, IgA and IgM are now available in a conjugated form it is possible to establish the class of immunoglobulin that is reacting with a viral antigen in an infected cell by the indirect immunofluorescence test. Here the patient's serum is allowed to react with the infected cells and after washing, the preparation is treated with the conjugated monospecific antiglobulin. Provided the appropriate controls are included, the specific class of immunoglobulin containing the antiviral antibody can be established.

RADIOIMMUNOASSAY METHODS

Increasing use has been made over the last few

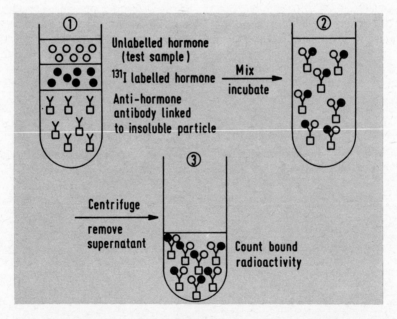

FIG 11.14

Illustration of the use of antihormone antibody linked to an insoluble particle for the assay of the amount of hormone in a test sample. The quantity of ^{131}I labelled hormone complexing with the antihormone antibody varies inversely with the amount of unlabelled hormone in the test sample. A standard curve can be prepared using known concentrations of purified hormone in the same way as illustrated in Fig. 11.13, this will enable the result obtained with the test sample to be plotted and its concentration obtained.

years of immunologically-based assay methods for the accurate quantitative estimation of polypeptide hormones. These methods offer a unique combination of specificity, precision and simplicity and are already available for the assay of some 14 of the 20 or so polypeptide hormones in man.

The principle of the assay methods is that radio-iodine labelled (purified) hormone competes with the non-labelled hormone of a sample under test for the antihormone antibody with which the labelled and non-labelled hormone are mixed. The more of the hormone there is in the test sample the less chance the labelled hormone has of combining with the limited number of antibody molecules that are available in the antihormone serum. Thus by measuring the quantity of labelled hormone combined with antibody (with isotope counting equipment) a measure of the hormone in the test sample can be obtained. The more labelled hormone combined with antibody the lower the hormone level in the test sample. The quantity of isotope-labelled hormone complexing with the antihormone antibody varies inversely with the quantity of unlabelled hormone in the test sample.

In order to measure the amount of labelled hormone attached to antibody it is necessary to separate the hormone-antibody complexes from the mixture. A variety of methods have been developed to achieve this, perhaps the most common being electrophoretic separation. Provided the *free* hormone has a different electrophoretic mobility from the antibody globulin, then separation of hormone *bound* to antibody is straightforward. Other methods of separation depend upon the antibody being linked to an insoluble support (e.g. cellulose). The insoluble complex is then mixed with labelled and test hormone (tube 1, Fig. 11.14), allowed to interact (tube 2, Fig. 11.14) and later the unreacted hormone is removed and the amount of labelled hormone attached to the insoluble complex is measured (tube 3, Fig. 11.14).

An assay for IgE levels in serum has been developed using iodine labelled IgE and anti-IgE linked to cellulose, and assays using these principles are being developed for the detection of Australia antigen in human serum.

REFERENCES

BARRETT, A. M. (1941) Serological diagnosis of glandular fever (infectious mononucleosis); new technique. *Journal of Hygiene (London)*, **41**, 330.

BRADSTREET, C. M. P. & TAYLOR, C. E. D. (1962) Technique of complement-fixation test applicable to the diagnosis of virus diseases. *Monthly Bulletin of the Ministry of Health Laboratory Service*, **21**, 96.

BYWATERS, E. G. L. & SCOTT, F. E. T. (1960) Rheumatism and connective tissues diseases. In *Recent Advances in Clinical Pathology*, p. 279. Edited by S. C. Dyke. London: Churchill.

CLARKE, D. H. & CASALS, J. (1958) Techniques for haemagglutination and haemagglutination-inhibition with arthropod-borne viruses. *American Journal of Tropical Medicine and Hygiene*, **7**, 561.

COONS, A. H. & KAPLAN, M. W. (1950) Localization of antigens in tissue cells. *Journal of Experimental Medicine*, **91**, 1.

CROWLE, A. J. (1961) *Immunodiffusion*. New York: Academic Press.

CSIZMAS, L. (1960) Preparation of formalized erythrocytes. *Proceedings of the Society of Experimental Biology (New York)*, **103**, 157.

DACIE, J. V. & LEWIS, S. M. (1968) Practical Haematology, 4th edn. Edinburgh: Churchill Livingstone.

DARTER, L. A. (1953) Procedure for production of anti-sheep haemolysis. *Journal of Laboratory and Clinical Medicine*, **41**, 653.

DERRIEN, Y., MICHEL, R. & ROCHE, J. (1948) Recherches sur la preparation et les proprietes de la thyroglobuline pure. *Biochemica et biophysica Acta (Amsterdam)*, **2**, 454.

FULTHORPE, A. J., ROITT, I. M., DONIACH, D. & COUCHMAN, K. (1961) A stable sheep cell preparation for detecting thyroglobulin auto-antibodies and its clinical application. *Journal of Clinical Pathology*, **14**, 654.

GELL, P. G. H. (1957) The estimation of individual human serum proteins by an immunological method. *Journal of Clinical Pathology*, **10**, 67.

GRASSET, E., BONIFAS, V. & PONGRATZ, E. (1958) Rapid slide precipitation micro-reaction of poliomyelitis antigens and antisera in agar. *Proceedings of the Society of Experimental Biology (New York)*, **97**, 72.

HEINER, D. C. (1958) Diagnosis of histoplasmosis using precipitin reactions in agar gel. *Paediatrics*, **22**, 616.

HOYLE, L. (1948) Technique of the complement fixation test in influenza. *Monthly Bulletin of the Ministry of Health Laboratory Service*, **7**, 114.

KABAT, E. L. & MAYER, M. M. (1961) *Experimental Immunochemistry*, 2nd edn., p. 476. Springfield, Illinois: Thomas.

LECOCQ, E. & LINZ, R. (1962) Agglutination d'hematies tannees traitees par deux antigens. *Annals Institute Pasteur, Lille*, **102**, 437.

LENETTE, E. H. & SCHMIDT, N. J. (1969) *Diagnostic procedures for rural and rickettsial infections*, 4th edn. American Public Health Association Inc.

NAIRN, R. C. (1969) *Fluorescent Protein Tracing*, 3rd edn. Edinburgh: Livingstone.

OAKLEY, C. L. & FULTHORPE, A. J. (1953) Antigenic analysis by diffusion. *Journal of Pathology and Bacteriology*, **65,** 49.

PREER, J. R. (1956) A quantitative study of a technique of double diffusion in agar. *Journal of Immunology*, **77,** 52.

PRICE, I. N. O. (1949) Complement-fixation technique; estimation of complement doses. *British Journal of Venereal Disease*, **25,** 157.

PRICE, I. N. O. (1950a) Complement-fixation technique; titration of Wassermann antigen. *British Journal of Venereal Disease*, **26,** 33.

PRICE, I. N. O. (1950b) Complement-fixation technique; Wassermann reaction. *British Journal of Venereal Disease*, **26,** 172.

RAYNER, A. G. (1943) A simple method for the preservation of cultures and sera by drying. *Journal of Pathology and Bacteriology*, **55,** 373.

REED, L. J. & MUENCH, H. (1938) A simple method of estimating fifty per cent end points. *American Journal of Hygiene*, **27,** 493.

RICHARDSON, G. M. (1941) The preservation of liquid complement serum. *Lancet*, **ii,** 696.

SAWYER, H. P. & BOURKE, A. R. (1946) Anti-sheep amboceptor production with elimination of rabbit shock. *Journal of Laboratory and Clinical Medicine*, **31,** 714.

SCHEIFFARTH, F. & GOETZ, H. (1960) Significance of immuno-electrophoresis in differentiation of pathological sera. *Archives of Allergy (New York)*, **16,** 61.

SEVER, J. L. (1962) Application of a microtechnique to viral serological investigations. *Journal of Immunology*, **88,** 320.

SINGER, J. M., ALTMAN, G., ORESKES, I. & PLOTZ, C. M. (1961) The mechanism of particle carrier reactions. *American Journal of Medicine*, **30,** 772.

SINGER, J. M. & PLOTZ, C. M. (1956) The latex fixation test. *American Journal of Medicine*, **21,** 88.

SMITH, J. W., LOWRY, S. P., MELNICK, J. L. & RAWLS, W. E (1972) Antibodies to surface antigens of herpesvirus type 1—and type—2 infected cells among women with cervical cancer and control women. *Infection and Immunity*, **5,** 305.

SONNENSCHEIN, C. (1930) Komplementkonservierung durch Natriumazetat und Borsaure. *Zeitschrift für Immunitätsforschung und experimentale Therapie*, **67,** 512.

SWAIN, R. H. A. & DODDS, T. C. (1967) *Clinical Virology*. Edinburgh: Livingstone.

TAKATSY, G. (1955) The use of spiral loops in serological and virological micro-methods. *Acta microbiologica Academiae Scientiarum hungaricae*, **3,** 191.

WILKINSON, A. E. (1950) Destructive effect of traces of zinc salts on complement. *Journal of Clinical Pathology*, **3,** 363.

FURTHER READING

HUMPHREY, J. H. & WHITE, R. G. (1969) *Immunology for Students of Medicine*, p. 348. Oxford: Blackwell.

WALLACE, A. C., OSLER, A. G. & MAYER, M. M. (1950) Quantitative studies of the complement-fixation. V. Estimation of complement-fixing potency of immune sera and its relation to antibody nitrogen content. *Journal of Immunology*, **65,** 661.

WEIR, D. M. (1973) *Handbook of Experimental Immunology*, 2nd edn. Oxford: Blackwell.

WILKINSON, A. E. (1970) The positive Wassermann reaction; investigation and interpretation. *British Journal of Hospital Medicine*, **4,** 47.

12. Bacteriology of Water, Milk, Food, Air

BACTERIOLOGICAL EXAMINATION OF WATER

Drinking-water supplies liable to contamination with sewage or other excreted matter may cause outbreaks of intestinal infections such as typhoid fever. In safeguarding public water supplies, health authorities and water engineers rely on information obtained from the results of frequent bacteriological tests. The demonstration of pathogenic bacteria, e.g. the typhoid bacillus, would obviously constitute the most direct proof of a dangerous impurity, but these pathogens, if present, are usually so scanty that the technical difficulty of their isolation makes the test impracticable for ordinary purposes. Instead we rely on tests that will reveal the presence of commensal bacteria of intestinal origin such as those of the coliform group, *Streptococcus faecalis* and *Clostridium welchii*. These do not themselves constitute a hazard, but they indicate that faecal matter has entered the supply and that the water is therefore liable to contamination with more dangerous organisms. The coliform bacilli are the most reliable indicators of faecal pollution. Although the presence of streptococci is strong evidence of faecal pollution, their absence does not exclude such impurity. The sporing anaerobes, on the other hand, being highly resistant, would in the absence of the other intestinal organisms indicate pollution of some remote period rather than one of recent occurrence.

Since the coliform group of bacteria may be derived from the intestines of various animals and birds they are likely to occur in small numbers even in water supplies far removed from the possibility of human contamination. Water grossly polluted with human excretal matter, e.g. sewage, contains them in larger numbers. The test for their presence as an index of the degree of pollution must therefore be carried out on a quantitative basis. The coliform group of lactose-fermenting Gram-negative bacilli includes a number of different organisms (Enterobacteriaceae). Those referred to as 'typical' or 'faecal' (e.g. *Esch. coli*) are essentially commensals of the intestine and are derived almost exclusively from this source. Others, known as 'atypical' (e.g. *Kl. aerogenes*), may grow also in the soil and on vegetation, and by derivation from these sources may often be present in waters that are not subject to excretal pollution. The typical faecal bacilli (*Esch. coli*) die in water during the course of several days or weeks after leaving the animal intestine; thus, their presence in water is an indication of recent faecal contamination, whereas the presence of the hardier atypical coliforms is not necessarily so. In carrying out the test for coliform bacilli in water it is therefore advisable to determine whether the strains present are typical or atypical.

A determination of the total number of viable bacteria in a water sample is a useful supplementary test, although of limited value by itself. It gives an indication of the amount and type of organic matter present in the supply. The test is carried out in duplicate at 37°C and 20°–22°C. The bacteria that grow at 37°C are those most likely to be associated with organic material of human or animal origin, whereas those growing at the lower temperature are mainly saprophytes that normally inhabit the water or are derived from soil and vegetation.

The routine tests generally used in bacteriological examination of water are:

1. A quantitative test for all coliform bacilli known as the *presumptive coliform count*.

2. A differential test for typical coliform bacilli (*Esch. coli*) known as the *differential coliform test*.

3. An enumeration of viable bacteria known as the *plate count*; this is done in duplicate, cultivating at 37°C and 22°C.

Chemical analyses are sometimes used for judging the quality of water supplies. They are not, however, as sensitive as bacterial tests for detecting dangerous pollution.

COLLECTION OF SPECIMENS

Specimens are taken in bottles, of *c.* 230 ml capacity, with ground-glass stoppers having an overhanging rim; they are sterilized by autoclaving, the stopper and neck of the bottle being covered over by two layers of kraft paper. Alternatively, 6-oz screw-capped bottles may be used. These are wrapped in kraft paper and sterilized in the autoclave. The opening and closing of the bottle in the process of collecting a sample must be carried out with meticulous care to avoid any bacterial contamination from an outside source. When water is drawn from a tap, the mouth of the tap should be flamed, e.g. with a blow-lamp or spirit lamp, and the water allowed to run for 5 min before filling the bottle. In the case of streams, rivers and lakes, the stopper should be removed carefully with one hand, and with the other the bottle held at its base should be inserted, mouth downward, a foot below the surface of the water; the bottle is then turned so that the mouth is directed to the current and water flows into the bottle without coming into contact with the hand. If there is no current the bottle should be moved horizontally, the mouth foremost, so that water flows into it. The bottle is then brought to the surface and the stopper is replaced. Care must be taken that the stopper is not contaminated during the sampling process. This method of sampling avoids the collection of surface water, which may contain a good deal of decomposing vegetable matter.

When a sample is to be obtained from a depth, a bottle weighted with lead is used, having two cords attached—one to the neck, the other to the stopper; the bottle is lowered to the required depth, and is filled by jerking out the stopper by means of the attached cord; the bottle is then quickly raised to the surface and re-stoppered.

When three hours or more must elapse before the laboratory examination can be carried out, the bottles should be kept on ice. Special insulated boxes for the purpose can be obtained and are essential where specimens have to be transported some distance.

Neutralization of Chlorine. If a sample is taken from a chlorinated water supply it is important that any traces of free chlorine should be neutralized immediately as otherwise killing of bacteria may proceed in the time elapsing before the specimen is examined in the laboratory. A crystal of sodium thiosulphate introduced into the sampling bottle prior to sterilization serves to effect neutralization.

Immediately before testing, the water sample should be mixed by inverting the bottle 25 times. Thereafter some of the contents are poured off, the stopper is replaced and the bottle is shaken vigorously 25 times with an up-and-down movement.

PRESUMPTIVE COLIFORM COUNT (MULTIPLE TUBE TECHNIQUE)

An estimation of the number of coliform bacilli in a water supply is usually made by adding varying quantities of the water (from 0·1 ml to 50 ml) to bile salt lactose peptone water (with an indicator of acidity) or in a chemically defined medium in which the bile salt has been substituted by glutamic acid, known as 'improved formate lactose glutamate medium' (see p. 145) contained in bottles with Durham tubes to show the formation of gas; acid and gas formation (a 'positive' result) indicates the growth of coliform bacilli. In this way it is possible to state the smallest quantity of water containing a coliform bacillus and thus to express the degree of contamination with this group of organisms.

This method requires examination by culture of several samples of several different quantities of the water so that an average result can be stated. It has been shown that if one 50 ml, five 10 ml and five 1 ml volumes, or five 10 ml, five 1 ml and five 0·1 ml volumes are tested, the probable number of coliform bacilli in 100 ml can be computed according to the various combinations of positive and negative results, tables compiled by McCrady being used for the purpose (p. 275). This is the method recommended for routine use.

Method. Measured amounts (see above) of single and double strength modified MacConkey's fluid medium are sterilized in bottles containing a Durham tube for indicating gas production. The size of the bottle varies with the quantity of medium and water to be added to it.

With sterile graduated pipettes the following amounts of water are added:

One 50 ml quantity of water to 50 ml double strength medium

Five 10 ml quantities each to 10 ml double strength medium

Five 1 ml quantities each to 5 ml single strength medium

Five 0·1 ml quantities each to 5 ml single strength medium

This range of quantities may be altered according to the likely condition of the water examined; thus, the 50 ml quantity is included when testing filtered or chlorinated water, and in this case it is unnecessary to examine 0·1 ml volumes. This amount i.e. 1 ml of the sample diluted 1 in 10 (for dilution technique see above), is tested only when the water supply is suspected of being highly contaminated.

The bottles are incubated at 37°C and examined after 18–24 h. Those that show acid and sufficient gas to fill the concavity at the top of the Durham tube are considered to be 'presumptive positive' as a result of the growth of coliform bacilli. Any remaining negative bottles are reincubated for another 24 h, and if acid and gas develop they too are regarded as being positive. In reporting the results of the presumptive test reference is now made to McCrady's probability tables. According to the various combinations of positive and negative results obtained the probable number of coliform bacilli in 100 ml of the water can be read.

DIFFERENTIAL COLIFORM TEST

To ascertain whether the coliform bacilli detected in the presumptive test are *Esch. coli.* the Eijkman test is usually employed. This depends on the ability of *Esch. coli* to produce gas when growing in bile-salt lactose peptone water at 44°C, and the inability of atypical coliform bacilli to do this. After the usual presumptive test, subcultures are made from all the bottles showing acid and gas into fresh tubes of single strength MacConkey's medium. It is advisable to heat the tubes to 37°C in a water-bath before inoculating them. They are then incubated at 44°C and examined after 24 h. Those yielding gas may be regarded as containing *Esch. coli* and a computation of the number in 100 ml of water can be made as before. This is the 'confirmed *Esch. coli* count'.

An alternative medium for use in the Eijkman test is *brilliant green bile broth* which

tends to suppress the growth of anaerobic lactose-fermenting organisms, such as *Cl. welchii*, that might otherwise give false positive

Probability Tables (according to McCrady)

Quantity of water	50 ml	10 ml	1 ml	
No. of samples of each quantity tested	1	5	5	
	0	0	0	0
	0	0	1	1
	0	0	2	2
	0	1	0	1
	0	1	1	2
	0	1	2	3
	0	2	0	2
	0	2	1	3
	0	2	2	4
	0	3	0	3
	0	3	1	5
	0	4	0	5
	1	0	0	1
	1	0	1	3
	1	0	2	4
	1	0	3	6
	1	1	0	3
	1	1	1	5
	1	1	2	7
	1	1	3	9
	1	2	0	5
	1	2	1	7
	1	2	2	10
	1	2	3	12
	1	3	0	8
	1	3	1	11
	1	3	2	14
	1	3	3	18
	1	3	4	20
	1	4	0	13
	1	4	1	17
	1	4	2	20
	1	4	3	30
	1	4	4	35
	1	4	5	40
	1	5	0	25
	1	5	1	35
	1	5	2	50
	1	5	3	90
	1	5	4	160
	1	5	5	180+

Left axis label: Number giving positive reaction (acid and gas)

Right axis label: Probable number of coliform bacilli in 100 ml of water

Quantity of water	10 ml	1 ml	0·1 ml	
No. of samples of each quantity tested	5	5	5	
	0	0	0	0
	0	0	1	2
	0	0	2	4
	0	1	0	2
	0	1	1	4
	0	1	2	6
	0	2	0	4
	0	2	1	6
	0	3	0	6
	1	0	0	2
	1	0	1	4
	1	0	2	6
	1	0	3	8
	1	1	0	4
	1	1	1	6
	1	1	2	8
	1	2	0	6
	1	2	1	8
	1	2	2	10
	1	3	0	8
	1	3	1	10
	1	4	0	11
	2	0	0	5
	2	0	1	7
	2	0	2	9
	2	0	3	12
	2	1	0	7
	2	1	1	9
	2	1	2	12
	2	2	0	9
	2	2	1	12
	2	2	2	14
	2	3	0	12
	2	3	1	14
	2	4	0	15
	3	0	0	8
	3	0	1	11
	3	0	2	13
	3	1	0	11
	3	1	1	14
	3	1	2	17
	3	1	3	20
	3	2	0	14
	3	2	1	17
	3	2	3	20
	3	3	0	17
	3	3	1	20
	3	4	0	20
	3	4	1	25
	3	5	0	25

Left column label (vertical): Number giving positive reaction (acid and gas). Right column label (vertical): Probable number of coliform bacilli in 100 ml of water

Quantity of water	10 ml	1 ml	0·1 ml	
No. of samples of each quantity tested	5	5	5	
	4	0	0	13
	4	0	1	17
	4	0	2	20
	4	0	3	25
	4	1	0	17
	4	1	1	20
	4	1	2	25
	4	2	0	20
	4	2	1	25
	4	2	2	30
	4	3	0	25
	4	3	1	35
	4	3	2	40
	4	4	0	35
	4	4	1	40
	4	4	2	45
	4	5	0	40
	4	5	1	50
	4	5	2	55
	5	0	0	25
	5	0	1	30
	5	0	2	45
	5	0	3	60
	5	0	4	75
	5	1	0	35
	5	1	1	45
	5	1	2	65
	5	1	3	85
	5	1	4	115
	5	2	0	50
	5	2	1	70
	5	2	2	95
	5	2	3	120
	5	2	4	150
	5	2	5	175
	5	3	0	80
	5	3	1	110
	5	3	2	140
	5	3	3	175
	5	3	4	200
	5	3	5	250
	5	4	0	130
	5	4	1	170
	5	4	2	225
	5	4	3	275
	5	4	4	350
	5	4	5	425
	5	5	0	250
	5	5	1	350
	5	5	2	550
	5	5	3	900
	5	5	4	1600
	5	5	5	1800+

reactions at 44°C. Positive results in this medium are indicated by gas production and turbidity. There is no colour change. In trial carried out by the PHLS Standing Committee on Bacteriological Examination of Water Supplies (1968) it was found that 1 per cent lactose ricinoleate broth gave better results than brilliant green broth and was less subject to variability of the bile or brilliant green.

Two types of atypical coliform bacilli are known to give rise to gas production at 44°C. They were classified as Irregular Type II and Irregular Type VI by Wilson *et al.* (1935) and these terms are still retained in water bacteriology since complete identification of the organisms is not necessary. Unlike typical coliform bacilli these types are unable to produce indole at 44°C. Although these irregular types rarely occur in water supplies in this country, the joints of water mains are sometimes packed with imported jute which may be contaminated with them; it is therefore advisable when carrying out Eijkman tests to inoculate at the same time tubes of peptone water from the positive 'presumptive' tubes. All tubes are incubated at 44°C.

The interpretation of results shown in Table 12.1 is given by Mackenzie *et al.* (1948).

It is very important that incubation at 44°C should be carried out in a thermostatically controlled water-bath that does not deviate more than 0·5°C from 44°C. An incubator is not satisfactory.

For fuller differentiation of the coliform group by means of the methyl-red, Voges-Proskauer, citrate-utilization and sugar fermentation reactions, reference should be made to Chapter 7.

The Plate Count (Colony Count)

With a sterile graduated pipette place 1 ml water in a sterile Petri dish (4 in diameter) and add 10 ml yeast extract agar, melted and cooled to 50°C; mix thoroughly and allow to solidify. The agar should be as transparent as possible.

If the water is suspected of being contaminated, plate out a smaller quantity, e.g. 0·1 ml, and in dealing with specimens which may be highly polluted it is advisable to make a series of plate cultures with further decreasing quantities of the water. Serial dilutions may be made from the sample, e.g. 1 in 10, 1 in 100, etc., using sterile quarter-strength Ringer's solution as a diluent. In preparing the 1 in 10 solution, 10 ml of the well-mixed sample is added to 90 ml of Ringer's solution contained in a screw-capped bottle of 120 ml capacity. After thorough mixing, further tenfold dilutions can be prepared by transferring 10 ml of the 1 in 10 dilution to a second bottle of 90 ml Ringer's solution and so on. One ml quantities of each dilution are then plated.

Prepare duplicate plates from each volume or dilution, and incubate one at 37°C for one day and the other at 20°–22°C for three days. Those organisms that grow rapidly at 37°C are mainly parasitic and are derived from excremental contamination, while those growing best at 20°–22°C are the natural saprophytes of water and soil. It is customary in some laboratories to extend the incubation period at 37°C to 48 h. This is not recommended since after two days certain saprophytic bacteria capable of growing more slowly at 37°C may have developed into visible colonies.

After incubation, the colonies that have developed in the medium are counted using a hand lens, if necessary, to detect small colonies. Each colony may be taken to represent one viable bacterium in the original specimen.

To facilitate the counting of colonies, to prevent eye-strain and to minimize inaccuracies, it is desirable that a special illuminated counting box fitted with a magnifying glass should be used and a mechanical hand tally counter. As

Table 12.1

Gas in brilliant green bile broth at 44°C	Indole production at 44°C	
+	+	Typical coliform bacilli
+	−	Irregular types of coliform organisms
−	+	
−	−	Other coliform organisms

each colony is recorded it should be 'spotted' by pen and ink on the under surface of the plate. If there are large numbers of colonies present divide the plate into sections by ruling lightly on the under surface with a grease pencil and count the colonies in each section. If the plates prepared from the undiluted water show between 30 and 300 colonies, these should be counted. If there are more than 300 colonies and the sample has been diluted, then the plates giving counts between 30 and 300 should be selected and the other discarded. If all plates show more than 300 colonies, then the result should be reported as more than 300 multiplied by the reciprocal of the highest dilution used; e.g. if the sample was diluted 1 in 100, the result would be given as 'more than 30 000'. Alternatively, provided no more than 500 colonies are present, a count of more than 300 colonies may be made as accurately as possible and the result given as an approximate one. Since only a proportion of the bacteria originally present in the water are capable of developing under the conditions of the test, the total colony count represents the number of organisms per ml of the sample, which have grown at the specified temperature (i.e. 37°C or 22°C) in the specified time (i.e. one day or three days). The result is expressed briefly as the plate count per ml at 37°C and 22°C.

INTERPRETATION OF RESULTS

It must be realized that it is not possible to lay down rigid bacteriological standards to which all drinking-water supplies should conform. The bacteriological flora of water varies widely according to the nature of the supply, i.e. whether it is derived from a well, river, lake or reservoir, and to the climatic conditions prevailing in the gathering grounds. The aim of the authorities should be to obtain a thorough knowledge of the topography of the catchment area and in the light of this to establish a standard for that particular supply, based on regular and frequent bacteriological examinations. Any later deviation from that standard should be viewed with suspicion.

Generally speaking, the results of plate counts are by themselves of little value in estimating the hygienic quality of a water supply, though where regular observations are made on the same supply, a high count on a particular occasion may draw attention to a fault requiring investigation. A slight rise in the colony count of water from a deep well which is normally very pure may be the earliest indication that a defect has occurred in the structure of the well, which is allowing its pollution from outside. The plate count is also of value in judging the efficacy of water treatment processes and in indicating whether a particular supply is suitable for use in the preparation of food and drink, where a high bacterial content may lead to food spoilage.

The test for coliform bacilli is of much greater value in assessing the quality of a water supply. In interpreting the results, however, the nature of the supply must still be taken into account. Heavy rain after a dry spell may cause flooding of the countryside carrying soil and vegetation into a water supply or give rise to flooding of drains and cesspools with the risk of more serious contamination. Bacteriological examination therefore should always be carried out after a sudden climatic change of this kind.

Chlorinated supplies. The water supplied to most large cities is treated by chlorination. In Report No. 71 (Department of Health and Social Security, 1969) it is recommended that if tests reveal the presence of coliform bacilli (of any kind) in 100 ml of chlorinated water as it enters the distribution system, the treatment should be considered inefficient. Since, however, spore-bearing bacilli such as *Cl. welchii* may survive chlorination and give a positive reaction in the presumptive test, it is advisable, before condemning the supply, to confirm the result by subculture to 1 per cent lactose ricinoleate broth or brilliant green bile broth for incubation at 37°C for 48 h. Production of gas in these media within 48 h confirms the presence of coliform organisms. The presumptive positive tubes should also be plated out on MacConkey agar so that if coliform organisms are present a pure culture may be obtained for further differential tests if necessary.

Non-chlorinated piped supplies. Non-chlorinated piped water supplies are not recommended. Where small supplies of this sort still exist it is not considered satisfactory if *Esch. coli* is present in 100 ml or if coliform organisms persist or increase to numbers greater than 3 per 100 ml in water entering the distribution system. It is considered that the presence of *Esch. coli* in 100 ml of water in a supply of this nature renders it unfit for drinking purposes. On the other hand, a certain degree of latitude with regard to the coliform count is permitted, since it is difficult to prevent the occasional presence of atypical coliform organisms in untreated water. For water taken in the distribution system the following standards are recommended: (1) 95 per cent should not contain any coliform organisms or *Esch. coli* in 100 ml; (2) no sample should contain more than 10 coliform organisms per 100 ml; (3) no sample should contain more than two *Esch. coli* per 100 ml; (4) no sample should contain 1 or 2 *Esch. coli* in conjunction with a total coliform count of 3 or more per 100 ml; (5) coliform organisms should not be detectable in 100 ml of any two consecutive samples.

It has been emphasized that the above standards only apply to the water as it enters the distribution system. Between that point and the consumers' premises there may be many sources of contamination (e.g. defective washers on taps, packing in joints of water pipes, service reservoirs or cisterns may all harbour coliform organisms). If a comparison of the water before and after distribution reveals wide differences in the quality, then steps should be taken without delay to detect and remove the cause. The WHO Report (1961) has recommended certain minimum requirements regarding the frequency of testing of water as it enters the distribution system depending on the size of population and whether or not the water requires to be treated. Samples collected from various points within the distribution system, whether or not the water is subject to chlorination, should be taken at the intervals shown in Table 12.2.

Unpiped rural supplies. In small rural communities where no piped water supply is available, a private supply, e.g. a shallow well adequately protected from obvious sources of pollution, should be considered adequate if the coliform count is less than 10 per 100 ml. If it fails repeatedly to keep within that limit, or if *Esch. coli* appears in more than minimal numbers, the supply should be condemned for drinking purposes.

Pollution resulting from heavy rain. It is particularly advisable to test all water supplies at short intervals after heavy rain follows a dry spell. A sudden increase in the number of coliform bacilli after rain might indicate flooding of the surrounding countryside and the potential danger of water-borne disease often associated with flood water.

Examination for Streptococci. The type of streptococcus indicative of faecal pollution is *Streptococcus faecalis.* This organism grows in the medium used for the test for coliform bacilli and by itself ferments the lactose but without gas production. Its presence in water can therefore be determined by further examination of the contents of the bottles showing acid or acid and gas fermentation in the presumptive coliform test.

In order to isolate *Strept. faecalis* from other organisms which may be present, several methods have been advocated. The Metropolitan Water Board have obtained the most satisfactory results from the use of a medium containing sodium azide (Hannay and Norton, 1947). Subcultures from all positive bottles in the presumptive coliform test are made into tubes containing 5 ml of sterile sodium azide medium. The presence of *Strept. faecalis* is indicated by the production of acid in the medium within 48 h at an incubation temperature of 45°C. Their presence in any tubes which become acid should be confirmed by plating out a heavy inoculum on MacConkey's agar.

Table 12.2

Population	Maximum interval between successive samples	Minimum number of samples from distribution system each month
Less than 20 000	1 month ⎫	
20 000 to 50 000	2 weeks ⎬	1 per 5000 of population per month
50 000 to 100 000	4 days ⎭	
More than 100 000	1 day	1 per 10 000 of population per month

Strept. faecalis produces characteristic minute red colonies.

The demonstration of *Strept. faecalis* is of value in confirming the faecal origin of coliform bacilli in cases where there may be difficulty in interpreting the results of the coliform test. *Examination for Clostridium welchii.* 50 ml of water are added to 100 ml of sterile milk (or litmus milk medium) in a stoppered bottle of suitable size. The bottle is then heated at 80°C for 15 min to destroy non-sporing organisms. Sterile liquid paraffin is run on to the surface of the medium to maintain anaerobiosis.

The tubes should be incubated for at least five days at 37°C, although the 'stormy clot' reaction which is indicative of the presence of *Cl. welchii* may develop within 24 to 72 h. If varying quantities of water are examined as in the presumptive coliform test, an estimate of the probable number of *Cl. welchii* in 100 ml of water can be made. This clostridium may be isolated from water more frequently by the use of differential reinforced clostridial medium (DRCM): 4 oz screw-capped bottles containing 50 ml double strength DRCM medium and 50 ml of water sample are incubated at 37°C for 48 h. A positive reaction is indicated by blackening of the medium. One loopful from each positive bottle is then inoculated into a tube of litmus milk and incubated at 37°C for 48 h for confirmation of the presence of *Cl. welchii* by the production of a 'stormy clot' reaction.

Although in recently contaminated water *Cl. welchii* occurs in much smaller numbers than *Esch. coli*, it is able to survive for much longer periods than the non-sporing bacteria of faecal origin. The chief value of the test therefore is in detecting pollution of some earlier date or to confirm the faecal origin of atypical coliform bacilli in the absence of *Esch. coli*.

BACTERIOLOGICAL EXAMINATION OF SEWAGE AND SEWAGE EFFLUENTS

The bacteriological examination of sewage may be carried out to determine the purity of an effluent from a sewage purification process. The procedure is the same as in water examination; an estimation of the viable bacteria present is made by plating and counting colonies, and the test for coliform bacilli is carried out as with a specimen of water; much smaller amounts, however, are tested than in the case of water, depending on the likely extent of pollution of the effluent. The numbers of bacteria per ml in crude sewage vary greatly, e.g. from 1 million to 100 million. Sewage may also be examined by the membrane filter technique.

For isolation of typhoid-paratyphoid bacilli from communal sewage either the sewer swab (Moore, 1948) or the membrane filter method is used.

BACTERIOLOGICAL CONTROL OF SWIMMING BATHS

Public swimming pools and indoor swimming baths may become infected with pathogenic organisms derived either from contaminated water entering the pool or from the bathers. Unless adequate means of purifying the water are provided, this contamination may lead to outbreaks of diseases, such as gastro-enteritis, infections of the respiratory tract, otitis media, infections of the conjunctiva and the skin.

Most modern swimming pools are operated on a system which provides a continuous circulation of the water from the bath at the deep end through a purification plant where it undergoes filtration, clarification and chlorination before entering the pool again at the shallow end. The amount of chlorine introduced into the water is accurately measured and controlled so that the free residual amount present in the bath is maintained between 0·2 and 0·5 parts/10^6 (Ministry of Health, 1951).

The results of bacteriological examinations of samples of water taken from the inlet and outlet of the bath give an indication of the effectiveness of the treatment in maintaining the water free from undesirable contaminants. The methods usually employed are those used for testing samples of drinking-water, viz. an estimation of the number of viable bacteria by the plate counts at 37°C and 22°C and the presumptive test for coliform bacilli followed by the differential tests for *Esch. coli*. The bacteriological quality of the water should approximate to that of high purity drinking-water.

The following standards for water purity were recommended by the Water Sub-committee of the Public Health Laboratory Service (Gray, 1969).

'No samples examined from a bath should contain any coliform organisms in 100 ml of water; and in 75 per cent of the samples examined from the bath the plate count at 37°C from 1 ml of water should not exceed 10 colonies and in the remainder should not exceed 100 colonies.'

Amies (1956) maintains that 'before a swimming pool can be pronounced as satisfactory, the surface water should be examined bacteriologically as well as the main body of the water', and describes a method for doing this. He presents evidence to show that oral or nasal bacteria collect in the surface film of fatty substances derived from the skin and hair of the bathers, and are protected by it from the action of the chlorine. He considers that this surface film may be a contributory factor in the spread of bacterial and viral diseases by swimming pools.

Swimming pools should be provided with overflow gutters into which the polluted film can drain. The method by which the surface film may be removed for bacteriological examination involves the use of calcium alginate gauze which is commercially available as sterilized surgical dressings measuring 4×7 in and weighing 1·2 g. The gauze is laid on the surface of the pool so that the layer of water beneath it is absorbed. It has been calculated that 8·8 g of water is absorbed in this way. The wetted gauze is then placed in a jar containing 50 ml 10 per cent aqueous solution of sodium hexametaphosphate in which it readily dissolves, thus liberating the bacteria. (In order to neutralize the effect of any residual chlorine, 0·1 ml of 10 per cent solution of sodium thiosulphate is added to the jar shortly before the sample is taken.)

The number of bacteria which were present in the surface film can be estimated by a viable count on the solution in the jar. The Miles and Misra technique is suitable for this purpose, blood agar and MacConkey's agar plates being inoculated with standard drops. If necessary the colonies which develop can be readily identified. For further details, reference should be made to the original paper.

THE MEMBRANE FILTER TECHNIQUE FOR THE BACTERIOLOGICAL EXAMINATION OF WATER AND SEWAGE

This method is based on the use of a highly porous cellulose membrane, the pore structure of which enables fairly large volumes of water or aqueous solutions to pass through rapidly under pressure, but prevents the passage of any bacteria present in the sample. These are retained on the surface of the membrane which is then brought into contact with suitable liquid nutrients. These diffuse upwards through the pores thereby inducing the organisms to grow as surface colonies which can be counted.

The technique was first described in this country by Windle Taylor et al., 1953. Since then much investigational work had been done in the laboratories of the Metropolitan Water Board in order to devise modifications suitable as standard techniques for the examination of water samples of all types, both treated and untreated. A review of the progress that has been made in membrane filtration technique has been published (Windle Taylor and Burman, 1964) and further progress described by Windle Taylor (1963–64). See also Report No. 71 (Department of Health and Social Security, 1969).

Membrane filters may also be used for the isolation of pathogens from water and sewage and for the demonstration of tubercle bacilli in cerebrospinal fluid and other fluid specimens including sputa from cases of tuberculosis. (Haley and Rosty, 1957.)

Apparatus

Various types of filtering apparatus suitable for water and sewage examination are now available. One of the most suitable consists of a cylindrical aluminium filter funnel graduated at 50 and 100 ml (A. Gallenkamp & Co. Ltd.) attached by means of a bayonet-locking device to the base of the apparatus which contains a disk of sintered glass on which the membrane is supported. The outlet is provided with a tap and fits into the rubber stopper of a suction jar. British-made membranes of 50 mm diameter marketed by Oxoid Ltd., have been found most satisfactory for the culture of the bacteria. Membranes that have been used for the coliform count may be washed in running water, dried between blotting-paper and sterilized for further use. This may be done up to twelve times, but damaged membranes should always be discarded.

Sterilization

The filtering apparatus is assembled without the membrane, wrapped in kraft paper and sterilized by autoclaving at 121°C for 15 min. Thereafter, between each test, it is sufficient to apply a jet of live steam, or to immerse the apparatus in boiling sterile distilled water for 1 minute. Both the inner and outer surfaces of the funnel as well as its base and the sintered glass disk require to be sterilized in this way. The routine examination of large numbers of water samples is facilitated by the use of several funnels for each piece of apparatus. While one sample is being filtered, the spare funnels for subsequent samples can be sterilized and cooled.

The membranes may be sterilized by one of two methods.

1. Gentle boiling in prefiltered distilled water on two occasions each of 20 min duration. Vigorous boiling tends to make the membranes buckle. This method not only sterilizes but washes out residual solvents and air present in the pores.

2. Autoclaving at 115°C for 10 min. For this purpose bundles of 10 membrane filters are interleaved with disks of good quality absorbent paper (subsequently to be used for holding the liquid medium). The bundles are secured between two pieces of thin card held in position by adhesive tape and the whole is wrapped in kraft paper and sterilized.

Media for Culture on Membrane Filters

1. *M-Yeast extract broth (for the enumeration of viable bacteria).*

In order to obtain results comparable with those of the agar plate count for all types of water, it is necessary to use nutrient broth of the following composition:

Yeast extract	.	.	.	.	6 g
Peptone	.	.	.	.	40 g
Distilled water	.	.	.	.	to 1000 ml
pH	.	.	.	.	.	7·4

2. *Membrane enriched Teepol broth* (0·4 *ET*) *(for estimations of Esch. coli).*

Modification of MacConkey broth previously used for estimating the number of coliform organisms has been replaced by media containing Teepol (0·4 per cent enriched Teepol broth—0·4 ET—see p. 125). This allows a count of coliform organisms and *Esch. coli* to be made in 18 hours and the use of a separate medium for resuscitation is unnecessary when this medium is used.

Method of Filtration

After sterilization, the filtering apparatus is inserted into the suction jar attached to the vacuum pump, the outlet tap being closed. The funnel is removed, and with sterile forceps one of the membranes is laid, grid-side up, on the top of the sintered glass disk. By turning on the pressure and opening the tap carefully, the membrane is sucked down and comes to lie quite flat against the disk. (In order to protect the membrane and hasten filtration, a disk of filter paper should be inserted between the supporting glass disk and the membrane.) After closing the tap and releasing the pressure, the funnel is screwed into place and a suitable amount of water to be examined is poured into it. The actual amount depends on the likely degree of pollution. If there is doubt about this, two or more different volumes of the sample should be filtered. The following amounts are recommended:

Purified tap water	.	.	250–500 ml
Well water	.	.	10 and 100 ml
River water	.	.	1 and 10 ml

Water which is highly contaminated should be diluted to 1 in 10, 1 in 100 and 1 in 1000 and each dilution filtered. Quantities smaller than 20 ml should be made up to that amount with sterile distilled water before being passed through the filter.

When the water has been filtered and a small

amount of sterile distilled water allowed to pass through as a final rinse the funnel is removed and the vacuum released. The membrane is then transferred with sterile flat-bladed forceps to a 2-in Petri dish containing a sterile absorbent pad (Whatman's No. 17 pads, 5 or 6 cm in diameter, are suitable), saturated with about 2 ml of the appropriate liquid medium. The membrane should be placed on the moist pad in such a way as to exclude any air bubbles. The Petri dish is then inverted with the pad and membrane adhering to the base and incubated in a moist atmosphere.

Incubation. For total colony counts at 37°C incubation for 18 h on yeast extract broth gives results that are comparable with the agar plate counts at that temperature. For colony counts at 22°C incubation for 3 days is necessary. All the colonies that develop on the membranes are counted and the number of bacteria per ml of undiluted water may then be calculated. For membrane coliform counts, the cultures on 0·4 per cent enriched Teepol broth are incubated for 4 h at 30°C followed by 14 h at 35°C. The number of yellow colonies is then counted. These merely represent lactose fermenting organisms that may or may not be gas producers. Their identity is presumed to be that of coliform bacilli for the purpose of routine water examination, but this can be confirmed by the usual tests if required.

For further studies on the Membrane Filter Technique reference should be made to the reports of the Metropolitan Water Board quoted above and to Department of Health and Social Security (1969) Report No. 71.

Isolation of Pathogenic Organisms from Water and Sewage

By Membrane Filter Technique. Relatively large amounts of the fluid to be tested, i.e. 500 ml or more, depending on the amount of suspended matter present, can be passed through the membrane filter fairly rapidly. If pathogenic organisms are present, even in small numbers, they will be retained on the surface of the membrane, and by transferring it to a suitable differential medium there is a reasonable chance of isolating them.

For isolating typhoid and paratyphoid bacilli Wilson and Blair's bismuth sulphite medium has been reported as giving satisfactory results by this method. The membrane may be placed directly on the agar medium in a small Petri dish, the proportion of agar having been reduced to 1·5 per cent, but Kabler and Clark (1952) recommend the use of absorbent pads impregnated with double-strength liquid medium (agar omitted). Characteristic convex black colonies with a paler periphery appear within 30 h at 37°C. If discrete, each one is surrounded by a halo, showing a metallic sheen. Blackening of the medium underneath the membrane is suggestive of typhoid colonies. In such a case, it is necessary to transfer the membrane to a tube or bottle of liquid medium such as tetrathionate broth or selenite enrichment medium subculturing from this after 18 to 24 h incubation at 37°C on desoxycholate citrate agar.

In order to isolate intestinal pathogens, other than typhoid and paratyphoid bacilli, Kabler and Clark recommend a preliminary incubation of the membrane for 3 h in contact with single-strength tetrathionate broth without chalk before transferring it to a differential medium. Incubation of the membrane for 3 h on this medium tends to inhibit coliform bacilli and enhances the growth of salmonellae other than *Salmonella typhi.* Characteristic colonies may then be recognized and subcultured for the usual confirmatory tests.

By a Concentration Technique, using a membrane filter apparatus with pulverized diatomaceous earth. The Metropolitan Water Board have reported satisfactory results from the use of a modification of the method of Hammerström and Ljutov (1954) and Ljutov (1954) for isolating pathogenic intestinal organisms from water and sewage. The technique is so simple and quickly carried out that its use is to be recommended rather than that mentioned above: Windle Taylor (1963–64).

A layer of diatomaceous earth (Hyflo Super-Cel) is substituted for the membrane at the bottom of the filter funnel, supported on a disk of stainless steel wire micro-mesh. After setting up the filtering apparatus with the micro-mesh in place, a small amount of sterile distilled water is poured into the funnel and to this is added a quantity of 1 per cent sterile Hyflo Super-Cel suspension to give the required thickness. The pressure is turned on and the measured sample poured in before all the sterile water has gone through. (Up to 100 litres of water can be filtered in thirty minutes, sewage from 3 to 10 ml suitably diluted, and effluent 50–500 ml.) After all the fluid has been sucked through, the wire-mesh support is lifted off with sterile forceps and the paste tipped into 100 ml selenite F medium in a screw-capped bottle (4 in in depth by 2 in in diameter). This is incubated at 42°C. After 18 h subcultures are made on selective media.

(Hyflo Super-Cel is a diatomaceous silica filter-aid preparation obtainable from the Johns-Manville Company Ltd., 20 Albert Embankment, London SW1.)

BACTERIOLOGICAL EXAMINATION OF MILK

In hygiene work the bacteriological examination of milk generally consists of:

1. An enumeration of viable bacteria present in a given quantity.

2. A quantitative estimation of contamination by coliform bacilli.

3. The determination of the presence of specific pathogenic organisms, e.g. *Myco. tuberculosis*.

Since 1936 the *methylene blue reduction test* has been used as a standard official method in England for gauging milk purity, i.e. as a substitute for the bacterial count. It depends on the reduction and decolourization of the dye by the bacteria in the milk, and the rate of reduction affords a measure of the degree of bacterial contamination.

As a check on the pasteurization of milk, the *phosphatase test* is now a standard procedure; it determines the inactivation by heat of the enzyme phosphatase, which is normally present in cow's milk. Activity of this enzyme implies that the milk has not been adequately heated for the destruction of pathogenic organisms present.

The *turbidity test* is the official test for 'sterilized' milk, i.e. milk that has been heated to 212°F (100°C) or over for such a period as to ensure that it will satisfy the turbidity test. The test depends on the fact that by heating to the degree necessary for sterilization the heat-coagulable proteins are precipitated, so that if ammonium sulphate is then added and the mixture filtered and boiled for 5 min no turbidity results. The test also distinguishes between pasteurized and 'sterilized' milk.

Under the Milk (Special Designation) Regulations, 1963 and 1965 of England, and the Milk (Special Designations) (Scotland) Order, 1965 and 1966, standard methods for testing milk have been prescribed in official memoranda. These should be consulted for full details of the methods recommended. Recently, a new special designation, '*Ultra Heat Treated*', has been prescribed in relation to milk that has been retained at a temperature of 270°F (132·2°C) for not less than one second.

BACTERIOLOGICAL STANDARDS

England and Wales

The following standards have been laid down under the Milk (Special Designation) Amendment Regulations, 1965 and 1972:

'*Untreated*' *milk* and '*Pasteurized*' *milk* when tested by the prescribed method at 9.30 a.m. on the day following that on which the sample was taken, must fail to decolourize methylene blue in 30 min. Before testing the samples must be maintained at atmospheric shade temperature when tested during the period 1st May to 31st October and at atmospheric shade temperature until 5 p.m. on the day of sampling and thereafter at a constant temperature of 17°C to 20°C when tested during 1st November to 30th April. The test is not carried out if the atmospheric temperature exceeds 21°C.

'*Pasteurized*' *milk* must also satisfy the phosphatase test (see above), i.e. when tested under the prescribed conditions the milk must give a reading of 10 μg or less of *p*-nitrophenol per ml of milk.

'*Sterilized*' *milk* must satisfy the turbidity test described above.

'*Ultra Heat Treated*' *milk* must satisfy a colony count test by yielding less than 10 colonies per standard loop (approx. 0·01 ml capacity) when grown in yeastrel milk agar at a preselected temperature of between 30°C and 37°C for 48 h.

Scotland

The special designations that may be used in Scotland are '*Premium*', '*Standard*', '*Pasteurized*', '*Sterilized*' and '*Ultra Heat Treated*'. The standards required by the Milk (Special Designations) (Scotland) Order when tested according to the provisions laid down in the Order are as follows:

'*Premium*' *milk* must contain not more than 15 000 bacteria per ml and no coliform bacteria in 0·01 ml.

'*Standard*' *milk* must not contain more than 50 000 bacteria per ml and no coliform bacteria in 0·001 ml.

'*Pasteurized*' *milk* must contain no coliform bacteria in 0·01 ml and on submission to the phosphatase test must give a reading not exceeding 10 μg of *p*-nitrophenol per ml of milk.

'*Sterilized*' *milk* must satisfy the turbidity test.

'*Ultra Heat Treated*' *milk* must contain not more than 1000 bacteria per ml.

SAMPLING. If the milk is contained in retail bottles, one unopened bottle delivered to the laboratory constitutes the sample. When the milk is in a bulk container it must be carefully mixed before a sample is taken. This can be done by means of a sterile plunger which is moved up and down several times in the milk. The specimen is then obtained with a sterile dipper from well below the surface of the milk and placed in a sterile 4 oz stoppered or screw-capped bottle. Bottles containing the milk samples should be dispatched to the testing laboratory without delay in an insulated box and should be examined as soon as possible after arrival except in the cases of 'Untreated' milk tested by the methylene blue test which requires special storage temperatures depending on the time of the year and 'Ultra Heat Treated' milk samples which are retained at 30°C for 24 h before being tested for the bacterial count.

TECHNIQUE OF ESTIMATING THE NUMBER OF VIABLE BACTERIA. The medium recommended in the regulations is yeast extract milk agar.

A series of dilutions of the milk sample is made up in sterile stoppered bottles with sterile tap water as follows:

1 in 10 90 ml water *plus* 10 ml milk
1 in 100 90 ml water *plus* 10 ml of the 1 in 10 dilution
1 in 1000 90 ml water *plus* 10 ml of the 1 in 100 dilution

Before these dilutions are made, the specimen should be carefully mixed by inverting the sample bottle about 25 times. The dilutions must also be mixed, but without vigorous shaking. The pipettes used should be straight-sided and appropriately graduated. For each dilution a separate sterile pipette should be used.

For testing *premium* milk under the Scottish regulations 1 ml of the 1 in 100 dilution is plated, duplicate or preferably triplicate plates being made; in examining *standard* milk 1 ml of the 1 in 1000 dilution is plated as above. The doluted milk is placed with a sterile pipette in a sterile Petri dish (4 in diameter) and 10 ml of melted agar cooled to 45°C is added and mixed with the milk by rotating the plate carefully first to the right, then to the left, so that the organisms are uniformly distributed throughout the agar.

The time between the preparation of the dilutions and the mixing with the medium should not exceed 15 min.

After the medium has solidified, the plates are incubated in the inverted position for 72 h at 30°C ± 0·5°C.

The number of colonies including 'pin-point' colonies, is counted in each plate and the mean calculated; this multiplied by the dilution is reported as the 'number of viable bacteria per ml'. The count is made as described above. If the number of colonies in a plate is over 300, a count may be made of those in a given part of the plate and the total is then calculated; but it is advisable in examining a milk of unknown quality to plate 1 ml of each dilution and use for the count those showing 30 to 300 colonies.

Ultra heat-treated milk samples are maintained in the unopened sample bottle in an incubator at a temperature of between 30°C and 37°C (in Scotland at 30°C ± 0·5°C) for 24 h. Under the Scottish milk regulations at the end of the 24 h incubation period, 1 ml of 1 in 10 dilution of the milk is plated as above and the Petri dish cultures are then incubated at 30°C ± 0·5°C for 48 h and the colonies counted. In England the milk is withdrawn from about 1 ml below the surface by means of a standard iridium platinum loop. (The loop has an internal diameter of 4 mm and is made of wire conforming to British Standard 19 containing 10 per cent iridium. It will withdraw about 0·01 ml milk.) The loopful of milk is transferred to 5 ml melted yeastrel milk agar cooled to between 45°C and 50°C contained in a test tube or screw-capped bottle of 1 oz capacity. The contents are carefully mixed and allowed to solidify in a sloping position. The bottle or tube is then incubated at a temperature of between 30°C and 37°C for 48 h after which time the colonies are counted.

Under the most favourable conditions a specimen of raw milk may contain at least 500 bacteria per ml; but under bad conditions the numbers may reach even several million per ml. The standards given below indicate the degree of bacterial contamination allowable in the case of designated milks.

Test for coliform bacilli. Varying amounts of milk are added to tubes or bottles of bile-salt lactose medium. The range of amounts that require to be tested depends on the likely degree of contamination. In the case of milk of unknown quality the following series is suggested:

1·0 ml of a 1 in 10   dilution of the milk
1·0 ml of a 1 in 100   dilution of the milk
1·0 ml of a 1 in 1000   dilution of the milk
1·0 ml of a 1 in 10 000 dilution of the milk

The decimal dilutions are prepared in series (see above).

The smallest amount that yields acid *and gas* is ascertained.

Under the Scottish regulations, for *premium* and *pasteurized* milk three tubes or bottles containing 10 ml of the above medium are inoculated (by means of a sterile pipette) each with 1 ml of the 1 in 100 dilution of the sample and incubated at 37°C for 48 h. For *standard*, three tubes are inoculated each with 1 ml of the 1 in 1000 dilution. The tubes are examined for acid and gas production; the milk is taken to have passed the test if acid and gas are absent from two of the three tubes.

Methylene blue reduction test. Standard methylene blue tablets must be used. (The names of manufacturers who supply such tablets are furnished by the Ministry of Health.) A standard solution is prepared as follows: one tablet is dissolved in 200 ml cold sterile glass-distilled water in a sterile flask with a rubber stopper. The solution is then made up to 800 ml with distilled water and stored in a cool, dark place. This solution gives a final concentration of methylene blue of approximately 1/300 000, and should not be used after two months.

Test-tubes conforming to the British Standards Specification 625:1959, nominal size 150 × 16 mm and a mark indicating 10 ml are used. They are stoppered with cotton-wool or aluminium caps and sterilized in a hot-air oven (160°C for 1 h). Rubber stoppers to fit the tubes are also required. These are sterilized in boiling water before use.

A thermostatically controlled, covered water-bath, with a rack to hold the tubes immersed in the water, is required; the water should be at 37°–38°C.

1-ml straight-sided pipettes are used for measuring the methylene blue solution (these should conform to a prescribed specification). They are sterilized in the hot-air oven.

The sample is mixed thoroughly, as prior to making the bacterial count (see above).

The milk is poured, with the usual aseptic precautions, into a test-tube up to the 10 ml mark, and 1 ml of methylene blue solution is carefully added. The tube is closed with a sterile rubber stopper which should be inserted with sterile forceps. It is then inverted slowly once or twice and placed in the water-bath.

The following controls should be put up: (1) 10 ml mixed milk *plus* 1 ml methylene blue solution; (2) 10 ml mixed milk *plus* 1 ml tap water. These control tubes are placed for 3 min in boiling water to destroy the natural reducing system of the milk. Comparison with (1) indicates when decolourization is beginning and with (2) when it is complete.

Decolourization is considered complete when the whole column of milk is decolourized or decolourized up to within 5 mm of the surface.

The time of complete decolourization is recorded. For the purposes of the Milk (Special Designation) Regulations *untreated* milk is considered satisfactory if it fails to decolourize methylene blue in 30 min.

RATIONALE OF THE VARIOUS BACTERIOLOGICAL TESTS USED FOR THE EXAMINATION OF MILK

Whichever test is adopted for the routine examination of milk it should be capable of indicating the degree of bacterial contamination and thereby of showing whether the conditions under which the milk is produced and handled are hygienically satisfactory.

The advantage of the plate count for this purpose is that it gives a direct assessment of the number of viable bacteria in the supply. The results are readily understood by the dairy-man, and since it is as suitable for milk of low bacterial content as for grossly contaminated supplies, it will indicate any changes in conditions of production leading to either an improvement or deterioration in quality. On the other hand, the plate count test is costly in time and material, the results are not available for 72 h and owing to the fact that a very small amount of milk is tested and that some of the bacteria are distributed in small clumps and chains, the error of sampling is high.

The coliform test is usually carried out in conjunction with the plate count. It indicates mainly the degree of contamination by coliform organisms arising from dust or unsterile utensils. Since adequate pasteurization destroys the majority of coliform bacilli, the presence of these in milk that passes the phosphatase test is an indication of contamination after pasteurization.

The methylene blue test is simple to carry out and requires a minimum of equipment. In general, the greater the number of bacteria in the milk, the greater their metabolic activity and consequently the shorter the reduction time.

However, milk heavily contaminated with inert bacteria may give a long reduction time, while short reduction times may be the result of non-bacterial reducing systems which are sometimes present in freshly produced milk,

milk obtained late in the lactation period and milk containing leucocytes or other cells.

The time required to reduce the dye is also dependent on the temperature at which the milk is held prior to testing; thus, in the winter, milk gives a longer reduction time than it would in the summer, with the same bacterial content. Allowance is made for this in the higher standard required in the winter time by the English regulations.

It is difficult to compare high-quality milks by means of the standard methylene blue test, since the reduction time is very long for all of them, but the test will readily detect milk of poor hygienic quality. With *pasteurized* milk, provided the milk is kept for at least 24 h at a temperature not exceeding 18°C (65°F) before being tested, the correlation between the reduction time at 37°C and the degree of bacterial contamination is fairly good. The test is of no value for freshly pasteurized milk.

The Resazurin Test. This test which is also a dye reduction test is sometimes used to determine the hygienic quality of a milk supply. One ml of a standard solution of resazurin is added to 10 ml of the well-mixed sample in a sterile test-tube which is then fitted with a sterile rubber stopper and placed in a water-bath at 37·5°C. Unlike methylene blue, the dye resazurin passes through a series of colour changes: blue, lilac, mauve, pink mauve, mauve pink, pink before it is finally reduced to the colourless state by bacterial action; thus a reading may be made at any specified time after the test has been set up and the milk graded according to the amount of reduction that has taken place. A set of colour standards are used in a Lovibond comparator against which the colour of the dye and milk mixture may be matched and the amount of reduction measured. Alternatively, the result may be expressed as the time required for complete reduction of the dye.

The Ten Minute Resazurin Test is used as a 'platform' test in creameries to detect unsatisfactory milk supplies as they arrive. Other modifications of the test are used for special purposes, e.g. the Temperature-Compensated Resazurin Test is used to off-set the effect of variations in atmospheric temperature on the metabolic activity of the bacteria prior to testing the milk. The time of incubation varies, according to the mean atmospheric shade temperature, from 120 min to 15 min for a temperature range of 40° and under to 4°–15·5°C (60°F). (For further details see Chalmers, 1962.)

PHOSPHATASE TEST FOR PASTEURIZED MILK

The statutory test for pasteurized milk is the Aschaffenburg and Mullen phosphatase test. This test determines inactivation of the enzyme phosphatase, normally present in cow's milk, by such degree and time of heating as to destroy non-sporing pathogenic organisms, e.g. 62·8°C (145°F) for 30 min or 71·6°C (161°F) for 15 s, as in the recognized methods of pasteurization. The standard method for detecting the presence of the enzyme is based on its ability to liberate p-nitrophenol from disodium p-nitrophenyl phosphate. This yields a yellow colouration and the result is expressed in arbitrary units that can be read by viewing the degree of colour in a Lovibond comparator.

Apparatus Required

A Lovibond 'all purpose' comparator complete with stand for work in reflected light and a comparator disc APTW or APTW 7. Two fused glass cells 25 mm deep.
A water-bath or incubator at 37·5°C ± 0·5°C.
A pipette to deliver 5 ml.
A supply of 1·0 ml straight-scaled pipettes of an accuracy equal to NPL grade B.
A 1000 ml graduated flask.
A 100 ml measuring cylinder.
A supply of test-tubes of British Standard 625:1959, nominal size 150×16 mm with rubber stoppers.

New glassware should be carefully washed in chromic acid solution and after use test-tubes and pipettes should be thoroughly washed in hot soda water, rinsed in warm water, and then distilled water, and dried. Glassware used for the test should not be used for any other purpose and should be stored separately from other laboratory apparatus.

Buffer-Substrate Solution

1. Buffer solution: 3·5 g anhydrous sodium carbonate and 1·5 g sodium bicarbonate are dissolved in distilled water and made up to one litre.
2. Substrate: 0·15 g disodium p-nitrophenyl phosphate is placed in a 100 ml measuring cylinder and made up to 100 ml with buffer solution.

Method

Five ml of the buffer-substrate solution is transferred to a test-tube which is then stoppered and brought to a temperature of 37°C by placing in a water-bath. One ml of the milk to be tested is added, the test-tube stopper is replaced and the contents shaken to mix. The test-tube is then replaced in the water-bath for exactly 2 h at 37°C. A blank prepared from boiled milk is incubated with each series of samples. Highly coloured milk such as that of Channel Island cows requires a separate blank of the same type of milk. After incubation the tubes are removed from the water-bath and their contents well mixed. The blank is placed on the left hand of the stand and the test sample on the right. Readings are taken in reflected light by looking down on the two apertures with the comparator facing a good source of daylight or a daylight type of artificial illumination. The disc is revolved until the test sample is matched. Readings falling between two standards are reported as plus or minus the figure of the nearest standard.

Interpretation

Milk that gives a reading of 10 μg or less of p-nitrophenol per ml of milk is considered to be properly pasteurized.

The turbidity test for sterilized milk. Add 20 ml of the well-mixed milk to a 50-ml conical flask containing 4 g ammonium sulphate (AR). Shake thoroughly for 1 min to dissolve all the ammonium sulphate. Allow to stand for 5 min and then filter into a test-tube through a Whatman No. 12 folded filter paper (12·5 cm in diameter). Collect at least 5 ml of clear filtrate and place the tube in a beaker of boiling water for 5 min. Cool in cold water and examine the tube for turbidity, holding it in front of an electric light suitably shaded from the eyes. It is advisable to compare it with a tube of milk heated in a boiling water bath for 20 min and then treated with ammonium sulphate in the same way.

An absence of turbidity indicates that the milk has been heated to at least (100°C) 212°F for a period of at least 5 min, which denatures the soluble proteins in the milk so that they can no longer be precipitated by ammonium sulphate. The test will detect the presence of 0·6 to 0·8 per cent raw milk, but owing to the heat resistance of some sporing organisms it gives no indication of the probable keeping quality of the 'sterilized' milk.

Examination for tubercle bacillus. The sample is thoroughly mixed and a quantity of 100 ml is divided into 50 ml amounts and centrifuged for 30 min at a minimum speed of 3000 rev/min. The sediment in each tube is suspended in 2·5 ml of sterile saline solution. It is advisable to add some of the cream to this inoculum. Two guinea-pigs are injected subcutaneously on the inner side of one thigh with the suspended sediment and kept under observation to ascertain whether tuberculosis lesions result. One guinea-pig is killed at the end of four weeks and an autopsy carried out; if it shows no tuberculous lesions, the other animal is kept for eight weeks, when it is killed and examined.

Lesions should be examined microscopically for the tubercle bacillus to confirm their tuberculous nature. (It has been shown that *Br. abortus* which may occur in cow's milk, produces tubercle-like lesions in guinea-pigs. It is advisable to inoculate at least two animals from one specimen, as inoculated guinea-pigs may die sometimes from infection with other organisms present in the milk, e.g. sporing anaerobic bacilli, or some intercurrent disease —e.g. pneumonia, enteritis, etc.—may also cause death before tuberculous lesions have developed and so nullify the test if only one animal is injected.

A direct microscopic examination of the deposit of centrifuged milk for tubercle bacilli may be made.

The absence of tubercle bacilli in films, however, does not exclude their presence in the specimen. On the other hand acid-fast bacilli other than the tubercle bacilli may be revealed. The microscopic test, therefore, is not a valid method of demonstrating tubercle bacilli.

The method of *direct cultivation* described in Chapter 6 can very suitably be applied to unmixed milk taken directly from the cow, but the animal inoculation test is the standard procedure for demonstrating tubercle bacilli in milk samples generally.

Examination for brucella infection in milk. In infected cows the brucella organisms tend to localize in the udder and to be excreted in the milk. They may be isolated by plating out thickly several loopfuls of cream taken directly from the top of the milk on to the surface of plates of glucose serum agar containing various antibiotics to inhibit contaminants (Jones and Brinley-Moyan, 1958). Alternatively, the milk may be centrifuged for 15 min at 1000 rev/min. The milk from below the cream is removed for the Whey Agglutination Test and the sediment mixed with some of the cream is plated out on the selective medium. One ml of the cream and sediment mixture may also be inoculated intramuscularly into two guinea-pigs. After six weeks both animals are killed. Blood is removed to provide serum for agglutination tests with *Br. abortus* suspension. This may give evidence of infection without the need to isolate the organism. The spleen is cut in two aseptically and the cut surface rubbed over a plate of serum dextrose agar. In infected animals the spleen is often considerably enlarged. Care should be exercised in handling the guinea-pigs at post-mortem since faulty technique may readily lead to accidental infection. Inoculated plates are incubated at 37°C in an atmosphere of 10 per cent CO_2 for at least five days. Colonies with the characteristics of brucella organisms should be subcultured on serum dextrose agar slopes and identified by the appropriate means. A slide agglutination test with standard brucella antiserum may be carried out in the first instance to identify the colonies as those of brucella organisms.

MILK RING TEST (MRT) FOR BRUCELLA. The milk of cows suffering from brucella infection of the mammary gland may contain brucella agglutinins. On the addition of a concentrated suspension of *Br. abortus* stained with haematoxylin the bacteria are agglutinated by the antibodies and rise up with the fat globules to form a deep blue ring in the cream layer. The test is very sensitive and may be applied to bulk milk of individual herds since a positive milk continues to give a blue ring reaction even when highly diluted with negative milk from non-infected cows. Care must be taken in interpreting a positive result, however, since the milk of animals immunized against brucellosis in adult life with the avirulent strain of *Br. abortus*, S19 may give a positive ring reaction for two years or more. On the other hand vaccination of calves during the sixth to eighth month does not interfere with this test although conferring a high degree of immunity to infection for several years.

The technique is as follows:

1. Mix the milk thoroughly and pour into a $3 \times \frac{3}{8}$ in test-tube sufficient to give a column of milk about 1 in high.

2. Add 1 drop of stained antigen and mix thoroughly by shaking. Avoid frothing which interferes with the reading of the test.

3. Incubate in a 37°C water-bath for about 40–50 min, i.e. sufficient time for the cream to rise.

The stained antigen* is prepared as follows:

Make a concentrated suspension of *Br. abortus* by washing off mass cultures of a smooth aerobic strain with 0·5 per cent phenol in saline; heat at 60°C for 30 min in a water-bath; wash the cells and pack by centrifuging; stain with haematoxylin diluted 1 in 5 (Ehrlich's or Delafield's) for 5 min; 10 ml of packed cells require 1200 ml of diluted stain; finally suspend the washed stained cells as a 4 per cent suspension in equal parts of glycerol and phenol-saline.

In milk containing brucella agglutinins the bacteria are agglutinated and rise with the cream, forming a blue cream line leaving the skim-milk white. In samples in which there are no agglutinins there is a white cream line and the rest of the milk remains blue.

The results may be interpreted thus:

Positive (+ + +). Cream layer forms a deep blue ring on top of a completely white column of milk. This indicates a high concentration of agglutinins.

Positive (+ +). Cream layer deeply coloured and milk column slightly blue.

Doubtful or weak positive (+). The cream layer has a definite blue ring but the column of milk is distinctly blue.

Negative (±). The cream layer is the same colour or slightly more coloured than the milk column.

Negative (−). The cream layer is white and the milk column blue.

WHEY AGGLUTINATION TEST. This is usually applied to the milk of individual cows. Since it is not considered to be influenced greatly by previous vaccination of the animals it is often used to confirm a positive Milk Ring Test.

A few drops of cheese-making rennet are added to 10 ml skim milk. The tube is incubated for 30 min at 37°C to hasten the coagulation of the casein and the liberation of the water-clear whey. Agglutination tests are carried out on the whey in the usual manner using a standard brucella suspension. A titre of 10 or more is considered diagnostic of udder infection.

Other pathogens in milk. The methods for demonstrating typhoid-paratyphoid bacilli and other pathogens correspond to those used for isolating those organisms from other infected material. The sediment after centrifugation is plated out on the appropriate media and some of the milk added to tubes of selective or enrichment broth. For the methods of identifying the organisms isolated by these means reference should be made to the relevant chapters dealing with the organisms being looked for.

BACTERIOLOGICAL EXAMINATION OF ICE-CREAM

The Ice Cream (Heat Treatment) Regulations 1947 and 1959, issued by the Ministry of Agriculture, Fisheries and Food and the Ministry of Health, require that the ingredients used in the manufacture of ice-cream must be

---

*Obtainable from the Ministry of Agriculture, Fisheries and Food, Central Veterinary Laboratory, New Haw, Weybridge, Surrey.

pasteurized. The general principles and methods applicable to milk can be adopted for the bacteriological examination of ice-cream. This subject has been reported on by the Public Health Laboratory Service Staff of the Medical Research Council (Gillespie *et al.*, 1947, 1948, 1949, 1950; and Lloyd, 1969).

Although no bacteriological standards exist for ice-cream in England and Wales, in a circular (No. 69/47) issued by the Ministry of Health attention is drawn to a form of the methylene blue reduction test for grading ice-cream from the hygienic standpoint. This is described in the first of the above reports.

The test should be commenced at 5 p.m. on the day on which the sample is taken. With a graduated pipette, 7 ml of one-quarter strength Ringer's solution are added to the reduction tube, as used for milk and 1 ml of standard methylene blue solution; the sample is then added up to the 10 ml mark (i.e. 2 ml and constituting a 1 in 5 dilution). With precautions to avoid bacterial contamination the tube is closed with a sterile rubber stopper and inverted once. The tube is placed in a water-bath at 20°C until 10 a.m. on the following day. It is then placed in a water-bath at 37°C and inverted once every half-hour until decolourization is complete, as compared with the control, the time for decolourization being recorded. This control consists of a tube to which are added 8 ml one-quarter strength Ringer's solution, and ice-cream to the 10 ml mark, and incubated at 20°C and 37°C as in the actual test. A methylene blue control should also be included as in milk testing.

According to the time taken at 37°C for complete decolourization the sample is graded provisionally as follows:

Grade 1   over 4 hours.
Grade 2 $2\frac{1}{2}$ to 4 hours.
Grade 3 $\frac{1}{2}$ to 2 hours.
Grade 4   decolourized at time of removal from the 20°C bath.

It is suggested that if ice-cream consistently fails to reach grades 1 and 2, it would be reasonable to regard this as indicating defects of manufacture or handling which call for investigation.

In Scotland the use of the plate count and the test for coliform bacilli are recommended for the bacteriological examination of ice-cream. According to the Ice-Cream (Scotland) Regulations of the Scottish Home and Health Department (SHHD) 1970, a bacterial count of 50 000 per g and over and the presence of coliform bacilli in 0·01 g are regarded as indicating faults in the manufacture and handling of ice-cream.

BACTERIOLOGICAL EXAMINATION OF SHELLFISH

The method used by Bigger (1934) for examining mussels is recommended with a few slight modifications. It may also be adapted to the examination of all types of shellfish including other bivalves such as oysters and univalves such as winkles and cockles.

Bigger's procedure for preparing the mussel emulsion is as follows:

1. Ten mussels of average size are selected.

2. These are washed with running tap water, using a boiled nail brush.

3. One is grasped with sterile ovum forceps, rinsed under the tap and then with sterile water.

4. It is placed on a piece of sterile parchment paper in which it is grasped with the left hand. The shell is held with the flat edge towards the body, the anterior (pointed) end to the left and the left valve of the shell upwards.

5. A small portion of the shell at the broad (posterior) end is nibbled away with sterile nibbling forceps, and through the opening the blade of a sterile scalpel is inserted. With this the posterior adductor muscle and the other attachments of the mussel to the left valve are cut, and, holding them with the paper interposed between them and the hands, the two valves of the shell are separated and the left one removed.

6. All the fluid in the shell is poured off and, with the help of the scalpel, the body is transferred to a small beaker provided with a graduation at the 25 ml level.

7. The body of the mussel in the beaker is thoroughly minced with a sterile pair of scissors. Sterile saline is added up to the 25 ml mark and mixed thoroughly with the minced body, the scissors being used for this purpose.

It has been found advisable to include the shell fluid in the test and to make up the volume to 25 ml with sterile water instead of saline in order to counteract the high salt content already present.

Varying amounts, viz. 0·5, 0·1 and 0·02 ml of the minced mussel emulsion are then added to tubes of bile-salt lactose medium. The following technique is suggested:

Add 25 ml sterile water to the beaker containing the 25 ml minced mussel emulsion, thus making a dilution of 1 in 2. With a sterile pipette, 1 ml of this dilution is added to 10 ml of bile-salt lactose medium; 2 ml of the dilution are next transferred with the same pipette to 8 ml sterile water in a test-tube giving a second dilution of 1 in 10. Using a fresh sterile pipette, 1 ml of the 1 in 10 dilution is added to a second tube of bile-salt lactose medium and 0·2 ml of the same dilution to a third tube of the medium. For greater accuracy duplicate tubes of bile-salt lactose medium are recommended for each dilution. This procedure is repeated with each mussel and the cultures are incubated at 37°C for 24 h when they are examined for acid and gas production. An additional reading is made after a further 24 h. When two tubes of medium are employed for each dilution, results are reported as positive only when acid and gas are produced in both tubes.

It has been found advantageous to use Eijkman's test to confirm the presence of typical or 'faecal' coliform bacilli. Subcultures are made from each 'positive' tube into fresh tubes of bile-salt lactose medium and are incubated at 44°C. The development of gas at this temperature within 24 h is considered to be evidence of the presence of *Esch. coli*.

Interpretation of results. According to Bigger's suggested standard, a batch of mussels should be considered undesirably contaminated if more than seven out of the ten tested have coliform bacilli in 0·5 ml of minced mussel emulsion or more than three in 0·1 ml or more than one in 0·02 ml.

Consignments of shellfish should not be condemned on the result of one examination alone, but only on a series of results combined with what is known of the condition of the source of the supply and the methods of treatment and handling after harvesting.

BACTERIOLOGY OF CANNED FOOD

Deleterious changes in canned food known as 'spoilage' may be brought about through the development of microorganisms. These may be present in the food either as a result of their resistance to the heating process or through being introduced after processing through defects in the structure of the can.

Heat-resistant organisms and the types of spoilage caused by them vary according to the nature of the food they infect. Foods preserved by canning can be divided broadly into two groups: (*a*) medium, low and non-acid foods with pH above 4·5, including meat, fish, vegetables, soup, milk and starch foods; (*b*) high acid foods with pH of less than 4·5. The border-line of pH 4·5 has been chosen because spores of the most heat-resistant of the food poisoning organisms, viz. *Clostridium botulinum*, will not germinate in conditions of acidity higher than this. For this reason it is not usual to heat the foods in group (*b*) above 100°C, which is sufficient to destroy all vegetative forms. Pressure heating on the other hand is necessary to render safe all foods with pH above 4·5. The actual amount of heating employed varies with the food to be processed and is determined by careful laboratory tests carried out by specialists in the canning industry, the main considerations being that although it should be sufficient to destroy spores of pathogenic organisms in the centre of the contents it should not be so great as to alter the appearance and palatability of the food in question.

The minimum degree of heat necessary to destroy the spores of *Clostridium botulinum* may not be adequate to sterilize completely the food and where extremely heat-resistant spores remain, and the temperature of storage is such that germination and growth of the organisms can take place, spoilage will occur.

Organisms that bring about spoilage of food as a result of their heat-resistance are aerobic and anaerobic spore formers of the genera *Bacillus* and *Clostridium*. Many are thermophilic, having an optimum temperature for growth of 55°C but have the ability to grow slowly at temperatures considerably below this. The type of spoilage gives an indication of the organisms responsible. The following are the main types of spoilage that may occur in group (*a*) foods.

(A) Saccharolytic Spoilage

1. Acid without gas, known as 'flat sour' spoilage, produced by certain species of the genus *Bacillus*, e.g. *B. megaterium*.

2. Acid with gas production sufficient to cause 'swelling' of the can, 'Hard Swell', due to saccharolytic species of the genus *Clostridium*, e.g. *Cl. multifermentans*.

3. Slight acid production with hydrogen sulphide. No 'swelling' occurs since the gas is soluble, but the contents become dark in colour. The organism usually responsible is *Clostridium nigrificans*.

(B) Putrefactive Spoilage

Digestion of the food with gas production results from the growth of putrefactive species of the genus *Clostridium*, e.g. *Clostridium botulinum* and *Clostridium sporogenes*.

Spoilage of acid foods of group (B) is brought about by acid tolerant bacteria and occasionally by yeasts and moulds, which survive the short periods of heating at temperatures below 100°C. The bacteria responsible include sporing aerobes and anaerobes as well as non-sporing species, all capable of developing in high concentrations of acid. Gas may or may not be produced. Examples are *Bacillus thermoacidurans*, *Clostridium pasteurianum*, *Lactobacillus lycopersici* and *Leuconostoc*.

Contamination after Processing

Microorganisms may enter leaking cans and infect the food after processing. They may include a variety of sporing and non-sporing bacteria, often derived from the water used for cooling the cans. If pathogenic organisms gain entrance in this way, cases of food poisoning will result. Staphylococci and organisms of the genus *Salmonella* have occasionally been incriminated in food poisoning outbreaks due to canned food, probably contaminated in this way.

Technique for Examining Canned Food

To test the sterility of canned food, and where spoilage has occurred or the food is suspected of causing food poisoning, the following procedure, based on that of Tanner (1944), is recommended for the isolation of the organisms responsible.

Unless the can shows visible signs of spoilage through 'swelling' it is advisable to stimulate the multiplication of heat-resistant organisms which may be present in only small numbers, and probably in a 'dormant' condition, by incubating it, before opening, at 37°C for at least one week for mesophilic and 55°C for thermophilic organisms. Acid foods should be incubated at 25°C for ten days.

Before being opened the can is carefully examined for physical defects, particularly round the seams. Any signs of 'swelling' are noted, and where rustiness or dents have occurred these are scrutinized for pin holes. After examination the can is scrubbed with soap and water and rinsed with alcohol or ether to remove the grease. The area where an opening is to be made is then sterilized by flaming or by treatment with 70 per cent alcohol. If heat is applied it should be carefully distributed in such a way as to avoid overheating the contents, which may then spurt out when the can is opened. If the can is swollen, it is advisable not to sterilize by heating but rather by the use of alcohol. The point of a sterile opener is then inserted into the sterilized area and an opening is cut sufficiently large to enable a portion of the food to be withdrawn in the following aseptic manner:

Liquid food is withdrawn with a sterile pipette or an untapered glass tube and inoculated directly into the culture medium. 15–20 ml should be tested in this way. Solid food is sampled with a modified cork borer, 10 in long and $\frac{3}{4}$ in in diameter, having a rod inserted to expel the contents. The sample should include food from the centre of the contents, where heat-resistant organisms are likely to occur, and from the surface, where contamination through leakage may have taken place. The solid food should then be thoroughly emulsified in sterile water by grinding with a sterile pestle and mortar or by shaking in a screw-capped bottle with pieces of broken glass (Baumgartner, 1945).

Technique for Culture

Tubes containing 10 ml amounts of suitable fluid media are inoculated with 1 ml of the liquid food and incubated at 37°C and 55°C, both aerobically and anaerobically. Cooked meat medium is recommended for culturing anaerobic bacilli, and glucose broth is suitable for aerobic mesophilic and thermophilic organisms. In order to culture spoilage organisms from acid foods, tomato glucose broth is recommended by Tanner. This consists of tomato juice and nutrient broth in equal parts with the addition of 1 per cent glucose. The tubes are examined after 24 and 48 h, and where growth has occurred the organisms may be identified by microscopic examination of stained films and by further culture tests. If the food is suspected of causing food poisoning through infection with organisms of the Salmonella and Staphylococcus groups, media selective for these organisms should also be inoculated with portions of the food. For salmonellae, tetrathionate broth and selenite medium are suitable; for staphylococci, cooked meat medium to which 10 per cent sodium chloride has been added is recommended.

Organisms developing in these selective media should be further examined by the methods described in the appropriate sections dealing with them.

It is advisable to make direct films of the food for microscopic examination although no significance should be attached to organisms seen unless the cultures confirm that they are viable.

After removing samples for culture, the food is turned out of the can and examined carefully for any abnormalities in appearance and smell. The inside of the can too should be inspected for defects in its manufacture.

The Bacteriological Examination of Milk Bottles

To test the adequacy of the cleansing and sterilization of milk bottles at farms and creameries, the following technique, based on the recommendations of the Ministry of Agriculture and Fisheries (1947) is advocated.

At least four bottles should be picked at random immediately after washing. They should be capped or fitted with a sterile rubber bung and sent immediately to the laboratory so that testing may be begun within 4 h of sampling.

To each bottle, irrespective of its size, 20 ml of sterile quarter-strength Ringer solution are added and the cap or bung replaced. The bottle is then laid horizontally on the bench and rotated by rolling so that the whole of the internal surface is rinsed with the solution. This process is repeated at intervals over a period of half an hour, the bottle being kept on its side during that time.

Five ml of the solution are then plated in duplicate using 20 ml yeast extract milk agar, this large amount being necessary to produce solidification. One plate is incubated at 37°C for 48 h and the other at 22°C for three days. (For greater accuracy duplicate plates may be prepared for both temperatures.) The results are reported as the colony count per bottle, i.e. the individual plate count multiplied by 4.

Based on the 37°C count, the following scheme of classification was suggested:

Average colony count per bottle	Classification
Not more than 200	Satisfactory
Over 200 to 600	Fairly satisfactory
Over 600	Unsatisfactory

In addition, a test for the presence of coliform bacilli should be carried out by inoculating each of two bottles containing 10 ml double-strength MacConkey's broth with 5 ml rinse solution. These are examined for acid and gas production after 48 h incubation at 37°C. If adequate methods are employed in cleansing and sterilizing the bottles, no coliform bacilli should be present.

THE BACTERIOLOGICAL EXAMINATION OF WASHED CROCKERY AND CUTLERY

The adequacy of washing-up methods employed in the kitchens of catering establishments, schools and other institutions may be tested by bacterial examinations of swabs taken from freshly washed crockery and cutlery.

Preparation of swabs. Absorbent cotton-wool swabs $\frac{3}{4}$ in long, as used for clinical purposes may be employed. It is more generally convenient to have them on wooden applicator sticks $6\frac{1}{2}$ in long than on wires, so that after the specimen has been collected the swab may be broken off above the cotton-wool and allowed to drop down into a container of quarter-strength Ringer's solution. The swabs are inserted into test-tubes 5 in by $\frac{1}{2}$ in plugged with cotton-wool and are sterilized by autoclaving at 115°C for 15 min.

Higgins (1950) obtained a greater recovery of organisms by using swabs made of calcium alginate wool instead of cotton-wool, the advantage being that the alginate swabs may be completely dissolved in Ringer's solution containing sodium hexametaphosphate. In this way all the bacteria contained in the swab are liberated into the solution. Not more than 50 mg of wool should be used for each swab to ensure complete solution even in cold weather, when larger amounts tend to form crystals. It is important that the calcium alginate wool should be declared by the manufacturer to be free from bactericidal substances such as 'Fixanol C', a quaternary ammonium compound which was originally impregnated into the wool for use in the manufacture of certain textiles.

Method of swabbing. One swab is used for five similar articles. It is first moistened by dipping in sterile quarter-strength Ringer's solution, the surplus liquid being squeezed out against the inside of the screw-capped container. The swab is then rubbed thoroughly over the whole of the appropriate areas, which are as follows:

the inner surfaces of plates and bowls that come in contact with food;

the inner and outer surfaces of cups, mugs and glasses to a depth of 3 cm below the rim;

bowls and the backs of spoons and the back and front surfaces of forks and between the prongs.

After swabbing five similar articles in this way, the swab is returned to the test-tube and sent to the laboratory without delay.

Method of Testing

1. If cotton-wool swabs have been used, the swab is broken off the wooden stick with sterile forceps and allowed to drop into a screw-capped bottle of 1 oz capacity containing 10 ml of sterile quarter-strength Ringer's solution. If delay in transporting the sample to the laboratory is unavoidable, this should be done by the person taking the sample. In the laboratory the bottle is shaken vigorously to disintegrate the swab and liberate as many as possible of the bacteria contained in it. One ml quantities of the test solution are plated out in duplicate on yeast extract agar, one plate of each being incubated at 37°C for 48 h and the other at 22°C for three days. The results are reported as the bacterial counts per utensil for each temperature (i.e. count per ml × 2).

2. If calcium alginate swabs are used, it is recommended by Higgins and Hobbs (1950) that two swabs should be employed for each test, one being moistened in Ringer's solution before use and the other used dry. The surfaces of five articles are rubbed over, first with the moistened swab and then with the dry one. Both swabs are then broken off the sticks with sterile forceps and allowed to drop into 9 ml quarter-strength Ringer's solution. One ml of 10 per cent sodium hexametaphosphate solution (sterilized by autoclaving) is then added and the bottle shaken until both swabs have dissolved. The solution is plated out either by the method described under (1) or by the Miles and Misra technique, using blood agar plates on which the test solution is inoculated in the form of drops of 0·02 ml volume delivered from a calibrated Pasteur pipette.

Standards

There is no standard officially recognized in Great Britain, but attention is drawn to the United States Public Health Standard (Tiedman *et al.*, 1944) for washed crockery. Based on the swabbing technique followed by the standard plate count test it allows a maximum of 100 colonies per utensil examined. If the Miles and Misra method is used, specimens giving 2 colonies or less per 6 drops of undiluted test suspension on blood agar plates may be considered to conform to the American standard.

EXAMINATION OF FOODSTUFFS IN OUTBREAKS OF FOOD POISONING

Bacterial food poisoning (acute gastro-enteritis) results from the consumption of food infected with certain pathogenic organisms which are capable of proliferating in food if conditions are favourable. They fall into two categories depending on the manner in which they produce their harmful effects: (*a*) those which infect the body (notably the salmonella group), and (*b*) those which produce a toxin during their growth in the food, the main cause of this type being certain coagulase-positive staphylococci. Certain types of *Clostridium welchii*, characterized by the heat resistance of their spores, are also responsible for a type of food poisoning but their mode of action has not yet been clarified.

Specimens of Food for Bacteriological Examination

Meat preparations (ham, brawn, sausages, etc.), and made-up dishes such as sandwiches prepared by hand, have been responsible for outbreaks of salmonella and staphylococcal food poisoning, and precooked meat, stews, beefsteak pies, etc., prepared the day before serving, frequently cause outbreaks of *Cl. welchii* food poisoning. Eggs used in the preparation of uncooked or only partially cooked foods, have caused salmonella infections, and unpasteurized milk and milk products have in the past been responsible for both staphylococcal and salmonella food poisoning. Any of the above foodstuffs should be viewed with suspicion if they have been eaten by the patients shortly before the commencement of symptoms, and samples should be examined bacteriologically for the three main food poisoning organisms.

For the methods of isolation and identification of the various specific bacteria, reference should be made to the appropriate sections in Chapter 7. The following points should be observed.

Non-specific contamination. The examination of food samples should commence with a careful inspection to determine if there are any abnormalities in appearance or smell. This is followed by a microscopic examination of stained preparations which will indicate any gross contamination. It is also useful to determine the total count of viable bacteria per gram of food at 37°C and 22°C by means of the *plate count method* applied to a suspension of 1 g of the food in 10 ml of sterile Ringer's solution. This test should be combined with an examination for coliform bacilli as in the examination of milk samples. These preliminary tests will indicate whether or not the food has been subjected to contamination of a non-specific nature arising from poor standards of kitchen hygiene.

Salmonella infection. In testing foodstuffs for organisms of the salmonella group, both direct culture and enrichment techniques should be carried out. Two 25 g amounts of the food are weighed in sterile jars with screw caps, and after the addition of 25 ml of quarter-strength Ringer's solution the mixtures are incubated for 1–2 h at 37°C before the addition of 50 ml double-strength selenite enrichment broth to one lot and 50 ml double-strength tetrathionate broth to the other. These enrichment cultures are incubated at 37°C and subcultured on to both desoxycholate citrate agar and Wilson and Blair's agar after 24 h and again after three days' incubation. Suspicious colonies are picked for identification.

This method may be applied to the examination of any liquid foods.

Staphylococcal intoxication. Although laboratory methods for identifying the enterotoxin of *Staphylococcus aureus* have been improved (Gilbert *et al.*, 1972), diagnosis of this type of food poisoning is best made if coagulase-positive staphylococci are isolated from the food. By the Miles and Misra counting technique, using 10 per cent salt milk agar as a selective medium, it is possible to determine the approximate number of staphylococci per g of suspected food. Although it is not known how many staphylococci are necessary to cause food poisoning, large numbers growing in direct culture from suspected food would be highly suggestive of their being the cause. In order to isolate *Staphylococcus aureus* from foodstuffs heavily contaminated with other organisms, the use of cooked-meat medium containing 10 per cent salt may be advantageous. Any coagulase-positive staphylococci isolated by the above methods should. be typed by bacteriophage or serological methods. In order to determine the source of the infection, all persons engaged in the preparation and handling of the food should be examined to determine whether they are harbouring the same organism in their noses or in skin lesions.

Cl. welchii food poisoning. This form of food poisoning, which has been increasingly recognized in recent years, is caused by a variant of Type A *Cl. welchii* that is feebly toxigenic. The organisms are usually non-haemolytic and have spores that can survive boiling for several hours but an appreciable number of haemolytic and non-heat resistant strains have also been incriminated in food poisoning (Sutton and Hobbs, 1968).

Anaerobic culture on blood agar plates inoculated by the Miles and Misra technique will indicate the degree of contamination by anaerobic or facultative anaerobic organisms. Unless they grow in relatively pure culture it may not be easy to distinguish the colonies of *Cl. welchii* from those of non-sporing organisms. They may be more readily isolated by inoculating small portions of the food into an enrichment medium such as cooked-meat medium and incubating for 18 h before culturing on blood agar, but it should be borne in mind that such indirect culture does not have the same significance as direct culture. Use may be made of the selective medium of Willis and Hobbs. The identity of any possible *Cl. welchii* colonies isolated by the above methods should be further confirmed (see Chap. 37 for further details).

Cl. botulinum intoxication. Botulism, a rare type of food poisoning, has an incubation period which varies from less than 24 h to 72 h. The highly potent exotoxin formed during the proliferation of *Cl. botulinum* in the food is absorbed through the gastric mucosa and affects the nervous system rather than the gastro-intestinal tract. This subject is dealt with more fully in Chapter 38.

Foods which have been incriminated include improperly processed canned and preserved meat, meat and game pastes, and vegetables that are eaten uncooked or only partially cooked (the toxin is destroyed by heating to 90°C). The spores of *Cl. botulinum* may survive boiling for several hours but are destroyed within 15 minutes by a temperature of 120°C. They fail to germinate if the pH of the food is less than 4·5.

Bacillus cereus food poisoning. *B. cereus* has been responsible for mild food poisoning in parts of Europe, Scandinavia and the U.S.A. In 1971 six food poisoning incidents of this nature were reported to the Public Health Laboratory Service in England (British Medical Journal, 1972). They were all associated with the consumption of fried rice from Chinese restaurants. It is likely that *B. cereus* originated from the uncooked rice and that spores that survived the initial boiling germinated, with the production of a toxin, during the interval of storage at room temperature prior to the rice being fried.

Vibrio parahaemolyticus. This organism has been incriminated in severe cases of gastro-enteritis in various parts of the world. It is usually associated with sea food. In 1972 it was encountered in England in travellers who became ill after eating crab meat on a flight from Bangkok to London (Peffers *et al.*, 1973).

BACTERIOLOGICAL EXAMINATION OF AIR

Settle Plates

In the past the procedure frequently adopted for determining the relative numbers and species of microorganisms present in air has been to expose open plates of culture medium for given periods of time, e.g. $\frac{1}{2}$ or 1 h. A count of the colonies after incubation of the plates for 24 h at 37°C yields a relative estimate of the number of organisms present, and if blood agar is used, the occurrence in the air of pathogenic staphylococci and streptococci can be determined. This method has proved valuable in demonstrating the presence of such organisms in the air and dust of hospital wards. Such findings have also thrown light on cross-infection in hospitals.

Slit Sampler

It is recognized that the simple method of exposing plates has certain limitations as a means of studying the bacteriology of air; for example, it is not a satisfactory method of detecting bacteria in very small suspended particles such as droplet-nuclei. More elaborate procedures have therefore been adopted. A technique introduced by Bourdillon, Lidwell and Thomas (1941) involves the use of a special instrument, the 'slit sampler', by which a known volume of air is directed on to a plate through a slit 0·25 mm wide, the plate being mechanically rotated so that the organisms are evenly distributed over it. One cubic foot of air per minute is allowed to pass through the slit, and samples of 1 to 10 cubic feet, or more, may be tested. More advanced models of the slit sampler have a timing arrangement that allows the number of colonies on each sector of the plate to be related to the number of bacteria-carrying particles sampled in a particular part of the sampling period. These instruments can be obtained commercially.

The slit sampler and other air samplers have been used in examining the amount of bacterial contamination in the air of hospitals, schools, factories and other places, with a view to determining the danger of air-borne infection and the factors that increase and decrease numbers of air-borne bacteria (Bourdillon *et al.*, 1948). Observations have been made in surgical operation rooms in relation to the efficacy of different ventilation systems in minimizing aerial contamination, and in schools, hospitals and other places in tests of the efficacy of ultraviolet irradiation and chemical vapours for air disinfection.

Cascade Impaction Sampler

Lidwell (1959) has described an impaction sampler that operates on the cascade principle and collects air-borne infected particles in four ranges of size on four separate culture plates. The size ranges (diameters) of the particles are: less than 4 μg, between 4 and 10 μg, between 10 and 18 μg and greater than 18 μg. In hospitals and other occupied places, the air-borne particles carrying pathogenic organisms such as *Staph. aureus*, *Strept. pyogenes*, *Candida albicans* and ringworm fungi, are mostly in the range of 10–18 microns in diameter (Noble, Lidwell and Kingston, 1963). Especial interest attaches, however, to the smaller proportion of infected particles (e.g. about 5 per cent) that are under 5 μg in diameter and are thus able to remain airborne for long periods (e.g. for more than 30 min) and, if inhaled, to penetrate deeply into the respiratory tract and reach the lung alveoli.

Levels of Air Infection

These are generally expressed in terms of the count of bacterial colonies of all kinds made on blood agar plates incubated for 24 h at 37°C. When plates are incubated for a much longer period at room temperature the counts are often very much higher as a result of the slow growth of saprophytic organisms that do not grow well at 37°C. The counts are expressed as the number of bacteria-carrying particles per cubic foot (28·3 litres) of air when the examination is made with a slit sampler, and as the number of bacteria-carrying particles settling on a $3\frac{1}{2}$ in (88 mm) Petri dish per minute, or per hour, when it is made with settle plates.

Since knowledge is still lacking of the relative dangers of infection that are presented by different levels of bacterial contamination of air, and since the levels of contamination vary very greatly from time to time and from place to place within occupied premises, it is not possible as yet to define the limits of the levels of contamination that may be regarded as acceptable.

Under conditions of normal occupation, the air in hospital wards, offices, schools, and private houses commonly shows levels of contamination in the range of 5 to 100 bacteria-carrying particles per cu ft, and in the range of 0·05 to 5 bacteria-carrying particles per $3\frac{1}{2}$ in (88 mm) settle plate per min; the higher levels are found when there is much bodily movement or other disturbance, such as bed-making, that is liable to raise dust into the air. Bourdillon *et al.* (1948) have suggested, as provisional standards of air hygiene, that the following may be regarded as the limits to the levels of infection that are acceptable: in factories, offices, homes, etc., 50 per ft³; in surgical operating theatres providing for most forms of surgery, 10 ft³; in surgical theatres where operations on the central nervous system or dressings of burns are done, about 1 per ft³. Peak levels of contamination limited to short periods of exceptional disturbance and movement are disregarded in applying these standards.

The great majority of the bacteria found in the air are harmless saprophytes or commensals, and even in hospital wards and other rooms occupied by patients and carriers, usually not more than 1 per cent, and commonly only 0·01–0·1 per cent, of the airborne bacteria are pathogens. *Staph. aureus* is the pathogen most commonly found in the air. It is present in most occupied premises. Occasionally up to 10, or more, *Staph. aureus*-carrying particles are found per ft³ of air, but much more commonly between 0·01 and 1·0 per ft³. *Strept. pyogenes* is sometimes found in large numbers (e.g. about 10 per ft³) in the air of rooms occupied by patients with tonsillitis, scarlet fever or infected wounds and burns, but usually the level of contamination is between 0·01 and 1 per ft³ in such places.

Whilst the higher levels of air contamination with pathogenic organisms are obviously the most dangerous, it should be noted that there is no level of contamination, however low, that can be regarded as certainly safe. Little is known about the minimum size of dose of organisms required to initiate infection on inhalation. It is quite possible that a man may be infected if he inhales only a single infected particle in the 500 or so ft³ of air that he respires in the course of a day. In an investigation described by Riley (1957) the number of tubercle bacillus-carrying particles present in the air in a tuberculosis hospital ward was calculated, from infection rates in guinea-pigs exposed to the ward air, to be on average only about 0·00008 per ft³. Such a level of contamination was considered to be sufficient to account for the infection of a considerable proportion of originally tuberculin-negative nurses during six months of duty in a tuberculosis hospital, since each nurse would in this time inhale a volume of air sufficient to contain one infective particle.

BACTERIOLOGICAL EXAMINATION OF ENVIRONMENTAL DUST

Sweep plates. The sweep plate method is used to examine personal clothing, bed-clothes, carpets, curtains, soft furniture and other domestic fabrics for the presence of pathogenic bacteria liable to be liberated in dust. An ordinary Petri dish containing nutrient agar, blood agar or a selective culture medium is removed from its lid and rubbed to and fro on the surface of the fabric. The medium faces the fabric and the edges of the plate are made to scrape the fabric so that dust is thrown up on to the medium. About 10 sweeps may be made with a plate of non-selective medium, and more with one of selective medium.

Dust on floors and hard surfaces. This may be collected on a cotton-wool swab moistened with broth and the swab is plated out in the usual way on a suitable medium. For large areas, a more representative sample may be obtained by sweeping the dust together and suspending a portion in broth and plating out different dilutions of the broth.

REFERENCES

AMIES, C. R. (1956) Surface film on swimming pools. *Canadian Journal of Public Health*, **47**, 93.

BAUMGARTNER, J. G. (1945) *Canned Foods*. London: Churchill Livingstone.

BIGGER, J. W. (1934) The bacteriological examination of mussels. *Journal of Hygiene (Cambridge)*, **34**, 172.

BOURDILLON, R. B., LIDWELL, O. M. & THOMAS, J. C. (1941) A slit sampler for collecting and counting airborne bacteria. *Journal of Hygiene (Cambridge)*, **41**, 197.

BOURDILLON, R. B., LIDWELL, O. M., LOVELOCK, J. E., CAWSTON, W. C., COLEBROOK, L., ELLIS, F. P., VAN DEN ENDE, M., GLOVER, R. E., MACFARLAN, A. M., MILES, A. A., RAYMOND, W. F., SCHUSTER, E. & THOMAS, J. C. (1948) Studies in air hygiene. *Special Report Series of the Medical Research Council (London)*, No. 262, H.M.S.O.

BURMAN, N. P. (1955) The standardization and selection of bile salt and peptone for culture media used in the bacteriological examination of water. *Proceedings of the Society of Water Treatment and Examination*, **4**, 10.

CHALMERS, C. H. (1962) *Bacteria in Relation to the Milk Supply*. London: Arnold.

DEPARTMENT OF HEALTH AND SOCIAL SECURITY (1969) The bacteriological examination of water supplies. Report No. 71. London: H.M.S.O.

EDITORIAL (1972) Epidemiology: Food-poisoning associated with *Bacillus cereus*. *British Medical Journal*, **i**, 189.

GILBERT, R. J., WIENEKE, A. A., LANSER, J. & SIMKOVIČOVÁ (1972) Serological detection of enterotoxin in foods implicated in staphylococcal food-poisoning. *Journal of Hygiene (Cambridge)*, **70**, 755.

GILLESPIE, E. H., KING, G. J. G., MOORE, B. & TOMLINSON, A. J. H. (1947); (1948); (1949); (1950) Bacteriological examination and grading of ice-cream. *Monthly Bulletin of the Ministry of Health Laboratory Service*, **6**, 60; **7**, 84; **8**, 155; **9**, 231.

GRAY, R. D., JEBB, W. H. H., McCOY, J. H., MORRISON RICHIE, J., KINGSLEY SMITH, A. J., WATKINSON, JOAN M., WINDLE TAYLOR, E. & SUTHERLAND, J. (1953) The choice of an indicator organism for the bacteriological control of swimming-bath purification. *Monthly Bulletin of the Ministry of Health Laboratory Service*, **12**, 254.

GRAY, R. D. (1969) Public Health Laboratory Service Standing Committee on the bacteriological examination of water supplies. *Journal of Hygiene (Cambridge)*, **62**, 195.

HALEY, L. D. & ROSTY, A. (1957) Use of millipore membrane filters in the diagnostic tuberculosis laboratory. *American Journal of Clinical Pathology*, **27**, No. 1, 117.

HAMMERSTRÖM, E. & LJUTOV, V. (1954) Concentration technique for demonstrating small amounts of bacteria in tap water. *Acta pathologica microbiologica Scandinavica*, **35**, 365.

HANNAY, C. L. & NORTON, I. L. (1947) Enumeration, isolation and study of faecal streptococci from river water. *Proceedings of the Society of Applied Bacteriology*, **1**, 39.

HIGGINS, M. (1950) A comparison of the pour plate and surface plate methods in estimating bacterial infection of table crockery and kitchen utensils. *Monthly Bulletin of the Ministry of Health Laboratory Service*, **9**, 52.

HIGGINS, M. & HOBBS, B. C. (1950) Kitchen hygiene: the effectiveness of current procedure in cleansing tableware. *Monthly Bulletin of the Ministry of Health Laboratory Service*, **9**, 38.

JONES, L. M. & BRINLEY-MOYAN, W. J. (1958) A preliminary report on a selective medium for the culture of Brucella, including fastidious types. *Bulletin of the World Health Organization*, **19**, 200.

KABLER, P. W. & CLARK, H. F. (1952) The use of differential media with the membrane filter. *American Journal of Public Health*, **42** (1), 390.

LIDWELL, O. M. (1959) Impaction sampler for size grading air-borne bacteria-carrying particles. *Journal of Scientific Instruments*, **36**, 3.

LJUTOV, V. (1954) Filtering methods for demonstration of Salmonella bacteria in water. *Acta pathologica et microbiologica Scandinavica*, **35**, 370.

LLOYD, T. P. (1969) Ice-cream. *Dairy Industries*, **34**, No. 4, 199; No. 5, 271; No. 6, 363.

MACKENZIE, E. F. W., TAYLOR, E. W. & GILBERT, W. E. (1948) Recent experiences in the rapid identification of bacterium coli Type I. *Journal of General Microbiology*, **2**, 197.

MINISTRY OF AGRICULTURE AND FISHERIES (1947) (National Milk Testing and Advisory Scheme). The bacteriological examination of milk bottles. Technique No. B743/TPB.

MINISTRY OF HEALTH (1947 and 1959) Ice-cream (Heat Treatment, etc.) Regulations.

MINISTRY OF HEALTH (1951) *The Purification of the Water of Swimming Baths*. London: H.M.S.O.

MOORE, B. (1948) The detection of paratyphoid carriers in towns by means of sewage examinations. *Monthly Bulletin of the Ministry of Health Laboratory Service*, **7**, 241.

NOBLE, W. C., LIDWELL, O. M. & KINGSTON, D. (1963) The size distribution of air-borne particles carrying micro-organisms. *Journal of Hygiene (Cambridge)*, **61**, 385.

PEFFERS, A. S. R., BAILEY, J., BARROW, G. I. & HOBBS, B. C. (1973) *Vibrio parahaemolyticus* gastroenteritis and international air travel. *Lancet*, **1**, 143.

PUBLIC HEALTH LABORATORY SERVICE STANDING COMMITTEE ON THE BACTERIOLOGICAL EXAMINATION OF WATER SUPPLIES (1968) *Journal of Hygiene* (Cambridge), **66**, 641.

RILEY, R. L. (1957) Aerial dissemination of pulmonary tuberculosis. *American Review of Tuberculosis*, **76**, 931.

SCOTTISH HOME AND HEALTH DEPARTMENT (SHHD) (1970) Ice Cream (Scotland) Regulations.

SUTTON, R. G. A. & HOBBS, BETTY C. (1968) Food-poisoning caused by heat-sensitive *clostridium welchii*. A report of five recent outbreaks. *Journal of Hygiene (Cambridge)*, **66**, 135.

TANNER, F. W. (1944) *Microbiology of Foods*, 2nd edn. Champaign, Ill.: Garrard Press.

TIEDMAN, W. D., FUCKS, A. W., GUNDERSON, N. O., HUCKER, G. J. & MALLMANN, W. J. (1944) A proposed method for control of food utensil sanitation. *American Journal of Public Health*, **34**, 255.

WILSON, G. S., TWIGG, R. S., WRIGHT, R. C., HENDRY, C. B., COWELL, M. P. & MAIER, I. (1935) The bacteriological grading of milk. *Special Report Series of the Medical Research Council (London)*, No. 206.

WINDLE TAYLOR, E. (1963–64) Progress with membrane filtration. 41*st Annual Report Dir. Water Exam. Met. Water Bd. London*, pp. 17–21.

WINDLE TAYLOR, E. & BURMAN, N. P. (1964) The application of membrane filtration techniques to the bacteriological examination of water. *Journal of Applied Bacteriology*, **27**, 294.

WORLD HEALTH ORGANIZATION (1961) *European Standards for Drinking-Water*. Geneva: Palais des Nations.

13. Centrifuges, Colorimeters, Bacterial Counts

CENTRIFUGES

The best method for the separation of a microorganism from its suspending fluid is that of centrifugation. This is carried out in the centrifuge, an apparatus for the separation of two substances of different density by centrifugal force.

The rate of settling r (cm/sec) of spherical particles of density dp and of radius a (cm) in a medium of viscosity η (cgs units) and of density dm is given by Stokes' law:

$$r = \frac{2a^2g(dp - dm)}{9\eta},$$

where g is the acceleration due to gravity (981 cm/sec^2).

From this equation, it is evident that the rate of settling of a particle will be increased by the following factors:

1. An increase in the size of the particle. Thus, larger microorganisms like yeast and fungi will sediment faster than bacteria which, in turn, will sediment faster than viruses. Note that the size of the particles is squared in the equation and thus an increase of the radius of the particles by a factor of 2 will increase the rate of settling by a factor of 4.

2. An increase in the difference between the density of the particles dp and that of the medium dm. Thus a capsulate bacterium will have a lower average density and be more difficult to sediment than its non-capsulate variant.

3. A decrease in the viscosity of the medium. For example, when defibrinated blood is being washed the first sedimentation of the corpuscles from the viscous serum takes much longer than when the corpuscles are suspended in saline.

4. An increase in the force due to gravity. This force is increased artificially in the centrifuge. The degree by which this force is increased is measured by the relative centrifugal force (RCF) which can be obtained by the following formula:

$$\text{RCF (in } g) = 1.118 \times 10^{-5} \times R \times N^2,$$

where R = the radius of the centrifuge in cm,

being the distance from the centre of the centrifuge shaft to the tip of the centrifuge tube: N = revolutions per minute (rev/min).

From this equation, it is evident that the speed of the centrifuge, being squared, is very important in determining the rate of sedimentation. Although an increase in the radius of the machine will increase the rate of sedimentation, it is more efficient and simpler practically to increase the speed. However, it is most important to express the efficiency of a centrifuge according to the maximum RCF rather than the speed itself, which, without specification of the radius of the centrifuge, is meaningless. The calculation is simple. Thus, a centrifuge with a radius of 10 cm and a speed of 4000 rev/min has an RCF of $1.118 \times 10 \times (4000)^2 \times 10^{-5} = 1788$ g, say 1800 times the force of gravity. Consequently, particles will sediment in this centrifuge at a rate 1800 times faster than in a tube on the bench.

Types of Centrifuges

A variety of centrifuges is now available and the choice of a suitable model depends upon the following factors.

1. The size of the particles to be sedimented. As shown previously, the smaller the particle, the greater will be the RCF and time required for centrifugation. Machines can be obtained commercially with speeds up to about 60 000 rev/min and RCFs of up to about 200 000 g. Generally speaking, yeasts and fungi require a centrifuge with a maximum RCF at least 1000–2000 g, bacteria about 2000–4000 g, and viruses about 50 000–150 000 g. At higher speeds (RCF above about 4000 g), glass tubes are apt to break even if surrounded by a rubber sleeve or a layer of water. Stainless-steel tubes may be supplied for the most exacting strength requirements, that is for the very highest speeds and centrifugal forces and for maximum resistance to corrosion. However, for most purposes, plastic tubes can be used. In order to prevent deformation of these tubes under high

centrifugal forces, caps should always be used and the tubes should be fully filled. The main disadvantage of plastic tubes in microbiological work is that they cannot be sterilized in a hot-air oven like glass tubes. Even boiling tends to cause deformation and it is recommended that the insides of the tubes and caps be exposed to ultra-violet light for sterilization.

2. The volume of material. Centrifuges can be obtained with capacities of up to at least 15 l. The fluid to be centrifuged is contained in tubes or buckets, the number and size of which is subject to a wide variation. For very large amounts of material, continuous-flow machines are available. The fluid to be centrifuged is normally continuously passed along the inside of a rotating tube. The particles sediment very quickly in the thin layer of liquid passing along the sides of the tube and the supernatant passes out of the machine to be collected. Continuous flow centrifuges (e.g. Sharples) of this type are common in industry, but are not often used in the laboratory.

3. The ease with which the particles form a hard pellet at the bottom of the tube. Many centrifuges are of the angle type in which the tubes, instead of being allowed to swing out and rotate in a horizontal plane, are fixed at an angle (from $20°-45°$) on the rotating head. The advantage of the angular position is that particulate matter is rapidly separated and concentrated, with consequent saving of time. This is because the particles have to traverse only a short distance before deposition on the sides of the tube, after which they slide to the bottom. The tubes are encased in a metal head, which in its rotation offers slight resistance to air and so obtains greater speed and is less liable to warm up due to friction. A disadvantage is that a 'line' of deposited material may remain adherent on the peripheral wall of the tube, and when the suspending fluid is removed it is difficult to avoid contamination caused by turbulence.

4. The temperature required for centrifugation. In most biological systems it is advantageous and often essential to centrifuge at low temperatures. This prevents metabolism, loss of viability or enzyme activity during centrifugation. Consequently, refrigeration units are built into many of the larger centrifuges. This is particularly important in high-speed centrifuges where the temperature may rise due to friction unless refrigeration is used. In many machines it is possible to obtain temperatures down to about $-15°C$.

For a routine bacteriological laboratory, a small bench centrifuge taking 10–20 tubes of capacity 10–30 ml at a maximum RCF of about 3000 g is essential. It is, however, convenient to have a centrifuge that will hold the standard 5-in test-tube and stopper used in routine bacteriological culture, thus avoiding the need for transference to a proper centrifuge tube. For more general and research purposes, larger machines are available, with or without refrigeration and with speeds up to about 6000 g. To centrifuge rickettsias and viruses and for special research purposes, speeds up to about 150 000 g are required. For such high-speed ultracentrifuges (above about 20 000 rev/min), the centrifuging compartment must be held *in vacuo* in order to reduce friction, and vacuum pumps are included.

Method of Using the Centrifuge

1. Tubes must be put in the centrifuge in pairs that have been accurately balanced. The members of a pair of tubes must be placed diametrically opposite each other. If there is an odd number of tubes, a balance tube containing water must be prepared. If the buckets are removable from the centrifuge, they should be balanced with the tubes. With a pipette or plastic washing bottle add a little water to the lighter bucket, not the tube, until the two sides are balanced.

2. Before putting tubes into the buckets, make sure that the rubber cushions or sleeves are in position at the bottom of the buckets. Otherwise breakages are liable to occur.

3. Precautions must be taken to ensure that the cotton-wool plugs of culture tubes are not forced down into the tube during centrifugation. In a swing-out head, fold the upper portion of the plug over the mouth of the tube and secure it with a rubber band. With an angle centrifuge, it is sufficient to splay out the top of the plug. However, even when the cotton-wool plug is secured in this way, cotton fibres become detached and can be seen micro-

scopically in the centrifugate. In order to avoid this, aluminium or stainless-steel caps can be used to keep the tubes sterile. Alternatively a screw cap without a washer can be placed over the mouth of the tube, the size being a loose fit. (For ordinary 15 ml tubes, the M2 screw cap of a $\frac{1}{4}$-oz 'bijou' bottle is convenient.)

4. After the tubes have been placed in position, make sure that the metal buckets in a swing-out head are properly seated on the rings and are free to swing.

5. Close the lid and make sure it is secure. The lid must not be removed when the centrifuge is running. Apart from the danger of an open lid, a decrease in speed due to 'winding' will ensue.

6. Make sure that the rheostat is back to the zero position. (Some centrifuges have an automatic switch-off unless this is so. This prevents strain by inadvertently switching on with the resistance out of circuit.)

7. Start the motor and *gradually* increase the speed by taking the resistance out by means of the rheostat. Pause at intervals to allow the machine to gather speed until the required rev/min are reached. Unless this process is carried out slowly, the life of the centrifuge will be considerably curtailed. Some machines have a built-in revolution counter, while in others the rheostat must be calibrated by placing a tachometer on the rotating spindle.

8. When the tubes have been centrifuged sufficiently, switch off the motor and *then* bring the rheostat back to the zero position. Some centrifuges have an automatic timer built in which will switch off after the required time-interval.

9. Allow the centrifuge to come to a stop. Never slow the rotating head with your hand as brake. This will tend to redisperse the centrifugate due to turbulence and may cause serious injuries. Wait until the machine has stopped before attempting to remove the tubes.

10. Periodically a centrifuge should be lubricated according to the maker's instructions.

The Washing of Bacteria and Other Cells: 'Washed Suspensions'

The cell suspension is centrifuged at a suitable speed and preferably at a low temperature. Microorganisms grown on a solid medium are first suspended in liquid by scraping off the surface of the agar with a curved glass rod into a small volume of a suitable suspending fluid. (This suspension may be contaminated with lumps of agar which can be removed by filtration through cheesecloth.) The pellet of cells at the bottom of the centrifuge tube is resuspended and centrifuged. This washing process is repeated once or more to free the cells from the original suspending medium. The cells are finally made up to the required volume in the required solution.

For metabolic experiments, the cells are washed in a medium similar in composition to the culture medium but with one or more components omitted so that growth does not occur. The 'washed suspension' so obtained is particularly suitable for experiments on catabolism; a substrate and buffer are added so that the breakdown of the substrate can be studied uncomplicated by growth processes or by the metabolism of other substrates. However, it must be realized that some activities 'decay' rapidly after, or during, the preparation of the washed suspension.

Density Gradient Centrifugation

In a normal centrifugation, the material being centrifuged is forced to migrate through a homogeneous liquid medium. In density-gradient centrifugation, a gradient of a suitable solute, such as sucrose or caesium chloride, is made in the tube in such a way that the density increases with the distance from the axis of rotation. Such a gradient may be formed during the centrifugation process itself (with caesium chloride) or, more commonly, it is prepared by layering or by a gradient machine.

Density-gradient centrifugation can be employed to analyse and separate subcellular particles or viruses. There are three main types of method.

1. *Stabilized moving boundary centrifugation.* By the use of a density gradient, the sedimentation constant of a substance can be found using a preparation centrifuge by a method analogous to classical analytical ultracentrifuge. The gradient is a shallow one which stabilizes the boundary which might otherwise be

destroyed by convection currents. The material to be centrifuged is distributed throughout the tube at the start of the experiment and, after centrifugation, the position of the band or bands is formed by separating and analyses fractions from the tube.

2. *Zonal centrifugation.* In this method, a concentrated preparation is layered on top of a fairly steep gradient in the tube prior to centrifugation. Each component in the preparation will then sediment at its own rate, forming bands or zones in the tube which are separated from each other by distances related to their sedimentation rates. In practice, this means a separation mainly according to their size. After centrifugation, the components can be removed separately from the tube according to their position.

3. *Isopycnic or equilibrium gradient centrifugation.* In this method, a steep gradient is produced to encompass the entire density range of the particles being separated. The preparation is layered on top of the tube as in zonal centrifugation, or is distributed evenly throughout the gradient, and centrifugation is continued until the particles reach positions at which the density of the surrounding liquid is equal to their own. Thus, separation is based solely on density.

PHOTOELECTRIC COLORIMETER AND SPECTROPHOTOMETER

One of the simplest and most accurate methods of measuring the quantity of a microorganism depends upon a turbidity measurement, just as many of the quantitative micro-methods used in biochemistry depend upon the measurement of the depth of colour in a solution. For such measurements, a photoelectric colorimeter or spectrophotometer is simpler and more accurate than visual comparison. It is also much quicker and free from many personal factors, such as eye fatigue, colour blindness, etc., which are inherent in visual methods.

The theory of the instrument as a colorimeter depends upon the application of Beer's Law, which states that the extent of diminution in light intensity on passing through an absorbing material depends upon the nature and concentration of the absorbing material and upon the length of the light path. This can be expressed as follows:

$$\log \frac{Io}{I} = acl$$

where I is the intensity of the beam after passing through the solution, Io is the incident intensity, a is the extinction coefficient depending upon the particular chromogen, c is the concentration of the chromogen and l is the length of the light path through the solution.

It is possible, therefore, to determine the concentration of a substance by measuring Io/I in a vessel of standard dimensions. In photoelectric colorimeters and spectrophotometers, light intensity is measured by photoelectric response which can be made directly proportional to the quantity of light falling on the photoelectric cell.

Two main types of instrument are available: (1) Single-cell apparatus (Fig. 13.1); (2) Twin-cell apparatus (Fig. 13.2).

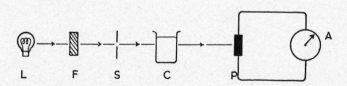

FIG. 13.1

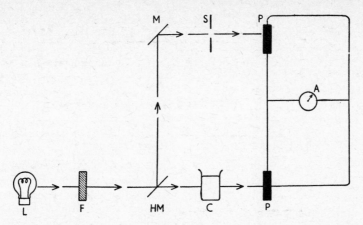

F<small>IG</small>. 13.2

The following points should be noted:

1. It is essential that the intensity of the source of light L should remain constant during a reading. A mains supply is subject to sudden changes of voltage and should be used only with a constant-voltage transformer. Alternatively, an accumulator can be used. With a twin-cell instrument, changes in light intensity affect both cells equally and therefore no error is involved. In a single-celled instrument it is necessary to check the reading with the blank solution after each determination.

2. The colour filter F isolates the part of the spectrum where absorption by the chromogen is greatest. A filter is selected that gives a colour of light complementary to the colour of the chromogen. Thus, if the solution is blue, a red filter should be used. The narrower the range of wavelength transmitted, the more can interference by other compounds be eliminated. In a spectrophotometer, a prism is built into the machine and selects light of a small wavelength band.

3. In the twin-celled instrument, a half-silvered mirror HM and a mirror M are used to split the light into two approximately equal beams.

4. There is an adjustable slit S in the light path.

5. The cuvette or tube C containing the solution should be of standard length of light path.

6. Light falls on the photoelectric cell or cells P and the current generated is measured by a microammeter A which is usually calibrated in a log scale permitting direct reading of log Io/I. In some two-celled apparatus, a calibrated slit is placed on one side of the slit and is adjusted to give no deflection on a galvanometer.

Directions for the use of a particular machine can be obtained from the makers. In all cases a blank solution is used in which the chromogen would be dissolved. A calibration curve should be constructed of the reading of the instrument (log Io/I) against known amounts of chromogen. If Beer's Law is obeyed, a straight line will be obtained. Unknown samples are compared with the plot.

The use of such instruments for turbidimetric measurements of bacterial numbers is considered later.

COUNTING BACTERIA AND MEASURING BACTERIAL GROWTH

The method used for determining the amount of a microorganism present in a suspension depends upon the kind of information required. In particular, since no constant relation exists between the ratio of increase in protoplasmic mass to rate of multiplication, it is necessary to distinguish clearly between methods which measure multiplication (e.g. total count) and those which measure growth (e.g. total nitrogen content, dry weight, etc.).

An evaluation of the methods that may be used to measure growth by physical and chemical means is given by Molette (1969).

1. *Total Count*

Microscopical Count

A total count of the living and dead bacteria in a liquid culture or suspension is made microscopically using a *slide counting chamber*. A suitable chamber (as supplied by Hawksley Ltd., London) consists of a thin glass slide with a flat, circular platform depressed exactly 0·02 mm below the surface and surrounded by a deeper 'trench'. An area of 1 mm^2 on the platform is marked with a Thoma-type grating of engraved lines into 400 small squares (each 0·0025 mm^2). The chamber is closed with a thick, optically-plane coverslip. When the space between platform and coverslip is filled with a bacterial suspension, the volume over each small square is 0·02 × 0·0025 mm^3, i.e. 0·000,000,05 ml. The average number of bacteria per square is calculated from counts made in sufficient squares (e.g. 100) to yield a significant total number of bacteria (e.g. 100–1000, preferably over 300). Counts are best made in preparations having between 2 and 10 bacteria per square (i.e. 40–200 million per ml). For bacteria occurring in pairs, chains or clusters, an 'individual cell count' may be made of all the cells, or a 'group count' of the groups plus any isolated single cells.

Procedure

1. Fix the bacterial suspension by adding 2 or 3 drops of 40 per cent formaldehyde per 10 ml. Mix thoroughly. If the suspension is too dense, prepare a measured dilution in the range 40–200 million bacteria per ml.

2. Wash, rinse, drain and dry the counting chamber and coverslip. Keep them covered until use, free from grit and dust.

3. Place a small drop or loopful of the suspension on the centre of the chamber platform and apply the coverslip. The size of the drop must be such that it will fill the whole space between platform and coverslip, yet not extend across the 'trench' to float the coverslip from the slide. The coverslip must be applied closely and evenly; it is pressed down until coloured 'Newton's rings' are seen uniformly distributed over the areas of contact.

4. Examine the preparation with a phase-contrast microscope, using the dry, $\frac{1}{6}$ in objective; this shows the unstained bacteria clearly and enables their distinction from detritus. Alternatively, a dark-ground microscope may be used, or an ordinary microscope with the iris diaphragm closed or the condenser slightly defocused (it may then be helpful to stain the bacteria by prior addition of freshly filtered methylene blue to a concentration of 0·1 per cent).

5. Count the bacteria in a sufficient number of squares to obtain a total of several hundred bacteria, selecting the squares in a pre-arranged pattern (e.g. all in every fifth row). Focus at different levels for the bacteria that have not settled; most settle on the platform in 5 or 10 min, but some adhere to the coverslip and a few remain in suspension.

6. Calculate the average number of bacteria per square. Multiply this by 20 000 000 and by the dilution factor, if any, to obtain the count per ml in the original suspension. Count two further preparations of the same suspension, and unless discordant, take an average of the three results.

If the original suspension contains much less than 40 000 000 bacteria per ml, a haemocytometer with a 0·1 mm chamber may be used so as to obtain a significant count in fewer squares. An ordinary microscope is used, the bacteria are stained and the preparation is left for twenty minutes before counting so that most bacteria may settle on the platform.

Total counts may be carried out automatically by means of the Coulter Counter (see Kubitschek, 1969).

2. *Viable Count*

Pour-Plate Method

The number of living bacteria or groups of

bacteria in a liquid culture or suspension is counted by a cultural method such as the *pour-plate method*. A measured amount of the suspension is mixed with molten agar medium in a Petri dish. After setting and incubation, the number of colonies is counted. As a compromise between sampling and overcrowding errors, counts of pure cultures should be made on plates inoculated to yield between 50 and 500 colonies (ideally 200–400).

Procedure

1. Prepare serial tenfold dilutions of the bacterial suspension over a range ensuring that one dilution will contain between 50 and 500 viable bacteria per ml. Use a diluent suitable for the organism concerned, e.g. buffered saline, Ringer or Locke's solutions. Pipette 9·0 ml amounts of diluent into each of several (6–9) sterile test-tubes. Mix uniformly the bacterial suspension (vigorous shaking may disrupt cell groups and increase the viable count). With a sterile 1-ml delivering pipette, transfer 1·0 ml suspension into the first tube of diluent (fill and empty the pipette with suspension several times before withdrawing from the original container, remove any excess drop from the outside of the pipette and then slowly deliver its contents into the tube of diluent, touching the wall of the tube but not dipping into the diluent). With a fresh sterile 1-ml pipette, mix the first dilution by filling and emptying several times, and then transfer 1·0 ml into the next tube of diluent. Make the remaining dilutions in the same way, using a fresh pipette for each.

2. Starting with the greatest dilution, pipette 1·0 ml amounts of each dilution into each of three 4-in Petri dishes. Then pour into each dish about 10 ml of clear nutrient agar, melted and cooled to 45–50°C. At once mix by rapidly moving the plate, while flat on the bench, in a combination of side-to-side and circular movements in different directions; continue for about ten seconds, taking care not to spill any of the contents. Allow the agar to set and incubate inverted for two days at 37°C, or as most suitable for the species examined.

3. Count the colonies in the three plates that were inoculated with the dilution giving between 50 and 500 colonies per plate (see above for counting methods). Multiply the average number per plate by the dilution factor to obtain the viable count per ml in the original suspension.

Surface Viable Count by Spreading Method

A surface viable count is made when the bacterium is best grown in surface culture or on an opaque medium. Prior to inoculation, the plate of medium is dried for at least two hours at 37°C with the lid ajar; it should then be able to absorb all the water of the inoculum within about fifteen minutes, i.e. before the bacteria can multiply. Tenfold dilutions of the bacterial suspension are made as for the pour-plate method. A suitable volume of each dilution, e.g. 0·1 ml, is pipetted on to the surface of each of three plates and at once spread widely with a fine wire loop. The viable count is calculated from the average colony count per plate.

Surface Viable Count by Miles and Misra Method

Alternatively, by the method of Miles and Misra (1938), the inoculum is deposited as drops from a calibrated dropping pipette. Each drop, 0·02 ml in volume, is allowed to fall from a height of 2·5 cm on to the medium, where it spreads over an area of 1·5–2·0 cm diameter. Each of six plates receives one drop of each dilution in separate numbered sectors. Counts are made in the drop areas showing the largest number of colonies without confluence (up to 20 or more); the mean of the six counts gives the viable count per 0·02 ml of the dilution.

Because of variations in average cell size, bacterial counts do not bear a constant relationship to the amount of protoplasmic growth. The amount of protoplasm is better gauged by an opacity measurement, weighing or a total nitrogen estimation.

A detailed description of methods to determine viability in cultures is given by Postgate (1969).

Methods of Measuring Growth

1. Centrifugation

A specified volume of the suspension is centrifuged in a special tube, usually a capillary tube. The height of the packed organisms provide a measure of the total protoplasmic mass. However, the method is only useful if very thick suspensions of cells are available.

2. Wet Weight

Amounts of culture for inoculation of animals are sometimes measured by wet weight. The moist surface growth on a solid medium is scraped from the medium and weighed at once. However, such estimations are inaccurate because of the difficulty of evaluating the relative contributions of water wetting the bacterial surface and intracellular water. Further, in bacteria forming capsules and slime, the wet weight may greatly overestimate the amount of protoplasm, since it includes the weight of these highly hydrated extracellular substances.

3. Dry Weight

The weight of the dried solid matter of bacteria affords a better measure of their protoplasm. The cells from a known volume of culture are washed free from soluble salts, nutrients and waste products by centrifugation in distilled water. It is assumed that no lysis occurs during this process. The whole or a known proportion of the washed cells is placed in a weighed vessel and weighed again after drying to a constant weight by heating in an oven, e.g. at 120°C for about three hours. Cool after each heating in a desiccator over P_2O_5 and weigh quickly to prevent absorption of water.

4. Total Nitrogen

One of the most reliable and constant methods of measuring the amount of bacterial protoplasm for metabolic measurements is by an estimation of the nitrogen present in the nitrogenous components of the cells, i.e. mainly proteins and nucleic acids (nitrogen content about 16 per cent). The cells from a known volume of culture are washed by centrifugation to free them from nitrogenous constituents of the medium and from extracellular excretion products. The total nitrogen of the cells is then estimated by the micro-Kjeldahl method. The cells are digested with sulphuric acid using a $CuSO_4$-K_2SO_4-selenium catalyst. The ammonia produced is removed after making the solution alkaline by steam distillation in a suitable still (e.g. a Markham still), trapped in 2 per cent boric acid and estimated either by titration or colorimetrically after the addition of a suitable reagent (e.g. Nessler reagent).

Instead of measuring the total nitrogen content of the cells, it may be preferable to measure the total non-dialysable nitrogen content. A measured volume of a washed bacterial suspension is placed in a length of dialysis cellophane tubing tied off at its lower end. The bacterial enzymes are inactivated and the cell membranes burst by immersing the sack in boiling water for a few minutes. The sack is then closed tightly on its contents by tying the upper end. It is placed for a period of 24 hours in a jar of running tap water, or in a large volume of distilled water. The fluid inside the dialysis sack is removed by cutting one end and the volume noted for any changes during dialysis. The nitrogen content is then determined as described.

5. Turbidity

Brown's opacity tubes. A simple method of determining the *approximate* number of bacteria in a suspension is by means of standard turbidity tubes such as the Brown series (Brown, 1919–20). This consists in comparing the opacity of the suspension with that of a series of ten standard tubes containing different dilutions of suspended barium sulphate. The suspension may be made up in liquid, in which case it must be well shaken before use. Alternatively a stable suspension in gelatin can be used provided a preservative is added. In making comparisons the bacterial suspension should, of course, be placed in a tube of similar dimensions to the standards. The matching is facilitated by reading printed letters through the suspensions.

The table gives the numerical equivalents of the opacity standards for certain organisms according to Cunningham and Timothy (1924).

It must be realized, however, that these figures may be inaccurate owing to the method of counting that was used. Further, the opacity of a bacterial suspension will depend not only on the number of bacteria and the species of bacterium but also on the strain and the conditions of growth, which both affect cell size and density. It is advised that if opacity tubes are used, they should be calibrated for the particular organism and growth conditions being studied.

Standard opacity tubes with the corresponding tables are supplied by Wellcome Reagents Co. Ltd.

USE OF A PHOTOELECTRIC COLORIMETER OR SPECTROPHOTOMETER. The turbidity of a suspension is caused by the light scattered by particulate matter during its passage through the suspension. Clearly, accurate measurements of turbidity and hence bacterial growth, can be obtained in two ways.

1. By measuring the amount of light scattered directly, a procedure occásionally called nephelometry. This is rarely used in practice.

2. By measuring the light lost from the beam by scattering. Light absorption is assumed to be absent. This loss can be measured accurately in a photoelectric colorimeter or spectrophotometer where a relation similar to Beer's Law applies. The expression is the same as that given above except that the term extinction coefficient is replaced by a constant called the turbidity coefficient. A standard plot can be made of log Io/I against either the total nitrogen content or the dry weight. The concentration factor applies mainly to protoplasmic mass as the size of the organism as well as their number determines turbidity.

The following points should be noted:

1. The calibration curve applies only to *a particular organism grown under a particular set of growth conditions*. A new curve must be prepared if a change is made in either of these. It should be noted that the shape of an organism as well as its size will alter turbidity. Further, cells grown in a medium to give a high carbohydrate or fat content generally have a high turbidity per cell.

2. Use a neutral or a blue filter. In a spectrophotometer use a wavelength of 5400 Å. Light

Table 13.1   Showing the relation of the opacity of Brown's Standards to the numerical equivalent of various bacteria estimated by means of the Haemacytometer Method

Opacity tube No.	Staphylococcus aureus	Streptococcus pyogenes	Pneumococcus	Gonococcus	Esch. coli	S. typhi	S. paratyphi B	N. catarrhalis	H. influenzae
10	3·8	3·0	7·1	3·6	3·8	4·6	4·2	3·6	11·4
9	3·4	2·7	6·3	3·2	3·4	4·1	3·8	3·3	10·3
8	3·0	2·4	5·6	2·9	3·0	3·7	3·3	2·9	9·1
7	2·7	2·1	4·9	2·5	2·7	3·2	2·9	2·5	8·0
6	2·3	1·8	4·2	2·1	2·3	2·7	2·5	2·2	6·8
5	1·9	1·5	3·5	1·8	1·9	2·3	2·1	1·8	5·7
4	1·5	1·2	2·8	1·4	1·5	1·8	1·7	1·4	4·6
3	1·1	0·9	2·1	1·1	1·1	1·4	1·3	1·1	3·4
2	0·8	0·6	1·4	0·7	0·8	0·9	0·8	0·7	2·3
1	0·4	0·3	0·7	0·4	0·4	0·5	0·4	0·4	1·1

The figures represent thousands of millions per ml.

scattering increases very greatly as the wavelength decreases, although it is not advisable to use too low a wavelength since light absorption will become increasingly apparent.

3. For the blank use the suspending fluid. The growth medium can be used provided the absorption is not altered by growth of the organisms. If it is altered, the cells must be washed and resuspended in fresh solutions.

4. At low concentrations, a linear calibration plot should be obtained, but at higher concentrations a considerable departure from a straight line will normally occur. High cell populations cannot be determined unless they are first diluted to a suitable range.

5. The suspending fluid must be the same as that used for the preparation of the calibration curve.

Turbidity estimations in this way are the easiest and the quickest way of calibrating a bacterial population and they are accurate for comparative studies provided the above points are borne in mind.

REFERENCES

BROWN, H. C. (1919–20) *Indian Journal of Medical Research*, **7**, 238.

KUBITSCHEK, H. E. (1969) In *Methods in Microbiology*, Vol. I, p. 593, edited by J. R. Norris and D. W. Ribbons. London: Academic Press.

MILES, A. A. & MISRA, S. S. (1938) *Journal of Hygiene (London)*, **38**, 732.

MOLETTE, M. F. (1969) In *Methods in Microbiology*, Vol. I, p. 522, edited by J. R. Norris and D. W. Ribbons. London: Academic Press.

POSTGATE, J. R. (1969) In *Methods in Microbiology*, Vol. I, p. 611, edited by J. R. Norris and D. W. Ribbons. London: Academic Press.

14. Biological Standardization

The microbiologist is obliged to make many measurements and comparisons in his routine and experimental work. At the simplest level, he is concerned with relative and absolute sizes of microscopically small objects. In some circumstances, it is quite sufficient to use relative terms and to relate the size of an observed bacterial rod in an exudate, for example, to the relatively 'standard' dimensions of a red blood cell observed in the same field. The fact that a red blood cell is subject to considerable variation in size depending upon osmotic factors, whereas a bacterial cell is rigid, is one of the reasons for regarding the red cell as a very poor standard. When it is necessary to determine cell dimensions accurately, various methods that employ the light microscope, electron microscope or other special equipment are available and these are described in Volume I (Chap. 1).

In this book, microscopical units of length are used. The micrometre (μm) is one millionth part of a metre or a thousandth part of a millimetre (0·001 mm); the term micron for this measurement is now obsolete. One thousandth of 1 μm was formerly referred to as 1 millimicron (mμ) but is now termed 1 nanometre (nm; 10^{-9} metre). The Angstrom unit (Å; 10^{-10} metre) should not be used now and measurements in this range should be expressed in nanometres (10Å = 1 nm). Thus: metre (m), centimetre (cm), millimetre (mm), micrometre (μm), and nanometre (nm) respectively denote 1, 10^{-2}, 10^{-3}, 10^{-6} and 10^{-9} metre. In general, the dimensions of protozoa, fungi and bacteria fall within the micrometre range and those of viruses are in the nanometre range.

In addition to being concerned with cell dimensions, the microbiologist is greatly concerned with cell numbers. Although a considerable proportion of the observations made in his routine work appear to be essentially qualitative, there are many in which a quantitative element is inferred or actually specified. For example, 'a scanty growth of *Escherichia coli*' isolated from a wound of the perineum may be regarded as less significant than a pure profuse growth of that organism in these circumstances. It must be acknowledged that such measures as 'profuse' and 'scanty' are subject to much observer bias.

Truly quantitative bacteriology had early application in blood culture work and is now practised as a routine in the diagnosis of urinary tract infections (Vol. I, Chap. 55) and in the testing of water supplies, etc. (Chap. 12). In the enumeration of cells, and particularly in relation to counts of viable cells in which colony-forming units are enumerated after incubation on a suitable medium (viable cell counts), it should be noted that a Poisson distribution is involved. In such circumstances —and always provided that no technical error is involved—the standard deviation, which is an index of the confidence limits of the count, is the square root of the number counted; it therefore follows that some hundreds of units should be counted if the range of error is to be kept reasonably small. These considerations and some others in this chapter are more fully discussed by Meynell and Meynell (1970). An important point is that the application of statistical concepts and rules cannot make amends for technical errors. For example, the errors associated with the preparation of dilutions for examination procedures are considered by Postgate (1967), and inevitable errors associated with certain counting chambers have been studied by Norris and Powell (1961) and Cook and Lund (1962).

Many methods of measurement in microbiology involve comparisons of the responses of sample groups of a test population of cells or animals or people to different stimuli or agents. If the responses are to be properly comparable, all of the samples or groups of the test population used in the experiment should be identical. It can be shown that haphazard selection of animals, for example, may result in the inclusion of a significantly higher proportion of more robust or less active animals in the early groups. There are also well recognized sources of observer and selector bias in unconscious preferences for certain numbers and other factors so that it is essential to adopt a correct *random sampling procedure* in selecting comparable population samples or groups.

Randomization affords some insurance against selecting unequivalent groups of individuals from a test population. Replication of observations increases the precision of the average values and gives some measure of the degree of random variation within the group. It may be that the effect of random variation can be reduced by making comparisons between subgroups that are more comparable. For example, animal experiments may be designed in which the responses of littermates to two different treatments are compared and, in this case, each of a pair of littermates of the same sex and similar weight may be randomly assigned to one treatment or the other.

Since variation between individual responses is inevitable there is bound to be unpredictable variation in the results of measuring any test sample. This variation is referred to as *sampling error* and the ways of measuring its effect are fully described elsewhere (see Hill, 1961). When several samples are tested from the same population it is useful to give the *mean* result, i.e. the arithmetic average of all the results. This value may, however, be affected considerably by the presence of a few extreme values, and where this is the case the *median* result may be given instead, i.e. the middle result of all the results when these are arranged linearly in ascending order. The median is not affected by a few extreme results. For a fuller discussion of these principles in relation to biological variation and measurement the reader is referred to Perry (1968).

BIO-ASSAY

Biological assay is the estimation of the amount of some material in a preparation by observation of its activity on a living population, usually laboratory animals, but occasionally microorganisms, plants, men or tissue cells. The procedure involves (1) a test preparation of unknown potency, (2) a reference prepara-

tion of known potency, (3) a test population, and (4) a detectable response that is specifically produced by the substance concerned in the assay. The potency of the test preparation is determined by ascertaining the mean response to a certain dose and comparing this dose with the amount of the reference preparation that produces the same mean response, or '*standard indicating effect*', under the same experimental conditions.

In assessing the potency of a biologically active substance, a *unit* of measurement must first be defined and the particular activity of the substance is then compared with that of a known standard preparation in terms of this unit.

A sample of a reference preparation is routinely included in each assay. Laboratories hold their own local reference materials and these are checked periodically against recognized standards that are held in stable form by a central laboratory. The International Laboratories for Biological Standards at the Statens Seruminstitut, Copenhagen, Denmark, and at the National Institute for Medical Research, London, England, hold all International Biological Standards and International Biological Reference Preparations. These include: (1) immunological substances such as tuberculin, tetanus toxoid, diphtheria toxoid, pertussis vaccine, tetanus antitoxin and diphtheria antitoxin; and (2) pharmacological substances such as antibiotics, hormones, vitamins and drugs. If no standard preparation exists, a stable form of the new preparation is submitted when possible and this may be regarded as a provisional standard, of which a fixed weight or volume is said to contain one unit of the particular activity. A unit is thus defined as the specific biological activity contained in a given weight or volume of the standard preparation. If it is attempted to define a unit otherwise, e.g. as the smallest amount of the substance producing a specified effect in an experimental animal, the wide variation in susceptibility between individual animals of the same species generally introduces many difficulties and sources of error. It will be evident that experiments involving such comparisons of test populations frequently demand a careful statistical approach and proper planning.

Assay Methods

Direct Assay. The amounts of the reference and test preparations required to produce a specified response are directly compared. For example, the dose of a substance that on average kills the test animal within a specified time (or that which, when infused at a constant rate, just kills the test animal) may be measured and compared with that of a standard preparation tested simultaneously. Since animals vary in susceptibility, the mean of several experiments is taken in each case and the potency of the test substance in relation to the standard is indicated by the ratio of the two means. Direct measurement of the critical dose required to elicit a particular response is frequently not possible and indirect assay methods are more usually employed.

Indirect Assay. Responses produced by different doses are observed. This type of assay may involve observations of: (1) the presence or absence of a typical response, such as death of the test animal. This 'all-or-nothing' result is referred to as a *quantal response*; or (2) degrees of magnitude of the response, such as increase of weight or time of survival of the test animal. This is a *quantitative response*.

When the responses of similar groups of the test population to graded doses of the standard and test preparations are measured in parallel and the means of each series are plotted against the logarithm of each dose (log. dose), a *dose-response curve* is obtained for each preparation. This is frequently linear in its midportion (see Wilson and Miles, 1964).

Microbiological Assay

Under appropriate conditions in a synthetic medium, the amount of bacterial growth (e.g. the number of cells when the growth is completed) is linearly proportional to the concentration of a growth factor or essential amino acid whose supply is deficient in relation to the other nutrients. Thus the amount of a growth factor or amino acid may be measured according to the amount of the growth that it supports, as in the assay of vitamin B_{12} using *Lactobacillus leichmannii*. The method has the advantage of specificity and high sensitivity.

In the case of vitamins it is possible to determine as little as 0·001 μg per ml, and in some cases (biotin and B_{12}) considerably less. It should be noted that the response in these assays, e.g. production of turbidity or acidity by a growing culture, is usually linearly related to the dose and not to the logarithm of the dose.

Microbiological assays are also of use in assaying antibiotics, and various methods have been devised. In these assays, the degrees of inhibition of growth of a culture of bacteria by different concentrations of the test preparation are compared with the degrees of inhibition produced by known concentrations of a standard preparation of the antibiotic.

Biologically active substances that can now be estimated quantitatively by physico-chemical methods may be assayed independently of biological methods. This is true of many substances that used to be assayed biologically, e.g. vitamin C, and some antibiotics. When a crude preparation of a newly discovered biologically active substance is assayed by a bio-assay method, it is initially necessary to establish a crude preparation as a provisional standard until purification procedures are developed. This was the case with benzyl penicillin, for example, and a unit of activity was defined in terms of a microbiological assay. As purer preparations were developed, these were adopted as standards; finally, pure salts of benzyl penicillin could be assayed chemically and the actual weight of benzyl penicillin present in any preparation could be determined. When the activity could be expressed in terms of weight of the pure substance, it became clear that the very small amounts required to produce an observed effect in the microbiological assay had influenced the choice of a unit. In fact, many thousands of units of benzyl penicillin constitute a clinical dose and it would have been more convenient in practice if the unit had been fixed at a much higher level. Thus, for preparations whose activity can be assayed in terms of the weight of a single pure substance, it is convenient to express dosages in terms of the weight of that substance rather than in units of activity. However, there are many biologically active substances that cannot yet be defined in strictly chemical terms and the potency of these substances continues to be expressed in terms of units in comparison with the activity of recognized standard preparations. Moreover, when dosages of a compound are initially expressed in units, the change to a weight basis is resisted by those who gained experience with the older system and, during the transition period, manipulations with conversion factors (e.g. units to micrograms) reflect the uneasiness with which a new dosage system is accepted.

MEASUREMENT OF VIRULENCE

The minimum lethal dose ('*MLD*'). This is the dose of a bacterial suspension or toxin that just kills the test animal (or all of several test animals) within a specified time after administration by a given route. The use of this measure assumes that all animals in the same species are equally susceptible, but since there may be differences in susceptibility between animals the accuracy of the determination is partly dependent upon the number of animals used. In a procedure recommended for the determination of diphtheria toxin in terms of MLD, final testing is considered probably correct within 10 per cent if at least three doses not differing more than $\pm$ 10 per cent are used with two guinea-pigs per dose (see Boyd, 1956); the smallest dose killing both guinea-pigs is the MLD.

LD50. The LD50 (50 per cent lethal dose) of a microbial culture or toxin is the dose that kills 50 per cent of the test animals within a specified time. In view of the variation in the susceptibility of different animals of the same species, the LD50 is usually a more practical and reliable measurement than the MLD. The LD50 of a particular preparation is usually estimated by reference to the linear mid-section of the dose-response curve in which percentage responses (deaths) between 25 and 75 are plotted against the logarithms of the doses administered. It should be stressed that this method of determining the LD50 involves assumptions regarding the linearity of the mid-section of the particular dose-response curve and ignores observations outwith the 25–75 per cent response range. Furthermore, misleading conclusions may be drawn if such an experimental determination is not performed with adequate numbers of animals in each group. The problems involved are discussed extensively by Boyd (1956).

The measurement of 50 per cent end-points. In testing the potency of a bacterial toxin, or the lethal dose or infective dose of a bacterial or viral suspension, varying amounts of the test preparation (differing by a constant dilution factor) may be inoculated into groups of susceptible animals. As described above, it is more accurate to take the end-point of the titration as that dilution at which 50 per cent of the animals react, and to work in terms of the LD50, ID50, etc. When the standard indicating effect is not death but some other response, the dose that is *effective* in 50 per cent of the test animals is referred to as the ED50. The dose *infecting* 50 per cent of animals is the ID50. The dose *protecting* 50 per cent, as in testing immunizing agents, is the PD50. In many virus titrations it is possible to use chick embryos or tissue cultures instead of animals. The TCD50 is the dose causing a *cytopathic effect* in 50 per cent of the challenged tissue cultures.

The most reliable assay method involves testing large numbers of animals or tissue cultures with many closely spaced dilutions near the value for 50 per cent reaction. Especially when animals are used, this is seldom economically possible and it is often necessary to use rather widely spaced dilutions (e.g. decimal or doubling dilutions) and groups of moderate numbers of animals.

The method of Reed and Muench (1938) allows a more precise determination of the 50 per cent end-point than is possible by simple interpolation between two critical dilutions and gives an effect as if larger groups of animals had been used than were actually inoculated. There is, moreover, a tendency to equalize chance variations.

Reed and Muench's Method for Estimation of LD50

In Reed and Muench's method it is assumed that animals dying at a stated dose would also have been killed by greater amounts of the agent and conversely that those surviving would also have survived smaller doses. An accumulated value for the animals affected is obtained by adding the number dying at a certain dilution to the number killed by lesser doses; a similar addition, but in the reverse direction, is made for the survivors (see example below.

The accumulated values of the two critical dilutions between which the 50 per cent end-point lies are now substituted in the formula and the LD50 is obtained.

In making these calculations it is assumed that the doses used are equally placed on the logarithmic scale, that the 50 per cent end-point falls somewhere in the middle of the range of dilutions used and that the same number of animals was used for each dilution.

Example:

Virus dilution	Mortality ratio	Died	Survived	Accumulated values			
				Died (D)	Survived (S)	Mortality Ratio	Per cent $\frac{(D)}{(D+S)} \times 100$
10^{-1}	10/10	10	0	31	0	31/31	100
10^{-2}	10/10	10	0	21	0	21/21	100
10^{-3}	8/10	8	2	11	2	11/13	85
10^{-4}	3/10	3	7	3	9	3/12	25
10^{-5}	0/10	0	10	0	19	0/19	0

The arrows indicate the direction of addition for the accumulated values.

In this titration the 50 per cent end-point is seen to lie between 10^{-3} and 10^{-4}. It will be located at the porportionate distance from 10^{-3}.

$$\frac{\text{Proportionate}}{\text{distance}} = \frac{\text{mortality above 50 per cent} - 50}{\text{mortality above 50 per cent} - \text{mortality below 50 per cent}}$$

$$= \frac{85-50}{85-25} = \frac{35}{60} = 0.58$$

$$\begin{array}{l}\text{Negative logarithm} = \text{Negative logarithm of dilution} + \text{proportionate} \\ \text{of LD50 titre} \qquad \text{above 50 per cent mortality} \qquad \text{distance} \end{array}$$
$$= 3.0 + 0.58$$
$$\text{LD50} = 10^{-3.58}$$

Note: Finney (1964) is not in favour of this method.

Käber's Method for Estimation of LD 50

An alternative and slightly simpler method is that of Kärber (1931):

$$\begin{array}{l}\log \text{LD50} = 0.5 + \log \text{ of greatest virus} \quad -\dfrac{\text{Sum of percentage of dead animals}}{100} \\ \text{titre} \qquad \text{concentration used} \end{array}$$

For the above example:

$$\log \text{LD50 titre} = 0.5 + (-1.0) - \frac{100 + 100 + 85 + 25}{100}$$
$$= 0.5 - 1.0 - 3.1$$
$$= -3.6$$
$$\text{LD50 titre} = 10^{-3.6}$$

Litchfield and Wilcoxon's Method for Estimation of LD50

This method (1949) is a rapid graphic procedure for estimating the median effective dose (ED50, LD50, etc.) and the slope of the dose-per cent effect curve. It gives confidence limits of both these parameters for 19/20 probability. It is highly recommended. The original paper should be consulted for detailed instructions.

For guidance in choosing methods of estimating the LD50 and ED50 with quantal response data, the reader is referred to the paper by Armitage and Allen (1950) and to the careful considerations of Meynell and Meynell (1970) of quantitative aspects of microbiological experiments.

TOXIN-ANTITOXIN ASSAY

The unit of diphtheria antitoxin was originally defined as that amount of antitoxin (or antitoxic serum) that just neutralizes 100 MLD of a certain diphtheria toxin. The MLD was defined as the minimum amount of toxin that kills a guinea-pig of 250 grams weight in four days. It is not feasible, however, to preserve a standard toxin for testing antitoxin, but by means of a preserved standard antitoxin any toxin preparation can be standardized by neutralization tests in guinea-pigs, and the value of a new antitoxin can then be estimated. The usual method is to ascertain first the '$L+$' dose of the toxin; this is the quantity of diphtheria toxin that, when mixed with 1 unit of standard antitoxin, is just sufficient to kill a 250-gram guinea-pig within four days. Varying dilutions of the new antitoxin are then mixed with the $L+$ dose and injected into guinea-pigs. In this way the neutralizing power of the new antitoxin can be compared quantitatively with the standard and the number of units in a given volume stated. Antitoxin may also be titrated by the neutralization of the *reaction* following the intracutaneous injection of mixtures of toxin and antitoxin in the guinea-pig or rabbit, using an 'Lr' dose of toxin. This is the amount of toxin that, when injected intradermally along with 1 unit of antitoxin, causes a localized erythema 5 mm in diameter within 36 hours. The amount of the unknown antitoxin producing the equivalent result when injected with the same dose of toxin will contain 1 unit of antitoxin. In practice, several skin tests may be done simultaneously on one animal and, in order to avoid injecting a lethal dose of toxin, these neutralization tests may be performed with dilutions equivalent to specified fractions of units (provided that the test dose of toxin injected is not diluted beyond its active titre).

It will be evident from the above example that in toxin-antitoxin testing, some effect such as death within a stated time, or production of a stated area of erythema or necrosis, is the specified response or *standard indicating effect*. Antiserum is routinely calibrated by determining the dilution that, when mixed with a fixed amount of the particular toxin (the *test dose*), just allows it to produce the standard indicating effect. In other words, the antitoxin in the serum is serially diluted in the presence of a test dose of toxin, the effect of which becomes demonstrable at the end-point of the titration. The amount of the test antiserum contained in the end-point dilution is then regarded as equivalent in the number of units to the amount of a standard antitoxin that allows the same standard indicating effect when mixed with a test dose of toxin in a parallel titration.

The test dose of toxin is determined by adding a constant volume of the standard antitoxin, containing x units, to graded doses of the toxin. The mixture that subsequently produces the standard indicating effect contains the test dose at the x-units level of testing. It is important that the proposed level of testing, i.e. the number of units contained in the fixed amount of standard antitoxin used, should be such that the appropriate test dose of toxin is indeed capable of producing the standard indicating effect. A simple control titration of toxin should always be included to demonstrate this.

The *Lo dose* of a toxin is the amount of toxin that is just neutralized by 1 unit of antitoxin. This is technically difficult to measure exactly and titrations are generally based instead on the *L+ dose*, i.e. the amount of toxin that, when mixed with 1 unit of antitoxin, produces the standard indicating effect.

Danysz phenomenon. Antibody and antigen combine in different proportions according to the amount of each in a mixture. The addition of a relatively small amount of toxin to a large amount of antitoxin results in the combination of many more antitoxin molecules per molecule of toxin than would occur if more toxin had been available in the initial mixture. Thus, if an amount of toxin and a minimum amount of antitoxin are chosen, such that they would give a non-toxic mixture if they were mixed together all at once, and if the toxin is split into several portions and these are added to the antitoxin one after the other, the final mixture will be found to be toxic. The initial combination of relatively large numbers of antitoxin molecules with relatively few toxin molecules leaves insufficient free antitoxin for the prompt neutralization of the fractions of toxin subsequently added. The final mixture therefore remains toxic, at least until a spontaneous rearrangement takes place in the combining ratio of the antibody and antigen molecules. For this reason, when mixtures of antitoxin and toxin are made in neutralization experiments, antitoxin is added to toxin and not *vice versa*.

In-vitro testing. Toxin and antitoxin may be assayed by in-vitro methods if an indicating effect of the toxin, such as haemolysis, can be specifically neutralized by the homologous antitoxin. The conditions under which such tests are performed may be critical and it is important to define them when reporting results. For example, the lecithinase (alpha toxin) of *Clostridium welchii* may be assayed in terms of its haemolytic activity. In this case, the species of red cell and the composition of the diluent greatly influence the result of the test.

Optimal proportions in precipitation or flocculation reactions. When a series of mixtures of antigen and antibody is set up in tubes with a constant amount of antiserum and increasing amounts of antigen, precipitation and flocculation occur most rapidly and most markedly in the tube in which antibody and antigen occur in *optimal proportions* (Dean and Webb, 1926). The ratio is constant for all dilutions of a given antiserum and antigen, and usually all of the antigen is precipitated at this point. The antibody content of different sera may therefore be compared by ascertaining the amounts required to produce most rapid and complete flocculation with a given antigen.

Thus antitoxin may be assayed *in vitro* by the Ramon flocculation method based on the rapid precipitation obtained when optimal proportions of toxin and antitoxin are mixed. The *Lf dose* of toxin is first determined as the amount of toxin that flocculates most quickly with 1 unit of antitoxin. The unknown antitoxin is then tested to find the dilution that flocculates most rapidly with 1 Lf dose of toxin. This dilution will contain 1 Lf unit of antitoxin.

Avidity of antiserum. In addition to the actual content of antitoxin in an antiserum, the combining power of the antitoxin in terms of rate and firmness of combination with toxin, i.e. its *avidity*, significantly influences its effective neutralizing power. The antitoxin in an avid serum combines quickly and firmly with toxin. The protective effect of an antiserum, as judged by animal experiments, may not always exactly parallel estimates of its potency based upon in-vitro experiments. One explanation for this is that slight differences may exist in a group of components that normally act as a single antibody complex but may consequently participate to different degrees in various in-vitro reactions. It is also clear that in-vitro procedures may not give a true estimate of the relative therapeutic values of two antisera containing equal amounts of antitoxin if one serum is much more avid than the other.

THE EVALUATION OF A PROTECTIVE ANTIGEN

Mouse protection test. In the evaluation of immunizing agents it is usual to give groups of animals graded doses of the test preparation and to give similar groups the same doses of a standard preparation. After a suitable period the animals in the two series are then challenged with, for example, a normally lethal dose (e.g. 100 LD50) of the bacteria or toxin against which they were presumably protected. The size of the challenge dose should be adjusted so that it is likely to produce a significant mortality but it must not be so great that there are no survivors in either of the series. The percentage of survivors in each group is subsequently recorded and the logarithms of the doses of the test and standard preparations associated with 50 per cent survival are estimated. The difference between these is the log. potency ratio, and the antilogarithm of this figure gives the actual potency ratio of the two preparations in terms of the amounts that produced 50 per cent protection (PD50) against the challenge dose.

In assessing the protective value of vaccines for human use, controlled field and laboratory studies should be done. The principles are discussed in Chapter 58, Volume I.

REFERENCES AND FURTHER READING

ARMITAGE, P. & ALLEN, I. (1950) Methods of estimating the LD50 in quantal response data. *Journal of Hygiene (London)*, **48**, 298.

BOYD, W. C. (1956) *Fundamentals of Immunology*. 3rd edn., pp. 642, 694. London and New York: Interscience Publishers.

COOK, A. M. & LUND, B. M. (1962) Total counts of bacterial spores using counting slides. *Journal of General Microbiology*, **29**, 97.

DEAN, H. R. & WEBB, R. A. (1926) The influence of optimal proportions of antigen and antibody in the serum precipitation reaction. *Journal of Pathology and Bacteriology*, **29**, 473.

FINNEY, D. J. (1964) *Statistical Method in Biological Assay*. 2nd edn. London: Charles Griffin & Co. Ltd.

HILL, A. B. (1961) *Principles of Medical Statistics*, p. 108. London: *Lancet*.

KÄRBER, G. (1931) Beitrag zur kollektiven Behandlung pharmakologischer Reihenversuche. *Archives of Experimental Pathology and Pharmacology*, **162**, 480.

LITCHFIELD, J. T. & WILCOXON, F. (1949) A simplified method of evaluating dose-effect experiments. *Journal of Pharmacology and Experimental Therapeutics*, **96**, 99.

MEYNELL, G. G. & MEYNELL, E. (1970) *Theory and Practice in Experimental Bacteriology*. 2nd edn., p. 173. Cambridge University Press.

NORRIS, K. P. & POWELL, E. O. (1961) Improvements in determining total counts of bacteria. *Journal of the Royal Microscopical Society*, **80**, 107.

PERRY, W. L. M. (1968) Biological variation and its measurement. In *A Companion to Medical Studies*, Vol. 1, Chap. 3, p. 31, edited by R. Passmore and J. S. Robson. Oxford and Edinburgh: Blackwell.

POSTGATE, J. R. (1967) Viability measurements and the survival of microbes under minimum stress. In *Advances in Microbial Physiology*, Vol. 1, p. 1, edited by A. H. Rose and J. F. Wilkinson.

REED, L. V. & MUENCH, H. (1938) A simple method of estimating fifty per cent end points. *American Journal of Hygiene*, **27**, 493.

WILSON, G. S. & MILES, A. A. (1964) *Topley and Wilson's Principles of Bacteriology and Immunity*. 5th edn., p. 1209. London: Arnold.

15. The Care and Management of Experimental Animals

Laboratory animals in Great Britain are protected by the Cruelty to Animals Act (1876), under which only workers who hold a licence granted by the Home Secretary are permitted to experiment on them. Advice on the procedure to obtain a licence may be got from the Research Defence Society, 11 Chandos Street, London W1. The licence authorizes the licensee to carry out experiments in the stated registered place only. All registered places are approved by the Home Office before registration is granted, and are thereafter visited from time to time without notice by the Home Office Inspector for the area. Depending on the scope of his experiments, the licensee may require a certificate (or certificates) in addition, for in any experiment authorized by licence alone, the animal must be anaesthetized before the experiment begins and must be killed before recovery from the anaesthetic. Certificate A must be obtained if no anaesthetic is to be used; this covers most of the bacteriologist's usual laboratory work with animals: namely, procedures that do not exceed the equivalent of injection or superficial venesection. It can authorize, for example, inoculation of the animal subcutaneously, intravenously, intraperitoneally, or by scarification. For experiments requiring procedures which exceed the equivalent of the above in severity, an anaesthetic must be used. Certificate B must be obtained to authorize any experiment whose object would be frustrated unless the animal is allowed to recover from the anaesthetic. Further certificates must be obtained to authorize experiments in which cats, dogs or the equidae are used. In all cases of doubt about animal experiments, and the law relating to them, the worker is strongly advised, in his own interest, to seek the advice of the Home Office Inspector for his area, whose name and address can be got by application to the Under Secretary of State, Home Office, London SW1.

GENERAL DIRECTIONS FOR THE CARE OF ANIMALS

The health and well-being of laboratory animals depend almost entirely on the care, humanity and watchfulness of the staff of the animal house. To keep laboratory animals healthy and contented requires a high degree of technical skill, a genuine liking for animals, and a full understanding of their ways of life. Animals in cages are deprived of their own ways of fending for themselves and they are completely dependent on their attendants for all their necessities and comforts; it is impossible for them to find their own food or water, to move to a cooler or a warmer place, to seek fresh air or to obtain exercise or companionship. To make good these deficiencies in their life a number of general principles must be observed in the day to day running of an animal house (Laboratory Animal Symposia, 1938; 1969).

Fluid

No animal should ever be deprived of a plentiful supply of fresh clean drinking water. It is wrong to assume that wet mashes and moistened diets supply enough fluid although it is true that in the case of guinea-pigs and rabbits, a plentiful supply of fresh cabbage or lettuce may obviate the need for drinking bottles. Animals kept short of water lose condition, eat less, waste, and are prone to cannibalize their young.

Drinking water can be conveniently supplied to the animals from a bottle attached to the outside of the cage. Suitable and inexpensive bottles are medical flats, blood transfusion bottles, ginger-beer bottles; wide mouthed pathological specimen jars are particularly recommended as being easily cleaned. The bottles should hold 250–500 ml of water, smaller bottles are more liable to leakage through agitation. The water is led in 6–9 mm glass tubing through a rubber bung to an accessible position inside the cage; the outlet of the tubing should be narrowed to about 3 mm.

Diet

A balanced diet which contains carbohydrate, fat, proteins, vitamins, mineral salts, and trace elements in appropriate proportions must be given regularly. Usually such a diet can be obtained commercially in the form of cubes or pellets and can be placed in hoppers attached to the sides of the cages so that food is available at all times to the animals. When cage hoppers are not available the pellets may be placed in dishes inside the cages or a dry or wet mash may be given in the same manner. The latter method, however, is time consuming and much foodstuff is wasted by spilling and contamination. The condition of many animals is improved by supplementing pellet diets with small quantities of greenstuffs.

Cleanliness

Animals will not thrive under dirty conditions and unless they are kept clean there is a considerable risk of epidemic disease. Once each week the animals should be transferred to clean cages and the dirty cages should be removed to a special room set aside for them where they should be scraped free from all litter and droppings, scrubbed thoroughly in soap and water and sterilized in the autoclave or hot air oven. The animals, especially when breeding, should not however have their cages changed too frequently because they are disturbed by the process and as a result often lose weight. With adequately absorbent litter such as peat moss the cages remain hygienic for a week. Where heat sterilizers are not available the cages can be boiled in soapy water or, failing that, immersed overnight in a solution of disinfectant such as 3 per cent lysol. Lysol, however, should not be used for rabbit cages because its smell distresses the animals. The cages should be perfectly dry before being used again. Clean cages should then be stacked on a trolley to be transferred for storage in a special clean room where clean litter can be placed in them and clean sterile hoppers or dishes of food and drinking bottles added to them before they are taken into use again. A special trolley should be reserved for the clean cages and another for dirty cages.

Litter

A layer of absorbent material should be spread to a depth of a half to one inch on the bottom of the cages. For this purpose fine soft wood sawdust, wood shavings, peat moss or sugar-cane pith are all satisfactory. Pregnant animals must also be supplied with nesting material; shredded paper is recommended for mice and clean hay for rabbits and guinea-pigs.

Cages

Each species of animal requires its own type of cage and the design must ensure that there is enough room to give free movement and space for resting when the animal lies down fully stretched out. The cage should be large enough for the animal to take some exercise; this is especially important for monkeys. To facilitate cleaning many cages are provided with coarse wire-mesh floors through which the excreta fall on to a tray which can easily be removed for cleaning without disturbing the occupants. Such cages do however inflict some discomfort on the animals and it is usually necessary to place some litter (e.g. paper shavings) within the cage in order to prevent the animals developing sores on the pads of the feet.

Labelling of Cages

Every cage should have attached permanently to it a socket or holder for a small card about $2\frac{1}{2} \times 3\frac{1}{2}$ in, on which is recorded the name of the experimenter, the identifying marks of the animals, the date, the nature of the experiment and any other relevant matter. The card must not be removed before the conclusion of the experiment and must be placed in such a position that it cannot be chewed or defaced by the animal. Breeding cages should also be labelled so that each animal can be identified especially if a breeding programme (e.g. inbreeding) is being carried out.

Ventilation

Ideally the animal house should be air-conditioned; at least ten changes of air in each hour are needed. When there is no air-conditioning adequate ventilation from windows must be ensured but great care must be taken not to expose the cages to draughts. Animals kept in badly ventilated rooms are more liable to respiratory diseases.

Temperature and Humidity

Each animal has its own optimum temperature and animal rooms must be kept close to this level if the stock is to remain healthy and able to breed. Sudden fluctuations of temperature must be avoided since they may result in the death of whole colonies of animals. If animals such as guinea-pigs or rabbits are kept in open runs, sufficient litter or hay must be provided for them to make nests in which to keep warm. The humidity of the animal house should range between 45 per cent for rabbits to 65 per cent for mice.

Handling

If animals are handled frequently and sympathetically they soon become tame and easily managed; it is only when they are frightened that they bite and then only in self-defence. Loud noises such as the clattering of metal cages and the slamming of doors must be avoided in the animal house which should be as quiet a place as possible. When it is necessary to handle an animal, place the cage on the bench and allow the creature to know what is happening; open the cage door gently, introduce the hands slowly and deliberately, and pick up the animal with firm unhurried movements. Give the animal a sense of complete security by fully supporting its weight and eliminating the risk of dropping it. Avoid all sudden grabbing movements and approach the animals with a steady confidence. It is seldom necessary to wear leather gloves when handling animals except when new stock is introduced into the colony and their confidence has not yet been won. An exception is made, however, with rats and monkeys, where a bite is accompanied by the risk of a severe infection to the handler.

Breeding

Porter and Lane-Petter (1962) give detailed instructions for the breeding of common laboratory animals.

Marking Animals

White or lightly coloured animals can be temporarily marked by staining the fur with a strong dye. Marking ink of the type contained in commercial glass ink-pens is very convenient and the dye persists on the fur for two months or more. Alternatively, strong carbol fuchsin can be used. Rabbits can be marked by tattooing the ears either with a special instrument designed for the purpose or with a needle dipped in India ink. For rats and mice ear punching is a simple method; a special ear punch can be obtained from veterinary instrument makers and this cuts holes about $\frac{1}{8}$ in in diameter in patterns arranged according to an identification code. For fowls, numbered metal tags are clipped through the loose skin of the wing.

The Detection of the Signs of Disease in Animals

It is easy to miss the early signs of illness in caged animals and in order to make sure that the stock is healthy a routine tour of inspection of the occupants of every cage should be made at least once a day but preferably twice, early in the morning and again in the evening. Attention must be paid to the general condition of the animals, the amounts of food and water consumed and the nature of the faeces. The position and movements of the animals should be noted and any animal that remains quiet and still or seems listless should be removed from its cage and exercised. A quiet animal left undisturbed may appear to be normal and yet may be found to be paralyzed or ataxic when made to move. The appearance of the fur is of particular importance; when the animal is generally in poor condition or is suffering from a chronic illness it lacks its normal lustre and when acutely ill the fur may be staring or ruffled. Acute illnesses are often accompanied by inflammation of the conjunctiva and nasal mucosa which often are also the sites of a muco-purulent discharge. Ulceration of the skin, the tail, and the pads may indicate ectromelia in mice, and localized lesions of this type may indicate parasite infestations. Full details of the commoner diseases of laboratory animals are given by Harris (1962), Worden and Lane-Petter (1957) and Parish (1950). Sometimes there may be no obvious clinical signs of illness and the only sign manifest in the animal is fever (e.g. rickettsial infections). Thus it may be necessary to record an animal's temperature daily or at more frequent intervals.

Taking an Animal's Temperature

An ordinary clinical thermometer smeared liberally with sterile petroleum jelly may be used though the blunt ended rectal thermometer is to be preferred as being less easily broken. It is introduced into the rectum or vagina to a depth of about three-quarters of an inch; the depth must be the same on every occasion and the mercury bulb must always be completely inserted. Whenever possible the animal's temperature should be taken before feeding and it must be remembered that the temperature of a frightened or struggling animal may be raised without any pathological cause being present.

Prevention of Disease

When new animals are purchased and introduced into the animal house they should be placed in a special quarantine room and kept there under observation for 10–14 days. If, during this period, any animals sicken or die the stock should be held in quarantine and necropsies must be made to investigate the cause of the trouble.

Animals infected experimentally with bacteria or viruses should be held in separate isolation rooms and full precautions taken to prevent the spread of infection to other animals. Bedding and unused foodstuffs from these animals should be removed and burned. The cages should be removed on a special trolley reserved for the purpose, handled separately, and autoclaved before being placed in contact with clean cages. People who have handled infected animals, cages, or any contaminated material should immediately wash their hands thoroughly with soap and water, and change to a clean coat before proceeding to handle clean animals.

Some potentially pathogenic organisms may be harboured by apparently healthy animals and can readily be transmitted to other animals whose resistance is lowered by overcrowding in cages, lack of ventilation, temperature fluctuation, or by inadequate diets. It is only by constant attention to all the rules of animal hygiene that infection can be prevented.

Insect Pests

Care must be taken in the animal house to control insect pests. General cleanliness, sterilization, and the proper design of cages and racks so that small crannies and crevices are eliminated are often sufficient, but special methods are occasionally needed. Bed bugs, fleas, lice, mites, ticks and flies, mosquitoes and cockroaches may all infest the animal house and can be controlled by the use of insecticidal sprays such as 0·5 per cent DDT or 10 per cent Lethane applied to focal points. To destroy fleas in the fur or feathers of animals an effective dusting powder containing 0·5 per cent of pyrethrin may be used. Insecticides such as dieldrin, aldrin, DDT or benzene hexachloride incorporated in a urea formaldehyde resin can be obtained in the form of a quick drying transparent lacquer. They can be sprayed or painted on to cages and racks and are very effective. Because the spray is inflammable great care is required in its use (Worden and Lane-Petter, 1972).

General Anaesthesia

Ether is one of the most satisfactory drugs for short periods of anaesthesia because its action is rapid and the depth of narcosis can be controlled from minute to minute. Chloroform has marked toxic properties for many species of animals, especially mice, and is best avoided. It is wise to fast animals for twelve hours before anaesthetizing them. For small animals a simple method is to place them on the wire tray of a glass desiccator which contains an ether-soaked pad in its lower compartment. Larger animals, such as rabbits may be placed in a box which has a hinged door and a glass inspection window; an ether-air mixture is pumped slowly into the box through a rubber tube leading from a wash bottle containing ether with rubber bellows attached to its inlet. Whatever method is used for anaesthesia great care must be taken that liquid ether does not touch the animal because mucous membranes can easily be burned in this way.

When the animal has lost consciousness and is lying quietly with deep, even respiratory movements it should be removed from the container without delay and placed on the bench. During the next 3–4 min simple inoculations or small operations can be carried out, but for more lengthy procedures the anaesthesia must be continued. For this purpose a suitable mask can be made by replacing the base of a conveniently sized tin with wire gauze and by shaping it to fit comfortably over the animal's nose. A pad soaked with ether is placed deep in the tin touching the wire gauze and the depth of anaesthesia is controlled by varying the distance between the mouth of the tin and the animal's nose.

For longer periods of anaesthesia barbiturate anaesthetics may be injected intraperitoneally or intravenously. The drug of choice is pentobarbitone sodium (Nembutal) and is usually used in a dose of 28 mg/kg body weight. A stock solution containing Nembutal 60 mg/ml is convenient and may be diluted to required strengths with 10 per cent ethyl alcohol. Thiopentone sodium (Pentothal sodium) may also be used but its action is less certain. Anaesthesia with these drugs may take 15–30 min to develop and lasts 1–2 h; complete recovery may take up to 12 h during which time the animal may pass through a phase of inco-ordination during which it may injure itself or tear out stitches if it is left unsupervized. It is important to keep the animal warm during the recovery phase (particularly mice) and the cage may be placed close to a radiator for this.

A useful introduction to anaesthetic methods for laboratory animals is given by Croft (1962).

Humane Ways of Killing Animals

Physical Methods

Most methods involve breaking the spinal cord in the cervical region or damaging the brain itself. They are used only for small animals which are easily handled and which have relatively thin skulls. Mice and guinea-pigs may be quickly and painlessly killed by bringing the head suddenly against a hard object such as the edge of a sink, but it is emphasized that this method requires some manual dexterity and must be learned from an experienced person. Birds can be killed by breaking the cervical cord; the legs are held in the left hand and the head in the right and the neck is then quickly extended and bent back with a sharp jerk.

Chemical Methods

Volatile Agents. An overdose of some volatile agent such as ether, chloroform, nitrogen, or coal gas is commonly employed for euthanasia. Ether alone, however, is not reliable; it is too irritant and excitant for large animals and very young mice and rats may recover many hours after appearing to die from its effects. Chloroform is suitable for most animals other than the dog in which it causes over-excitement. For small animals a pad of cotton-wool soaked in chloroform is placed in the lower compartment of a desiccator and the animal is placed on a wire mesh tray above the pad. For larger animals the chloroform may be applied on an anaesthetic mask but care must be taken that it does not actually touch the face of a conscious animal because the liquid is irritant. If coal gas is used an easy death is achieved but only if it is introduced slowly into the chamber.

Non-Volatile Agents. Where the intravenous route of injection is practicable animals can be quickly and painlessly killed by the injection of a saturated solution of magnesium sulphate but it must be remembered that this substance is lethal only if injected into a vein. Pentobarbitone sodium (e.g. Nembutal) or thiopentone (e.g. Pentothal sodium) can also be used to kill animals but is rather expensive; the dose is three to four times that required for anaesthesia and the drugs may be injected by the intravenous, intraperitoneal or intramuscular routes.

Disposal of Dead Animals

The best way to dispose of animal carcases is to burn them in the incinerator, but before this can be carried out it is absolutely essential to be sure that the animal is dead. *In order to ensure against the possibility of accidentally burning a live animal no carcases should be put in the incinerator unless one of the following conditions applies*: (1) The body is cold, still and rigor mortis has set in. (2) The animal has been decapitated. (3) A complete necropsy has been performed. (4) The heart has been removed.

Fuller details of the care and manipulation of laboratory animals are given by Smith (1931).

MATERIAL INOCULATED

Urine, cerebrospinal fluid, blood and *serous fluids* are easily inoculated with a medium-bore needle. Tenacious material such as *pus* and *sputum* is injected through a wide-bore needle.
CULTURES. Fluid cultures are easily drawn through a medium-bore needle. It may be found advantageous first to pour the culture into a small (2-in) Petri dish, or a wide-mouthed 1-oz screw-capped bottle. Growths on solid media may be scraped off and suspended in broth or saline, or the diluting fluid may be poured on the culture which is then emulsified with a wire loop.
TISSUES. Small fragments of soft tissues such as brain, liver, spleen and kidney are readily homogenized by crushing them with a suitable diluent in a Ten Broeck grinder. If larger volumes of tissue suspensions are needed or if firmer tissues such as muscle or lung have to be used, an electrically powered blender of the Waring type is recommended. Tough and fibrous tissues such as skin or chronically inflamed lymph glands should be cut into small pieces in a sterile porcelain mortar by means of scissors sterilized by boiling. Some clean, coarse sand, previously washed with acid to remove carbonates, or fine powdered sintered glass, contained in a stoppered bottle and sterilized by hot air, is then added to the mortar and the whole thoroughly ground with the pestle. When the tissue has been well ground up, saline is added and the mixture further triturated. On standing for a short time, the sand and tissue rapidly settle to the bottom

of the mortar and the supernatant fluid can be drawn into the syringe. When intravenous inoculation of a tissue suspension has to be employed, care must be taken that no large particles are injected. To avoid this, the suspension must be centrifuged at low speed and only the supernatant fluid used.

NECROPSY

All experimental animals, whatever the cause of death, should be examined *post mortem* as a routine. When a virulent organism such as the bacillus of plague or of anthrax has been used, special care must be taken, otherwise the infection may be disseminated, with danger to the operator and other workers.

Details will be given of the procedure in conducting a necropsy in the usual manner, and also the method used when dealing with highly infectious organisms.

As a primary reason for the necropsy is to recover organisms previously injected into the animal, the examination must be conducted with strict aseptic precautions.

Materials Required

A suitable animal board or *table*, on which the carcase can be fixed in the supine position.
Instruments. Three scalpels; scissors, ordinary size, four pairs; mouse-toothed forceps, four pairs; small bone forceps, if the skull is to be opened; a searing iron—a 4-oz soldering bolt is suitable for the purpose; sterile capillary pipettes; sterile Petri dishes; sterile test-tubes, and tubes, bottles or plates of media.

The knives are sterilized in strong lysol (about 20 per cent) and then placed in a weaker solution (2 per cent), and the metal instruments by boiling in a sterilizing bath, e.g. an enamelled 'fish-kettle'. When ready for use, the tray of instruments is lifted out of the sterilizer and laid on a spread towel which has previously been soaked in 1:1000 solution of mercuric chloride.

It is a useful practice, where cultures have to be made, first to immerse the animal completely in weak lysol solution (3 per cent) for a few moments. This not only destroys most of the surface organisms, but prevents the dust in the fur from getting into the air and contaminating other materials. The animal is now fixed to the board and towels moistened with antiseptic are placed over the head and lower extremities.

The instruments are removed from the sterilizer. A long median incision through the skin of the abdomen and chest is now made and the skin widely dissected, exposing the abdominal and chest muscles. With another set of instruments the peritoneal cavity is opened and the abdominal wall is reflected to each side. With fresh instruments the spleen is removed and placed in a sterile Petri dish. Other organs such as the liver and kidneys may be similarly removed. The ensiform cartilage is now tightly gripped with a pair of strong forceps, and by means of a sterile pair of strong scissors a cut is made on either side of the chest through the costal cartilages. The sternum is raised and pulled towards the head. The heart is now exposed. A sterile capillary pipette, furnished with a teat, is passed through the heart wall. Blood can thus be withdrawn and inoculated into various media. If the necropsy has been properly performed, it is not necessary to sear the surface of the heart. The lungs are then removed with fresh instruments by cutting each organ free at the hilum. Care must be taken not to open the oesophagus if the lungs are to be used for cultivation.

After the organs to be used for culture have been removed and placed in separate Petri dishes, the necropsy can be completed.

While the instruments are again being boiled the naked-eye appearances of the organs should be studied. For culture the spleen gives the best results, but the other solid viscera may similarly be used. The organ is cut with sterile instruments and a small portion is taken up with a stiff wire and smeared on the surface of solid media. Liquid media are inoculated with a small fragment of the tissue.

In conducting post-mortem examinations, various animal diseases, such as worm infestation, coccidiosis, pseudotuberculosis, etc., may be noticed, and the worker should be familiar with their appearances.

When the animal is infected with highly pathogenic organisms the worker *must* wear rubber gloves. The carcase is soaked in antiseptic solution as before and nailed to a rough piece of board of the appropriate size. This board is then placed in a large enamelled iron tray. The necropsy is carefully performed in the usual way. The carcase is finally covered with 10 per cent lysol, which flows over the board and into the tray. The whole contents of the tray—board and carcase—are then destroyed in a furnace or incinerator. The rubber gloves, instruments and tray are thoroughly sterilized. When performing animal necropsies we strongly advise the wearing of a large overall made of waterproof material, and in addition, the use of some form of glasses or goggles to protect the eyes.

RABBITS

Data

Rectal temperature	$38 \cdot 7°-39 \cdot 1°C$; $101 \cdot 6°-102 \cdot 4°F$

(No temperature below 40°C or 104°F is regarded as pathological.)

Normal respiration rate	55 per min
Pulse rate	135 per min
Gestation period	28–31 days
Weaning age	6–8 weeks
Mating age	6–9 months
Litters	4 yearly; average litter, 4
Room temperature	$15 \cdot 5°-18 \cdot 5°C$; $60°-65°F$
Humidity	40–45 per cent
Weight—adult	$0 \cdot 9-6 \cdot 75$ kg

Cages

Individual cages are best made of galvanized iron. The minimum size for a medium sized rabbit is $2 \times 2 \times 1\frac{1}{2}$ ft, but larger cages may be needed for the bigger breeds. Young rabbits up to three months of age may be housed together but after that time the sexes should be separated. From 8 to 10 young rabbits may be kept together in a pen similar to that used for guinea-pigs.

Feeding

The pelleted diet 18 of Bruce and Parkes (1947) or commercial breeders pellets are suitable for rabbits. Alternatively a daily supply of 2·5 oz (72 g) of a mixture of one part oats and three parts bran may be fed as a slightly moist mash. Either diet may be supplemented with greenstuffs or root vegetables and hay. A liberal supply of clean drinking water is essential at all times.

Handling

Smooth the ears of the rabbit back and then pick up the ears and the loose skin at the back of the neck with one hand in a firm grip, place the other hand under the hind quarters to support the weight and lift gently. A rabbit must never be lifted by the ears alone. When a rabbit is removed from its cage it should always be placed on a non-slippery surface because otherwise it feels insecure and becomes frightened; for this purpose the bench may be covered with a piece of sacking. Most rabbits remain quiet and still if they are handled by people they know; if restraint is required during anaesthesia or inoculation, they can be wrapped in a roller towel or placed in a special box so constructed that the head only protrudes at one end.

Breeding

When the doe is on heat the vulva becomes moist, red and swollen. At this time she is taken to the buck for mating; do not introduce the buck into the doe's cage as she may attack and injure him. Small-size strains of rabbits may be mated for the first time at the age of six months, larger strains at about nine months. The gestation period is 28 days and at about the 24th day the doe is transferred to a clean breeding cage, preferably with a screened breeding compartment where the animal can produce its young in seclusion. Liberal bedding and hay must be provided for nesting. In order to avoid the risk of cannibalism the doe and her new litter should be disturbed as little as possible during the first ten days. The young are weaned at six to eight weeks, sexed, and then separated into male and female pens.

Common Diseases

Coccidiosis is a common disease of rabbits taking two forms, hepatic and intestinal. The symptoms are a ravenous appetite with diarrhoea, progressive emaciation, and gradually increasing weakness of the hind limbs. The diagnosis is easily confirmed by the finding of the oocysts of *Eimeria stediae* in wet films of the faeces. In fatal cases yellowish white nodules and haemorrhages are seen at necropsy in the liver and intestine. Treatment with sulphadimidine included in a mash in a concentration of 1 per cent is effective if given within ten days of infestation.

Pseudotuberculosis is a chronic infection with *Pasteurella pseudotuberculosis* and is characterized by loss of weight, emaciation and eventually by death. At necropsy primary caseous nodules are present in the intestine and are most marked in the caecum; metastatic lesions are seen as well defined yellow areas, like those of miliary tuberculosis, in the liver, spleen, and lymph glands.

Respiratory tract infections. The most common is 'Snuffles', which is so-called from the characteristic nasal discharge. The disease is due to *Pasteurella septica* and is highly infectious; animals suffering from this infection should be removed from the animal house and destroyed at once. Rabbits are also liable to infection with pneumococci and streptococci which may cause a rapidly fatal pneumonia with pericarditis.

Intestinal infections. Mucoid enteritis, a disease of obscure origin may be responsible for epizootics in the animal house. Severe diarrhoea and marked emaciation are the principal symptoms and the condition may be mistaken for coccidiosis. The mortality of very young rabbits is 100 per cent, that of adults about 30 per cent. Diarrhoea may also be caused by organisms of the *Salmonella* group, e.g. *S. typhimurium*.

Rabbit syphilis. A relatively common condition characterized by papules or discharging ulcers on denuded areas of the genitalia. It is caused by *Treponema cuniculi*, a spirochaete very similar to *Treponema pallidum*. The condition reponds well to treatment with penicillin.

Ear canker is the commonest form of mange in the domestic rabbit. It is caused by two species of mites, *Psoroptes communis* and *Chorioptes communis*. The condition can be easily cleared up by softening the scabs with vegetable oil, removing them and then applying a 20 per cent emulsion of benzyl benzoate (National Formulary).

Worms. The cysticercus stage of the dog tapeworm, *Taenia pisiformis*, is a common type of infestation and is characterized by numerous cysts in the omentum and liver.

Experimental Procedures

The chief use of the rabbit lies not so much in diagnostic work as in its value for experimental purposes. It is, also, extensively used for the production of immune sera, such as agglutinatting and neutralizing sera, which are used in diagnostic work.

Antisera. There is no agreement on the best inoculation schedule for the production of antisera in rabbits. One method employs four to six intravenous injections of gradually increasing amounts of the antigen spaced at two to three day intervals. (Many workers complete the course within ten days to minimize the risk of anaphylactic shock.) A sample of blood should be taken before beginning the course and a second six to eight days after finishing it. The antibody titres of both samples are estimated and if that of the second sample has not risen to a high level further injections may be given. Although this method gives good results (e.g. in the preparation of antisera to salmonellae) many other schedules using other routes of inoculation in various combinations, different doses of antigen, longer or shorter time intervals, may all give equally satisfactory results. It is, however, wise to reduce the number of inoculations to the minimum needed to produce the required antibody titres because a prolonged series of injections may harm the animal and may also result in the appearance of unwanted or non-specific antibodies. In general, the worker will be guided in the choice of a schedule by such factors as the toxicity and purity of the antigen, whether living or dead microorganisms are to be injected, and by the condition of the animal being immunized.

It is possible to produce high levels of antibodies with a single subcutaneous inoculation if the antigen is mixed with Freund's complete adjuvant. Freund's adjuvant (Difco) can be obtained commercially with or without (in-complete) added mycobacteria; it comprises nine parts of an oil, Bayol F, and one volume of an emulsifying agent, Arlacel A, with the addition, if required, of 2 mg per ml of heat-killed *Mycobacterium butyricum*. Equal volumes of a saline suspension of the antigen and Freund's adjuvant are mixed to make a water in oil emulsion. In making the emulsion successive small amounts of the antigen are squirted below the surface of the adjuvant with a syringe and the mixing is continued by filling and emptying the syringe through the needle until the emulsion has assumed an opaque appearance and a syrupy consistency. Considerable care must be taken to obtain the correct consistency to give a *water in oil emulsion*, which is achieved when a drop let fall on the surface of a beaker of water remains as a discrete drop. Oil in water suspensions, which are not so effective antigenically, are detected when a drop allowed to fall on the surface of water spreads out to form a diffuse film.

Anaesthesia. Short-acting—Ether; Long-acting—Pentobarbitone sodium 28 mg/kg body-weight intravenously.

With pentobarbitone, anaesthesia develops rapidly and there are 45–60 minutes of unconsciousness followed by some abnormality of the central nervous system lasting up to 24 hours.

Scarification. The hair is removed from the flank of the animal by first clipping and then shaving, or by means of the depilating mixture described on page 331. The skin is cleansed with alcohol, which is allowed to evaporate. A number of parallel scratches are made with a sharp sterile scalpel, just sufficiently deep to draw blood. The infective material is rubbed into the scarified area with the side of the scalpel. This method is mainly used for the propagation of vaccinia virus.

Subcutaneous inoculation may be made either into the abdominal wall or into the loose tissue about the flank or at the back of the neck. The hair is clipped, the skin is sterilized with iodine and then pinched up, and the needle is inserted. The technique is the same as that for the guinea-pig.

Intravenous inoculation is employed when material has to be introduced directly into the circulation. The marginal vein of the ear is the most convenient site. The rabbit may be held by an assistant or placed in a special box so that only its head protrudes. The hair over the vein may be dry-shaved with a sharp razor. The vein may be distended for ease of inoculation either by vigorous rubbing with a piece of cotton-wool or by holding the ear over an electric-light bulb, when the heat causes a dilatation of the blood vessels. According to the amount of material to be injected, a suitable sterile syringe is selected. The operator faces the animal and the ear is held horizontally by means of the left hand. The needle is kept as nearly parallel as possible to the vein and the point inserted towards the head of the animal. When the injection is completed, the needle is withdrawn and a small piece of cotton-wool placed on the vein, which is then compressed between the thumb and finger.

Intraperitoneal inoculation is carried out as in the guinea-pig.

Intracerebral inoculation. The animal is anaesthetized with ether, the hair over the head shaved, and the skin disinfected with alcohol and tincture of iodine. A short incision is made through the scalp at a point situated 2 mm lateral to the sagittal suture and 1·5 mm anterior to the lambdoidal suture. The skull is then perforated with a trephine or a mechanical drill, and the needle, which is cut down to 6–8 mm long, introduced through the opening. About 0·45 ml of material can be inoculated into the occipital lobe of a large rabbit. After injection the needle is rapidly withdrawn, the skin sutured and the area covered with collodion solution.

Rabbits may also be inoculated in the frontal lobe, at a point situated 2 mm lateral to the median plane on a line joining the two external canthi of the eyes.

Intra-testicular. If the testes are not palpable in the scrotum they are made to descend from the abdominal cavity by steady pressure on the belly while the animal lies on its back. Under anaesthesia they are then fixed by an assistant who places a finger over each abdominal ring. The scrotal skin is cleansed with methylated spirit and is stretched tightly over one of the testicles. A hypodermic needle is now plunged directly into the centre of the organ and 0·2–0·4 ml of inoculum can be injected.

Ophthalmic. Material may be dropped into one eye from a Pasteur pipette leaving the other untreated as a control. Under anaesthesia the cornea of one eye may be scarified before the instillation of infected material. Only one eye is inoculated as the procedure should never give any risk of blinding the animal.

Collection of blood. From the ear vein of a large rabbit 20–30 ml of blood may be obtained easily and without causing any distress to the animal. The ear is shaved and sterilized with sterile gauze soaked in 70 per cent alcohol. Meanwhile a small vessel containing petroleum jelly has been heated over the Bunsen to render it sterile, and when cool, but still fluid, the petroleum jelly is painted over the vein, and on the margin and under-side of the ear. The ear is held forward and the vein is made prominent by means of a small spring clip at the base of the ear, and then incised with a small sharp sterile scalpel. The blood flows over the petroleum jelly, and is allowed to drop into a sterile flask containing glass beads or a suitable anticoagulant according to requirements. The vessels of the ear can be dilated by holding an electric bulb below it or by rubbing the part not covered by petroleum jelly with a pledget of wool moistened with xylol. When sufficient blood has been obtained the clip is removed and a piece of cotton-wool pressed firmly over the cut in the vein. The xylol is removed from the ear with alcohol, and some petroleum jelly then lightly smeared on. *Water should always be provided in the cage of the animal after bleeding.*

Larger amounts of blood can be obtained by *cardiac puncture.* The anaesthetized animal is fastened to a board with the body axis quite straight and the fur clipped over the left side of the chest; the area is shaved and then sterilized with alcohol and ether. A 100 ml bulb pipette (see Fig. 15.1) is cut down at both ends to 9 in in length, one end being slightly tapered and the other end stoppered with cotton-wool. It is wrapped in kraft paper and sterilized in the hot-air oven. A wide-bore transfusion needle is fitted into a short length (1½ in) of thick rubber tubing and sterilized by boiling. When the animal is anaesthetized, the rubber tubing is attached to the tapered end of the pipette and to the other end is fitted a mouth-piece such

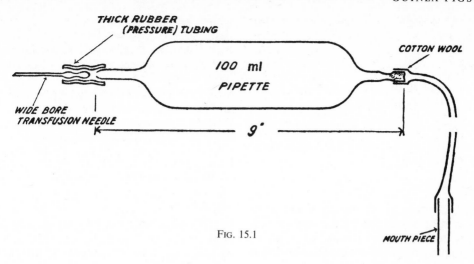

THICK RUBBER
(PRESSURE) TUBING

COTTON WOOL

100 ml
PIPETTE

WIDE BORE
TRANSFUSION NEEDLE

9″

MOUTH PIECE

Fig. 15.1

as that used in pipetting. The needle is inserted into the left side of the chest and suction applied. The needle should lie in the right ventricle of the heart, and blood rapidly flows into the pipette. About 50 ml of blood per kg of body-weight can be obtained. The blood is then transferred to a sterile 500-ml flask or bottle containing glass beads for defibrination.

GUINEA-PIGS

Data

Rectal temperature	37·6°–38·9°C; 99·6°–102°F
Normal respiration rate	80 per min
Pulse rate	150 per min
Gestation period	59–72 days; average 63 days
Weaning age	14–21 days
Mating age	12–20 weeks
Litters	3 yearly; average litter, 3
Room temperature	18·5°–21°C; 65°–70°F
Humidity	45 per cent
Weight—weaning	120 g
adult	200–1000 g

Cages

Stock runs should be about 4 × 6 ft and 1 ft 8 in high. One square foot of space should be allowed for each animal and not more than 25 animals should be kept in any one pen.

For experimental animals galvanized-iron cages are recommended as they can be readily cleaned and sterilized. A convenient size is 14 × 9 × 8 in fitting in a tray 1½ in deep.

Feeding

A diet in pelleted form is recommended in preference to mashes. Pellets are placed in a hopper in the animal cage and provide a continuous source of food. Diet 18 of Bruce and Parkes (1947) contains balanced proportions of protein, fat and carbohydrate with added vitamins, salt and trace elements. This diet is recommended and to it must be added 2 oz of cabbage or kale and 2 oz hay daily for each animal. In winter, carrots, swedes or mangold may be substituted for the green food. Fresh water must be provided from a bottle attached to the cage.

If, however, a mash is to be used instead of pellets, the following simple formula may be of value:

Crushed oats	2 parts
Broad bran	1 part

It may be fed dry or slightly moistened with water. This mash lacks sufficient protein to maintain reproduction and the growth of young animals. It must be supplemented with cabbage and hay as above and it may be necessary to add protein concentrates such as fish or meat meal.

Handling

Place one hand across the back of the animal with the thumb behind the shoulders and the other fingers well forward on the opposite side; lift the animal gently and support its weight with the other hand placed palm uppermost under the hind quarters.

Breeding

The boar is fertile at the age of 8–10 weeks when it weighs about 500 g; the sow can be mated for the first time at the age of 12 weeks when it weighs about 450 g. One boar is placed in a breeding pen with 5–10 sows and one square foot of space allowed for each animal. As the sows approach parturition they are isolated in individual cages. After weaning at 14–21 days the young are weighed, sexed and the sows and boars are placed in different pens. The mother is then returned to the breeding pen.

Common Diseases

PSEUDOTUBERCULOSIS. May be either acute or, more commonly, chronic. In the acute type the animal dies in a few days. In the chronic type the liver, spleen and mesenteric glands show very numerous yellowish-white areas scattered through them, somewhat suggestive of tuberculosis. Often a whole stock becomes infected, and experimental animals frequently die before the experiment is completed.

ABSCESSES IN LYMPHATIC GLANDS, due to haemolytic streptococci of group C, are not uncommon. (These organisms may also produce septicaemia.)

RESPIRATORY TRACT INFECTIONS. Guinea-pigs are liable to pneumonia and pleurisy, often haemorrhagic, and septicaemia due to such organisms as the pneumococcus, pneumobacillus, haemolytic streptococcus, *Pasteurella* group.

INTESTINAL INFECTIONS. Organisms of the *Salmonella* group, e.g. *S. typhimurium*, are the cause of the most lethal of all guinea-pig diseases. Explosive epizootics may occur in

which practically the whole of a colony is destroyed.

PROTOZOAN DISEASES. Coccidiosis is of common occurrence. Toxoplasmosis is found infrequently.

VIRUS DISEASES, such as guinea-pig paralysis and pneumonia, may be met with.

Experimental Procedures

For general purposes an adult guinea-pig weighing about 400 g is satisfactory.

Anaesthesia

Short acting: Ether. Excessive post-operative mucous secretions are common but can largely be prevented by the use of 0·5 ml of a 0·5 per cent solution of atropine sulphate (2·5 mg) given at least half an hour preoperatively by the subcutaneous route.

Long acting: Pentobarbitone sodium 28 mg/kg body-weight intraperitoneally. 56 mg/kg body-weight is the fatal dose.

With pentobarbitone sodium anaesthesia may take about 15 minutes to develop, lasts 1–2 hours, and complete recovery may take up to 12 hours during which time the animal must be kept warm.

SUBCUTANEOUS INOCULATION. An assistant holds the animal during the operation, and the injection is made under the skin of the flank. The animal is grasped across the shoulders in one hand, with the thumb curved round the animal's neck so that it rests on the lower jaw. The hind legs are secured between the first and second, and second and third fingers of the other hand, the knuckles being uppermost, and the animal is held so that the flank is presented for inoculation. The skin may be disinfected with tincture of iodine. The operator picks up a fold of skin and introduces the point of the needle into the base of the fold so that it lies in the subcutaneous tissue. Amounts up to 5 ml can be introduced. A 2-ml or a 5-ml syringe is convenient for the purpose.

Some workers inoculate by picking up a fold of skin about the mid-abdomen. The needle is introduced into the base of the fold and passed down in the subcutaneous tissue until it reaches the groin, where the injection is made. This method obviates superficial ulceration when tuberculosis material is injected.

INTRACUTANEOUS INOCULATION. This method is used in testing cultures of the diphtheria bacillus for virulence. The hair is removed from the flanks of the animal by plucking or alternatively by means of a fresh 5 per cent solution of sodium sulphide or a depilating powder. White guinea-pigs (300–400 g weight) are used, as the skin is unpigmented and the results of the test can easily be read.

The depilating powder is made as follows:

Barium sulphide, commercial
powder . . . . . 7 parts
White household flour . . 7 parts
Talcum powder . . . 7 parts
Castile soap powder . . 1 part

Remove the hair from the flanks as closely as possible with hair clippers. Make up the depilating powder into a smooth paste with water, and rub into the animal's hair with a wooden spatula or toothbrush. Allow the paste to act for one minute and renew the application. After two minutes remove the paste with the spatula or handle of the toothbrush. Now wash the animal's skin and surrounding hair with warm water and dry with a cloth. The depilated surface should be quite smooth and white. It is advisable not to leave the paste on too long as the skin becomes red and excoriated in patches, making the subsequent observation of reactions very difficult. The depilating powder should be used at least one hour before the intracutaneous injection is carried out.

For the test a 1-ml all-glass tuberculin syringe, fitted with a short needle of No. 25 or 26 gauge (exactly as used for Schick and Dick tests), is employed. The skin of the animal is pinched up between the thumb and forefinger, and the point of the needle is inserted at the top of the fold so that the bevel of the needle is towards the surface of the skin. The needle passes only into the dermis, as near the surface as possible, *and not into the subcutaneous tissue*; when the injection has been correctly made a definite and palpable bleb appears in the skin. The usual amount injected is 0·2 ml and when several tests are to be made the injections should be about one inch apart

and not too near the middle line of the abdomen. No more than ten injections should be made on one animal. The results are read 24–48 h later.

Intraperitoneal inoculation. The animal is held in a similar manner. The inoculation is made in the mid-line in the lower half of the abdomen. The assistant holds the animal with its head downwards, so that the intestines fall towards the diaphragm. The skin is pinched up, the point of the needle is first passed into the subcutaneous skin tissue and then downwards through the abdominal wall into the peritoneal cavity. There is no risk of damage to the intestines. Not more than 5 ml can safely be inoculated intraperitoneally.

Collection of blood. Small amounts, up to 0·5 ml, may be taken by simple incision of the marginal ear vein. Cardiac puncture is, however, the only satisfactory way of obtaining larger volumes. The animal is lightly anaesthetized with ether and then laid on its back with its front limbs drawn forwards. An area over the fourth and fifth left intercostal spaces is plucked and the skin painted with tincture of iodine. The position of the apex beat of the heart is defined by digital palpation and at this point a needle (No. 20 gauge mounted on a syringe) is inserted between the ribs. A sharp downward movement inclined towards the mid-line then takes the needle point through the ventricular wall. As much as 15 ml of blood may be obtained from a 350–400 g animal, though smaller amounts are advisable if the guinea-pig is to survive. Very sharp needles are essential for the success of this operation.

MICE
Data

Normal temperature .	37·4°C; 99·3°F
Pulse rate . .	120
Oestrous cycle .	4–5 days
Gestation period .	19–21 days
Weaning age .	19–21 days
Mating age .	6–8 weeks
Litters . .	8–12 yearly; average litter, 7–8
Room temperature .	20°–21°C; 68°–70°F
Humidity . .	50–60 per cent
Weight—weaning	7 g
adult .	25–28 g

Cages

There are many different designs of mouse cages and no one pattern is the standard. A common form is an aluminium box approximately $6 \times 12 \times 6$ in deep, with tapering sides to facilitate stacking. The lids are made of sheet metal or of strong wire mesh and are designed so that a food hopper is built into them and accommodation provided to hold the drinking bottle. The cages are light, durable and easily sterilized by dry or moist heat. Similar cages made of polypropylene are now available and are quieter to handle and, since the plastic material is not a good conductor of heat, are warmer for the animals. Plastic cages are less expensive than metal and appear to be equally satisfactory; they can be sterilized in the autoclave but not in the hot air oven. Up to six mice can be housed in cages of this type which are suitable for breeding purposes. Larger cages to hold up to 100 mice approximately $30 \times 18 \times 6$ in can be used for stock rearing or holding purposes but overcrowding in such cages carries a great risk of epidemic disease.

Feeding

Pelleted diets such as diet 86 of Howie (1952) or diet 41 of Bruce (1950) are satisfactory. Fresh water in drinking bottles must be provided *ad lib*.

Handling

An assistant takes a grip on the middle of the tail of the animal with the left hand and gently raises the hind limbs from the floor of the cage. A mouse held in this position cannot turn round and bite. Then with the right finger and thumb a fold of skin is taken up as close as possible to the head. The animal can now be lifted into a convenient position for the operator to carry out simple inoculation procedures. When an assistant is not available a mouse can be manipulated single handed: place the animal on a rough surface and hold it by its tail with the right hand, then pick up the loose skin at the base of the neck with the left forefinger and thumb, lift and turn the left hand palm uppermost at the same time catching the tail and pressing it against the palm with the left little finger. The right hand is now free to pick up a syringe.

Breeding

Two methods may be used: (1) *Monogamous mating* when one male and one female aged 8–12 weeks are placed permanently in a cage together. Three to four weeks later the first litter is produced and mating occurs again in the immediate post-partum period. The young mice must be weaned just before the next litter is expected. Thus litters may be expected every 3–4 weeks. (2) *Polygamous mating* when one male is placed in a cage with up to four females. When it is established that a female is pregnant she is transferred to a separate cage and allowed to nest and nurse her young until they are weaned at the age of three weeks, after which she is mated again. Both systems have advantages and disadvantages; the first produces double the number of mice but the young mice produced by the second method are heavier and reach maturity and suitability for experimental use in a shorter time.

Common Diseases

SALMONELLOSIS. Intestinal infections termed 'Mouse typhoid' are common and are usually caused by the Salmonella group (e.g. *S. typhimurium* and *S. enteritidis*).

Severe epizootics may follow the introduction of new stock into a colony especially when the animals are overcrowded or where animal hygiene is inadequate. It seems impossible to control an epizootic with chemotherapy and the only satisfactory procedure is to destroy existing animals, sterilize their cages, and then to obtain a fresh clean stock.

ECTROMELIA (Mouse pox) is the most troublesome of mouse diseases; it takes two forms: (*a*) the acute form characterized by necrosis of the liver and spleen with a rapidly fatal result; (*b*) a chronic form with generalized skin eruption and characterized by ulcers which are covered by crusts of dried serous discharges. These lesions may occur anywhere on the body but are most obvious on the tail. In the most chronic form there is enlargement of one of the foot pads due to oedema and scab formation followed by gangrene either of a digit or the whole foot. The disease is caused by a pox virus related to the vaccinia virus. When this infection is established it is extremely difficult to control and may necessitate the destruction of the whole colony. If valuable stocks are threatened by ectromelia it is, however, possible to protect them by vaccination on the tail with the calf lymph used against human smallpox.

STREPTOBACILLUS MONILIFORMIS infection may be epizootic or sporadic. The acute form of the disease has no characteristic lesions but the organism can readily be recovered from the blood and organs. The chronic form is commoner and is characterized by swelling of the ankles and tail with ulceration of the foot. The condition may closely resemble ectromelia.

MISCELLANEOUS VIRUS INFECTIONS. Among the many virus infections affecting mouse colonies are the pneumonia virus of mice (PVM of Curnan and Horsfall, 1946), Nigg's pneumonitis virus (Nigg and Eaton, 1944), and the lymphocytic choriomeningitis virus (Traub, 1939; Haas, 1954).

WORMS. Occasional infestation with the tapeworm *Taenia taeniae-formis* may occur with large cysts formed in the liver. The primary host of this helminth is the cat which should be excluded from mouse rooms. Cats may infect oats, maize and pellets with tape-worm ova in the mill and these feeding stuffs should not be purchased unless they have been sterilized and packed in paper bags by the makers.

Experimental Procedures

Anaesthesia

Short acting: Ether.

Long acting: Pentobarbitone sodium stock solution 60 mg/ml diluted 1 in 25 with 10 per cent ethyl alcohol 0·8 ml per 100 g body-weight intraperitoneally.

Mice are particularly sensitive to cold while they are unconscious, and it is important that the animals be kept warm until they have returned to consciousness.

Subcutaneous inoculation. An assistant grasps the loose skin at the nape of the neck in one hand and the tail in the other. In this manner the animal is held in a fixed position while the needle is introduced under the skin near the root of the tail. Amounts up to 1 ml may be injected.

Intraperitoneal inoculation may be carried out if the animal is similarly held and then turned over. For steadiness, the assistant's arms should rest on the table. The injection is made to one side of the middle line in the lower half of the abdomen and amounts up to 2 ml can be introduced.

Intravenous inoculation may be made into a vein at the root of the tail if a fine needle be used and the vein dilated by placing the tail of the animal in water at about 45°C. The maximum amount that can be injected is 0·5 ml for a mouse of 20 g. A small cylindrical cage made of perforated zinc, and just large enough to hold the mouse with its tail protruding, is useful for this procedure.

Intracerebral inoculation. The skin over the head is cleansed with 70 per cent alcohol and the animal is lightly anaesthetized with ether for the inoculation. A fine-bore needle attached to a 1-ml syringe (as used for intracutaneous inoculation) is employed and easily penetrates the skull. The site of injection is midway between the outer canthus of the eye and the point of attachment of the pinna of the ear at about 3 mm from the mid-line. The point of the needle is carried through the skull for 3–6 mm. Up to 0·03 ml of fluid can be injected with safety.

Intranasal inoculation. This should if possible be carried out in an inoculating chamber designed for the purpose for there is a risk that the operator may himself inhale infective material. Failing this, a mask should be worn. The mouse is lightly anaesthetized with ether and as soon as its breathing has become deep and automatic 0·1 ml of the inoculum is introduced into the anterior nares on *one side only*.

Collection of blood. Under deep anaesthesia the animal is pinned out and the skin over the thorax and abdomen is reflected as for necropsy. The great vessels in the axilla are incised and the blood which wells out is taken up in a sterile Pasteur pipette. An alternative and less time-consuming method is to displace the globe of the eye forwards and to puncture the retro-orbital plexus of veins with the tip of a fine Pasteur pipette which is then used to take up the free-flowing blood. About 1·0 ml may be obtained and the mouse may be permitted to recover from the anaesthetic and to survive. Small samples of blood can be obtained by clipping the tail as in the rat.

Inoculation of infant mice. Suckling mice no older than 48 hours are used for the isolation of the herpes simplex, coxsackie and arboviruses. Great care and cleanliness is required in handling the litters if cannibalism by the mothers is to be avoided. The following injections can be used: 0·03 ml subcutaneously, 0·05 ml intraperitoneally, 0·03 intracerebrally. Sometimes the intraperitoneal and the intracerebral routes are used together in the same animals.

Snell (1941) gives full details of the biology of the laboratory mouse.

RATS

Data

Normal temperature	.	37·5°C; 99·5°F
Normal respiration rate	.	210 per min
Oestrous cycle	.	4–5 days
Gestation period	.	21–23 days
Weaning age	.	23–28 days
Mating age	.	70–84 days
Litters	.	7–9 yearly; average litter, 7
Room temperature	.	18·5°–21°C; 65°–70°F
Humidity	.	45–55 per cent

Cages

Rats can be housed in cages similar to those used for guinea-pigs. For details of stock and breeding cages see the UFAW Handbook (Worden and Lane-Petter, 1972).

Feeding

The dry pellet diet No. 86 (Howie, 1952) used for mice can be used without supplementation. A plentiful supply of drinking water is essential.

Handling

Docile rats can be handled by an experienced operator in exactly the same way as guinea-pigs. Wild or vicious rats, however, should be handled with the hand covered by a leather glove because the sharp incisor teeth can inflict a deep wound. Alternatively, the animal may be picked up by gripping the loose skin at the base of the neck with tongs or broad bladed forceps.

Breeding

As in mice monogamous mating may be practised or alternatively polygamous mating used when two males which have been living together for some weeks are placed in a breeding cage with six females; the animals should be 10–12 weeks old. Each female, when pregnant, is removed to a separate cage where she nests and nurses her young until they are weaned at the age of 3–4 weeks. After resting for two weeks the female may be mated again.

Common Diseases

Bronchopneumonia and more rarely suppurative otitis may occur due to *Bord. bronchiseptica*, *Streptobacillus moniliformis*, streptococci, *diphtheroids*, etc. Salmonellosis (often due to *S. typhimurium* or *S. enteritidis*) causes a severe form of enteritis which may spread rapidly in a colony. Mange is a common parasitic infestation and is characterized by brownish scales on the skin of the ears and tail which are often encrusted with dried blood.

Anaesthesia

Short acting: Ether.
Long acting: Ether or
  Adult rats: Pentobarbitone sodium stock solution (60 mg/ml) diluted 1 in 10 with 10 per cent ethyl alcohol. 0·75 ml per 100 g body-weight intraperitoneally.
  Young rats: Pentothal sodium stock solution (under 50 g body-weight) (60 mg/ml) diluted 1 in 25. 1 ml per 100 g body-weight intraperitoneally.

Experimental Procedures

Inoculation by the subcutaneous and intraperitoneal routes is made in a manner similar to those described for the guinea-pig. Intravenous inoculation may be made into the vein at the root of the tail. The vein should be dilated by immersing the tail in warm water. Blood may be collected by cardiac puncture as in the guinea-pig. Small samples of blood can be obtained on repeated occasions, by snipping off with very sharp scissors or a razor blade a very small portion of the tip of the tail.

HAMSTERS
Data

Rectal temperature	.	36·7°–38·3°C; 98°–101°F
Oestrous cycle	.	4–5 days
Gestation period	.	16–17 days
Weaning age	.	3–4 weeks
Mating age	.	7–9 weeks
Litters	.	3–4 yearly; average litter, 6
Room temperature	.	20°–22°C; 68°–72°F
Humidity	.	40–50 per cent

Cages

Galvanized-iron cages in sheet metal or mesh are satisfactory. A convenient size is $17 \times 7 \times 9$ in. Cages of aluminium, zinc or wood are not suitable as hamsters may gnaw through them.

Feeding

Commercially available cubed diets for mice, rats or guinea-pigs are satisfactory for the basic diet but better health results when daily supplements of fresh green foods are given. Milk added to a bran and oats mash is valuable as an additional supplement for pregnant or lactating females. Fresh drinking-water must always be available.

Breeding

The mating of animals is best carried out under observation for the female after coitus may often attack the male and injure him severely.

Diseases

Golden hamsters are remarkably free from spontaneous disease. They may, however, acquire salmonella infections and mange in the animal-house.

The golden hamster (*Mecocricetus auratus*) is susceptible to many bacterial and viral infections. The animals should be handled gently and carefully, for they can inflict a deep biting wound if they are suddenly disturbed. *Intraperitoneal* and *subcutaneous inoculation* may be carried out in the manner used for rats or guinea-pigs. The susceptibility of the hamster to bacterial and viral infection is often markedly increased by the injection of cortisone acetate in a dose of 2 mg per kilo body-weight prior to inoculation.

Anaesthesia

Short acting: Ether.
Long acting: Pentobarbitone sodium stock solution (60 mg/ml) diluted 1 in 10 with 10 per cent ethyl alcohol. 1 ml per 100 g body-weight intraperitoneally.

Experimental Procedures

Inoculation and bleeding is carried out in the manner used for guinea-pigs.

FERRETS
Data

Normal temperature	.	37·8°–39·2°C; 100°–1·2·5°F
Gestation period	.	41–42 days
Weaning age	.	6–8 weeks
Mating age	.	6–9 months
Litters	.	2 yearly; average litter, 7–8
Room temperature	.	15·5°–18·5°C; 60°–65°F
Humidity	.	50–60 per cent
Weight at birth	.	10 g

Cages

A common form is a wooden hutch 3 ft by 1 ft 6 in by 1 ft 6 in high; it is divided into two compartments by a partition through which a circular hole 4 in in diameter is cut. The inner compartment, which is for sleeping and breeding, is kept dark. The outer compartment serves as an exercise run and is provided with a hinged door with vertical metal bars. The hutch will house three adult ferrets. Individual animals under experiment may be housed in metal cages constructed of sheet zinc forming an 18 in cube with a perforated lid for ventilation.

Feeding

Each ferret requires 4 oz of raw meat (horse flesh, lights, etc., are satisfactory) and 4 oz fresh milk daily.

Breeding

The oestrous condition is easily recognized by the redness, moisture and tense swelling of the vulva. At this time the bitch is brought to the dog for mating; if fertilization occurs the vulvar swelling subsides in about a week, if not the mating should be repeated. As soon as it is certain that the bitch is pregnant she is isolated in a separate hutch. After the birth of the litter the animals should on no account be disturbed for the fear that the mother will eat her progeny. After five to six weeks when the young are able to move out into the exercise compartment it is safe to handle the animals.

Precautions against Infection

Because ferrets are highly susceptible to the influenza and canine distemper viruses, great care is needed to prevent their accidental infection. Those who work with ferrets must be constantly aware of the possibility of the risk of transferring on their persons the distemper virus from infected canine pets and of themselves infecting the ferrets with influenza during the early stages of an illness. The risk of the worker himself being infected from the ferrets must also be borne in mind.

There is a very great risk of cross infection in experimental animals inoculated with these two viruses and special measures required to prevent this occurring include the use of special isolation cages with solid walls and the use by the worker of rubber boots, waterproof overalls and rubber gloves all of which are washed down with lysol after use.

Handling

It is advisable for beginners to wear leather gloves, but once the confidence of the animals has been won they can be picked up with the bare hands. A ferret should be lifted with a steady and firm grip with the fingers encircling the neck, shoulders and fore limbs while the other hand supports the rump.

Common Diseases

DISTEMPER. Ferrets are highly susceptible to distemper and the mortality is almost 100 per cent. The manifestations of the disease are similar to those in the dog. If distemper is accidentally introduced into the animal house all infected ferrets should be destroyed and the premises should be vigorously disinfected.

FOOT ROT is caused by mites and occurs only if the ferrets are kept in dirty conditions. It can be treated by cutting back the claws, bathing off the crusts on the swollen feet with warm soap and water, and by applying a 20 per cent emulsion of benzyl benzoate (National Formulary) or a 10 per cent sulphur ointment.

Staphylococcal and streptococcal infections and toxoplasmosis also occur.

Experimental Procedures

Anaesthesia

Short acting: Ether.
Long acting: Pentobarbitone sodium stock solution (60 mg/ml) diluted 1 in 10 with 10 per cent ethyl alcohol. 1 ml per kg body-weight intraperitoneally.

Intranasal inoculation. Under light ether anaesthesia, as soon as regular respiration is established, 1–2 ml of material can be introduced into the nares from a Pasteur pipette. Other methods of inoculation are those described for the guinea-pig.

FOWLS

Data

Rectal temperature	.	41·6°C; 106·9°F
Normal respiration rate	.	12 per min
Normal pulse .	.	140 per min

Cages

Galvanized-iron wire cages about 24 in tall and 20 × 20 in are suitable for individual birds.

For further information on the breeding and care of poultry the reader is referred to Ministry of Agriculture Bulletins Nos. 54 and 56.

Feeding

One of the pellet diets ('breeding' or 'laying' diets) available commercially can be used; it should be properly balanced and contain vitamins and trace elements. Green foods may be fed two or three times a week and grit and fresh water must be provided *ad lib*.

Common Diseases

Intestinal infections due to salmonellae of various types (e.g. *S. typhimurium*) are not uncommon. *S. pullorum* is the cause of bacillary white diarrhoea of young pullets and *S. gallinarum* causes outbreaks of 'Fowl typhoid'. Coccidiosis is another cause of acute enteritis in young chicks. *Tuberculosis* due to the avian type of *M. tuberculosis* is now relatively uncommon.

Parasitic infections due to lice and red mites may be controlled by the use of an aerosol spray of 2·0 per cent piperonyl hydroxide + 0·4 per cent pyrethrum. Two applications spaced seven to ten days apart should be used.

Avian leucosis of three different types, lymphoid leucosis, myeloid leucosis and erythroleucosis, is a very common cause of loss in poultry.

Virus diseases include infectious laryngotracheitis, fowl pest due in Great Britain to the Newcastle virus and also, elsewhere, to the fowl plague virus and fowl pox. In the preparation of prophylactic vaccines for poultry flocks it is essential that the material is proved to be uncontaminated by viruses of these types.

Experimental Procedures

The red blood cells, serum and plasma of the domestic fowl are frequently required in virological work and it is often necessary to keep a number of cockerels in the animal house. For certain types of work hens' blood is unsuitable. Turkeys, ducks, geese and pigeons are occasionally used and the day-old domestic chicken is a valuable experimental animal in some types of infectivity studies. The use of the chicken embryo is described in Chapter 10.

ANAESTHESIA. It should be noted that *ether anaesthesia is seldom satisfactory* in birds and that the injection of pentobarbitone sodium in a dose of 25 mg per kg body-weight intramuscularly in the thigh region gives better results. The anaesthetic should be given about half an hour in advance.

SUBCUTANEOUS INOCULATION is carried out in the pectoral or thigh regions.

INTRAPERITONEAL INOCULATION is carried out in the mid-line between the vent and the posterior end of the sternum.

INSUFFLATION. Infective material is dropped from a Pasteur pipette into the nostril.

COLLECTION OF BLOOD. If clear plasma is required, the bird should be deprived of food for about eight hours before bleeding.

From the wing vein. A 10- or 20-ml syringe with a No. 21 or 22 gauge needle is required and it is usually necessary to treat it and the tubes into which the blood is to be placed with a solution of heparin. The bird is placed on its side and the upper wing is fanned out to expose its under-surface. Feathers are then plucked from an area over the 'elbow' and the large brachial vein can be seen running over the bone and just beneath the skin. The area is cleaned with 70 per cent alcohol, and when dry the vein is gently pierced with the needle. Great care must be taken to avoid passing the needle too deep and on through the far side of the vein for if this happens a large haematoma results and it becomes impossible to obtain any blood.

Cardiac puncture: Method (1). The bird is anaesthetized and placed on its right side. The needle is inserted over the heart between the second and third ribs at a point close to where the edge of the breast muscle can be felt. At a depth of 38–40 mm the needle enters the ventricle. This method carries a risk of lung puncture and requires experience before it can be used with confidence. *Method* (2) is perhaps easier. Place the bird on its back, ventral side uppermost, and stretch its neck over the edge of the table. Pluck the base of the neck and clean the skin with alcohol as before. A 20-ml syringe with a No. 17 or 18 gauge needle 50 mm long is inserted horizontally just deep to the sternum; it should be tilted very slightly downwards and will enter the heart at a depth of about 38 mm.

MONKEYS

Data

Normal temperature	. 38·3°C; 101·0°F
Normal pulse rate .	. 100 per min
Normal respiration rate	. 20 per min
Gestation period .	. 5½–6 months
Room temperature	. 20°–22°C; 68°–72°F

Cages

A galvanized-iron cage having a floor space of approximately 3×4 feet and a height of 4 feet is required to give the animal sufficient space for exercise. A pair—male and female—can be kept together in such a cage. The floor may be of wire mesh with a tray fitted beneath it to catch the excreta. A wooden board may be fitted halfway up the cage for the monkey to perch and sleep on. The door fitted to the cage should be of the sliding type and it should contain at its base a small hinged door through which food trays can be put into the cage. Both the doors should be fitted with padlocks. A convenient addition to this cage is the fitting of a movable screen or false back to the cage which can be adjusted in position so that the monkey can be brought very close to the bars of the cage to receive a sedative injection before handling.

Feeding

A basic diet of boiled potatoes and a slice of bread covered with Bemax (vitamin B) is fed once a day and vegetables such as carrots, lettuce, turnips or parsnips are added *ad lib.* Alternatively, a pellet diet may be used (Short and Parkes, 1949). A lump of sugar soaked in a solution of vitamins A, C and D is given daily. Monkeys love oranges, bananas, grapes and tomatoes, and these may be fed several times a week. Fresh water is placed in a hopper high up on the side of the cage so that it escapes fouling.

Handling

Monkeys can be caught directly with the gloved hands, and are held with their arms clasped firmly behind their backs just above the elbows. Often, however, it is necessary to catch them with a net. The use of barbiturate drugs concealed in foodstuffs or given by injection to the animal pressed against the side of the cage has much to recommend it (Laboratory Animal Symposia, 1969).

Common Diseases

The commonest diseases that monkeys contract in captivity are tuberculosis, bacillary dysentery, measles and pneumonia. Newly arrived animals should be kept apart for several weeks and observed carefully for signs of disease; they should be tuberculin tested and their faeces should be examined for the presence of pathogenic bacteria. Tuberculous monkeys constitute a considerable risk to their attendants and if the disease is suspected on clinical grounds or because the tuberculin reaction is positive the diagnosis should be checked by X-rays and if confirmed the animal should be destroyed painlessly without delay. Bacillary dysentery may be treated by incorporating sulphaguanidine in the diet or by injecting streptomycin. Pneumonia, which is the least common of the diseases, can be treated with sulphadiazine.

REFERENCES

BRUCE, H. M. (1950) Feeding and breeding of laboratory animals. *Journal of Hygiene (London)*, **45,** 70.

BRUCE, H. M. & PARKES, A. S. (1947) Observations on the feeding of guinea-pigs. *Journal of Hygiene (London)*, **47,** 70.

CROFT, P. G. (1962) *An Introduction to the Anaesthesia of Laboratory Animals.* London: The Universities Federation of Animal Welfare.

CURNEN, E. C. & HORSFALL, F. L. (1946) Studies on pneumonia virus of mice (P.V.M.). *Journal of Experimental Medicine*, **83,** 105.

HAAS, V. H. (1954) Some relationships between lymphocytic choriomeningitis virus (L.C.M.) and mice. *Journal of Infectious Diseases*, **94,** 187.

HARRIS, R. J. C. (1962) *The Problems of Laboratory Animal Disease.* London: Academic Press.

HOWIE, J. W. (1952) Nutrition experiments in laboratory animals. *Journal of the Animal Technicians Association*, **2,** 7.

LABORATORY ANIMAL SYMPOSIA (1938) Vol. 1. *The Design and function of laboratory animal houses.*

LABORATORY ANIMAL SYMPOSIA (1969) Vol. 2. *Dietary standards for laboratory rats and mice.*

LABORATORY ANIMAL SYMPOSIA (1969) Vol. 4. *Hazards of handling simians.*

MINISTRY OF AGRICULTURE, FISHERIES AND FOOD. *Bulletin Nos.* 54 *and* 56. London: H.M.S.O.

NIGG, C. & EATON, M. D. (1944) Isolation from normal mice of pneumotropic virus which forms elementary bodies. *Journal of Experimental Medicine,* **79,** 497.

PARISH, H. J. (1950) *Notes on Communicable Diseases of Laboratory Animals.* Edinburgh: Livingstone.

PORTER, G. & LANE-PETTER, W. (1962) *Notes for Breeders of Common Laboratory Animals.* London: Academic Press.

SHORT, D. J. & PARKES, A. S. (1949) Feeding and breeding of laboratory animals. X. A compound diet for monkeys. *Journal of Hygiene (Cambridge),* **47,** 209.

SMITH, W. (1931) The breeding, maintenance and manipulation of laboratory animals. *A System of Bacteriology,* Vol. 9, 236. London: H.M.S.O.

SNELL, G. D. (Ed.) (1941) *The Biology of the Laboratory Mouse.* Philadelphia: Blakiston.

TRAUB, E. (1939) Epidemiology of lymphocytic choriomeningitis in mouse stock observed for four years. *Journal of Experimental Medicine,* **69,** 801.

WORDEN, A. N. & LANE-PETTER, W. (Eds.) (1972) *The UFAW Handbook on the Care and Management of Laboratory Animals,* 4th edn. Edinburgh: Livingstone.

16. Safety in the Microbiology Laboratory

Teachers, students, technicians, research workers and other staff in microbiology laboratories are exposed to the danger of infection from clinical specimens and laboratory cultures as well as to non-infective hazards such as cuts with broken glass, shocks from electrical apparatus, fire and explosion of gases and solvents, burning with corrosive chemicals, and poisoning by ingestion or inhalation of toxic chemicals. Infections and other accidents take place from time to time even in well regulated laboratories, but their frequency is minimized by the taking of careful precautions based on an understanding of the risks.

Immunity acquired naturally by clinical or subclinical infection with pathogens endemic in the community outside the laboratory, or artificially by vaccination, gives a valuable protection to workers handling the same pathogens in the laboratory. Such protection, however, is likely to be absent in the case of exotic and unusual pathogens, which, therefore, need to be handled with special care.

Besides the need to protect themselves, microbiologists have a duty to guard against disseminating infection into the community at large, whether by the careless disposal of contaminated material without prior disinfection, or by the occurrence of infection in a laboratory worker who may transmit it to persons outside the laboratory. Precautions against the 'escape' of virulent exotic pathogens such as the smallpox virus are particularly important (Wedum, 1953).

Occurrence of Laboratory Infections

Although many instances are known in which microbiologists have been infected with the organisms they were handling, the true prevalence of laboratory infections is unknown because there is no comprehensive system for their recording. Many laboratories do not keep records of such infections, so that surveys have depended mainly on information given from memory. Sulkin and Pike (1951) sent questionnaires to about 5000 laboratories in the USA, including those of hospitals, public health departments, medical and veterinary schools, research institutes and manufacturers of biological products. They obtained information about 1342 cases of laboratory-acquired infection, 39 of which were fatal. Sulkin (1961) later described a total of 2348 laboratory infections, of which 107 were fatal.

Sulkin and Pike's series of 1342 cases included 775 bacterial infections (the commonest were brucellosis 224, tuberculosis 153, tularaemia 65, typhoid fever 58, streptococcal infection 55, shigellosis 31, anthrax 30 and erysipeloid 27); 265 viral infections (hepatitis 95, psittacosis 44); 200 rickettsial infections (Q fever 104, typhus 64); 63 fungal infections (49 coccidioidomycosis) and 39 protozoal and helminthic infections. The great majority were in trained scientists, graduate students and technicians (1010) and only relatively few in students doing classwork but not research (63), animal caretakers, janitors and dish-washers (132) and clerical and maintenance staff (86). Clinical microbiology gave rise to the largest number of infections, research to the next largest, but classwork and the manufacture of biological products to relatively few (less than 5·3 and 5·6 per cent respectively).

Known accidents accounted for only 16 per cent of the infections, the common ones being self-inoculation with a syringe needle, spilling or spattering of cultures and infective fluids, pipetting by mouth, injuries with broken glass and bites from experimental animals. A further 10 per cent of the infections were in persons who were in contact with infected animals, 7 per cent in persons who performed a human necropsy and 1·5 per cent in persons handling discarded laboratory materials. The handling of clinical specimens accounted for 13 per cent of infections, including 80 of the 95 cases of viral hepatitis, most of which arose from the handling of specimens of blood submitted for chemical or serological examinations. In the remaining 52 per cent of cases the mode of infection was unknown, but in some was thought to have been airborne.

Tuberculosis in Laboratory Workers

Information about the frequency of laboratory infections has also been obtained from surveys comparing the incidence of a particular disease in laboratory staff with that in the community at large. In Britain the survey by Reid (1957) provided the first convincing evidence that tuberculosis was often acquired in the micro-biological laboratory. Rates of claims for occupationally-acquired tuberculosis in 1953–55 were eight times higher among pathologists and bacteriologists and six times higher among chest physicians and chest surgeons than among other hospital consultants. They were nearly three times higher among medical laboratory technicians than among other medical auxiliaries. In a special survey of staff in hospital and public health laboratories for the period 1949–53, the attack rate of pulmonary tuberculosis severe enough to cause absence from work was about three times greater in pathologists, bacteriologists and technicians who handled human necropsy material, tuberculous experimental animals, tuberculous sputum or cultures of tubercle bacilli than in laboratory staff who were not in contact with such infected material. The rates in laboratory staff of the latter, unexposed group were similar to those in socially comparable groups of Post Office professional engineers and clerical staff of the same age. In the survey by Koch (1951) in Dusseldorf the frequency of tuberculosis was four times higher among pathologists than among bacteriologists, but in Reid's survey the attack rate was not appreciably higher in those handling necropsy material than in those handling sputum or cultures.

Serum Hepatitis in Laboratory Workers

Hepatitis, presumed to be due to the virus B of serum hepatitis, has frequently been reported as occurring in the staff of laboratories where specimens of human blood are subjected to chemical, haematological or serological tests. In a survey of 51 laboratories with 731 personnel in the USA and 38 laboratories with 883 personnel in other countries, LoGrippo and Hayashi (1973) recorded an incidence of hepatitis (icteric and non-icteric) of 7·4 per cent in personnel in the USA and 5·2 per cent in other countries, and an incidence of Australia antigenaemia of 2·5 per cent in the USA and 2·7 per cent in other countries. These rates of clinical infection and antigenaemia in laboratory staff are considerably higher than those reported for the general population in the countries concerned and are evidence that many of the infections were acquired during work in the laboratory.

ROUTES OF INFECTION IN THE LABORATORY

The main mechanisms by which infection may be acquired from pathological specimens and laboratory cultures are: (1) soiling or inoculation of the skin or conjunctiva; (2) ingestion into the mouth, and (3) inhalation into the respiratory tract. The relative importance of these routes is uncertain. It has been possible to infer the route of infection from the preceding circumstances only in the minority of cases (16 per cent of Sulkin and Pike's series) attributable to known accidents such as self-inoculation with a syringe, injury with contaminated broken glass or contamination of the mouth in pipetting. The likelihood of infection taking place by a particular route depends on the tissue preferences of the micro-organism and the pathology of the disease. Thus it is reasonable to assume that most laboratory cases of cutaneous sepsis, anthrax and erysipeloid are contracted through the skin, most cases of typhoid fever and dysentery through the mouth and most cases of pulmonary tuberculosis, rickettsial infection, psittacosis and coccidioidomycosis through the respiratory tract. Certain other infections, such as brucellosis, may readily be acquired by any of the three routes.

Infection Through the Skin and Conjunctiva

Because the intact skin is a highly effective barrier against microorganisms, infection is likely to be acquired through it only when there is an accidental inoculation with a contaminated syringe, sharp instrument or fragment of glass. Great care must be taken in the handling and disposal of such objects. Wounding with a needle during inoculation into an animal or disposal of a used syringe is one of the commonest of laboratory accidents.

Although the soiling or splashing of intact skin with infective material is much less dangerous than inoculation through it, the microorganisms deposited on the surface may be able to pass through small, unperceived lesions or else be transferred by the hands into the mouth or by airborne dust into the respiratory tract. Contamination of the skin and clothing should therefore be avoided by the practice of proper bench technique, particularly by avoiding or disinfecting spillages of infective materials, preventing contact of contaminated equipment with the skin, clothing or bench, safely disposing of infective materials and contaminated equipment into 'discard' containers which are disinfected or sterilized, wearing a rear-opening protective gown and washing the hands after work.

The conjunctiva is a much less effective barrier to infection than the intact skin and it is probable that many bacteria and viruses can cause infection if deposited or splashed into the eye. In experimental animals, for instance, the intestinal-pathogenic salmonellae can cause systemic infection from much smaller inocula when placed on the conjunctiva than when given by mouth. Bench workers should avoid touching their eyes with their fingers, which may be contaminated, and should take care not to splash infective material into their eyes. When working with virulent pathogens they should wear glasses, safety spectacles or a vizor.

Infection Through the Mouth

The danger of infection being acquired through the mouth is greatest with organisms that are natural parasites either of the intestine, e.g. typhoid and dysentery bacilli and enteroviruses, or of the throat, e.g. *Strept. pyogenes* and *C. diphtheriae*, but probably many other kinds of pathogens can occasionally infect by the oral route. The procedure most likely to cause ingestion of a large dose of organisms, and so to pose the greatest risk of infection, is the use of the mouth in pipetting cultures and other infective fluids. In a microbiological laboratory the mouth should *never* be used for pipetting. A plug of cotton-wool is commonly inserted in the upper end of the pipette to prevent the entry of contamination before use, but fluid may readily be sucked through the plug into the mouth. In pipetting by mouth the upper end of the pipette and the finger controlling it are placed between the lips and this act is itself a hazard because the end of the pipette and the tip of the finger may be contaminated. It is imperative, therefore, that pipettes should be used with a rubber teat or some other manual or automatic suction device.

Other modes of infection are less likely to introduce large numbers of microorganisms into the mouth. The commonest hazard to be avoided is that of touching the mouth with the fingers or other objects such as pencils which may, unsuspectedly, have become contaminated. Eating and smoking in the laboratory and the licking of adhesive labels carry the same kind of danger.

Infection Through the Respiratory Tract

Many common laboratory procedures produce an inapparent contamination of the air with infective aerosols or dusts, which are liable to be inhaled into the upper and lower respiratory tracts (Darlow, 1972). Effective precautions against such airborne infection are difficult and laborious, but are essential in any work with virulent pathogens that are infective by the respiratory route, e.g. tubercle, anthrax, brucella, plague and tularaemia bacilli, rickettsiae, smallpox virus and many other viruses.

An *aerosol* is a spray or cloud of small droplets of liquid. Those droplets initially smaller than 0·1 mm in diameter rapidly dry and become solid droplet-nuclei so small, e.g. 1–20 μm in diameter, that they remain floating in the air for several minutes to several hours. Invisible aerosols are produced by almost any action that breaks the continuity of the surface of a liquid. For instance, the simple withdrawal of a loopful from a broth culture draws out filaments of liquid which break up into chains of droplets. Droplets are given off when a film of culture bursts in an inoculating loop, when a charged loop vibrates vigorously or sputters during flaming, when a loop is used to mix a suspension and when a hot wire touches broth or agar. Moderate numbers of droplets are discharged when a wet screw-cap or wet cotton-wool stopper is removed from a container. Large numbers may be discharged when a residue of fluid is expelled from a pipette or syringe or when liquid from a pipette or bottle is allowed to fall in drops into a container instead of being run gently down its side. Very large amounts of aerosol are generated in vigorous shaking or high-speed mixing of liquids, in dropping and breaking tube or plate cultures, and in centrifuging, especially when tubes break or when overful tubes or tubes with wet rims are centrifuged in an angle-head centrifuge.

Infective *dusts* consist of dry solid particles that are small enough to float in the air for several minutes or several hours. They are readily produced in the laboratory when cultures or other infective liquids are spilt on the skin, clothing, bench or floor. The spilt fluid dries and is then readily broken up into small dust particles which are raised into the air by almost any, even minor movement. When a cotton-wool stopper becomes moistened with the contents of a tube and then dries on standing, its subsequent removal disseminates dust from the dried crust. Clouds of infected dust or spores may be liberated during the opening of ampoules of freeze-dried cultures or containers of spored fungal cultures (Tomlinson, 1957).

Within one or two minutes after their liberation the airborne droplet-nuclei and dust particles are disseminated widely throughout the laboratory by convectional air currents. When inhaled, the particles larger than 5 μm are deposited in the nose and throat, whilst many of those smaller than 5 μm reach the bronchi and lungs.

Care should always be taken to minimize infection of the laboratory air by the practice of safe and gentle techniques, but the modes of aerial infection are so diverse and inapparent that it is necessary to adopt the additional precaution of using a *safety cabinet* for all manipulations of materials known or thought to contain virulent pathogens that are infective by the respiratory route. The safety, or 'exhaust protective' cabinet encloses sufficient space for ordinary bench procedures and has a front port through which the worker introduces his arms and which may either be open (Williams and Lidwell, 1957) or be occupied by rubber gauntlets (Darlow, 1967a,b). It is ventilated by exhaustion of air through a microfilter to outdoors at a rate sufficient to ensure that infected particles will not escape through the arm-port or any other opening into the air of the laboratory.

SAFETY ORGANIZATION

LABORATORY FACILITIES

The director of the laboratory has overall responsibility for safety. He should set up a safety organization and do his best to provide the facilities necessary for its implementation. Thus he should ensure that the workload is not so great that the staff have insufficient time to practise safe techniques, that the laboratory is not overcrowded and that ample supplies of protective materials are available. Wash-hand basins and disposable towels should be provided in each room in which cultures, clinical specimens or other infective materials are handled. Benches should have a smooth, impermeable surface. A special room or area should be provided for the receipt and opening of clinical specimens. Centrifuges with windshields and swing-out heads should be provided in preference to open or angle-head centrifuges, and either a special area screened against coarse spraying or a safety cabinet to contain aerosol should be provided for their use. Arrangements should be made for the regular servicing of centrifuges by the manufacturers or their agents. Separate rooms with exhaust ventilation to outdoors and proper facilities for disinfection of cages and safe disposal of litter must be provided for work with animals infected with dangerous pathogens such as the tubercle bacillus.

Safety Cabinets

Exhaust protective cabinets should be provided for all work with tubercle bacilli and other dangerous respiratory pathogens. They must be of an approved design (e.g. see *Hospital Building Note No. 15* (revised 1971) (DHSS, 1971)). The inward air-flow through the arm-port should be not less than 0·6 m/s and the exhaust should vent through a 5 μm filter to outdoors away from open windows, otherwise through an absolute filter after the 5 μm filter. The rate of air-flow should be checked weekly with an anemometer and the filters changed when it becomes less than 0·6 m/s. Before filters are changed or other maintenance work done, the cabinet, filter and trunking should be disinfected by boiling 100 ml formalin (40 per cent formaldehyde) or 10 per cent glutaraldehyde on an electric heater in the cabinet while the exhaust fan is running and the arm-port almost occluded. For further information see Evans, Harris-Smith and Stratton (1972).

Disinfectants

Each workplace in the laboratory should be provided with one or more deep plastic jars filled with disinfectant for the disposal of contaminated pipettes, slides, infective residues, etc., and a bottle of disinfectant to pour on spillages. One of the best disinfectants for general laboratory use is *sodium hypochlorite*. It is rapidly lethal to most bacteria and viruses, is relatively cheap, and is free from any marked or persistent irritant or toxic effect. Its main disadvantages are that it is ineffective against tubercle bacilli, readily inactivated by blood, pus and other organic materials, and corrosive to metals. 'Chloros', a proprietary preparation, is a 10 per cent solution of sodium hypochlorite which yields about 100 000 parts of available chlorine per million of solution. *Strong hypochlorite solution* yielding 10 000 parts per million of available chlorine (e.g. Chloros diluted 1 in 10) is used for equipment visibly soiled with blood or other organic material and *weak hypochlorite solution* yielding 1000 parts per million of available chlorine (e.g. Chloros diluted 1 in 100) is used for equipment not so soiled. The solutions must be made up freshly each day in carefully cleansed containers (Kelsey and Maurer, 1971) and may be tested at intervals with starch-iodide paper which turns blue if they are still active.

Alternatively, *phenolic disinfectants* such as 'Hycolin' or 'Sudol' may be used at 1 or 2 per cent concentration, the higher where there is much soiling with blood, pus or other organic matter. These disinfectants are less liable to inactivation than hypochlorite and are effective against tubercle bacilli, but are less actively cidal against some viruses and are less readily removed by rinsing from equipment, especially rubber. It is preferable not to use caustic phenolic disinfectants such as Lysol.

Formaldehyde 4 per cent solution (formalin 10 per cent) and glutaraldehyde 2 per cent buffered with 0·3 per cent sodium bicarbonate are actively cidal to viruses, vegetative bacteria and bacterial spores, and may be used to disinfect centrifuges and other metal equipment liable to be corroded by hypochlorite. They are, however, too irritant for general use in the laboratory.

For *skin disinfection*, a supply of 70 per cent ethanol containing 0·5 per cent chlorhexidine (tincture of hibitane) should be available. For repeated use, the addition of 1 per cent glycerol as an emollient is recommended. This disinfectant is non-irritant, though less effective than hypochlorite and phenolic disinfectants which must be rinsed from the skin after a brief contact. It may be used in preference to the latter for swabbing skin contaminated with microorganisms that are not highly virulent.

Safety Officer and Safety Code

Attention to safety precautions is best fostered among staff if the laboratory has a formal safety organization. A senior member of staff should be appointed as Safety Officer and representatives of different grades as a Safety Committee. The Officer and Committee should formulate a Safety Code, explain it to other staff and supervise its implementation. The Officer should keep an accident book and record details of every laboratory accident or infection.

The Safety Code should be drawn up to suit the special conditions in the particular laboratory, but might well be based on the recommendations given in the handbook *Safety in Pathology Laboratories* (DHSS, 1972a). If blood or other material from cases or carriers of serum hepatitis is dealt with, the laboratory code in the reports *Hepatitis and the Treatment of Chronic Renal Failure* (DHSS, 1972b) and

Viral Hepatitis (WHO, 1973) should be consulted. For work with tuberculous materials and cultures of tubercle bacilli the recommendations in the leaflet *Precautions Against Tuberculous Infection in the Diagnostic Laboratory* (HM(70)60) (DHSS, 1970) should be followed. The Code should include instructions on the following points.

1. *Mishaps.* Wash any cuts or pricks at once with soap and water. If the eye is splashed with infective material, rinse it at once with tap water. If the mouth is contaminated, spit and rinse with water before swallowing. If the skin is soiled with blood, exudate or culture, rinse it with strong hypochlorite and then wash it with soap and water. Alternatively, if it is contaminated with a culture that is not highly virulent, swab it with tincture of hibitane. If the clothing is contaminated, moisten the affected area with hypochlorite or phenolic disinfectant and then rinse well in water. Pour strong hypochlorite or phenolic disinfectant on any spillage of blood, clinical material or pathogenic culture and leave it for at least 10 min before wiping with a disposable cloth or paper tissue; discard the latter into a container for autoclaving. Report any mishap to the Safety Officer for recording and seek a decision about possible prophylaxis with an antibiotic, vaccine or gamma-globulin where appropriate.

2. *Personal hygiene.* Do not smoke, eat or drink in the laboratories or adjoining corridors. Do not lick labels. Do not put fingers, pencils or other objects into the mouth. Do not finger the eyes. Wash the hands after any procedure in which they may have become contaminated with traces of infective material, and always before leaving the laboratory. When in a working area, always wear a protective gown with a back opening or a coat with an overlapping (double-breasted) front opening. When opening or processing clinical specimens or dangerous cultures, wear also a waterproof plastic apron and disposable plastic gloves; if there is danger of splashing into the eye, wear spectacles or a vizor. Before leaving the laboratory for any purpose, remove the gown, apron and gloves; leave the gown and apron on their proper pegs and discard the gloves for disposal.

3. *Collection of clinical specimens.* Collect specimens of blood, exudate, etc. only into containers supplied by the laboratory, e.g. screw-capped bottles of a pattern known not to leak When introducing the specimen, avoid overfilling or soiling the rim and outside of the container. Close the container tightly. Write the patient's name on the label already attached to the container and send the container to the laboratory in a metal rack which holds it in the upright position. Send the request forms with the particulars of the patient and the examination required in a separate packet; do not attach the form to, or wrap it round the container.

When receiving and unpacking clinical specimens in the laboratory, wear disposable plastic gloves. Examine the containers to confirm that they have been properly closed. Show soiled and leaking containers to the Safety Officer, who may decide that they should be discarded without examination. When opening containers, do so slowly and carefully to avoid spurting and the formation of aerosol.

4. *Care of the workplace.* Ensure that disinfectants, discard jars and disposal bins are present. Keep the workplace tidy, for mistakes and accidents are most likely to happen when the bench is overcrowded with equipment and materials. Place tubes and containers in suitable racks or trays, never directly on the bench. Quickly pour strong hypochlorite or phenolic disinfectant over any spillage of infective material and leave for at least 10 min before wiping with disposable tissue. Wipe bench with hypochlorite at the end of each day's work.

5. *Discard jars with disinfectant.* At the start of each day empty the contents from the previous day, carefully clean the jar, preferably disinfect it by heating at 65°C for 10 min, and refill with fresh disinfectant diluted accurately to the correct concentration, e.g. hypochlorite to give 1000 or 10 000 parts per million of available chlorine or phenolic disinfectant, e.g. Hycolin at 1 or 2 per cent. Use hypochlorite for viruses and phenolic disinfectant for tubercle bacilli, the higher concentrations for heavily soiled and the lower for relatively clean equipment. Carefully introduce the used pipettes, slides and infective fluids into the disinfectant in such a way as to avoid splashing. Once or twice in the day, test hypochlorite with starch-iodide paper to confirm that it is still

active. At regular intervals, e.g. fortnightly, check the adequacy of the disinfectant and concentration used by making an 'in-use' test on the contents of the jar at the end of a day's work (Maurer, 1972).

6. *Discard bins.* Place all glass equipment such as tubes, culture plates and specimen containers, into a metal bin for autoclaving. Preferably dispose of plastic articles, including tubes, culture plates, containers, gloves and syringes into a separate bin for autoclaving. Alternatively, place plastic plates, containers and disposable gloves, but not syringes with needles, into a waterproof paper or plastic bag, seal it and incinerate it. Only members of the laboratory staff should be entrusted with the transport of bags of undisinfected material to the incinerator and plastic equipment should be incinerated only if it is known that the incinerator is of a type and size that will not be clogged by the molten plastic.

7. *Bench technique.* Take care to avoid spilling or splashing cultures or other infective material on to the hands, face, clothing or bench. Discard infective materials, cultures and contaminated equipment only into the proper discard jars and bins. After pouring an infected liquid, e.g. in discarding the supernatant from a centrifuged culture or sputum into disinfectant, remove any residual drop of liquid from the rim of the container with a strip of sterile blotting paper and discard the strip into disinfectant.

Carry out all procedures with cultures and infective materials in a gentle manner, taking care to avoid any unnecessary production of aerosol. Use a short inoculating wire with a small loop to avoid the risk of droplets being projected by vibration of the wire. Always flame the inoculating wire to red heat along its whole length before laying it on a rack or the bench. After inoculating dangerous, e.g. tuberculous, material that is liable to sputter when flamed, either dip the loop in boiling water or strong disinfectant for about 5 s before flaming or flame it in a hooded device (e.g. that described by Darlow, 1959).

8. *Pipetting.* Use a rubber teat or automatic suction device, *never the mouth.* Take care not to draw fluid up as far as the top of the pipette. When transferring fluid to another container,

first place the tip of the pipette well inside the mouth of the receptacle in contact with its wall and then allow the contents to run gently down the wall. Do not let drops or a jet of fluid fall from the pipette and do not blow out the residual fluid. Do not place the contaminated pipette in a rack or on the bench. At once lower it gently into a jar of disinfectant until it is completely submerged.

9. *Hypodermic syringes.* Preferably use disposable plastic syringes. Before use, ensure that the needle is tightly attached. When expelling air bubbles, embed the needle in a sterile swab or wad of paper tissue to soak up any escaping fluid. When emptying the contents of the syringe into a container or their residue into a jar of disinfectant, do so very slowly to avoid the formation of an aerosol. After emptying the syringe, at once place the used syringe with the needle attached or the detached needle into a rigid (e.g. metal) container for autoclaving or incineration so as to avoid the danger of anyone pricking himself with the exposed point.

10. *Safety cabinet.* Carry out all procedures with clinical specimens and cultures containing tubercle bacilli, brucellae, coxiellae, rickettsiae chlamydiae and other dangerous airborne pathogens in a safety cabinet. Before using the cabinet, switch on the ventilating fan. After use, switch on the ultraviolet lamp in the cabinet and leave on for 2 h. Once a week test the air intake flow rate with an anemometer to confirm that it is at least 0·6 m/s. If it is less, arrange to have the filter changed.

11. *Centrifuging.* Use the centrifuge strictly according to the operating instruction posted beside it. To avoid breakages by vibration or unseating of buckets, balance the loads accurately and symmetrically and take care to fit the buckets and trunnions properly in place. To balance loads, add water to the tubes, not directly into the buckets; include a blank set of tubes in each opposing set of carriers to receive the balancing water if it is desired to avoid adding it to the specimens. Use only stout glass or plastic containers that are unlikely to break, preferably screw-capped bottles of the Universal (28 ml), McCartney (28 ml) and bijou (6 ml) series. When filling the bottle, take care not to soil its rim or cap. Do not overfill,

e.g. not more than three-quarters full. Cap the tube or bottle firmly, preferably by tight application of a screw-cap over a good rubber washer. Before placing the tube or bottle in the centrifuge bucket, make sure that the supporting rubber pad is correctly in place at the bottom of the bucket and that it is free from fragments of grit or broken glass. When the tube or bottle is in place, make sure that it is supported at its foot, not by the projecting rim of its cap. After centrifugation, turn the speed controller to zero and allow the centrifuge to come slowly to rest; do not brake it violently or touch the rotor with the hand. Open the lid only after the rotor is at rest. Use the centrifuge only in its proper place, e.g. behind a screen or in a safety cabinet.

If a breakage occurs during centrifugation, switch off the centrifuge and leave it closed for 10 min after it has stopped to allow the aerosol to settle. Remove the buckets with their contents and place them in a container for autoclaving or into phenolic disinfectant, formaldehyde or glutaraldehyde, but not into hypochlorite which corrodes metal. Leave a swab soaked in 40 per cent formaldehyde (undiluted formalin) in the closed centrifuge bowl overnight, then swab the bowl with disinfectant and wash with water.

12. *Immunization*. Staff of laboratories dealing with infective materials should be immunized against diphtheria, tetanus, poliomyelitis, tuberculosis, typhoid fever, smallpox and, in the case of women of childbearing age, rubella. A full course of inoculations should be given for any infection for which immunization was not begun in childhood. Smallpox vaccination should be repeated every three or four years. Tuberculin-negative staff must not work with tuberculous materials or cultures until they have been rendered tuberculin-positive by BCG vaccination. Where Q-fever coxiella and typhus rickettsia are handled, staff should be vaccinated against these organisms; the Q-fever vaccine should be given only after skin testing to those found non-immune.

USE OF PATHOGENS IN TEACHING

A special responsibility falls on teachers to minimize the risks of infection to students doing practical classwork with pathogenic microorganisms. They must make a careful choice of the types of experiments and species of pathogens to be used and thoroughly train the students in safe techniques. It is, of course, possible for medical, dental, veterinary and science students to learn the principles of microbiology from practical work with harmless saprophytes and from demonstrations of killed pathogens, but properly organized work with live pathogens carries relatively little risk, even to beginners, and the slight element of danger brings a sense of reality into training in safe technique. After qualification, doctors, dentists and veterinarians are often required to handle infective materials from their patients, and science graduates may at some stage in their careers wish to work with pathogens. They can best be trained in safe technique while they are still undergraduate and impressionable.

Compared with the number of laboratory infections reported in trained scientific staff engaged in research or clinical microbiology, infections in students doing classwork have been relatively few. Thus, in Sulkin and Pike's survey of 5000 laboratories only 63 (4·7 per cent) of 1342 infections were in students working with pathogens in the classroom. These infections in students were mostly cases of typhoid fever, brucellosis, erysipeloid and localized bacterial sepsis. The relatively low risk in classwork is probably due to the conscientious adherence of students to their working instructions and the limitation of their work to pathogens of low virulence and to simple experiments involving a minimal risk of microbial dissemination.

Work with Pathogens for Beginners

If pathogens are to be used in practical work for large classes of beginners in open classrooms without safety cabinets, the following precautions should be taken.

1. The students should be instructed and supervised in the rigorous application of conventional aseptic techniques, particularly not to spill or splash cultures or allow them to come into contact with the hands, face or clothing; promptly to apply disinfectant to spillages; to flame the inoculating wire before

laying it down; to avoid pipetting by mouth; to discard pipettes directly into disinfectant; to avoid eating, smoking, fingering the mouth or eyes, or placing any object in the mouth; and to wash the hands before leaving the laboratory.

2. Experiments should be limited to procedures of a relatively simple, closely circumscribed type, e.g. the making and staining of films and the simple inoculation of cultures. They should not involve the preparation of bulk cultures of pathogens, or centrifugation, homogenization, ultrasonication or chemical extraction.

3. As far as possible, old stock cultures should be used, e.g. from a collection maintained by repeated subculture on Dorset's egg, in agar stabs or in cooked meat broth. Many such cultures are probably much attenuated in virulence, but it should be realized that some old laboratory cultures, e.g. a line of the LT2 strain of *Salmonella typhimurium*, have been found still virulent and have caused infections in laboratory workers.

4. The species of pathogens selected for class-work should be confined to those that are *commonly endemic* in the community at large. Exotic or highly virulent species should not be used. Students are likely to have been exposed during their childhood to most of the pathogens endemic in the community and either to have demonstrated an innate resistance to them or to have acquired immunity to them as a result of clinical or subclinical infection. At least, they are no more likely to become infected with such organisms in the laboratory than outside it.

Pathogenic bacteria suitable for practical classes in Britain might include: *Staph. aureus*; *Strept. pyogenes*; pneumococcus; meningococcus; diphtheria bacillus; *H. influenzae*; *Bord. pertussis*; *Esch. coli*; *K. aerogenes*; proteus; *Ps. pyocyanea*; salmonellae (but not *S. typhi*); shigellae (but not *Sh. dysenteriae* or *Sh. boydii*); pasteurellae (but not plague or tularaemia bacilli); *Bacillus* spp. (but not *B. anthracis*); clostridia (but not *Cl. botulinum*); mycobacteria (but not *Myco. tuberculosis* or *Myco. bovis*); actinomycetes; nocardiae and *Mycoplasma pulmonis*. Classwork should not be done with brucella, listeria, erysipelothrix, *V. cholerae*, rickettsiae, coxiellae, chlamydiae or pathogenic spirochaetes.

Among pathogenic fungi, *Candida albicans*, *Microsporum* spp. (e.g. *M. gypseum*) and *Trichophyton* spp. (e.g. *T. mentagrophytes*) may be used, but not the exotic fungal pathogens. Among viruses, work may be safely done with vaccinia virus (or rabbit-pox or ectromelia if the students have not been vaccinated), an egg-adapted strain of influenza virus type A, a vaccine strain of poliovirus type 1, and late tissue-culture passage lines of adenovirus and echovirus.

Senior Students and Trainee Technicians

Advanced students in medical microbiology and medical laboratory technology require to learn to work with every kind of pathogen liable to be encountered in the community, e.g. in Britain, the tubercle, typhoid and brucella bacilli. They should, therefore, be taught with these more dangerous pathogens, but only in laboratories that normally handle them, e.g. hospital and veterinary laboratories. They should practise procedures under individual supervision and should do this in the appropriate diagnostic laboratory, not in a practical classroom. They should use the protective equipment, e.g. a safety cabinet, and other precautions used routinely by the diagnostic staff and should be protected by the same immunization programme (Moore, 1971).

Live preparations of virulent exotic pathogens such as the smallpox virus should *never* be used in teaching.

REFERENCES

DARLOW, H. M. (1959) a device for flaming platinum loops. *Lancet*, **2**, 651.

DARLOW, H. M. (1967a) The design of microbiological safety cabinets. *Chemistry and Industry*, 1914.

DARLOW, H. M. (1967b) Safety in the microbiological laboratory. In *Methods in Microbiology*, edited by J. R. Norris and D. W. Ribbons, Vol. 1, pp. 168–204. London and New York: Academic Press.

DARLOW, H. M. (1972) Safety in the microbiological laboratory: an introduction. In *Safety in Microbiology*, edited by D. A. Shapton and R. G. Board, pp. 1–20. London and New York: Academic Press.

DHSS (1970) Precautions Against Tuberculous Infection in the Diagnostic Laboratory. HM(70)60. London: Department of Health & Social Security.

DHSS (1971) Hospital Building Note No. 15 (Revised 1971). Pathology Department, paragraphs 105–106. London: Department of Health & Social Security.

DHSS (1972a) Working Party of the Central Pathology Committee. Safety in Pathology Laboratories. London: Department of Health & Social Security; Cardiff: Welsh Office.

DHSS (1972b) Report of the Advisory Group. *Hepatitis and the Treatment of Chronic Renal Failure.* London: Department of Health & Social Security.

EVANS, C. G. T., HARRIS-SMITH, R. & STRATTON, J. E. D. (1972) The use of safety cabinets for the prevention of laboratory acquired infection. In *Safety in Microbiology,* edited by D. A. Shapton and R. G. Board, pp. 21–36. London & New York: Academic Press.

KELSEY, J. C. & MAURER, ISOBEL M. (1971) *Health Trends,* 3, 47.

KOCH, O. (1951) *Tuberkulosearzt,* 5, 498.

LOGRIPPO, G. A. & HAYASHI, H. .(1973) Incidence of hepatitis and Australia antigenemia among laboratory workers. *Proceedings of the Laboratory Section of the American Public Health Association,* 10, 157.

MAURER, ISOBEL M. (1972) The management of laboratory discard jars. In *Safety in Microbiology,* edited by D. A. Shapton and R. G. Board, pp. 53–59. London & New York: Academic Press.

MOORE, B. (1971) The handling of infectious material in the laboratory. *Annals of Clinical Biochemistry,* 8, 136.

REID, D. D. (1957) Incidence of tuberculosis among workers in medical laboratories. *British Medical Journal,* 2, 10.

SULKIN, S. E. (1961) Laboratory-acquired infections. *Bacteriological Reviews,* 25, 203.

SULKIN, S. E. & PIKE, R. M. (1951) Survey of laboratory-acquired infections. *American Journal of Public Health,* 41, 769.

TOMLINSON, A. H. (1957) Infected air-borne particles liberated on opening screw-capped bottles. *British Medical Journal,* 2, 15.

WEDUM, A. G. (1953) Bacteriological safety. *American Journal of Public Health,* 43, 1428.

WILLIAMS, R. E. O. & LIDWELL, O. M. (1957) A protective cabinet for handling infective material in the laboratory. *Journal of Clinical Pathology,* 10, 400.

WHO (1973) World Health Organization Technical Reports, Series No. 512. *Viral Hepatitis,* Geneva.

Volume II: Part 2
Identification of Specific Microbes.
Laboratory Diagnosis of Specific Infections

17. The Role of the Laboratory in the Diagnosis and Control of Infection

The staff of microbiological laboratories serve three main functions in medicine: (1) They help their clinical colleagues in the diagnosis and effective treatment of sick patients in institutions or at home; (2) they collaborate with medical, nursing and administrative staff in monitoring nosocomial infections and the procedures devised to control these infections, e.g. proper functioning of sterilizing equipment, sterility of hospital supplies and the control of infection in special care units; and (3) they may collaborate with public health staff and family doctors in tracing the sources and modes of spread of endemic and epidemic infection in the community and in testing and monitoring measures, e.g. prophylactic vaccination, aimed at the control of these community infections. For the effective performance of these functions, the laboratory staff must act as a team of which the leader will usually be a medically qualified microbiologist. The team includes laboratory assistants and domestic staff engaged in the preparation of culture media and of the appropriate swabs and containers for collecting specimens, technical staff concerned with the receipt, identification and primary culture of specimens, clerical staff to record the request forms and prepare and file the reports of the laboratory findings, and a combined professional and technical group who identify any pathogens present in the specimens and carry out serological or other tests which are needed for the laboratory diagnosis of specific infections and for epidemiological investigations. A strong esprit de corps and high morale are essential to maintain the effective performance of the team, each member of which must feel that he or she is playing an important part in the care of sick patients or in the control of infection in institutions and/or in the general community.

Specimens from Sick Patients

In the laboratory examination of specimens from sick patients, the first requirement is to check the identity of the patient on the request form and the specimen, e.g. that both the christian name and surname of the patient (or a specific number) is clearly written (preferably in printed letters) on the request form which must contain all relevant data likely to help the microbiologist, e.g. age, sex, clinical symptoms, duration of illness, antibiotics used (if any), previous reports (if any), and must be signed by a medical officer responsible for the care of the patient. If there is any ambiguity about the information given or examinations requested, the microbiologist should, where possible, contact his clinical colleague and ask for elucidation. In attempts to minimize the occurrence of these deficiencies, it is customary in many hospitals for a senior microbiologist to meet each new group of junior medical staff and explain to them the requirements and need for effective liaison between the ward and the laboratory. However, in practice, the collection of specimens and the filling in of request forms is often done by nursing staff although this is not formally part of their duties. In these circumstances, arrangements should, if possible, be made through the Matron's office for instructions about laboratory specimens to be given either verbally to groups of senior nurses or by the issue of an explanatory pamphlet.

Where there is urgency in receiving the laboratory findings, a provisional report should be given, either personally or by telephone, to the medical officer in charge of the case. For example, examination of a Gram stained smear of a purulent CSF will often allow a presumptive diagnosis of the infecting pathogen to be made so that the physician may immediately prescribe the most appropriate antimicrobial drug. Again, positive cultural findings after overnight incubation, e.g. numerous colonies of β-haemolytic streptococci from a throat swab or a positive slide agglutination of lactose non-fermenting colonies, e.g. *Shig. sonnei* in a case of diarrhoea should be urgently telephoned to the doctor in charge, and a confirmed report sent later. Written laboratory

353

reports should be as informative as possible and often require careful formulation based on experience and good judgment before they are sent to the clinician. The author was once telephoned by an angry and perplexed physician who had received a report '*S. thompson* present' in a case of diarrhoea.

Many laboratories now have arrangements for an emergency 24-hour service and, although much of this emergency work is handled by experienced technical staff, a qualified microbiologist must always be available for consultation. For routine work, the most satisfactory arrangement is that in which there is close collaboration and frequent consultations between laboratory and clinical staff with visits in both directions, including invitations to the microbiologist to ward rounds and bedside consultations. This kind of personal contact becomes increasingly difficult when laboratory services are being centralized and specimens are collected by van from outlying hospitals and health centres. In these circumstances, the consultant microbiologist should plan regular visits to the hospitals where he can discuss technical and professional problems with the clinical staff who, in turn, should be encouraged to visit the laboratory. This kind of close liaison maintains a high standard of laboratory collaboration and avoids the danger of the 'slot-machine' impersonal service. It also helps to reduce the number of ill-considered requests from junior staff and improves the quality of collected specimens, e.g. sputum instead of saliva, faeces instead of anal swab, or freshly voided rather than stale specimens of urine.

The most suitable containers for specimens of sputum, faeces, urine, CSF, pus, etc., the best kind of swabs, and the procedures of handling specimens after receipt in the laboratory are described in Appendix 1.

SPECIMENS IN EPIDEMIOLOGICAL INVESTIGATIONS

The staff in some laboratories are primarily concerned with the examination of specimens from cases and contacts of infection, occurring sporadically or in families or as larger outbreaks in the community or in institutions. In efforts to discover sources and modes of spread of the infection, investigations must often extend to the examination of water, milk, foodstuffs and other possible vehicles, to establishments where food is sold or consumed, and to possible animal reservoirs in the zoonoses. These epidemiological investigations are carried out as joint exercises by the laboratory staff working in close concert with public health officers and general practitioners. When a presumed common pathogen has been isolated from various sources, its precise identity may require the expert services of a Reference Laboratory where detailed serotyping, phage-typing, bacteriocin typing and other specialized tests are carried out. The Public Health Laboratory Service (PHLS) of England and Wales with its network of area, regional, central and reference laboratories is admirably organized and equipped to perform these epidemiological services (Howie, 1965, 1972a, 1972b). However, the PHLS recognizes the need to be engaged in hospital diagnostic services if it is to collect reliable information about the extent and nature of different infections in the whole community so that any one PH laboratory, often sited in hospital grounds, will be engaged in both diagnostic services to the hospital and public health services to the community. In addition, over 400 hospital laboratories, working under the National Health Service in England and Wales, supply positive laboratory findings for incorporation in the weekly Communicable Diseases Report (CDR) which collates the relevant data from all contributing laboratories for analysis and quick distribution to laboratory staff and health administrators.

In Scotland, there is no separate Public Health Laboratory Service, but many laboratories are carrying out work for both institutions and the general community. Again, a weekly digest of the collected data (Communicable Diseases, Scotland or CDS), together with veterinary information on zoonoses, reports on outbreaks, summaries of monthly or quarterly reports on venereal diseases, specific virus infections, tuberculosis, etc., is distributed to all cooperating and interested bodies.

When a laboratory performs the double role of diagnostic services to hospitals and public health services to the general community, including the bacteriological examination of water, milk, foodstuffs, etc., there is a risk that the demands for the hospital services may be so pressing and apparently so much more important—and interesting—that the public health laboratory services will suffer. There is the further difficulty for a small hospital laboratory in coping with a sudden increase in work following an outbreak of infection. It may be prudent in such circumstances to have regional public health laboratories with adequate and experienced staff geared to handle a sudden influx of specimens and to collaborate actively with public health officers in the epidemiological investigations that may be needed. In small countries like Scotland, facilities of this kind can be organized in some of the larger cities or in University Departments; similarly, regional laboratories are available to deal with more detailed virological examinations or the precise identification of microorganisms, e.g. atypical mycobacteria or pathogenic fungi, that the ordinary laboratory cannot tackle.

An increasingly important function of the microbiological services is collaboration with public health staff in the surveillance of certain infections, e.g. poliomyelitis, influenza, which may flare up nationally or locally, and in the assessment of the safety and efficacy of prophylactic vaccines against such common infections as whooping-cough, measles and rubella.

The establishment of epidemiology committees comprising laboratory staff, health administrators, general practitioners and specialists in paediatrics and infectious diseases, serving a population of 3–5 millions and meeting at regular intervals, has proved a useful forum for the discussion of matters of common interest and for the organization of collaborative studies.

TRAINING OF MICROBIOLOGISTS

Professional staff in medical laboratories have a structure, status and salary scale similar to staff in clinical departments. To be effective as consultant colleagues in the diagnosis and treatment of sick patients and in the epidemiological study and control of infection in a community, the medical microbiologist should have had a good training in clinical medicine, preferably including experience in paediatrics and infectious diseases, after the statutory pre-registration appointments. If his interests incline towards the laboratory diagnosis of sick patients in hospital, he will benefit from a trainee period of 2–3 years, covering all the pathological disciplines, but specializing in his chosen subject in the latter part of the traineeship. If, on the other hand, he is more interested in public health microbiology, he should take an academic course for the Diploma in Bacteriology which includes some basic training in epidemiology and statistics and thereafter continue his training in a regional public health laboratory. For more senior appointments in either branch of microbiology, membership of the Royal College of Pathologists is a useful qualification for advancement.

REFERENCES AND FURTHER READING

HOWIE, J. W. (1965) The Public Health Laboratory Service. *Lancet*, **i,** 501.

HOWIE, J. W. (1972a) A microbiology service for communicable disease epidemiology. *Lancet*, **i,** 857.

HOWIE, J. W. (1972b) Medical microbiology for patient and community. *Journal of Clinical Pathology*, **25,** 921.

THOMSON, W. A. R. (1971) *Calling the Laboratory*, 3rd edn. Edinburgh: Churchill Livingstone.

WHO REPORT (1969) *Communicable Diseases: Methods of Surveillance.* Report of a Seminar; World Health Organization Regional Office for Europe. Copenhagen: Limited distribution.

18. Staphylococcus and Other Cluster-Forming Gram-Positive Cocci

Introduction

The cluster-forming Gram-positive cocci belong to the genera *Staphylococcus*, *Micrococcus*, *Gaffkya*, *Sarcina*, *Peptococcus* and *Aerococcus*, the distinguishing features of which are given in Table 18.1. *Gaffkya* and the aerobic species of *Sarcina* are classified by some authors in the genus *Micrococcus*.

These organisms include only one important pathogenic species, namely *Staphylococcus aureus*, which causes a variety of superficial and deep infections, in most cases pus-forming. Other staphylococci, namely *Staph. albus* (*Staph. epidermidis*), and members of the other five genera are commonly present either as commensals or contaminants on the surfaces of the body, but lack virulence and primary pathogenicity. They are frequently found as contaminants in clinical specimens taken from the body surfaces, e.g. swabs from skin, nose, throat, wounds, burns and bed-sores, where their presence should not be regarded as being clinically significant. Occasionally, however, *Staph. albus* and *Micrococcus* spp. act as opportunistic pathogens and cause infections of the urinary tract or, rarely, more serious, e.g. bacteriaemic, infections in debilitated patients. *Gaffkya tetragena* is a rare cause of suppurative lesions in the mouth, neck or respiratory tract.

The characters of *Staph. aureus* that are absent from most or all strains of *Staph. albus*, and thus useful for the identification of *Staph. aureus*, are: golden colony pigmentation, the production of coagulase, deoxyribonuclease, phosphatase, alpha, beta and delta haemolytic toxins, leucocidin, fibrinolysin and hyaluronidase, the anaerobic fermentation of mannitol,

Table 18.1 Distinguishing characters of six genera of the family Micrococcaceae, the cluster-forming Gram-positive cocci

Genus	Predominant grouping of cocci	Atmospheric requirements	Catalase production	Breakdown of glucose	Ecological character
Staphylococcus	Irregular (grape-like) clusters	Aerobic and facultative (aerobic growth greater than anaerobic)	+	Fermentative (acid formed under either aerobic or anaerobic conditions)	Pathogenic and commensal parasites
Micrococcus	Irregular or rectangular clusters and tetrads	Aerobic (no growth in absence of O_2)	+	Oxidative (acid formed only under aerobic conditions) or inactive	Free-living saprophytes
Gaffkya	Tetrads	Aerobic and facultative	...	Fermentative	Pathogenic parasites
Sarcina	Cubical packets of eight cocci	(1) Anaerobic	...	Fermentative or inactive	Free-living saprophytes
		(2) Aerobic	+	Oxidative	Free-living saprophytes
Peptococcus	Clusters and tetrads	Strictly anaerobic	+	Fermentative or inactive	Commensal parasites
Aerococcus	Small clusters	Facultative	− or weak	Fermentative	Free-living saprophytes

susceptibility to phages of the *Staph. aureus* phage-typing set, and agglutinability by *Staph. aureus* typing antisera.

STAPHYLOCOCCUS AUREUS

Morphology and staining. Spherical, diameter 0·8–1·0 μm. In films of pus or from solid culture medium: grape-like clusters with some single and paired cocci. In broth: small groups, pairs, singles and *short* chains (less than five cocci in line). Gram-positive, non-sporing, non-motile and, except for rare strains, non-capsulate.

Cultural characters. Facultative anaerobe. Temperature for growth; range 12°–44°C, optimum 37°C. Optimum pH, 7·4–7·6.

1. NUTRIENT AGAR. Colonies after aerobic incubation at 37°C for 24 h are 2–3 mm in diameter, have a smooth glistening surface, entire edge, butyrous consistency and an opaque, pigmented appearance. In most strains, the pigmentation is golden (orange, yellow and cream-to-buff varieties) but in a few it is white (the white-colonied variety of *Staph. aureus* is fully virulent). Colonies are smaller and pigmentation is absent on plates incubated anaerobically.

2. MILK AGAR (see below). Colonies as on nutrient agar but more intensely pigmented, with clearer distinction between orange, yellow and cream-buff strains. Zones of clearing around colonies due to digestion of heat-coagulated casein by staphylococcal proteases.

3. MACCONKEY'S AGAR. Colonies pinkish and very small to normal in size depending on the batch of medium.

4. BROTH. Uniform turbidity with some powdery deposit.

5. GELATIN STAB after 5 days at 22°C: filiform growth with liquefaction from top. Coagulated serum slopes slowly liquefied.

Pigmentation and pigment-enhancing media. The observation of golden (orange, yellow or cream-buff) pigmentation is an important diagnostic step because it makes possible the provisional identification of *Staph. aureus* colonies in mixed primary cultures. Pigmentation is often poorly developed in 24 h on nutrient agar or blood agar and it is then best seen by viewing in daylight the aggregated

material scraped up from several colonies on to an inoculating wire. It is enhanced by prolongation of incubation to 48 h or by the use of a special pigment-enhancing medium such as *milk agar* (33 per cent full fresh milk, Christie and Keogh, 1940), *cream agar* (10 per cent cream), or *glycerol monoacetate agar* (1 per cent, Jacob, Willis and Goodburn, 1964; Willis, O'Connor and Smith, 1966).

Phenolphthalein phosphate agar. This indicator medium (Barber and Kuper, 1951) allows easy provisional identification of colonies of *Staph. aureus* in mixed cultures. The inoculum is plated out to yield discrete colonies and the plate incubated for 18 h at 37°C; 0·1 ml ammonia solution (SG 0·88) is placed in the lid of the Petri dish and the dish with the culture is placed over it for a minute or so. All strains of *Staph. aureus* form phosphatase and so liberate phenolphthalein which reacts with the ammonia to give the colonies a bright pink colour. Few strains of coagulase-negative staphylococci are phosphatase-positive; the majority form colonies that remain uncoloured on exposure to ammonia. For avoidance of false-positive reactions medium should be newly made with a fresh solution of phenolphthalein diphosphate. A parallel control plate should be set up with inocula of known positive (*Staph. aureus*) and negative (*Staph. albus*) cultures.

Selective culture media. (*a*) *Salt media*. Staphylococci tolerate higher concentrations of sodium chloride than many other kinds of bacteria and salt-containing media are therefore useful for the selective culture of *Staph. aureus* from faeces, foodstuffs, dust, clothing and other materials likely to contain a predominance of other bacteria; e.g. milk agar plus 7–10 per cent NaCl, glycerol monoacetate agar plus 5 per cent NaCl, and cooked meat broth plus 10 per cent NaCl. (*b*) *Polymyxin agar* (Finegold and Sweeney, 1961) is selective specifically for *Staph. aureus* and it inhibits *Staph. albus* as well as Gram-negative bacilli and other bacteria.

Coagulase production. Since, for practical purposes, *Staph. aureus* is defined as the species consisting of the coagulase-positive strains of staphylococci, the test for coagulase production is the conclusive identifying test for the species.

Most strains of *Staph. aureus* form both *free coagulase*, which reacts in the tube coagulase test, and *bound coagulase* (clumping factor) which reacts in the slide coagulase test. A small minority of strains form only the one or other type of coagulase.

The reagent for the test is human or rabbit plasma. If human plasma is used it should, as a precaution against laboratory infections with serum hepatitis, be prepared from blood collected from a donor who has been shown to be free from Australia antigen. Small volumes of plasma are obtained by centrifugation of blood to which sodium oxalate has been added to a concentration of 0·2–0·3 per cent. Larger volumes are conveniently collected from out-dated (e.g. 3-week-old) human blood containing trisodium citrate, approx. 0·33 per cent, which has been discarded by the blood transfusion service. After the suitability of the plasma for the coagulase test has been confirmed in slide and tube tests with standard positive and negative cultures, a batch may be stored in 20-ml volumes at −20°C for many months and an in-use volume may be stored for a week or so in the refrigerator at 4°C.

1. SLIDE COAGULASE TEST (Williams and Harper, 1946). Place a drop of saline (0·85 per cent NaCl) solution or water on a clean microscope slide. With the minimum of spreading, emulsify a small amount of solid culture, e.g. one or two colonies, in the drop of saline to form a smooth milky suspension. If the strain is autoagglutinable and a smooth suspension cannot be obtained, do not proceed with the slide test. Dip an inoculating loop or straight wire into *undiluted plasma* warmed to room temperature and stir the adhering traces (not a loopful) of plasma into the drop of bacterial suspension on the slide. Coarse clumping becoming visible to the naked eye within 5–10 sec is a positive result. A slower reaction is a negative result but the strain giving a slow reaction should always be examined by the tube test.

The slide test gives 'false-negative' reactions with about 5 per cent of coagulase-positive strains, so that when a negative slide reaction is obtained with a strain thought likely, on account of its source or pigmentation, to be *Staph. aureus*, the strain should be retested by

the tube method or by an alternative identifying test such as the deoxyribonuclease test.

2. TUBE COAGULASE TEST (Gillespie, 1943). Prepare a 1 in 10 dilution of the plasma in saline (0·85 per cent NaCl) solution and place 1 ml of the *diluted plasma* in a small tube. Inoculate the strain under test into the tube preferably by adding 0·1 ml of an 18–24 h broth culture (about 10^8 cocci). A more convenient but less reliable method of inoculation is to emulsify the material of a few colonies (e.g. 10^9 cocci) in the plasma and to add a drop of broth. Incubate the tube at 37°C and examine for coagulation at 1, 3 and 6 h. Leave the negative tubes at room temperature overnight and re-examine. The conversion of the plasma into a soft or stiff gel, best seen on tilting the tube to the horizontal position, is a positive result. Since the coagulum may be liquefied sometime after it has been formed, it is necessary to examine the tubes at each of the times prescribed above.

Control tests of known coagulase-positive and coagulase-negative cultures and a tube of uninoculated plasma should be set up with each batch of tests.

Coagulase-negative strains of Staph. aureus. Rare strains are encountered of apparently pathogenic *Staph. aureus*, either golden- or white-colonied, which nevertheless give negative reactions in both the slide and tube coagulase tests. Except for their negative coagulase reaction, these strains show the biochemical characters typical of *Staph. aureus* (*Staphylococcus* subgroup 1, Table 18.2), and in many cases also form deoxyribonuclease, alphatoxin, staphylokinase (fibrinolysin) and hyaluronidase, and are typable with *Staph. aureus* phages and *Staph. aureus* agglutinating antisera (Choudhuri and Chakrabarty, 1970; Bayston, 1972). They are probably best detected by the DNase test.

Deoxyribonuclease (DNase) production. All coagulase-positive strains of staphylococci hydrolyse DNA, whereas only a minority (about 25 per cent) of coagulase-negative strains do so; a test for DNase can therefore be used to screen out coagulase-negative organisms (Blair, Emerson and Tull, 1967).

Prepare tryptose agar medium containing deoxyribonucleic acid 2 g per litre, autoclave at

Table 18.2 Distinguishing characters of species and subgroups of *Staphylococcus* and *Micrococcus* (Baird-Parker, 1966)

Character	Staphylococcus subgroups						Micrococcus subgroups							
	1 *S. aureus**	2	3	4	5 *S. albus (S. epidermidis)*	6	1 *M. luteus*	2	3	4	5	6	7	8 *M. roseus**
Acid from glucose:														
(1) aerobically	+	+	+	+	+	+	+	+	+	+	+	+	W	W
(2) anaerobically	+	+	+	+	+	+	−	−	−	−	−	−	−	−
Coagulase	+	−	−	−	−	−	−	−	−	−	−	−	−	−
Phosphatase (3–5 days)	+	+	+	−	−	+	+	+	+	+	−	+	−	−
Acetoin (Voges-Proskauer)	+	+	+	+	+	+	+	+	+	+	−	+	−	−
Acid aerobically from:														
(1) arabinose	−	−	d	−	d	d	−	−	−	+	d	+	−	−
(2) lactose	+	+	d	−	+	+	d	+	d	+	+	+	−	−
(3) maltose	+	+	−	d	+	+	d	+	+	+	+	+	−	W
(4) mannitol	+	−	−	−	+	+	−	−	+	+	+	+	−	−

W = Weak or negative.
d = Different reactions (+ or −) in different strains.
* = Aureus pigment in most strains of *S. aureus* and some strains in each subgroup of *S. albus*. Pink pigment in *M. roseus*. White, yellow or orange pigment in different strains in other subgroups of *Micrococcus*.

121°C, mix well and pour in plates. Inoculate material from a colony on the primary culture plate by spotting it on a small area of the DNA plate and incubate for 18 h. Then flood the DNA plate with Normal HCl, which precipitates the DNA and turns the plate cloudy. The appearance of a zone of clearing (absence of turbidity) round the colony denotes DNase production and a positive result.

Opacity reaction in egg yolk. Many coagulase-positive staphylococci of human origin, but only a few such strains from animals, produce a dense opacity due to lipolytic activity when grown in glucose egg-yolk broth; coagulase-negative strains do not give the reaction (Gillespie and Alder, 1952).

Haemolysin production. Nearly every strain of *Staph. aureus* forms one, other or more than one of three haemolytic exotoxins, alpha, beta and delta, which are antigenically distinct and differ in their action on the red blood cells of different animal species, thus:

Species	Alpha	Beta	Delta
Horse	−	−	+
Man	−	+	+++
Rabbit	+++	+	+
Sheep	+	+++	∓

Most coagulase-positive human strains form both alpha and delta toxins and a few also form beta toxin, whereas most coagulase-positive strains from animals form beta as well as alpha and delta toxins. Coagulase-negative strains (*Staph. albus*) do not form alpha, beta or delta toxin, but most of them form another haemolysin, epsilon, which acts on rabbit and sheep cells and is uninhibited by antiserum to the *Staph. aureus* toxins. For details and references see Elek and Levy (1950), Elek (1959), Arbuthnott (1970) and Wiseman (1970).

Though the effects of these haemolysins may often be seen in the production of zones of partial or complete haemolysis on blood agar plates, their reliable demonstration and identification requires the use of different bloods and the observation of specific prevention by *Staph. aureus* antitoxic serum. It is therefore too laborious for use in the routine identification of *Staph. aureus*.

Elek and Levy (1950) described a method for the identification of alpha, beta, delta and epsilon haemolysins by growing cultures for 48 h at 37°C on plates of sheep and rabbit blood agars containing strips of filter paper soaked with antiserum. To ensure maximal toxin production, the plates are incubated in air containing 30 per cent CO_2.

The best method of demonstrating the production of haemolysin is by growing the culture in soft nutrient agar (0·35 per cent New Zealand agar) for 24 h at 37°C in an atmosphere of air plus 20–30 per cent CO_2. To harvest the toxins, break up the culture medium, freeze at $-40°C$, thaw rapidly and centrifuge to yield a clear toxin-containing supernate. Test this fluid by mixing doubling dilutions of it with equal volumes of washed red blood cells suspended to 2 per cent (v/v) in 0·01 M phosphate-saline buffer pH 7·0, and incubating for 1 h at 37°C. Use rabbit cells to demonstrate alpha toxin and sheep cells to demonstrate beta toxin. The sheep cell suspension should contain 0·001 M Mg^{2+} and after incubation at 37°C the tests should be held overnight at 4°C to demonstrate the great intensification of haemolytic effect produced by this procedure with the 'hot-cold' beta haemolysin. Tests may be done with horse or human red cells to demonstrate delta toxin.

Enterotoxin production. A proportion, probably over 50 per cent, of strains of *Staph. aureus* form enterotoxin and thus are capable, by growth and toxin production in a foodstuff, of causing staphylococcal food-poisoning. Different strains of *Staph. aureus* produce five antigenically distinct forms of enterotoxin, A–E, recognized by their specific precipitation reactions with antisera (Bergdoll, 1970). Except for rare strains of doubtful status, coagulase-negative staphylococci do not form enterotoxin.

The ingestion of as little as 1 μg enterotoxin may cause the onset of nausea, vomiting, abdominal pain and diarrhoea within 1–6 h. The enterotoxin is relatively heat-stable and may remain active despite heating at 100°C for several minutes to half an hour. Food-poisoning may, therefore, be caused by food that has been cooked and in which the heat of cooking has killed all the staphylococci. In such cases a laboratory diagnosis cannot be made by cultural demonstration of *Staph. aureus* in the food remains, but must be made by identifying enterotoxin extracted from the food.

Methods for extracting and concentrating enterotoxin from food and for identifying it by reactions with specific antisera are reviewed by Bergdoll (1970). Casman and Bennett's slide agar-gel double-diffusion method modified by Gilbert *et al.* (1972) detects as little as 0·02 μg toxin per g food. No convenient laboratory animal is susceptible to the toxin, but the effects are demonstrable in rhesus monkeys given the toxin by mouth or by tube into the stomach.

PV leucocidin, hyaluronidase and fibrinolysin. Methods for demonstrating the production of these products of *Staph. aureus* are reviewed by Elek (1959).

Biochemical reactions. Acid, no gas from glucose, maltose, lactose, sucrose and, usually, mannitol. *S. aureus*, like other staphylococci, forms acid from glucose when tested under either aerobic or anaerobic conditions; micrococci ferment glucose only under aerobic conditions (Table 18.2); for method, see below under 'Other cluster-forming Gram-positive cocci'. Most strains of *Staph. aureus* from human sources ferment mannitol and since few strains of *Staph. albus* and *Micrococcus* do so, mannitol fermentation may be used for the provisional identification of human *Staph. aureus*. Catalase positive on media with 1 per cent glucose. Oxidase negative. Nitrates reduced to nitrite. Methyl red and Voges-Proskauer tests positive. Lipase activity against tributyrin and some other lipids. Indol negative. Most strains are proteolytic on gelatin, coagulated serum and coagulated casein; they hydrolyse urea and produce ammonia from peptone.

Sensitivity to physical and chemical agents. Laboratory cultures survive for months, and in some cases for years. The cocci withstand moist heat at 60°C for 30 min but are killed in 1 h. Moderately resistant to natural drying and, in the absence of direct sunlight, survive in dust for several days, weeks or months. Fairly readily killed by common disinfectants used at proper concentration, e.g. in a few minutes by 2 per cent phenol or a hypochlorite solution containing 1000–10 000 parts/10^6 available chlorine. Strains may be distinguished as mercury-resistant or mercury-sensitive according to whether or not they will grow on peptone agar containing 1 in 27 500 mercuric chloride; mercury resistance is a 'marker' character that has been found to be associated with antibiotic resistance and infectivity in hospitals (Moore, 1960).

Antibiotic sensitivity. The majority (e.g. 50–75 per cent) of strains of *Staph. aureus* isolated outside hospital are sensitive to benzyl penicillin (Minimum Inhibitory Concentration 0·03 µg/ml), phenoxymethyl penicillin (0·03 µg/ml), ampicillin (0·1 µg/ml), cloxacillin (0·12 µg/ml), methicillin (2 µg/ml), cephaloridine (0·12 µg/ml), streptomycin (2 µg/ml), kanamycin and neomycin (0·5 µg/ml), chloramphenicol (8 µg/ml), tetracycline (0·12 µg/ml), fucidin (0·06 µg/ml), erythromycin (0·12 µg/ml), novobiocin (0·12 µg/ml) and vancomycin (1 µg/ml). A large proportion (e.g. 75 per cent) of hospital strains are penicillinase-producing and thus resistant to benzyl penicillin, phenoxymethyl penicillin and ampicillin (e.g. MIC > 1000 µg/ml) and many of these penicillin-resistant strains are also resistant to tetracycline and a number of other antistaphylococcal antibiotics. The latter, 'multi-resistant' strains, are usually sensitive to the penicillinase-resistant penicillins, e.g. cloxacillin (0·25 µg/ml) and methicillin (2 µg/ml), and to the cephalosporins (cephaloridine 5 µg/ml), fucidin (0·06 µg/ml), vancomycin (1 µg/ml) and cotrimoxazole (Septrin). However, a small proportion of these strains are 'methicillin-resistant', being able to grow in the presence of low therapeutic concentrations of methicillin and cloxacillin as well as in those of other penicillins. In cultures at 37°C the MIC of methicillin for methicillin-resistant strains is only about 5 µg/ml, but at 30°C it is about 100 µg/ml.

Antibiotic disk diffusion tests should be done on nutrient or blood agar with an appropriate selection of disks, e.g. disks containing benzyl-penicillin 1·2 µg (2 units), methicillin 10 µg, tetracycline 10 µg, erythromycin 15 µg, fucidin 5 µg and kanamycin 30 µg. A control test should be done with the Oxford strain of *Staph. aureus* (National Collection of Type Cultures No. 6571) which is sensitive to all these drugs. *Penicillinase-producing staphylococci* may show a fairly large inhibition zone round a penicillin (or ampicillin) disk but are easily identified by their growth forming a heaped-up edge (or large colonies) bordering the zone; this form of edge differs from the smooth, tapering edge given by the control, penicillin-sensitive culture. Organisms showing such an edge should be reported as 'penicillin-resistant' regardless of the size of the zone. *Methicillin-resistant staphylococci* often appear sensitive after incubation for 24 h at 37°C and incubation should be continued for 48 h when growth may appear within the early-inhibited zone. It is preferable, however, to perform a separate test for methicillin sensitivity either by incubating a culture with a 10 µg disk overnight at 30°C or by incubating a culture on agar containing 10 µg methicillin per ml and 5 per cent added NaCl for 18 h at 30°C (Hewitt, Coe and Parker, 1969).

Serotyping. Slide agglutination tests with absorbed antisera distinguish three major serotypes, I, II and III, of *Staph. aureus* (Cowan, 1939) and a number of minor types. Hobbs (1948) recognized 13 types. Oeding (1953) identified nine antigenic factors with selectively absorbed 'factor sera'; these characterized four groups, three of which corresponded with Cowan's types, and some relatively uncommon subtypes. Torres Pereira (1961) observed that two major agglutinating antigens (13 and 17) of freshly isolated strains tended to be lost and replaced by others (antigens 3 and 1, respectively) on continued subcultures in the laboratory. Haukenes (1967) described technical developments of Oeding's methods that identify 18 agglutinin-specific antigens. Serotyping has been used in epidemiological studies of *Staph. aureus*, but the information obtained has been less satisfactory than that obtained by phage-typing.

Phage-typing. Several hundred different phage-types of *Staph. aureus* are distinguished according to the pattern of susceptibility of strains to an internationally recognized set of about 24 standard phages. The majority of the phages belong to one or other of four groups of related phages. The staphylococci are designated by the group and types of the phages that lyse them, as shown in Table 18.3.

The typing phages are grown on susceptible host strains of *Staph. aureus* (propagating strains) designated by the number of the phage

Table 18.3

Phage group	Individual phages	Common phage-types of staphylococci
I	29; 52; 52A; 79; 80	29; 52/52A; 52/52A/80/81; 80
II	3A; 3B; 3C; 55; 71	3A/3B/3C; 3C/55, etc.
III	6; 7; 42E; 47; 53; 54; 75; 77; 83A; 84; 85	6/7/47/53/54/75/77 and many others, usually complex
IV	42D	
Unclassified	81; 187	

and the prefix PS, e.g. strain PS52 is used to propagate phage 52. The propagating strains and the phages are obtainable by accredited laboratories from the Cross-infection Reference Laboratory, Central Public Health Laboratories, Colindale Avenue, London. Digest broth plus 400 mg $CaCl_2$ per litre is used for propagation. To avoid variation, both phage and propagating strain are started on each occasion from freeze-dried stock.

The simple broth propagation method of Blair and Williams (1961) gives suitable titres of most phages. Grow the propagating strain overnight in digest broth at 37°C and add an inoculum of this culture to fresh broth in the proportion of 1 to 100. Add phage, reconstituted in broth, to give a dilution equivalent to the RTD (see below) in the culture. Incubate with shaking at 37°C for 6 h. Centrifuge the lysate and collect the supernate.

Titrate the supernate by placing 0·02 ml drops of decimal dilutions in peptone water on the surface of a digest agar plate previously seeded by flooding with a 4–5 h or overnight culture of the propagation strain (as for typing). Incubate at 30°C overnight or at 37°C for 6 h. The highest dilution of phage giving lysis with almost confluent plaques is the Routine Test Dilution (RTD).

If the titre is satisfactory, i.e. > RTD × 1000, filter the phage preparation through a 5/3 sintered glass filter to remove remaining bacteria, re-titrate the sterile filtrate to check on loss of potency during filtration, and confirm the lytic spectrum (host range) of the phage by spotting drops of undiluted filtrate on plate cultures of a set of indicator (propagation) strains. Store the undiluted phage filtrate at 4°C and freeze-dry samples for future propagation.

When sufficiently high titres of phage cannot be obtained by the broth propagation method, particularly with phages 29, 42D, 47, 52, 52A, 79, 80 and 187, the freeze-and-thaw agar method of Williams and Rippon (1952) should be used.

For typing purposes, prepare dilutions of phage at RTD and RTD × 1000 weekly and store in the refrigerator.

Typing method. Flood the surface of a nutrient agar plate with a 4–5 h or overnight broth culture of the strain of *Staph. aureus* to be typed, drain off excess fluid with a pipette and dry plate on the bench with lid ajar. Apply the typing phages in 0·01 ml drops from capillary pipettes in a constant order over the squares of a grid marked on the bottom of the Petri dish. Avoid touching the plate with the pipette lest bacteria contaminate the phage before its application to the plate of another strain of staphylococcus. A more rapid method of applying phage is by the use of a machine such as that obtainable from Messrs. Biddulph and Son, Manchester, which delivers the set of phages simultaneously in a fixed pattern on to the plate via a battery of wire loops which are sterilized by flaming between applications.

Allow the inoculated plates to dry and incubate overnight at 30°C or for 6 h at 37°C. Next day examine the plates in a good light against a dark background and record the reaction for each phage as follows:

+ + + confluent lysis with or without phage-resistant growth;

+ + 50 or more plaques;

+ up to 50 plaques.

Combine the designations of each phage giving a reaction to give the phage-type of the staphylococcus. If no reaction is obtained at RTD, repeat the typing at RTD × 1000 and if still no reaction is obtained, designate the staphylococcus as untypable.

Animal pathogenicity. Strains from human lesions are pathogenic to rabbits; a small quantity of culture produces an abscess when injected subcutaneously and leads to septicaemia, pyaemia and renal abscesses when injected intravenously. Mice and guinea-pigs may be infected but are less susceptible. Animal tests are not used for diagnosis and identification.

Laboratory diagnosis of infections. Specimens collected from patients may include pus or wound exudate (in a tube or on a swab), blood for culture (e.g. from a patient with pyrexia of uncertain origin), mid-stream urine, sputum from a patient with bronchopneumonia, and faeces, vomit and food remains (from food-poisoning). Nasal and perineal swabs may be collected from suspected carriers. The main task of the bacteriologist is to determine whether or not *Staph. aureus* is present in the specimen. The organism is generally first recognized by the golden pigmentation of its colonies on a nutrient or blood agar plate and its identity must then be confirmed by the demonstration that it gives a positive coagulase reaction.

1. Examine a Gram-stained smear for Gram-positive cluster-forming cocci suggesting the presence of a *Staphylococcus* sp. Do not make smears from blood culture bottles before incubation and do not smear swabs on unsterile slides.

2. Inoculate the specimen (or a sample from the blood culture after daily periods of incubation) on a plate of nutrient, blood or milk agar and inspect for characteristic golden or white staphylococcal colonies after 24 h at 37°C and note whether they are scanty or numerous. If the specimen is faeces or food, use a plate of selective, salt or polymyxin agar.

3. Perform the slide coagulase test on golden colonies, if present, otherwise on any white colonies. If the result for either golden or white colonies is positive, report the presence of *Staph. aureus*. If it is doubtful or negative in cases in which a positive result is expected, perform the tube coagulase test or the DNase test before reporting the absence of *Staph. aureus*.

4. Perform a disk-diffusion antibiotic sensitivity test either on a primary plate culture inoculated confluently from the specimen or on a plate subculture from a coagulase-positive colony.

5. Determine the phage-type of an isolate of *Staph. aureus* only if the information is required for epidemiological purposes.

6. If *Staph. aureus* is not isolated, consider the possible clinical significance of any coagulase-negative staphylococcus isolated (see end of succeeding section) and if it is thought possible that such an organism may have a pathogenic role in the patient under examination, test and report its antibiotic sensitivities.

7. *Serological diagnosis.* Normal serum frequently agglutinates staphylococci in low titre and many sera contain low titres of antibodies to staphylococcal toxins, e.g. 0–2 units anti-staphylolysin (anti-alpha-haemolysin). In staphylococcal infections the titres may be greatly raised, but the absence of antibody does not exclude staphylococcal disease and serological tests, therefore, are little used. (See 11th edition of this book, p. 142, for a method of performing the anti-staphylolysin test.)

OTHER CLUSTER-FORMING GRAM-POSITIVE COCCI

Separation of Staphylococci from Micrococci

As shown in Tables 18.1 and 18.2, the staphylococci are distinguished from the micrococci and aerobic sarcinae by their ability to form acid from glucose fermentatively, i.e. under anaerobic conditions. Baird-Parker (1966) describes the method for testing this property, which is based on the modified Hugh and Leifson test proposed by the International Subcommittee on Staphylococci and Micrococci (1965).

Medium for test for fermentative acid production. Dissolve in distilled water (per cent w/v) Difco tryptone 1·0, Difco yeast extract 0·1, glucose 1·0, bromocresol purple 0·004, Difco agar 0·2; pH 7·2. Dispense in 10-ml amounts into 6 in × $\frac{1}{2}$ in test-tubes and sterilize by autoclaving for 20 min at 115°C. If stored, steam before use and cool rapidly in iced water.

Preparation of inoculum. Check that the organism to be tested is a Gram-positive coccus and produces catalase on nutrient agar containing 1 per cent glucose. Grow for 24 h at 37°C on medium containing (per cent w/v): Difco tryptone 1·0, Difco yeast extract 0·1 and agar 1·5.

TEST. With a long wire loop, heavily inoculate the culture to be tested throughout the length of duplicate tubes of the glucose-tryptone agar, cover one tube of the pair with a layer of sterile liquid paraffin at least 1 in in depth and incubate both tubes for 5 days at 37°C. If acid production (yellow colour) is seen throughout both tubes the organism attacks glucose fermentatively and is a *Staphylococcus* sp. If acid is seen only in the unsealed tube, e.g. near the surface (and sometimes also a little at the surface of the sealed tube) or if no acid is formed in either tube, the organism is a *Micrococcus* sp.

G+C ratio. Species of *Micrococcus* are distinguished from other Gram-positive cocci by their high percentage G+C, which is in the range 55–75. The percentage G+C of *Staph. aureus* and *Staph. albus* is 30–40.

IDENTIFICATION OF SUBGROUPS OF STAPH. ALBUS AND MICROCOCCUS

Subgroups of *Staph. albus* and *Micrococcus* are distinguished in a scheme described by Baird-Parker (1963, 1965, 1966) and shown in Table 18.2. In addition to tests already described, the scheme relies on tests for phosphatase activity, acetoin production from glucose, acid production from arabinose, lactose, maltose and mannitol, and pink pigmentation on plates incubated 3 days at 30°C. Test for *phosphatase production* after incubation for 3 days at 30°C on Barber and Kuper's phenolphthalein phosphate agar.

Acetoin production. Inoculate organism into a screw-capped bottle containing 5 ml of medium (per cent w/v): tryptone 1·0, Lab-Lemco meat extract 0·3, yeast extract 0·1, glucose 2·0; pH 7·2. Incubate for 14 days at 30°C. Test for acetoin by Barritt's method; add 1 ml 40 per cent KOH and 3 ml of a 5 per cent solution of alpha-naphthol in absolute ethanol, shake vigorously for at least 30 sec and examine after 1 and 2 h at room temperature for the development of a pink colour denoting a positive reaction.

Acid production from sugars. Medium (per cent w/v): $NH_4H_2PO_4$ 0·1, KCl 0·02, $MgSO_4.7H_2O$ 0·02, bromocresol purple 0·004, agar 1·5; pH 7·0. Autoclave 95-ml amounts for 15 min at 121°C, add 5 ml of a 10 per cent Seitz-filtered solution of arabinose, lactose, maltose or mannitol and pour plates. Inoculate from broth cultures up to four isolates as streaks on each plate, incubate at 30°C and examine for acid production (yellow colour change) daily for 7 days.

SIGNIFICANCE OF COAGULASE-NEGATIVE STAPHYLOCOCCI AND MICROCOCCI IN CLINICAL SPECIMENS

Since *Staph. albus* and micrococci are commonly present on the skin (Noble, 1969), in the alimentary canal and in dust, they commonly appear as contaminants or commensals in clinical specimens collected from skin lesions, burns, open wounds, nose or throat, and in sputum and faeces. Their finding in cultures of these specimens is generally regarded as having no clinical significance; it is not reported to the physician in charge of the patient and the organism is not tested for antibiotic sensitivities. During the procedure of specimen collection, coagulase-negative cocci sometimes gain access, as contaminants, to blood cultures (e.g. in 1 per cent), and specimens of cerebrospinal fluid, pleural fluid, pus from closed abscesses and other fluids from deep areas. In most cases, therefore, their finding in such specimens is probably without any clinical significance, but the possibility of their having a pathogenic role in special cases should not be ignored.

Staph. albus coagulase-negative sometimes causes chronic septicaemia or subacute bacterial endocarditis, e.g. in patients subjected to cardiac surgery or fitted with artificial heart valves. It also causes meningeal and bacteriaemic infections in patients fitted with ventriculo-venous cerebrospinal fluid shunts (mainly subgroup-2 strains, Holt, 1969), and deep or septicaemic infections in immunosuppressed or immunodefective patients (Andriole and Lyons, 1969). The finding of *Staph. albus* in the blood, cerebrospinal fluid and other specimens from deep sites should therefore be reported to the physician, though with a caution that the organism may be present only as a contaminant. The isolate should be tested for antibiotic sensitivities. The finding of *large numbers* of cocci in the specimen (e.g. more than five colonies in a poured-plate blood culture) or their finding in *repeated specimens*, e.g. in three successive blood cultures, is suggestive of their presence being due to infection rather than contamination.

Staph. albus derived from the urethral orifice is commonly present in small or moderate numbers as a contaminant in mid-stream specimens of urine, and, where their viable count is $< 10^5$ per ml, they may be disregarded. However, in many patients with urinary-tract infection and intense pyuria, *Staph. albus* is found in large numbers in almost pure culture in repeated specimens, so that it appears to be the true cause of the infection. When, therefore, it is found in numbers $> 10^5$ per ml urine, its antibiotic sensitivities should be tested and the results reported. In certain series of urinary-tract infections with coagulase-negative cocci, strains of a particular type, which may have a special affinity for the urinary tract, have been mainly implicated, e.g. novobiocin-resistant cocci of *Micrococcus* subgroup 3 with agglutinating antigen 51 (Torres Pereira, 1962; Roberts, 1967; Mitchell, 1968). *Staph. albus* strains of *Staphylococcus* subgroup 2 appear to be the commonest coccal contaminants of urine.

Antibiotic sensitivity. When a coagulase-negative isolate is thought possibly to be acting as a pathogen, its sensitivities to the series of antibiotics commonly used for *Staph. aureus* should be tested. Isolates from hospital sources show a greater frequency of resistance and width of resistance spectrum to different antibiotics than isolates from sources outside hospital (Corse and Williams, 1968). Many strains of *Staph. albus* are resistant to penicillin, methicillin and novobiocin. The cephalosporins, gentamicin and vancomycin have been found to be the most commonly effective drugs.

REFERENCES

ANDRIOLE, V. T. & LYONS, R. W. (1969) Coagulase-negative staphylococcus. *Annals of the New York Academy of Science*, **161,** 533.

ARBUTHNOTT, J. P. (1970) Staphylococcal α-Toxin. In *Microbial Toxins* Vol. III, p. 189, edited by T. C. Montie, S. Kadis and S. J. Ajl. New York and London: Academic Press.

BAIRD-PARKER, A. C. (1963) A classification of micrococci and staphylococci based on physiological and biochemical tests. *Journal of General Microbiology*, **30,** 409.

BAIRD-PARKER, A. C. (1965) The classification of staphylococci and micrococci from world-wide sources. *Journal of General Microbiology*, **38,** 363.

BAIRD-PARKER, A. C. (1966) Methods for classifying staphylococci and micrococci. In *Identification Methods for Microbiologists*, edited by B. M. Gibbs and F. A. Skinner. Part A. The Society for Applied Bacteriology Technical Series No. 1, p. 59. New York and London: Academic Press.

BARBER, MARY & KUPER, S. W. A. (1951) Identification of *Staphylococcus pyogenes* by the phosphatase reaction. *Journal of Pathology and Bacteriology*, **63,** 65.

BAYSTON, R. (1972) Coagulase-negative strains of *Staphylococcus pyogenes*. *Journal of Clinical Pathology*, **25,** 62.

BERGDOLL, M. S. (1970) Enterotoxins. In *Microbial Toxins*, Vol. III, p. 265, edited by T. C. Montie, S. Kadis and S. J. Ajl. New York and London: Academic Press.

BLAIR, E. B., EMERSON, J. S. & TULL, A. H. (1967) A new medium, salt mannitol plasma agar, for the isolation of *Staphylococcus aureus*. *American Journal of Clinical Pathology*, **47,** 30.

BLAIR, J. E. & WILLIAMS, R. E. O. (1961) Phage-typing of staphylococci. *Bulletin of the World Health Organization*, **24,** 771.

CHOUDHURI, K. K. & CHAKRABARTY, A. N. (1970) Relationship of staphylococcal toxins and enzymes with serological and phage types. *Journal of Clinical Pathology*, **23,** 370.

CHRISTIE, R. & KEOGH, E. V. (1940) Physiological and serological characteristics of staphylococci of human origin. *Journal of Pathology and Bacteriology*, **51,** 189.

CORSE, JEAN & WILLIAMS, R. E. O. (1968) Antibiotic resistance of coagulase-negative staphylococci and micrococci. *Journal of Clinical Pathology*, **21,** 722.

COWAN, S. T. (1939) The classification of staphylococci by slide agglutination. *Journal of Pathology and Bacteriology*, **48,** 169.

ELEK, S. D. (1959) *Staphylococcus Pyogenes and its Relation to Disease*. Edinburgh: Livingstone.

ELEK, S. D. & LEVY, E. (1950) The distribution of haemolysins and pathogenic and non-pathogenic staphylococci. *Journal of Pathology and Bacteriology*, **62,** 541.

FINEGOLD, S. M. & SWEENY, E. E. (1961) New selective and differential medium for coagulase-positive staphylococci allowing rapid growth and strain differentiation. *Journal of Bacteriology*, **81,** 636.

GILBERT, R. J., WIENEKE, A. A., LANSER, J., SIMKOVICOVA, M. (1972) Serological detection of enterotoxin in foods implicated in staphylococcal food-poisoning. *Journal of Hygiene (Cambridge)*, **70,** 755.

GILLESPIE, E. H. (1943) The routine use of the coagulase test for staphylococci. *Monthly Bulletin Emergency Public Health Laboratory Service*, **2**, 19.

GILLESPIE, W. A. & ALDER, V. G. (1952) Production of opacity in egg-yolk media by coagulase-positive staphylococci. *Journal of Pathology and Bacteriology*, **64**, 187.

HAUKENES, G. (1967) Serological typing of *Staphylococcus aureus*. 7. Technical Aspects. *Acta Pathologica Microbiologica Scandinavica*, **70**, 590.

HEWITT, J. H., COE, A. W. & PARKER, M. T. (1969) The detection of methicillin resistance in *Staphylococcus aureus*. *Journal of Medical Microbiology*, **2**, 443.

HOBBS, BETTY C. (1948) A study of the serological type differentiation of *Staphylococcus pyogenes*. *Journal of Hygiene (London)*, **46**, 222.

HOLT, R. (1969) The classification of staphylococci from colonized ventriculo-atrial shunts. *Journal of Clinical Pathology*, **22**, 475.

INTERNATIONAL SUBCOMMITTEE ON STAPHYLOCOCCI AND MICROCOCCI (1965) Recommendations of subcommittee. *International Bulletin of Bacteriological Nomenclature and Taxonomy*, **15**, 109.

JACOB, S. I., WILLIS, A. T. & GOODBURN, GILLIAN M. (1964) Pigment production and enzymatic activity of staphylococci: the differentiation of pathogens from commensals. *Journal of Pathology and Bacteriology*, **87**, 151.

MITCHELL, R. G. (1968) Classification of *Staph. albus* strains isolated from the urinary tract. *Journal of Clinical Pathology*, **21**, 93.

MOORE, B. (1960) A new screen test and selective medium for the rapid detection of epidemic strains of *Staph. aureus*. *Lancet*, **ii**, 453.

NOBLE, W. C. (1969) Skin carriage of the Micrococcaceae. *Journal of Clinical Pathology*, **22**, 249.

OEDING, P. (1953) Serological typing of staphylococci III. Further investigations and comparison to phage-typing. *Acta Pathologica Microbiologica Scandinavica*, **33**, 324.

ROBERTS, A. P. (1967) *Micrococcaceae* from the urinary tract in pregnancy. *Journal of Clinical Pathology*, **20**, 631.

TORRES PEREIRA, A. (1961) Antigenic loss variation in *Staphylococcus aureus*. *Journal of Pathology and Bacteriology*, **81**, 151.

TORRES PEREIRA, A. (1962) Coagulase-negative strains of staphylococcus possessing antigen 51 as agents of urinary infection. *Journal of Clinical Pathology*, **15**, 252.

WILLIAMS, R. E. O. & HARPER, G. J. (1946) Determination of coagulase and alpha-haemolysin production by staphylococci. *British Journal of Experimental Pathology*, **27**, 72.

WILLIAMS, R. E. O. & RIPPON, J. E. (1952) Bacteriophage typing of *Staphylococcus aureus*. *Journal of Hygiene (London)*, **50**, 320.

WILLIS, A. T., O'CONNOR, JEAN J. & SMITH, J. A. (1966) Colonial pigmentation of *Staphylococcus aureus*. *Journal of Pathology and Bacteriology*, **92**, 97.

WISEMAN, G. M. (1970) The Beta- and Delta-Toxins of *Staphylococcus aureus*. In *Microbial Toxins*, Vol. III, p. 237, edited by T. C. Montie, S. Kadis and S. J. Ajl. New York and London: Academic Press.

19. Streptococcus

The genus *Streptococcus*, chain-forming and Gram-positive cocci, is first divisible into aerobes (or facultative anaerobes) and obligate anaerobes. The aerobes are further divisible into two groups: (1) those which produce soluble haemolysin and usually cause a definite zone of clearing or haemolysis around colonies on plates of blood agar (beta (β)-haemolytic), e.g. *Streptococcus pyogenes*; and (2) those which do not produce soluble haemolysin; some species cause partial clearing and often green colouration around colonies on blood agar (alpha (α)-haemolytic), e.g. *Strept. viridans*: others cause no obvious change when grown on blood agar: these are sometimes called gamma (non-haemolytic) streptococci, e.g. *Strept. salivarius*, but this is a misnomer and should not be used.

STREPTOCOCCUS PYOGENES

Identification

The beta-haemolytic streptococci have been divided into serogroups, based on antigenic differences in the group-specific polysaccharide or similar antigens present as structural components of the cell wall; these group antigens can be extracted in soluble form and identified by precipitation reactions with the specific group antisera. On this basis, Lancefield identified different groups of beta-haemolytic streptococci and labelled them A, B, C, etc.: there are now 17 serological groups with sequential letters A–S in the alphabet (except I and J) (see tests for Lancefield grouping). The majority of beta-haemolytic streptococci causing infections in man belong to group A and are given the generic name *Streptococcus pyogenes*. This pathogen is directly responsible for a variety of inflammatory and suppurative conditions, e.g. sore throat, scarlet fever, adenitis, cellulitis, erysipelas, impetigo, puerperal sepsis, vaginitis, otitis media, arthritis, meningitis, wound infections, etc., and is indirectly associated with rheumatic fever, glomerulo-nephritis and erythema nodosum.

Morphology and staining. Gram-positive spherical cocci 0·7–0·9 μm occurring in chains of varying length, best demonstrated in smears of pus or in liquid medium cultures: non-motile, non-sporing: capsulate in very young cultures.

Cultural characters. Facultative anaerobe: optimum temperature for growth 37°C (range 22°–42°C): grows on ordinary nutrient agar but growth is better on blood or serum-agar, small semi-transparent low convex discrete colonies (0·5–1 mm diameter after 24 h): matt surface when freshly isolated: after subculture surface may become smooth or glossy with change from S → R form: mucoid colonies may occur when strain is obviously capsulate: clear, often wide, zone of haemolysis around colonies on horse or sheep blood agar; variable haemolysis with human or rabbit blood agar: granular growth and powdery deposit in broth culture: poor growth and no liquefaction in gelatin: selective media, blood agar with 1 in 500 000 crystal violet: Pike's medium.

Sensitivity to physical and chemical agents killed by 54°C for $\frac{1}{2}$ h: may resist natural drying for weeks if protected from daylight: laboratory cultures should be stored at 3–5°C in blood broth or cooked meat medium: or freeze-dried: sensitive to most antiseptics but more resistant than staphylococci to high dilutions (1:500 000) of crystal or gentian violet: sensitive to a wide range of antimicrobial drugs but resistance to sulphonamides and less commonly to tetracyclines, lincomycin and the macrolides has developed. *Strept. pyogenes* is more sensitive to bacitracin than other haemolytic streptococci and this phenomenon is utilized as a screening test in serogrouping.

Biochemical activities: ferments a number of sugars with production of acid only: fermentation reactions are rarely used in diagnosis but help in subdivision of species: MB−: VP−: nitrate not reduced: catalase−: not bile soluble (Chap. 7).

Biological activities: *Strept. pyogenes* produces several exotoxins and enzymes which may contribute to pathogenicity and identification.

1. STREPTOLYSINS O AND S. Oxygen-sensitive (SLO) and stable haemolytic (SLS) exotoxins responsible for β-haemolysis and also toxic to leucocytes and other tissue cells: SLO can be reactivated by reducing agents and is produced in serum-free broth: SLS cannot be so produced.

SLO, also formed by C and G strains, is antigenic and neutralized by its antitoxin: SLS is non-antigenic, but is responsible for the soluble haemolysin test: leucocidin may be identical with SLO.

2. ERYTHROGENIC TOXIN. Produced only by certain strains ('scarlet fever strains') that are lysogenic for specific phages. A heat-stable component causes the skin rash in non-immune patients with a throat or, rarely, wound infection. A heat-labile component is pyrogenic, enhances susceptibility to SLO and Gram-negative endotoxins, and depresses RE function. The exotoxin is antigenic (groups A, B, C) and is neutralized by its antitoxin.

Dick test demonstrates susceptibility to the toxin and thus to scarlet fever. Erythrogenic toxin 0·2 ml is injected intradermally in the forearm. Erythema at least 1 cm in diameter within 12–24 h is a positive result indicating susceptibility.

3. STREPTOKINASE (fibrinolysin) present in culture filtrates of recently isolated strains: causes rapid lysis of human fibrin.

4. HYALURONIDASE (spreading factor): hydrolyses hyaluronic acid binding tissue cells together: and also streptococcal capsules.

5. DESOXYRIBONUCLEASE (DNAase) splits DNA and liquefies pus: 4 antigenically distinct DNAases have been identified (A, B, C, D): DNAase B is most commonly present in group A strains.

NICOTINAMIDE ADENOSINE-DINUCLEO-TIDASE (NADase) or diphosphopyridine nucleotidase (DPNase) which is antigenic and leucocidal.

For details of tests for, and the significance of, specific antibodies to these enzymes, see Wannamaker and Ayoub (1960).

Cellular antigens. In addition to the division of β-haemolytic streptococci into serogroups, *Strept. pyogenes* (serogroup A) is divisible into more than 50 serotypes related to the M protein, a surface antigen and the main viru-lence factor: specific anti-M antibodies develop after infection but tests for their demonstration are complicated. Another surface antigen, T protein, which may be shared by different serotypes, is used as a marker in epidemio-logical studies of streptococcal infections (see tests for serotyping). A third antigen (R) is present in a few types (e.g. 28) but its signifi-cance is unknown.

Tests for specific antibodies to streptococcal exotoxins and enzymes which are antigenic and are liberated during infection may be used in laboratory diagnosis (see below).

Animal pathogenicity. Recently isolated cul-tures, in practice, matt-glossy variants, are usually pathogenic to rabbits, mice and guinea-pigs, producing local inflammatory and suppurative lesions after subcutaneous inoculation, and septicaemia or pyaemia after intravenous injection.

Laboratory Diagnosis

Throat and nose swabs from cases of sore throat or from suspected carriers, high vaginal swabs from cases of puerperal pyrexia, pus (or pus-coated swab) from suppurative infections and blood-culture from cases of systemic infec-tion are the usual specimens received in the laboratory. If there is likely to be delay of more than 6–8 h before a swab is inoculated on to culture media, use should be made of a holding medium: or a serum-coated swab may be used. In children over three years of age with sore throat, a specimen of saliva expec-torated into a sterile container may be prefer-able to a throat swab.

Throat and other swabs are inoculated on to horse or sheep blood-agar plates and incubated aerobically, and anaerobically to improve haemolytic activity: Gram-stained smears of pus are prepared and if a mixed flora is present, e.g. from ear or vaginal swabs, the specimen may also be inoculated on to crystal violet blood agar and preferably incubated anaerobi-cally. Haemolytic colonies are examined for morphology and staining since haemolytic *Haemophilus influenzae* colonies may closely resemble those of *Strept. pyogenes* but the former do not produce haemolysis on sheep blood agar. Antibiotic sensitivity tests with disks may be necessary to detect tetracycline or sulphonamide resistant strains.

Specific sensitivity of *Strept. pyogenes* to bacitracin may be similarly demonstrated.

Lancefield serogrouping may be done routinely or in special circumstances, e.g. identification of carriers in paediatric or maternity units. Serotyping is done mainly for epidemiological purposes as in tracing the source and spread of an outbreak of streptococcal infection.

Serological tests, if possible with paired sera, may be used to identify or confirm infection with *Strept. pyogenes* in primary infections, e.g. sore throat, but more often in cases of rheumatic fever and acute glomerulonephritis when isolation of haemolytic streptococci from the primary lesion may not be possible. The antibody which is most commonly sought is antistreptolysin O which may show a significant rise in titre or a sufficiently high titre (over 200 units) with a single specimen to corroborate recent streptococcal infection in around 80 per cent of cases. The measurement and significance of ASO serum titres in the diagnosis of rheumatic fever etc. are described and discussed in a pamphlet issued by Burroughs, Wellcome & Co. Demonstration of some other antibodies, e.g. anti-DNAase and anti-hyaluronidase, antistreptokinase and anti-NADase will increase the proportion of confirmed streptococcal infections to nearly 100 per cent (see Wannamaker and Ayoub, 1960; WHO Report, 1968).

Other Lancefield Groups of β-haemolytic Streptococci

Of Lancefield groups other than A, groups B, C, D and G are of particular medical interest because they are frequently isolated from human secretions and excretions and may cause infections such as sore throat, puerperal pyrexia, erysipelas, bacterial endocarditis and septicaemia. Group B streptococci may be present in the oropharynx and usually appear as small colonies on blood agar, often with little surrounding haemolysis and, therefore, liable to be misdiagnosed; this streptococcus is an important cause of systemic infection in infants and occasionally of bacterial endocarditis. *Strept. agalactiae*, a common cause of bovine mastitis, belongs to group B. Group C streptococci appear as small colonies with a wide zone of β-haemolysis and are pathogenic in both man, e.g. erysipelas, endocarditis, and animals, e.g. strangles in horses: in this group are included types 7, 20 and 21 of Griffith's original series of pathogenic streptococci: more human and animal types have been described and fermentative action of group C strains on trehalose and sorbitol serves to subdivide them into three subgroups. Group G streptococci also produce a wide zone of haemolysis on blood agar, share a protein antigen with group C strains and ferment trehalose but not sorbitol: like group C streptococci they are pathogenic to both man and animals.

Lancefield group D streptococci include all strains (haemolytic and non-haemolytic) of *Strept. faecalis:* and may cause urinary tract infections and bacterial endocarditis in man (see Vol. 1, Chap. 16).

More detailed descriptions and the possible pathogenicity of these and other β-haemolytic streptococci are given in *Principles of Bacteriology and Immunity* (Wilson and Miles, 1964).

STREPTOCOCCUS VIRIDANS

A group of non-haemolytic streptococci, most of which produce partial haemolysis (alpha-haemolytic) and green colorization around colonies on blood-agar plates are constantly present in the bacterial flora of the mouth and oropharynx ($10^8/10^9$ per ml): various attempts using biochemical tests and antigenic analysis have been made to subdivide this group, e.g. Colman and Williams (1972) recognize six species (based on various characters), viz. *salivarius*, *mitis*, *milleri*, *sanguis*, *mutans* and *pneumoniaes*. In this book the pneumococcus is classified with the *Lactobacillaceae* as *Diplococcus pneumoniae*.

The medical importance of the *viridans* group is their association with dental sepsis and dental caries and as the most common infecting organism in subacute bacterial endocarditis (see Vol. 1, Chap. 16).

Morphologically, they resemble *Strept. pyogenes* but sometimes may be more ovoid: culturally they usually grow well on nutrient agar: because of the green colorization on blood agar they may have to be distinguished from pneumococci (see table): slightly granular growth in broth with short chains as a rule: killed by heat at 55°C for half-an-hour: strains may be more resistant to antimicrobial drugs, e.g. penicillin, than *Strept. pyogenes* so that isolates from blood in cases of bacterial endocarditis should always be tested for their antibiogram.

STREPTOCOCCUS FAECALIS
(ENTEROCOCCUS)

This streptococcus, usually in the non-haemolytic form, is constantly present as a commensal in the intestine and therefore in the faeces: it is sometimes present in the oral flora. It may be associated with urinary tract infections and is a causal organism in subacute bacterial endocarditis, particularly in older patients.

Morphologically, it appears characteristically in ovoid pairs or in short chains: rather larger than *Strept. pyogenes*: non-motile, noncapsulate: grows readily on ordinary culture media: it also grows on MacConkey's agar as minute (0·5–1·0 mm) pink coloured colonies and on media with a high salt content: uniform turbidity in broth: withstands heat at 60°C for 30 min, a distinguishing feature from other streptococci and also grows within a wider temperature range (10°–45°C): ferments man-

nitol with gas production: some variants liquefy gelatin and produce H_2S: VP+. Strains may be subdivided into specific types according to biochemical and other activities.

Moderately resistant to penicillin and to streptomycin, but cases of bacterial endocarditis due to *Strept. faecalis* usually respond to high doses of both drugs combined.

ANAEROBIC STREPTOCOCCI

Obligate anaerobic streptococci are commonly present as commensals in the female genital tract but they may be associated with puerperal infections, in particular pelvic infection and suppurative thrombophlebitis.

Peptostreptococcus putridus is the best documented species: very small Gram-positive cocci (0·5 μm) occurring in short chains and exhibiting pleomorphism on culture: after 48 h cultivation, colonies on blood agar are smooth low convex, 1–2 mm in diameter: no alteration in the blood medium: in cooked meat broth, cultures produce proteolysis and give off a very offensive odour: various sugars fermented (in the presence of 0·1 per cent sod. thioglycollate) with abundant gas formation: strains are sensitive to penicillin. For details of cultural and biochemical activities of anaerobic streptococci see the papers of Hare *et al.* (1952) and Thomas and Hare (1954).

Table 19.1.   Biochemical 'types' of Group D. streptococci

Type	Sorbitol	Arabinose	Gelatin liquefaction	Growth at pH 9·6	Haemolysis on horse-blood agar
Strept. faecalis var. *faecalis*	A	–	–	+	–
var. *liquefaciens*	A	–	+	+	–
var. *zymogenes*	A	–	+	+	β
Strept. faecium	–	A	–	+	α
Strept. durans	–	–	–	–	α or β
Strept. bovis	–	A	–	–	α

Key: Fermentation Reaction: A = acid produced; – = no fermentation.

Serologic Identification of β-haemolytic Streptococci

LANCEFIELD GROUPING. Extraction of group-specific polysaccharide can be undertaken by one of the following methods:

1. Acid extraction

The centrifuged deposit from 50 ml of overnight culture in Todd-Hewitt broth is harvested in a $3 \times \frac{1}{2}$ in test-tube. The deposit is thoroughly resuspended in 0·4 ml of 0·2 N HCl. Place tube in a boiling water-bath. After ten minutes' exposure, remove tube from bath and allow to cool. Add 1 drop of 0·02 per cent phenol red. Neutralize carefully with 0·5 N and 0·2 N NaOH. The clear supernatant obtained by centrifugation is the extract.

2. Enzyme extraction

Suspend a loopful of growth from an eighteen-hour blood-agar culture in 0·25 ml enzyme solution (see below) contained in a flocculation tube. Place tube in 50°C water-bath. Inspect tube at one, one and a half and two hour periods, and when contents are clear, use as extract.

The enzyme is produced from a *Streptomyces albus* (obtainable from NCTC, Colindale Avenue, London) growing in the following medium.

NaCl	.	.	.	.	5 g
K₂HPO₄	.	.	.	.	2 g
MgSO₄, 7H₂O		.	.	.	1 g
CaCl₂	.	.	.	.	0·04 g
FeSO₄, 7H₂O	.	.	.	.	0·02 g
ZnSO₄, 7H₂O	.	.	.	.	0·01 g
Yeastrel	.	.	.	.	5 g
Agar powder	.	.	.	.	11 g
Distilled water		.	.	.	1 l

Place suitable amounts (75–100 ml) in Roux bottles, sterilize and add aseptically glucose and casamino acids, each in a final concentration of 0·5 per cent, pH should be 7·0–7·4.

1. Inoculate the surface of above medium by flooding with *Streptomyces albus* glucose-broth culture.

2. Incubate at 30°–37°C for four to five days.

3. Place Roux bottles in a −10°C refrigerator and then allow to thaw out; the fluid expressed on thawing is the enzyme solution.

4. Adjust pH to 7·5 by adding 1 N HCl; filter through a Seitz disk.

5. Test for potency of the filtrate by adding 0·1 ml of a heavy suspension of heat-killed group A streptococci to 0·4 ml of the enzyme preparation. Place in a 50°C water-bath along with a tube containing a control mixture in which the enzyme has been destroyed by heating. An active preparation will lyse the streptococcal suspension in one-half to one hour.

6. Stored in the cold with 0·5 per cent phenol as preservative, the preparation keeps well and is active over a pH of 5·6–9·6.

The enzyme extraction method is reliable for streptococci in groups A, C or G; for other groups the acid (Lancefield, 1933) or formamide (Fuller, 1938) methods are preferred as less likely to give minor cross-reactions occasionally encountered with acid extracts. Group-O polysaccharide is sensitive to formamide so that such extracts do not react with O antiserum. Acid extracts can also be used for identification of type-specific M antigens.

Precipitation test for grouping of Strept. pyogenes. This may be performed in the narrowing neck of small Pasteur pipettes. A small volume of group A antiserum is placed in the pipette and the antigenic extract carefully superimposed. If the extract contains polysaccharide specific for group A, then precipitation will be observed at the interface with the serum within five minutes; reactions appearing after this time should not be regarded as positive. Extracts should also be tested with antisera for groups C and G routinely, and if necessary with other group sera.

In order to conserve serum, tests may be performed in capillary tubes; a $\frac{1}{2}$-in column of serum is run into the tube, the exterior of which is carefully wiped before an equivalent volume of antigen extract is introduced. The contents are allowed to run well up the tube and the upper end is then occluded with the forefinger until the tube has been placed in a plasticine block. Macroscopic precipitation should be evident within the time limits stated above if the reaction is positive.

Type identification of group A strains. All strains should be tested for type both by agglutinating (T) and precipitating (M) antisera, since a smaller percentage of strains will thus be regarded as untypable than when either method is employed alone.

1. Slide agglutination test. The strain is grown in 5 ml of Todd-Hewitt broth at 28°C for 18–24 hours and the centrifuged deposit thoroughly resuspended in 0·5 ml of supernatant broth. Provided that the suspension is not granular, 6 loopfuls are placed on a clean glass slide and each then mixed with a small (1 mm) loopful of pooled antisera and the slide rocked to and fro for one minute. Agglutination may be noted with one of the pooled antisera and fresh loopfuls of suspension should then similarly be tested with all the specific sera comprising that particular pool. Strains may react in more than one type-specific serum, but the pattern of such reactions is epidemiologically significant.

Granular suspensions and those that react with many sera should be treated as follows: Add 1 drop of BDH Universal Indicator and 2 drops of pancreatic extract to the suspension; adjust the pH to 8–8·5 with 0·2 N NaOH and place in 37°C water-bath for one hour, shaking the tubes every fifteen minutes. On retesting with pooled and specific antisera as above, many such strains will react normally; if results are still unsatisfactory, a further period of fifteen minutes in a 50°C bath may be tried.

2. Precipitation test. Acid extracted antigen prepared for group determination is used. Using the results of slide agglutination as a guide, the extract is tested against the relevant antisera by the capillary tube method. The mixtures are incubated for two hours at 37°C and results noted; after overnight refrigeration the tubes are again examined for a white precipitate at the interface.

REFERENCES AND FURTHER READING

COLMAN, G. & WILLIAMS, R. E. D. (1972) Taxonomy of some human viridans streptococci. In *Streptococci and Streptococcal Diseases*. New York and London: Academic Press.

FULLER, A. T. (1938) The formamide method for the extraction of polysaccharides from haemolytic streptococci. *British Journal of Experimental Pathology,* **19,** 130.

HARE, R., WILDY, P., BILLETT, F. S. & TWORT, D. N. (1952) The anaerobic cocci: gas formation, fermentation reactions, sensitivity to antibiotics and sulphonamides. Classification. *Journal of Hygiene (Cambridge),* **50,** 295.

THOMAS, C. G. & HARE, R. (1954) The classification of anaerobic streptococci and their isolation in normal human beings and pathological processes. *Journal of Clinical Pathology,* **7,** 300.

UHR, J. W. (1964) *The Streptococcus, Rheumatic Fever and Glomerulonephritis.* Baltimore: Williams and Wilkins Co.

WANNAMAKER, L. W. & AYOUB, E. M. (1960) Antibody titres in acute rheumatic fever. *Circulation,* **21,** 598.

WANNAMAKER, L. W. (1970) Differences between streptococcal infections of the throat and of the skin. *New England Journal of Medicine,* **282,** 23, 78.

WHO REPORT (1968) Streptococcal and staphylococcal infections. *World Health Organization Technical Report Series,* No. 394.

WILSON, G. S. & MILES, A. A. (1964) *Principles of Bacteriology and Immunity.* 5th edn. London: Arnold.

20. Diplococcus Pneumoniae (Pneumococcus)

The main causative organism of lobar pneumonia: also commonly associated with acute and chronic bronchitis: bronchopneumonia: suppurative sinusitis: otitis media: meningitis, peritonitis, arthritis, etc.

Morphology and staining. Gram-positive diplococcus, 0·8–1·0 μm, ovoid or lanceolate with blunt ends opposed: capsulate in infective material but tends to lose capsule on repeated subculture when cocci become more rounded and may occur in short chains in liquid media: non-motile, non-sporing.

Cultural characters. Facultative anaerobe: optimum temperature 37°C: may need 5–10 per cent CO_2 for primary culture: 0·1 per cent glucose or 5–10 per cent blood or serum in nutrient agar facilitates growth: colonies on blood agar, small (1 mm diameter) flat: smooth surface: later develop raised rim (draughtsman colony): partial clearing of blood around colony (alpha-haemolysis) with green colouration which is best seen on heated blood agar (chocolate agar) like that around *Strept. viridans* (see Table 20.1 for differential features): colonies of type 3 pneumococcus are larger and mucoid with glistening surface, associated with large capsule: uniform turbidity in broth: non-capsulate mutant (R) strains from rough, irregular colonies and give more granular growth in broth than capsulate S forms.

Sensitivity to physical and chemical agents killed at 52°C for 15 min: tends to die out on repeated subculture, when R mutants tend to replace the parental S form: may be maintained in semi-solid blood agar: freeze-drying is recommended for maintenance in smooth form: sensitive to a wide range of anti-microbial drugs including the penicillins, tetracyclines, cotrimoxazole: tetracycline resistant strains and, rarely, penicillin resistant strains occur: sensitive to optochin (see below).

Optochin sensitivity test. Disks of filter paper, 8 mm in diameter, sterilized by dry heat at 160°C are impregnated with a 1 in 4000 aqueous solution of optochin (ethyl hydrocuprein hydrochloride) each disk containing approximately 0·02 ml. The solution can be sterilized in the autoclave at 121°C for 30 minutes without appreciable effect on its potency. Organisms are tested by making radial stroke cultures on a blood agar plate, a disk being placed in the centre of the plate: a known sensitive strain is included in each set of tests. Pneumococci are inhibited in a zone of at least 5 mm from the circumference of the disk, whereas strains of *Strept. viridans* grow up to the disk margin: occasionally a few colonies of pneumococci, resistant to optochin, will be noted in the zone of inhibition: an optochin disk may be incorporated in the multi disk used for testing drug sensitivities.

Biological activities. Pneumococci are soluble in bile: the test consists of adding one part of 10 per cent sodium taurocholate to ten parts

Table 20.1 Pneumococcus v Streptococcus viridans: differential characters

	Pneumococcus	Strept. viridans
Morphology	Lanceolate diplococci	Short chains of rounded cocci
Capsule	+	–
Cultural characters		
(a) blood-agar	Flat: draughtsman Partial haemolysis with green colouration	Raised Partial haemolysis with green colouration
(b) broth	Uniform turbidity	Granular growth
Bile solubility	+	–
Inulin fermentation	+	–
Optochin sensitivity	+	–
Mouse virulence	+	–

of a uniformly turbid broth culture: or 0·1 ml of 10 per cent sodium deoxycholate may be added to 5 ml broth culture which should have pH lower than 6·8: lysis with complete clearing of broth culture occurs within 15 min at 37°C: various sugars are fermented but are not used in diagnostic tests: inulin fermentation may be used to differentiate from *Strept. viridans* on freshly isolated strains: tests are performed in Hiss's serum water or on serum-agar slopes as for neisseriae.

Antigenic characters. Pneumococci may be subdivided into some 80 serotypes on the basis of the chemically specific polysaccharides in the capsular substance: serotyping may be done by *slide agglutination*, using first pooled and then single type-specific sera: or by demonstration of 'capsule-swelling' (the Quellung reaction) either directly in the specimen of sputum or pus or in a young broth or blood agar culture: a loopful of antiserum (pooled, then single) is added to the specimen or to a smooth suspension of the pneumococcus on a glass slide, the mixture is covered with a No. 1 coverslip and examined with the oil-immersion lens, with suitably dimmed lighting: a positive reaction occurs when the margin of the capsule becomes distinct giving a false appearance of capsule swelling. A set of pooled and type specific sera may be purchased from the State Serum Institute, Copenhagen (Lund, 1970).

Animal pathogenicity. The pneumococcus, in particular strains from infective conditions, is highly virulent for the mouse: intraperitoneal inoculation (0·5 ml) of a homogenized specimen of sputum from a case of pneumonia or other respiratory infection will result in death within 1–3 days with pneumococci predominant in the peritoneal exudate and heart-blood: rabbits are also highly susceptible.

Laboratory Diagnosis

In lower respiratory tract infections, coughed-up sputum should, whenever possible, be used and should be cultured within 4–8 h. Sputum should be homogenized by agitating the specimen for 30 min in a mechanical shaker with an equal quantity of distilled water and a small number of glass beads: Gram-stained smears are prepared and examined from the homogenized sputum which is inoculated on to plates of blood agar and heated blood agar and incubated in 10 per cent CO_2 for 18–24 h. If sputum is unobtainable, as in young children, a laryngeal swab is taken and inoculated on to blood agar and heated blood agar. Blood-culture may be taken before antimicrobial therapy is begun.

For other suspected pneumococcal infections, e.g. otitis media or sinusitis, swabs are commonly used and inoculated on blood agar and on crystal violet blood agar which is selective for pneumococci and streptococci. Further tests for differentiating pneumococci from *Strept. viridans* are as listed in Table 20.1.

To detect very small numbers of pneumococci in material containing a predominance of other bacteria, the material (e.g. nasopharyngeal swab or sputum) should be inoculated into blood broth and after 24 h incubation of 0·5 ml of the culture is injected subcutaneously into a mouse; heart blood is cultured after death or killing within 5 days.

REFERENCES

LUND, ERNA (1970) On the nomenclature of the pneumococcal types. *International Journal of Systematic Bacteriology*, **20**, 321.

21. Bordetella

The genus *Bordetella* comprises three species: *Bordetella pertussis*, *Bord. parapertussis* and *Bord. bronchiseptica*. The first two are human pathogens responsible for a common childhood infection, whooping cough which sometimes affects adults; the third is primarily an animal pathogen, causing respiratory infections in rodents and rabbits and occurring as a secondary bacterial pathogen in canine distemper. It is occasionally isolated from the human respiratory tract.

BORDETELLA PERTUSSIS

Morphology and staining. Small ovoid Gram-negative cocco-bacilli, mostly uniform in size, but longer bacillary forms appear, particularly on repeated culture: non-motile, non-sporing. Capsules may be demonstrable in young freshly isolated cultures. In films from cultures, loose clumps of bacilli with clear spaces between give the so-called 'thumb-print' appearance.

Cultural characters. Aerobe: optimum temperature 35°–36°C: primary cultivation requires an enriched medium, containing catalase and a substance, e.g. albumin or charcoal, which absorbs toxic products (possibly unsaturated fatty acids). Bordet-Gengou medium—a potato-glycerol-agar medium with a high content of blood (33 per cent) or some modification of it is commonly used for primary isolation. The medium is made more selective by the addition of penicillin (0·25 units per ml) and diamidine, M and B 938 (see Chap. 5, Vol. II and Lacey, 1954). On a medium freshly prepared and with a moist surface, typical whitish highly refractile colonies appear after 2–3 days incubation. The colonies, which have been compared to mercury drops or bisected pearls, are small (0·5–1·0 mm in diameter), smooth, raised and cohesive and may be picked off entire for film preparation or slide agglutination (but see Preston, 1970).

Subsequent cultures may be obtained on non-blood-containing nutrient agar to which charcoal or starch has been added—or on semi-synthetic liquid media (Cohen and Wheeler, 1946). On repeated subculture, *Bord. pertussis* may change from the *smooth* to the *rough* phase with longer bacillary and filamentous forms and a tendency to auto-agglutination and granular growth in liquid media.

Sensitivity to physical and chemical agents. Die within a few days on culture or on drying: killed by heat at 55°C for half-an-hour: retains viability at low temperatures (0°–10°C): sensitive to tetracycline, ampicillin and erythromycin but relatively resistant to penicillin.

Biochemical and biological activities. *Bord. pertussis* has no significant fermentative activities. It contains or produces a number of toxic and enzymic factors: e.g. heat-labile toxin, endotoxin (lipopolysaccharide), histamine sensitivity factor and the lymphocytosis factor, all or some of which may be associated with its pathogenesis.

Antigenic characters. All smooth strains of *Bord. pertussis* have a common, dominant surface antigen which gives the organisms considerable antigenic homogeneity so that all strains are agglutinated or fix complement when mixed with a smooth strain antiserum. There are, in addition, agglutinating factors labelled 1–6 present in variable degree in different strains, which allow recognition of three main serotypes: 1,2; 1,2,3; and 1,3. Other antigenic fractions are haemagglutinin and protective antigen, the latter being closely associated with the histamine sensitizing factor (see Pittman, 1970).

Animal pathogenicity. Intranasal inhalation of *Bord. pertussis* by mice results in a severe interstitial pneumonia. Mice are also highly susceptible to small intracerebral inoculations with virulent strains. A syndrome resembling whooping cough has been produced in monkeys after respiratory infection with whole cultures of *Bord. pertussis*.

Laboratory Diagnosis

The most suitable specimen for isolation of *Bord. pertussis* from a suspected case of whooping cough is obtained on a pernasal swab; or a post-nasal swab passed through the mouth to the nasopharynx may be used (see Plates 21.1 and 21.2). In either case, the swab must be inoculated within 3–4 h. Less conveniently, the cough-plate may be used when a plate of Bordet-Gengou medium is held 4 in in front of the mouth of the patient while coughing; inoculated plates are incubated for at least three days (preferably in a plastic bag) and examined for the typical metallic colonies, which are picked for slide-agglutination. More detailed antigenic analysis may be done in a reference laboratory (Preston, 1970).

The diagnostic value of immunofluorescence tests (IF) in detecting *Bord. pertussis* in the secretions of clinically suspect cases, or of close contacts of cases, or in later confirmation (or otherwise) of clinical whooping cough by specific antibody, has been examined in a number of laboratories. In general, it may be concluded that: (a) IF techniques are not likely to give a higher proportion of positive, al-

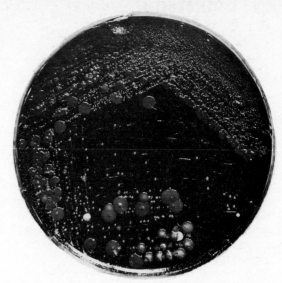

PLATE 21.2

Culture from a post-nasal swab on Bordet-Gengou medium after 72 h. Note the growth of bacteria other than *Bord. pertussis*.

though immediate, results in the identification of *Bord. pertussis* than are cultural methods, and may often give false-positive findings (Kendrick, Elderling and Eveland, 1961; Linneman, Bass and Smith, 1968); and (b) tests for specific pertussis antibodies developing rather late in a clinical infection give comparable results by the IF and CF tests (Bradstreet *et al.*, 1972).

BORDETELLA PARAPERTUSSIS

Bord. parapertussis grows more quickly than *Bord. pertussis* on Bordet-Gengou medium so that pearly colonies are seen after two days incubation. The underlying medium becomes greeny-black due to the production of a brown pigment. It actively produces catalase and on subculture grows readily on ordinary culture media. Antigenically distinct from *Bord. pertussis* and specifically identified by agglutination with absorbed antiserum.

BORDETELLA BRONCHISEPTICA

This organism is related antigenically and in toxin production to *Bord. pertussis* but has also

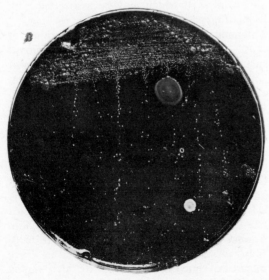

PLATE 21.1

Culture from an early case of whooping-cough of a pernasal swab after 72 h incubation on Bordet-Gengou medium. The colonies of *Bord. pertussis* in almost pure culture are small, raised and highly refractile (like a mercury drop).

some relationship with brucella. It is motile with peritrichous flagella and grows on ordinary culture media without the addition of blood. It may cause a secondary respiratory infection in canine distemper, it is frequently responsible for secondary broncho-pneumonia in rodents and may be a cause of snuffles in rabbits.

REFERENCES AND FURTHER READING

BRADSTREET, C. M. P., TANNAHILL, C. J., EDWARDS, J. M. & BENSON, C. F. (1972) Detection of *Bordetella pertussis* antibodies in human serum by complement fixation and immunofluorescence. *Journal of Hygiene, Cambridge*, **70**, 73.

COHEN, S. M. & WHEELER, W. M. (1946) Pertussis vaccine prepared with phase I cultures grown in fluid medium. *American Journal of Public Health*, **36**, 371.

KENDRICK, P. L., ELDERLING, G. & EVELAND, W. C. (1961) Fluorescent antibody techniques: methods for identification of *Bordetella pertussis*. *American Journal of Diseases of Children*, **101**, 149.

LACEY, B. W. (1954) A new selective medium for *Haemophilus pertussis* containing a diaminidine, sodium fluoride and penicillin. *Journal of Hygiene (London)*, **52**, 273.

LINNEMAN, C. C., BASS, J. W. & SMITH, M. H. D. (1968) The carrier state in pertussis. *American Journal of Epidemiology*, **88**, 422.

PITTMAN, M. (1970) *Bordetella pertussis:* Bacterial and host factors in the pathogenesis and prevention of whooping cough. In *Infectious Agents and Host Reactions*. Edited by Stuart Mudd. Philadelphia, Toronto, London: W. B. Saunders.

PRESTON, N. W. (1970) Technical problems in the laboratory diagnosis and prevention of whooping-cough. *Laboratory Practice*, **19**, No. 5.

22. Haemophilus

The genus *Haemophilus* is so called because of inability to grow on culture media without the addition of whole blood or of certain growth promoting factors (called X and V) present in blood (but which may also be derived from other sources). Whilst *Haemophilus influenzae* and certain other haemophilic species require both factors for growth, others require only one or other of the two factors. *H. influenzae* and associated species are common commensals in the upper respiratory tract: the common non-capsulate (R) strains act as secondary opportunistic pathogens on mucous membranes with lowered resistance from antecedent virus infection or respiratory pollutants. The rarer capsulate (S) strains act as causal organisms of acute purulent meningitis and laryngoepiglottitis (croup).

HAEMOPHILUS INFLUENZAE

Morphology and staining. A small Gram-negative bacillus showing considerable pleomorphism from the cocco-bacillary form in purulent, sputum and in recently isolated young cultures to larger bacillary filamentous forms in older cultures and sometimes in purulent CSF. Because the bacilli do not show up well with weak stains, dilute carbol-fuchsin is recommended as a counterstain in the Gram method. Most strains are non-capsulate (R) but the rarer (S) strains are capsulate. Non-motile, non-sporing.

Cultural characters. Aerobe: optimum temperature 37°C. Whole blood or blood extracts are the best sources of both X and V factors. X factor, heat resistant, is present in haemin; V factor, a respiratory coenzyme, is destroyed by heat at 120°C for a few minutes, but is released from blood cells by heating at 70°–80°C so that heated blood agar (chocolate agar) or a transparent medium containing blood extracts is preferred to fresh blood agar (see Chap. 20, Vol. I and Chap. 5, Vol. II). After 24 h incubation, colonies of the common non-capsulate strains are small (0.5–1.0 mm), trans-

parent, smooth and low convex or flat: colonies of capsulate strains are larger (1–2 mm), more opaque, mucoid and when viewed by oblique light characteristically iridescent on a transparent medium. Colonies of *H. influenzae* grow to a larger size in the neighbourhood of certain other bacterial colonies, e.g. of staphylococci which secrete V factor, a phenomenon known as 'satellitism' (Plate 22.1). Cleared zones of β-haemolysis occur around colonies of certain strains on fresh blood agar (haemolytic *H. influenzae*), giving a close resemblance to *Strept. pyogenes*. Some strains require only V factor for growth and are designated *H. parainfluenzae* (Table 22.1).

Sensitivity to physical and chemical agents. Killed at 55°C for 30 min and dies quickly at refrigerator temperature (0°–4°C), *H. influenzae* is sensitive to a wide range of antimicrobial drugs including sulphonamides, penicillin, ampicillin, streptomycin, tetracyclines and chloramphenicol. The last of these is recommended for the treatment of *H. influenzae* meningitis because of its diffusibility into the CSF. Ampicillin, tetracyclines and cotrimoxazole are used in acute and chronic respiratory infections.

Biochemical reactions. Glucose and other carbohydrates are fermented with acid production only: some strains produce indole.

Antigenic characters. Capsulate strains of *H. influenzae* are divisible into six serotypes, labelled *a–f* based on the chemical constitution of the capsular substance. Type *b* is responsible for most of the cases of meningitis and laryngo-epiglottitis. Non-capsulate strains of *H. influenzae* are antigenically heterogeneous.

Animal pathogenicity. Mice may be infected by intraperitoneal injection of strains suspended in mucous. *H. suis* has been associated with an influenza A virus in an influenza-like infection of pigs: it has no fermentative activities.

Laboratory Diagnosis

Great urgency is needed in the diagnosis of acute purulent meningitis, due to different

Table 22.1 Growth requirements, etc., for *Bordetella pertussis* and *Haemophilus spp.*

	Bord. pertussis	H. influenzae	H. haemolyticus	H. parainfluenzae	H. suis	H. canis	H. aphrophilus	H. paraphrophilus
Bordet-Gengou medium (growth)	+	−	−	−	−	−	−	−
Fildes digest agar growth	−	+	+	+	+	+	+	+
Requires X factor	−	+	+	−	+	+	+	−
Requires V factor	−	+	+	+	+	−	+	+
Indole	−	+	d	d	+	d	−	−
Nitrate reduction	−	+	+	+	+	+	+	+
Haemolysis on blood agar	NG	−	+	−	−	−	−	−
Requires 5–10 per cent CO_2	:	−	−	−	−	−	+	+

NG = No growth; d = Different reactions in different strains.

pathogens, so that the appropriate antimicrobial drug is given as early as possible. Gram-stained smears of the CSF deposit, with dilute carbol-fuchsin used as the counter stain, and methylene-blue stained smears will often give a quick diagnosis. Confirmation may be obtained in the case of *H. influenzae* meningitis by the use of type *b* antiserum to show capsule swelling in a fresh smear. Or the CSF may be layered on top of the antiserum in a capillary tube to elicit a precipitin ring at the interface. The deposit is cultured on fresh blood agar and chocolate agar of *good nutrient quality*. Capsulation and serological type can be confirmed from the culture by the use of specific a–f antisera.* Blood culture is usually positive in cases of *H. influenzae* meningitis and laryngoepiglottitis and is essential in the latter infection since it is difficult to isolate the organism from the local lesion.

Sputum from cases of acute respiratory infection and chronic bronchitis must first be

* See footnote to p. 380.

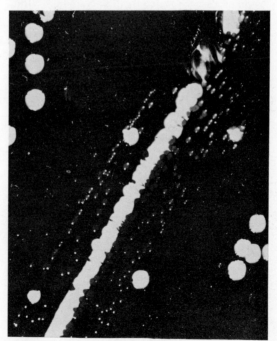

PLATE 22.1

Satellitism enhancement of colonial size of *Haemophilus influenzae* from proximity to streak culture of staphylococcus.

homogenized by mechanical shaking for 30 min with a few glass beads and then inoculated on blood agar and chocolate agar plates. Suspected haemophilus colonies may be confirmed on subculture on which disks containing X or V factor or both are placed* or by demonstrating 'satellitism' with a streak culture of staphylococcus. Similar procedures are used with specimens from cases of sinusitis, conjunctivitis, otitis media, vaginitis etc., in which *H. influenzae* may be a causal pathogen.

OTHER HAEMOPHILI

Haemophilus aegyptius (Koch-Weeks bacillus) is associated with acute infectious conjunctivitis and is biologically very similar to *H. influenzae*. *Haemophilus ducreyi* (Ducrey's bacillus) is associated with chancroid or soft sore. Gram-negative rod ($1 \cdot 5 \times 0 \cdot 4$ μm): occurs in pairs or short chains: non-motile, non-sporing, non-capsulate: isolation on artificial media is difficult: requires X but not V factor: growth may be obtained by inoculating pus from the lesion or juice aspirated from a secondary bubo, on to nutrient agar containing 20–30 per cent defibrinated rabbit blood in sterile tubes and then incubated at 35°C. Strains are all agglutinated by a specific antiserum. *H. aphrophilus* requires both X and V factors and also 5–10 per cent CO_2 for growth (Khairat, 1940)

* Specific a–f haemophilus antisera are available from Wellcome Reagents Ltd, and details of tests for X, V or X + V factors are described in the *Oxoid Manual*, 3rd edn, p. 284.

H. paraphrophilus requires V factor and CO_2 (Zinnemann et al, 1968).

Moraxella lacunata (Morax-Axenfeld bacillus) is associated with a subacute or chronic conjunctivitis perhaps secondary to a primary virus infection: morphologically, large Gram-negative rods (2 μm × 1 μm) in pairs: non-motile, non-sporing, non-capsulate.

Aerobic: requires whole blood or serum for growth, e.g. Loeffler's serum on which it causes liquefaction so that colonies develop 'pits' or 'lacunae' on the surface of the medium: optimum temperature 37°C: no growth at temperature of 20°–30°C in contrast to *Moraxella liquefaciens* which grows well on ordinary nutrient media over a wide range of temperature and liquefies gelatin at 22°C: this latter organism is associated with a conjunctivitis in which the cornea may be involved.

REFERENCES and FURTHER READING

KHAIRAT, O. (1940) Endocarditis due to a new species of Haemophilus. *Journal of Pathology and Bacteriology*, **50**, 497.

SIMS, W. (1970) *Oral haemophili. Journal of Medical Microbiology*, **3**, 615.

TURK, D. C. & MAY, J. R. (1967) *Haemophilus influenzae: Its Clinical Importance*. London: English Universities Press.

ZINNEMANN, K., ROGERS, K. B., FRAZER, Joyce & BOYCE, J. M. H. (1968) A new V-dependent *Haemophilus* species preferring increased CO_2 tension for growth and named *Haemophilus paraphrophilus*, nov. sp. *Journal of Pathology and Bacteriology*, **96**, 413.

23. Corynebacterium: Erysipelothrix: Listeria

The genus *Corynebacterium* contains many species, some of which are pathogenic to man and animals and others non-pathogenic commensals, commonly called diphtheroids. Some diphtheroid bacilli have, like *Staphylococcus albus*, been implicated in the colonization of Spitz-Holter valves. *Corynebacterium diphtheriae* is the principal human pathogen and owes its pathogenicity to the production of a potent diffusible exotoxin with an affinity for certain tissues such as heart muscle and peripheral nerves. These infections are typically associated with a local inflammatory lesion with membranous exudate affecting mucous membranes of the upper respiratory tract but they may occasionally give rise to wound infections or to chronic skin infections.

Another species, *Corynebacterium ulcerans*, commonly causes localized throat ulceration although rarely it may give rise to a clinical picture indistinguishable from diphtheria. Evidence has accumulated in recent years that *Corynebacterium haemolyticum* is sometimes the cause of severe sore throat often associated with an itching scarlatiniform rash (Ryan, 1972). Other species such as *Corynebacterium ovis* and *Corynebacterium pyogenes* are associated with suppurative or granulomatous lesions in various domestic animals.

CORYNEBACTERIUM DIPHTHERIAE
(Klebs-Loeffler bacillus)

Morphology and staining. Gram-positive rods of varying length (average measurements, $3.0 \mu m \times 0.3 \mu m$) occurring in obtuse angled pairs or parallel rows of 3-4 bacilli (palisade formation) and giving an overall picture likened to Chinese lettering: considerable pleomorphism in older cultures—club shaped, oval and globular forms: stain rather irregularly with Gram's method: easily decolourized: special stains (Neisser, Albert) pick out the volutin granules and give the bacilli a beaded or barred appearance: the granules are polar in short bacilli and absent from most non-pathogenic short diphtheroids. The microscopic morphology of the corynebacteria is very dependent on the medium employed. The same organism may show classical metachromatic granules in films from a moist Loeffler slope and no granules at all in films from a dry one. Morphology in films prepared from tellurite containing media is quite atypical. *C. diphtheriae* is non-motile, non-sporing, non-capsulate.

Cultural characters. Facultative anaerobe: optimum temperature 37°C (range 20°–40°C): grows best on blood or serum containing culture media, e.g. Loeffler's serum, fresh, laked or heated blood agar: the addition of potassium tellurite (0.04 per cent) to serum or blood agar inhibits most pathogenic or commensal species other than corynebacteriae: the shape, size and colour of colonies on tellurite blood agar (e.g. Hoyle's medium) helps in the differentiation of *C. diphtheriae* into three main biotypes which were labelled *gravis*, *intermedius* and *mitis* because differences in the severity of the clinical infection were often related to the biotype: gravis strains produce relatively large, greyish black, lustreless colonies which in old cultures may show atypical 'daisy-head' appearance: growth in broth is granular: colonies of *mitis* strains are convex, greyish-black, with ground glass but glistening surface: uniform turbidity in broth: colonies of *intermedius* strains are small, grey-black, lustreless with a remarkable uniformity in size which is in contrast to other types which may show considerable colonial variation (for more detailed description of colonial appearances on tellurite blood agar, see Cruickshank, 1968).

Sensitivity to physical and chemical agents. Killed by heat at 60°C in 10 min: resists natural drying and may remain viable in dust, etc., for weeks if protected from daylight.

Antibiotic sensitivity. *C. diphtheriae* is sensitive to penicillin, erythromycin, lincomycin and clindamycin, the last three antibiotics being useful for the treatment of patients who are allergic to penicillin. In addition to their role in the treatment of chronic carriers, antibiotics

381

have an invaluable synergistic role with anti-toxin in the treatment of diphtheria as they have the immediate effect of 'switching off' further toxin production.

Biochemical reactions. Ferments glucose, galactose, maltose and dextrin with acid production only but not lactose, mannitol or sucrose (except rarely): *gravis* strains also ferment starch and glycogen and produce H_2S: fermentation tests are usually done in Hiss's serum medium but serum-free fermentation media can be prepared and have certain advantages (Zamiri, personal communication).

Toxigenicity. The biotypes were named according to the clinical severity of the disease with which they were associated. Such distinctions now have little clinical validity in the U.K. Today the most commonly isolated strain is *mitis*, of which only 10–12 per cent of all isolates are toxigenic. Both *gravis* and *intermedius* strains have been only rarely isolated in Great Britain in recent years.

All toxigenic strains are lysogenic; if they are 'cured' of their lysogenicity they cease to be toxigenic but can be made to revert to toxin production by reinfection with prophage.

Tests for toxigenicity may be carried out by guinea-pig inoculation or *in vitro* by a gel precipitation test (Elek, 1949). The serological tests may be difficult and unreliable (Bickham and Jones, 1972). In view of the relative rarity of diphtheria and the importance of an early and accurate assessment of the potential danger of a new isolate, the guinea-pig method should be preferred. A simple lethal test carried out by injecting a large subcutaneous dose of test organisms (e.g. 0·5 ml of a dense suspension) into protected and unprotected animals is

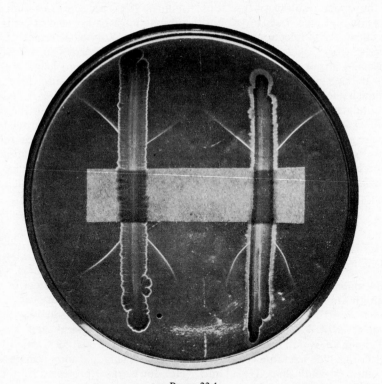

PLATE 23.1

Photograph showing the recognition of toxigenic strains of the diphtheria bacillus by Elek's method. In the centre is the horizontal strip of filter paper containing the anti-toxin with the growths of the diphtheria bacillus at right angles to it. The fine white lines showing a positive reaction are well defined.

best for fresh isolates. To economize in the use of animals, subsequent strains from contacts may be tested by intradermal inoculation into either protected and unprotected guinea-pigs or into the same animal in parallel before and after antitoxin administration (Cruickshank, 1968, p. 181). The intradermal test has the added advantage that it may help in the recognition of atypical or unsuspected strains of *C. ulcerans*. In addition to the classical diphtheria toxin, these strains produce an antigenically distinct toxin of the *ovis* type. As *C. ulcerans* may produce both types of toxin it can give rise to classical diphtheria, with a typical lethal reaction in a guinea-pig. On *intradermal* inoculation *C. ulcerans* will produce skin necrosis in both protected and unprotected guinea-pigs (because the diphtheria antitoxin does not cross-protect against the ovis toxin).

Antigenic characters. By agglutination tests, *gravis* strains were divided into 13 serotypes, *intermedius* into four types and *mitis* into 40 types. Serotyping was never fully developed as an epidemiological method. The phage-typing method (Saragea and Maximescu, 1966) was developed in Rumania during a time when epidemic *gravis* strains were common. It is applicable mainly to *gravis* strains and is less valuable in the tracing of the *mitis* strains which are predominant today in Britain. Bacteriocine typing shows promise as a method for the epidemiological tracing of strains of significant corynebacteria (Zamiri, personal communication).

Laboratory Diagnosis

Swabs are taken from the local lesion (including skin lesions when appropriate) or from the nose and throat of contacts or suspected carriers. The swabs are inoculated on to moist Loeffler slopes, blood agar and tellurite plates. Jellard (1971) suggests that the use of Tinsdale's medium is a help in identifying diphtheria bacilli especially when experienced staff are not available. The production of an opalescent halo around suspected colonies (due to the action of cysteinase) helps identification.

Films are made from the Loeffler slope after 6 h or overnight incubation, stained by one of the special methods for the characteristic morphology of *C. diphtheriae*. Tellurite-medium cultures should be examined at 18, 24 and 48 h and the results considered in relation to the biochemical reactions.

Early identification of the type of diphtheria bacilli is greatly facilitated by the use of a plate microscope. When diphtheria-like colonies are seen on blood agar but not on tellurite-containing media, the presence of *C. haemolyticum* should be considered. This organism is inhibited by tellurite in normal concentration and may not produce significant haemolysis until incubated for 48 hours (Ryan, 1972). Films from Loeffler slopes may be the first indication of the presence of a diphtheria bacillus. Fresh slopes should be inoculated from single colonies of any suspected strains and the cultures used for guinea-pig inoculation and for fermentation reactions. Gelatine liquefication is best tested at room temperature on gelatine slope cultures—with a stroke inoculum; charcoal—gelatine 'tablets' are unreliable for this test.

As glandular fever may give rise to a sore throat with membrane formation, it may be useful to carry out a Paul-Bunnell test if the diagnosis is in doubt (Christie, 1969). Direct smears from throat swabs should also be examined for Vincent's organisms.

Corynebacterium Ulcerans

Associated with exudative or ulcerative throat lesions which resemble diphtheria: morphologically, pleomorphic with clubbed, coccoid or filamentous forms, particularly in older cultures: stains irregularly with Gram's method and is easily decolourized: fermentation reactions similar to *gravis* strains of *C. diphtheriae* but in addition ferments trehalose and liquefies gelatin: a narrow zone of haemolysis is seen around colonies on blood agar.

Corynebacterium Haemolyticum (C. pyogenes var. hominus/C. haemolyticum group)

Organisms of this type have been reported for some years in the United States and in Europe but only recently in Great Britain. With increasing interest it is likely that this organism will be found more commonly. Its failure to grow on standard tellurite media is an obvious source of error and it is hoped that a suitable selective media may be developed. The organism is described by Ryan (1972) as Gram-positive with some resemblance to *C. diphtheriae* but no metachromatic granules. Enriched medium is required for growth but tellurite is inhibitory; growth is equally good aerobically or anaerobically. Colonies on horse blood agar are about 0·5 mm at 24 h, later reaching 1–1·5 mm. No haemolysis is seen on horse or sheep blood after 24 h aerobic incubation: on human blood agar there may be partial haemolysis after 24 h with β-haemolysis after 48 h.

Catalase, oxidase, urease, indole production, H₂S production and nitrate reduction all negative: weakly proteolytic: acid produced from glucose, lactose and starch: non-lethal to guinea-pigs but may cause local abscess production.

Diphtheroid Bacilli

These are non-toxigenic corynebacteria with little or no pathogenicity.

Corynebacterium Hofmannii

A commensal of the throat.
MORPHOLOGY AND STAINING. Gram-positive short rods or cocco-bacilli with Loeffler's methylene blue, an unstained bar in the middle of the organism is a frequent character and renders it not unlike a diplococcus. Usually no volutin granules are detected by Neisser's or Albert's stains.
CULTURAL CHARACTERS. Grows aerobically on ordinary media; the colonies are larger and more opaque. For appearances on one of the tellurite media, see above.
BIOCHEMICAL REACTIONS. No fermentation of glucose or sucrose.

It is non-pathogenic to laboratory animals.

Corynebacterium Xerosis

A commensal in the conjunctival sac; originally thought to be the cause of xerosis conjunctivae. Closely resembles the diphtheria bacillus, and may show volutin granules but differentiated by its production of acid in sucrose as well as in

glucose and by its non-pathogenicity to laboratory animals.

Corynebacterium Acnes (Propionibacterium Acnes)

An organism associated with acne, but its aetiological relationship to the disease is doubtful. It is Gram-positive, rod-shaped, and measures about 1·5 μm by 0·5 μm. It is markedly pleomorphic and frequently shows a beaded appearance: Micro-aerophilic.

Other Diphtheroid Species

Certain diphtheroids are morphologically similar to the diphtheria bacillus, and may exhibit the characteristic volutin granules by Neisser's staining method, though differing in fermentative reactions, e.g. by fermenting sucrose. They are mostly non-pathogenic, and have been isolated from the secretions of the nose and nasopharynx, the external ear, conjunctival sac, the skin, lymph glands (apart from disease) and other tissues, pus, wounds, etc.

Corynebacteria Pathogenic in Animals

Brief descriptions of corynebacteria pathogenic to various domestic animals, e.g. *C. ovis*, *C. pyogenes*, *C. equi* and *C. renale* are given in Cruickshank, 1968, pp. 189–190.

Erysipelothrix: Listeria

These two genera are members of the family Corynebacteriaceae and share many biological characters: they are primary pathogens of both domestic and wild mammals and birds and sometimes infect man.
Erysipelothrix Rhusiopathiae (Ery. insidiosa). The causative organism of swine erysipelas.

Morphologically slender, Gram-positive, non-motile, rod-shaped bacilli 1–2 by 0·2–0·4 μm, occurring singly and in chains. In culture media, longer and filamentous forms are observed. True branching has been described.

Culturally micro-aerophilic when first isolated: in agar-shake cultures grows best just below the surface: later facultative anaerobe: optimum temperature 37°C but grows about room temperature on ordinary nutrient agar. In gelatin-stab culture, growth along the wire track with lateral spikes or disks radiating from the central growth. Two types of surface colonies on nutrient agar plates: (*a*) exceedingly minute and dewdrop-like, with a smooth surface; (*b*) larger with granular appearance. Various carbohydrates are fermented (without gas production), e.g. glucose, lactose, sucrose, but mannitol not fermented. Antigenically, different groups have been recognized.

Animal pathogenicity. Mice, rats, rabbits and pigeons can be infected experimentally: mice and pigeons usually die with septicaemia within 4–5 days. Subcutaneous injection in rabbits produces a spreading inflammation and oedema with a fatal result. Experimental inoculation in swine reproduces the natural disease: smooth-colony type is the more pathogenic.

A similar, possibly identical organism, *Erysipelothrix muriseptica,* is responsible for epizootic septicaemia in mice.

Ery. rhusiopathiae may occur in apparently healthy pigs, and has been isolated from the tonsils, intestines and faeces. It has a wide distribution in other animals and in birds. It is also found, apparently as a commensal, on the skin and scales of many fish (particularly members of the perch family).

Laboratory Diagnosis

The most satisfactory method for isolation is from a biopsy of the actively growing edge of the lesion: incubate for 48 h in 1 per cent glucose broth, subculturing on to blood agar: lesion swabs give poor results: blood culture may be made in acute cases. Infective material may also be inoculated into mice or pigeons. An agglutination test is applicable.

LISTERIA MONOCYTOGENES

The disease, listeriosis, now has a world-wide distribution, affecting many species of wild and domestic animals (foxes, dogs, gerbils, chinchillas, etc.), birds and fish. Transmission from animal to man is often difficult to demonstrate:

in man, rare cases of meningo-encephalitis in older adults: a generalized infection (granulomatosis infantiseptica) may occur in neonates following a symptomless infection in the mother.

Morphologically *Listeria monocytogenes* is a Gram-positive straight or slightly curved non-sporing rod, 2–3 by 0·5 μm (average), often in pairs, end to end at an acute angle: sometimes elongated filaments particularly in solid medium at room temperature: feebly motile at 37°C, but more active in young broth cultures at 25°C: exhibits up to four flagella. In older cultures, the bacilli are mostly Gram-negative.

Culturally, aerobic; optimum temperature 37°C; grows on ordinary media but growth improved by media containing liver extract, blood, serum or glucose. After 24 h incubation colonies are very small and droplet-like; larger after a few days' growth (diameter 2 mm), at first smooth and transparent: later more opaque: narrow zone of complete haemolysis on blood agar. Gelatin and Loeffler's serum not liquefied. In glucose, maltose and certain other common sugars acid is promptly produced without gas: lactose and sucrose are fermented slowly, but mannitol is not fermented.

Listeria is susceptible to penicillin, streptomycin, the tetracyclines, chloromycetin and erythromycin, but resistant to sulphonamides, bacitracin and polymyxin.

Listeria produces a haemolysin which probably plays little part in pathogenicity: experimentally, pathogenic for rabbits, mice and guinea-pigs, but not for rats and pigeons: focal lesions on the chorio-allantoic membrane of chick embryo.

Laboratory Diagnosis

Isolation of the organism is made by culture of the blood or lesions in generalized infections in infants and of spinal fluid in cases of meningitis. The pathogen may be misdiagnosed as a contaminating diphtheroid. The CSF in cases of meningitis, is slightly turbid (300–2000 cells/ml polymorphs and lymphocytes): the diphtheroid-like bacilli may be seen in a stained film of the centrifuged deposit. Leucocyte counts of the blood show a relative monocytosis.

REFERENCES and FURTHER READING

BICKHAM, S. & JONES, W. (1972) Problems in the use of the *in vitro* toxigenicity test for *C. diphtheriae*. *American Journal of Clinical Pathology*, **57**, 244–246.

CRUICKSHANK, R. (1968) *Medical Microbiology*, 11th edn., revised, pp. 181, 186, 189–190. Edinburgh: Livingstone.

CHRISTIE, A. B. (1969) In *Infectious Diseases, Epidemiology and Clinical Practice*, p. 913. Edinburgh: Livingstone.

ELEK, S. D. (1949) The plate virulence test for diphtheria. *Journal of Clinical Pathology*, **2**, 250–258.

JELLARD, C. H. (1971) Comparison of Hoyle's medium and Billing's modification of Tinsdale's medium for the bacteriological diagnosis of diphtheria. *Journal of Medical Microbiology*, **4**, 366–369.

RYAN, W. J. (1972) Throat infection and rash associated with an unusual Corynebacterium. *Lancet*, **ii**, 1345–1347.

SARAGEA, A. & MAXIMESCU, P. (1966) Phage-typing of *Corynebacterium diphtheriae*. *Bulletin of the World Health Organization*, **35**, 681–689.

ZAMIRI, I. (1973) A Study of Diphtheria. Thesis presented for degree of M.D., Sheffield University.

24. Mycobacterium

Mycobacteria are widely distributed in nature. There are two main pathogenic species: (1) *Mycobacterium tuberculosis* associated with tuberculosis affecting man and certain mammals; and (2) *Myco. leprae* the cause of leprosy, a chronic disease of man only. Man may also be affected by *Myco. bovis*, a primary pathogen in cattle and other mammals and, very rarely, by *Myco. avium*, pathogenic to birds and some animals, e.g. the pig. A group of 'atypical mycobacteria' with which may be included two species causing skin ulceration (*Myco. ulcerans* and *Myco. marinum*) may cause clinical or latent infections in man.

MYCOBACTERIUM TUBERCULOSIS

Morphology and staining. Typically slender, straight or slightly curved rods (average 3.0×0.3 μm), occurring singly, in angled pairs or in small bundles of parallel bacilli (cf *C. diphtheriae*) but size may vary from cocco bacilli to long bacilli ($0.8–5.0 \times 0.23–0.6$ μm). Non-motile, non-sporing, non-capsulate: filamentous forms may be seen in older cultures.

Because of a waxy material (containing mycolic acid) in the cell wall, *Myco. tuberculosis* resists staining by ordinary dyes: stain penetration requires a strong mordanted dye in the presence of heat: carbol-fuchsin is most commonly used: after staining, the bacilli resist decolourization with 20 per cent sulphuric acid and with alcohol—or a combination of acid and alcohol: methylene blue or malachite green is used as a counterstain (Ziehl-Neelsen method): staining may be irregular giving beaded or bipolar forms: tubercle bacilli may also be stained with auramine and/or rhodamine and the smears examined by fluorescence microscopy under low magnification. Mycobacteria are Gram-positive but in most species it is difficult to stain the organisms by Gram's method.

Cultural characters. Aerobe: optimum temperature 35°–37°C (range 30°–41°C): primary isolates do not grow on ordinary nutrient media: growth occurs on blood or serum agar but is better on media containing whole egg or egg-yolk, sterilized at low temperature (e.g. Dorset and Löwenstein-Jensen media): alternatively, a semi-synthetic medium containing mixtures of organic or inorganic salts, oleate, albumin, glucose and glycerol (Middlebrook and Cohn modified from Middlebrook and Dubos medium), solidified with agar and poured in plastic plates may be used: Stonebrink's medium is recommended for the growth of bovine tubercle bacilli and for isolation of human strains from patients on antimicrobial therapy: growth is slow (mean generation time 1–3 days) so that primary cultures may not be macroscopically visible until 10–14 days after incubation—or as late as 6–8 weeks (see Chapter 5).

Colonies on Löwenstein's medium gradually increase in size and coalesce into a raised dry wrinkled or mamillated growth, at first whitish, later buff-coloured or yellowish: friable, tenacious and granular when picked for film examination: colonial morphology on transparent media (e.g. Middlebrook and Cohn) is often distinctive for different species of mycobacteria (see U.S. Public Health Series Publication, 1970) a fragment of culture on solid media when floated on the surface of glycerol broth in a shallow flask grows as a whitish wrinkled pellicle: submerged growth at first rather granular but later more uniformly turbid, is obtained in Dubos liquid medium containing a surface-wetting agent 'Tween 80' (polyoxyethylene sorbitan mono-oleate): the addition of glycerol (2–5 per cent) to egg or serum media increases the growth of *Myco. tuberculosis* and certain other mycobacteria, but not *Myco. bovis*.

Sensitivity to physical and chemical agents. Killed by heat at 60°C for 15–20 min: may resist natural drying for several weeks if protected from daylight: relatively resistant to various chemical disinfectants, e.g. infected sputum may require several hours' exposure to 5 per cent phenol for disinfection: highly susceptible to sunlight and daylight, even through glass: sensitive to a wide range of antimicrobial drugs of which the most important for clinical use are streptomycin, isoniazid, para-amino salicylic acid (PAS), ethambutol, pyrazinamide, prothionamide, rifampicin and thiocetazone (see Chap. 22, Vol. I).

Biochemical reactions are not ordinarily used in the identification or differentiation of mycobacteria: no detectable acid production in sugar containing media: catalase+.

Antigenic characters. Four serological groups of mycobacteria—mammalian, avian, reptilian and saprophytic: human, bovine and murine species indistinguishable antigenically: phage-typing has been used as a research tool to differentiate species of mycobacteria.

Animal pathogenicity. The guinea-pig is highly susceptible to experimental infection: after subcutaneous injection with tubercle bacilli in infected specimens or from culture, a local swelling appears in 3–5 days, consisting of small nodules which coalesce, caseate and finally ulcerate: neighbouring and later more distant lymph nodes are involved: infection spreads to spleen, liver, peritoneum, etc., but lungs and kidneys have few lesions: mice are much less susceptible but after intraperitoneal or intravenous injection of relatively large doses develop progressive generalized infection. Rabbits are much less susceptible to *Myco. tuberculosis* than to *Myco. bovis,* the difference between the two species can be demonstrated by an intravenous injection into a rabbit of an emulsion in saline of 0·01–0·1 mg (dry wt) of a solid medium culture. The bovine species produces an acute generalized tuberculosis and the rabbit usually dies within 3–6 weeks; with the human species the animal survives or dies after several months with chronic lesions in the lungs and kidneys. Chick embryos may be infected: monkeys, cattle, pigs, dogs and cats may become naturally infected (for more detailed discussion of experimental tuberculosis in animals, see Wilson and Miles, 1965).

LABORATORY DIAGNOSIS

The specimen most commonly examined is *sputum,* which is mixed pus and mucous secretion coughed up from the lungs. Saliva or throat secretion spat from the mouth is not an adequate specimen, and if the specimen submitted is clean and does not have the opaque-yellow or greenish appearance indicating a content of pus, another specimen should be requested. Normally, several successive specimens are examined from the same patient before a negative result can be accepted.

Three main methods are used to detect tubercle bacilli in sputum and other materials: (1) microscopic examination for acid-fast bacilli in a Ziehl-Neelsen or fluorochrome stained film of concentrated or unconcentrated material; (2) culture on egg medium after decontamination and concentration, and (3) inoculation into guinea-pigs.

Microscopic examination has the advantage of giving a result at once, but is likely to be successful only if large numbers of bacilli are present, e.g. 10^5/ml or greater. Culture and guinea-pig inoculation are much more sensitive methods and may detect as few as 1–10 bacilli/ml, but owing to the slow growth of the bacillus, give their results only after several weeks. Cultural isolation is, moreover, necessary if drug-sensitivity tests are to be carried out on the patient's strain.

Sputum: Z-N Film

Tubercle bacilli are usually present in considerable numbers in the sputum of chronic cavitated cases of pulmonary tuberculosis: they may be demonstrable in the deposits of urine and CSF in cases of urinary tuberculosis and tuberculous meningitis respectively: they are usually scanty in pus from lymph nodes and in the respiratory secretions of cases of primary pulmonary and miliary tuberculosis and Z-N stained smears from such material require prolonged microscopic examination. A direct film of sputum or a film from the deposit of a homogenized specimen (see Petroff's method) is stained by the Z-N method. Care must be taken not to contaminate such films with saprophytic acid-fast bacilli from a cold water tap or with stained tubercle bacilli on blotting paper used to dry a previous film. The presence of numerous acid-fast bacilli in purulent sputum from suspected cases of pulmonary tuberculosis may be reported as presumptive confirmation: scanty acid-fast bacilli in only one specimen of sputum or in specimens of urine, CSF or pus should be reported as such: for colour-blind microscopists who fail to see the bacilli stained red, a blue-green filter should be placed in front of a highly intense illuminant when the tubercle bacilli appear black against a homogeneous background if malachite green is used as the counterstain: a 1/7 (3–6 mm) fluorite oil immersion lens should be used to allow rapid screening of smears. Positive findings on specimens stained with fluorochrome agents (auramine, rhodamine) should be confirmed with Ziehl-Neelsen staining: fluorescent staining of smears is recommended when large numbers of specimens have to be examined: a high dry lens (magnification 400X) is used after preliminary screening with a low power lens (100X).

Laryngeal Swab; Gastric Lavage

Where sputum is absent or, if present, is being swallowed, material for culture may be obtained either by the laryngeal swab or by stomach wash-out.

The laryngeal swab consists of a piece of nickel or 'Nichrome' wire 9 in long and $\frac{1}{16}$ in in diameter, bent at an angle of 120° an inch and a half from the end. Cotton-wool is wrapped round this end of the wire, which has been flattened and spirally twisted to hold the cotton-wool firmly. Each swab is placed in a boiling-tube (7×1 in) the open end of which is plugged with cotton-wool. The tubes with swabs in position are sterilized in the autoclave. Immediately before use the swab is moistened with sterile distilled water.

The swab may be passed into larynx either with the guidance of a laryngeal mirror, or blindly. For both methods the patient is seated and supplied with a piece of gauze with which to hold his tongue fully protruded. The operator, if using a mirror, sits opposite the patient and with the aid of the mirror guides the tip of the swab over the epiglottis into the larynx. Without a mirror the operator stands at the side of the patient and passes the swab through the mouth backwards and downwards strictly in the mid-line; the manoeuvre is facilitated by asking the patient to take

panting breaths. Reflex cough usually develops as the swab enters the larynx, and absence of cough suggests that the swab has not entered the larynx. Two consecutive swabs should be taken from each patient.

In the laboratory sufficient 10 per cent H_2SO_4 (v/v) is added to the boiling-tube to cover the cotton-wool on the swab. After five minutes in acid the swab is removed, excess of fluid is expressed on the side of the tube, and the swab is transferred for a further five minutes to a second boiling-tube containing a similar amount of 2 per cent NaOH. The swab is again drained of excess fluid and is rubbed over the surface of a slope of Löwenstein-Jensen medium. The inoculated medium is incubated at 37°C for 6–8 weeks and examined at weekly intervals.

An alternative procedure is to immerse the swab in a saturated solution of trisodium phosphate and incubate at 37°C overnight. The swab is then removed and the fluid centrifuged at 3000 rev/min for 20 min. The supernatant is decanted and the deposit is inoculated on to two Löwenstein-Jensen slopes.

It is inadvisable to leave a long delay between the collection of the swabs and inoculation on to culture medium.

Fasting stomach contents may be aspirated with a Ryle tube in the morning after a period of coughing and swallowing. The material should be despatched to the laboratory as quickly as possible, or if there is likely to be a long delay, the contents should be neutralized with caustic soda. The deposit is homogenized by either the modified Petroff or the modified Jungmann method and inoculated on two slopes of Löwenstein-Jensen medium. Patients prefer the laryngeal swab to gastric lavage, which, however, may give at least as high a proportion of positive results. Neither of these methods will give as good results as scanty expectoration.

Specimens from Other Sources

Urine, pleural and peritoneal fluids are centrifuged, films are made from the deposit and stained by the Ziehl-Neelsen method. As tubercle bacilli are often scantily present in these fluids, the deposit from 50–100 ml should be used for both direct microscopic examination and for culture; or the cultural method recommended by Ives and McCormick (1956) may be used, i.e. 100 ml of pleural fluid is added directly to 100 ml of double-strength Sula liquid medium.

With all urinary specimens it is essential to treat the film with alcohol (two minutes) after decolourization with acid in the Ziehl-Neelsen process, in order to exclude smegma bacilli. In examining urine it is advisable to obtain the sediment from three consecutive morning specimens because of intermittency of excretions. Alternatively the deposit from a 24-h collection may be examined.

Cerebrospinal fluid is allowed to stand in a stoppered tube for an hour or longer, when a 'spider-web' coagulum usually forms in the fluid. The clot is carefully transferred to a slide, the preparation is dried, fixed by heat and stained by the Ziehl-Neelsen method. In the absence of clotting the fluid is centrifuged and the deposit examined in the usual way.

Cultural Methods

Microscopic examination of direct sputum smears will not ordinarily detect tubercle bacilli if the numbers are less than 50 000 per ml. Because of this limitation and because cultural isolation of *Myco. tuberculosis* confirms the diagnosis and allows further identification tests with atypical cultures and sensitivity tests to anti-tuberculous drugs, specimens of sputum and other materials from suspected cases of tuberculosis should be cultured on two tubes of Löwenstein-Jensen medium and/or on plates of the Middlebrook-Cohn medium.

When the specimen, as in the case of sputum, is contaminated with other bacteria, a process of preliminary homogenization and decontamination is necessary. Various methods have been advocated: those most generally used are the modified Petroff alkali method with 4 per cent sodium hydroxide or the more slowly acting trisodium phosphate (12–24 h): Nassau's modification of Jungmann and Grushka's acid method and the use of quaternary ammonium compounds and mucolytic enzymes, singly or in combination (Saxholm, 1958).

1. *Petroff's method (modified)*. Sputum is mixed thoroughly with an equal volume of 4 per cent sodium hydroxide and placed in the incubator at 37°C for 30 min, the container being shaken every five minutes. The mixture is centrifuged at 3000 rev/min for 30 minutes and the supernatant fluid poured off. The deposit is neutralized with 8 per cent hydrochloric acid, which is added drop by drop, the reaction of the mixture being tested by adding a drop of phenol red solution to the tube. The deposit is examined microscopically and is then inoculated on Löwenstein-Jensen medium. Solidified Dubos medium or some modification of it can also be used.

2. *Nassau's modification of Jungmann and Grushka's method*. Prepare the following solutions:

Solution A
  Ferrous sulphate .   .   .   20 g
  Sulphuric acid 20 per cent v/v 100 ml
Solution B
  Hydrogen peroxide   .   . 0·3 per cent
                                    (1 vol)

Solution A can be made up in bulk and keeps indefinitely. Solution B must be made up fresh on each occasion from a standard pharmacopoeal 6 per cent w/v solution kept in the dark. For use place 2 ml of sputum in a universal container. Add 1·2 ml solution A and 1·2 ml solution B. Shake the container for thirty seconds and allow to stand on the bench for twenty minutes, shaking at intervals. Centrifuge at 3000 rev/min for thirty minutes and discard the supernatant fluid. Fill the container to the shoulder with 5 per cent sterile sodium citrate, shake vigorously, and again centrifuge. Decant the supernatant fluid and inoculate the deposit on two slopes of Löwenstein-Jensen medium.

pH and gaseous requirements. The culture medium should have a slightly acid pH (6·5–7·0) and must be kept moist. Both O_2 and CO_2 are required for growth. If Löwenstein-Jensen slopes in screw-capped containers are used, the cap should be loosened once weekly at the time of inspection for growth. If a solid modified Dubos medium is used, the plates should be incubated in a jar with 2–10 per cent CO_2; on this medium small colonies may be seen within 7–10 days and reach optimum size in 2–3 weeks. Records should be kept of the presence, character, pigmentation, etc., of growth on Löwenstein-Jensen medium at weekly intervals for 6–8 weeks.

Drug sensitivity. The methods and interpretation of tests for the sensitivity of tubercle bacilli to different antimycobacterial drugs are described in Chapter 8.

Serology. Serological tests for specific antibodies in human sera after tuberculous infection are not ordinarily used for diagnostic purposes. The haemagglutination test of Middlebrook and Dubos (1948) has not been found to be sufficiently specific or sensitive to be of clinical value (Hilson and Elek, 1951).

Guinea-pig inoculation. About 0·5 ml of the neutralized deposit after decontamination by Petroff's or another method is injected intramuscularly or deeply subcutaneously in the thigh in two guinea-pigs. The animals are examined weekly by palpation for the development of a local tuberculous abscess and enlarged inguinal lymph nodes. One is killed as soon as lesions are felt, otherwise one is killed at 6 weeks and the other at 8 weeks or later. At necropsy, each animal is examined for a local abscess and enlarged inguinal and abdominal lymph nodes, and for the presence of yellowish tubercles of 1–2 mm in diameter in the viscera, particularly the liver and spleen. Small portions of tissue containing suspected tubercles and portions of enlarged lymph nodes are excised aseptically and used to prepare Ziehl-Neelsen films and, if required for sensitivity tests, cultures on Löwenstein-Jensen medium.

MYCOBACTERIUM BOVIS

Morphologically, the bovine species of tubercle bacilli tend to be straight and stubby but otherwise resemble the human species. Culturally, the two species cannot be readily differentiated on media containing no glycerol (e.g. Dorset's egg medium) but on glycerol enriched media, e.g. Löwenstein-Jensen, the human species grows well as a thick, confluent, wrinkled culture with buff or yellow colouration (eugonic) whereas the bovine species grows poorly as discrete, flat, whiting colonies with smooth or ground glass surface (dysgonic). Since some human strains may also be dysgonic differentiation of the two species is best made by virulence tests on rabbits injected intravenously with a saline suspension (0·01–0·1 mg dry weight) of a culture on solid medium. The bovine bacillus produces acute generalized tuberculosis with death in 3–6 weeks: with the human bacillus the rabbit is not obviously ill and either survives or dies after several months with localized tuberculous lesions in lungs and kidneys.

The differentiation of the mammalian mycobacteria from atypical, avian and skin mycobacteria is discussed in Chapter 25.

Safety in laboratory. Laboratory workers have commonly been infected with tuberculosis as a result of working with pathological specimens and cultures of tubercle bacilli. Infection is most probable by the inhalation of airborne particles or droplets. Dangerous infected aerosols may be liberated in simple inoculation procedures with infected fluids and, particularly, liquid cultures. All such manipulations should be done in an exhaust-ventilated safety cabinet of approved design (Chapter 16).

REFERENCES AND FURTHER READING

HILSON, G. R. F. & ELEK, S. D. (1951) The haemagglutination reaction in tuberculosis. *Journal of Clinical Pathology*, **4**, 158.

IVES, J. C. J. & MCCORMICK, W. (1956) A modification of Süla's medium for the cultivation of tubercle bacilli from pleural fluid. *Journal of Clinical Pathology*, **9**, 177.

MIDDLEBROOK, G. & DUBOS, R. J. (1948) Specific serum agglutination of erythrocytes sensitized with extracts of tubercle bacilli. *Journal of Experimental Medicine*, **88**, 521.

SAXHOLM, J. (1958) *An Experimental Investigation of Methods for the Cultivation of Mycobacterium Tuberculosis from Sputum*. Oslo: Oslo University Press.

U.S. PUBLIC HEALTH SERIES NO. 1549 (1970) *Laboratory Methods for Clinical and Public Health: Mycobacteriology*. Georgia: U.S. Public Health Service.

WILSON, G. S. & MILES, A. A. (1965) *Principles of Bacteriology and Immunology*, 5th edn. London: Arnold.

25. Atypical Mycobacteria: Myco. Leprae

Atypical mycobacteria resemble tubercle bacilli but seldom cause disease in man. The most important and widely distributed species in Britain are *Mycobacterium kansasii*, *Myco. intracellulare*, *Myco. avium* and *Myco. marinum*. The first three may be isolated from lymph nodes and lungs; *Myco. intracellulare* and *Myco. avium* may, rarely, spread from the lungs to other tissues. *Myco. marinum* is limited to abraded skin. *Myco. ulcerans*, another skin pathogen, is not found in Britain but occurs in warm-climate countries.

MYCOBACTERIUM KANSASII

These organisms are acid-fast, long rods larger than tubercle bacilli, with marked beading and banding. Films from cultures show the organisms arranged in bundles and cords, although this feature is not as pronounced as in *Myco. tuberculosis*.

On Löwenstein-Jensen medium at 37°C colonies appear in several weeks. They grow more slowly at 25°C. The colonies resemble those of *Myco. tuberculosis* but are relatively soft and can be spread quite easily on a slide. The colour of the growth is slightly yellower than that of tubercle bacilli, but after exposure to light and overnight incubation, the colonies become canary yellow.

Myco. kansasii does not produce niacin but it is strongly catalase-positive. It is, unlike other atypical mycobacteria, susceptible to 10 μg/ml of thioacetazone in Löwenstein-Jensen medium.

Myco. kansasii does not cause progressive disease in guinea-pigs or rabbits.

Laboratory Diagnosis

Films of sputum or homogenized lymph node stained by Ziehl-Neelsen's method show the presence of acid-fast bacilli, which cannot be distinguished from tubercle bacilli.

The specimen is treated as for the cultural isolation of tubercle bacilli. Growth is slow, and the colonies resemble those of *Myco. tuberculosis*, but they are soft in consistency and spread as a greasy smear on a slide instead of being granular like the colonies of *Myco. tuberculosis*. Their content of large, acid-fast bacilli should be confirmed. Exposure of a young culture to either natural or artificial light for 1 hour while the cap of the container is loosened to allow access of air and a further period of incubation overnight deepens the colour to canary yellow. The niacin test is negative, catalase activity is vigorous, and the organism is resistant to PAS and isoniazid, and susceptible to thioacetazone 10 μg/ml in Löwenstein-Jensen medium.

MYCOBACTERIUM INTRACELLULARE AND *MYCO. AVIUM*

These mycobacteria are acid-fast, stubby cocco-bacilli. Films from cultures show tiny, single, short rods grouped irregularly into small, loose clumps. They are not arranged in cords or skeins.

Both organisms grow slowly and poorly on Löwenstein-Jensen medium. Growth is enhanced on Stonebrink's pyruvate medium. If the inoculation is heavy, a nearly colourless film of growth is produced. The colour is not altered by exposure to light. *Myco. intracellulare* grows slowly at 25°C but not at 45°C, whereas *Myco. avium* grows at the latter temperature but not at the former.

These mycobacteria do not produce niacin, and catalase activity is slight. *Myco. intracellulare* produces arylsulphatase (after incubation for 2 weeks it releases phenolphthalein from 0·001 M potassium phenolphthalein disulphate in liquid medium) and *Myco. avium* does not.

Intravenous inoculation of a newly isolated culture of *Myco. avium* into a chicken causes progressive tuberculosis; and in the rabbit it causes arthritis. *Myco. intracellulare* does not cause progressive disease in these animals.

Laboratory Diagnosis

Films of sputum, pus or homogenized tissue may reveal the presence of tiny, acid-fast bacilli. The specimen is treated as for the isolation of tubercle bacilli; growth on Löwenstein-Jensen medium is slow and poor but may be enhanced on pyruvate medium. The colourless growth, which is unaffected by exposure to light, is soft and spreads easily on a slide, where its content of small acid-fast bacilli should be confirmed. The niacin test is negative, the catalase test weakly positive. *Myco. intracellulare* produces arylsulphatase and does not cause progressive disease in chicken or rabbit, whereas *Myco. avium* does not produce arylsulphatase, and newly isolated cultures cause progressive tuberculosis in the chicken and arthritis in the rabbit.

Both organisms are resistant to antituberculosis drugs.

MYCOBACTERIUM MARINUM

These organisms are long, beaded rods larger than tubercle bacilli and resembling *Myco. kansasii*, but films from cultures do not show alignment into cords.

On Löwenstein-Jensen medium incubated at 30°C to 33°C colonies of *Myco. marinum* appear in two to three weeks. They are smooth, round, convex and yellowish. After exposure to light for an hour followed by overnight incubation, they become deep yellow. Subcultures grow rapidly and profusely at 30°C; they also grow at 37°C but not luxuriantly. *Myco. marinum* does not produce niacin but is strongly catalase-positive.

Intradermal inoculation in the rabbit produces a lesion resembling swimming-pool granuloma. In the footpad of the mouse inflammation and abscess-formation occur in a few days after inoculation.

Laboratory Diagnosis

The homogenized biopsy specimen or pus is treated as for the isolation of tubercle bacilli. If the specimen is not heavily contaminated exposure to sodium hydroxide may be reduced to 15 or 20 minutes. Slopes of Löwenstein-Jensen and pyruvate media are inoculated in pairs and incubated at 37°C and 30°C. Growth appears at the lower temperature in two to three weeks; if growth occurs at 37°C it will be poor on primary isolation. After subculture the organism grows at 30°C in several days; it also grows at 37°C.

The organisms spread readily on a slide, and when stained with Ziehl-Neelsen stain appear as large, acid-fast rods. After exposure to light and re-incubation the culture becomes yellow. It does not produce niacin, but catalase activity is vigorous.

MYCOBACTERIUM ULCERANS

Myco. ulcerans is found in tropical and subtropical zones and does not occur in Britain. It resembles *Myco. marinum*.

These organisms are slender, strongly acid-fast bacilli. Films from cultures show some organisms aligned into cords although this feature is not marked.

On Löwenstein-Jensen medium incubated at 32°C growth is scanty and slow, the colonies appearing in the course of 8 weeks. They are colourless or slightly yellow, matt in texture, convex or flat, and never more than 3 mm in diameter. *Myco. ulcerans* does not grow either primarily or on subculture at 25°C or at 37°C. It does not produce niacin but possesses moderate catalase activity. Inoculation of the footpad of a mouse gives rise to a slowly progressing oedema of the limb and ulceration at the site of injection.

Laboratory Diagnosis

Smears from the spreading edge of the ulcer show masses of strongly acid-fast bacilli. Homogenized curettings from the edge are treated with 4 per cent sodium hydroxide and inoculated on to slopes of Löwenstein-Jensen medium, some of which are incubated at 32°C and some at 37°C. A scanty growth appears on the slopes incubated at 32°C in the course of 8 weeks; there is no growth at the higher temperature. Films of the cultures show strongly acid-fast bacilli. The cultures do not produce niacin and show only moderate catalase activity. Inoculation of the footpad of the mouse causes slowly progressing oedema and ulceration.

SCOTOCHROMOGENS

The scotochromogens are important only as transient commensals in the patient or contaminants of specimens. They appear on cultures from time to time because they are isolated in the same way as other mycobacteria. They grow slowly at 37°C to produce smooth, domed, orange-coloured colonies. Exposure to light increases the depth of colour. The organisms spread easily on the slide; they vary in appearance, are arranged singly or in loose clumps, and are not aligned in cords. They are niacin-negative, strongly catalase-positive, and do not cause disease in laboratory animals.

MYCOBACTERIUM LEPRAE

Leprosy is a very chronic disease affecting skin, mucous membranes and peripheral nerves and is manifest in two main clinical forms: lepromatous leprosy in which skin and mucous membrane lesions and granulomata cause much disfigurement, and tuberculoid or maculoanaesthetic leprosy in which infiltration of nerves results in subcutaneous nodules, anaesthesias, and blanching of the skin followed by trophic ulcers, burns and various deformities. *Morphology.* The leprosy bacillus, recognized inside cells from leprosy nodules in 1874 by Hansen, a Norwegian doctor, was the first bacterial pathogen to be described.

It is a straight or slightly curved slender bacillus, about the same size as the tubercle bacillus, with pointed, rounded or club-shaped ends; non-motile and non-sporing. With the Ziehl-Neelsen stain, it is less strongly acid-fast than the tubercle bacillus but it resists decolorization with 5 per cent H_2SO_4; the bacilli stain evenly in material from active lesions but usually show marked beading in smears from patients on effective chemotherapy; the proportion of solid-staining to irregular-staining bacilli is known as the 'morphological index'. The organism is Gram-positive and can be stained fairly readily by Gram's method.

Cultivation. This organism has not been grown successfully on any artificial culture media despite claims to the contrary; nor has it been possible to infect laboratory animals by conventional inoculation procedures. Much progress has been made in recent years in growing the leprosy bacillus in the footpad of the mouse, presumably facilitated by temperatures below 37°C. The bacilli survive well in wet-ice refrigeration so that suspected scrapings or tissue may be sent by air to laboratories equipped to do mouse-pad tests. The rate of division is very slow and numbers in the inoculated mouse footpad are limited to c. 10^6 bacilli; thymectomized, irradiated mice provide a host that develops generalized infection with invasion of nerves, skin and other tissues.

Laboratory Diagnosis

Films are made from any ulcerated nodule on the skin, or a non-ulcerated nodule may be punctured with a needle and squeezed until lymph exudes, from which films are made. Films may also be prepared from scrapings from a skin incision, particularly of the ear lobe, which may yield a positive result even when there is no obvious local lesion. Or a piece of skin (about 2 mm deep) overlying a nodule may be removed with curved scissors and smears prepared from the deep surface. Films should be made in all cases from scrapings or secretions from the nasal mucosa, as diagnostic information may be obtained in this way even when skin lesions are not obvious.

Films or sections are stained by the Ziehl-Neelsen method, with 5 per cent instead of 20 per cent sulphuric acid. The presence of the characteristic acid-fast bacilli, especially when they occur in large numbers inside cells, is diagnostic.

When the lungs are affected the bacilli may be demonstrated in the sputum, and may be differentiated from the tubercle bacillus by decolorizing with both 5 and 20 per cent H_2SO_4 in the Ziehl-Neelsen stain, and by guinea-pig inoculation.

Infection of the mouse footpad, which can be initiated with even a few leprosy bacilli, is followed by the production of characteristic leprosy lesions. This model is also useful in testing strains for drug resistance and in studying the antimicrobial activity of new drugs against the leprosy bacillus. Thus, in clinical trials, the viability of the leprosy bacilli can be assessed more reliably by the mouse footpad test than by the morphological index.

For an assessment of the Mitsuda skin reaction with lepromin (a boiled extract of lepromatous tissue) in the diagnosis of leprosy, see Volume I, Chapter 23.

FURTHER READING

HOBBY, GLADYS L., REDMOND, W. B., RUNYON. E. H., SCHAEFER, W. B., WAYNE, L. G. & WICHELHAUSEN, RUTH H. (1967) A study of pulmonary disease associated with mycobacteria other than *Mycobacterium tuberculosis*: identification and characterization of the mycobacteria. *American Review of Respiratory Diseases*, **95**, 954.

REES, R. J. W. & WEDDELL, A. G. M. (1970) Transmission of human leprosy to the mouse. *Bulletin of the World Health Organization*, **64**, 31.

SELKON, J. B. (1969) Atypical mycobacteria: a review. *Tubercle*, London, Supplement, **50**, 70.

W.H.O. REPORT (1970) Fourth report of expert committee on leprosy. *World Health Organization Technical Report Series*, No. 459.

26. Actinomyces: Nocardia

ACTINOMYCES

Actinomyces is a genus of anaerobic or micro-aerophilic, non-acid-fast organisms within the family Actinomycetaceae.

There are three species in this genus; *Actinomyces israelii* which is primarily commensal and occasionally pathogenic in man, *Actinomyces bovis,* which causes infection in bovines, and *Actinomyces baudetii,* the causal agent of actinomycosis in dogs and cats.

ACTINOMYCES ISRAELII

Morphology and staining. In pus the organism forms colonies that can be seen with the naked eye, e.g. 0·3–1 mm in diameter, and are referred to as *sulphur granules;* in early infections they are white and semi-transparent but develop a yellow colour later and eventually, in long-standing infections become dark brown.

Under the microscope a crushed granule is seen as a mycelium, or felted mass of branching filaments 1 μm thick; centrally, filaments irregularly interlaced, but at periphery of colony filaments arranged radially; true dichotomous branching, but rapid break up of central filaments into coccal and bacillary fragments so that extensive branching rare. Club-shaped structures of lipoidal material around colonies are rare in *Actino. israelii* infections but common in *Actino. bovis* infections.

In cultures, typical mycelium is incomplete; there are short bacillary forms resembling diphtheroid bacilli and some branching filaments.

Staining. Filaments are Gram-positive but show Gram-negative areas. Clubs are Gram-negative and stain acid-fast when 1 per cent instead of 20 per cent H_2SO_4 is used for decolourization in the Ziehl-Neelsen method.

Cultural characters. Anaerobic or micro-aerophilic conditions required; 5 per cent CO_2 assists growth; optimum temperature 37°C; growth enhanced by addition of blood, glucose or serum.

1. BLOOD AGAR. Colonies raised, nodular, cream-coloured and opaque; pleomorphic and firmly adherent to medium.
2. SHAKE CULTURE IN NUTRIENT AGAR. Colonies characteristically distributed in a zone 10–20 mm below surface; deeper colonies larger and knobby.
3. BROTH. Growth in bottom of tube of knobby white granules, supernatant clear.

Biochemical reactions. Saccharolytic anaerogenic fermentation of a wide range of substrates; no action on starch; non-haemolytic; non-proteolytic; no soluble pigments on solid media.

Antigenic character. Strains antigenically homogeneous and different from *Actino. bovis* and *Actino. baudetii.*

Animal pathogenicity. Circumscribed tumour-like granulomatous lesions containing colonies of the organism are produced in rabbits and guinea-pigs; lesions are not always produced and are never extensive or fatal.

LABORATORY DIAGNOSIS

The pus from the lesion, usually in the cervico-facial region but sometimes from abdominal infections, should be submitted to the laboratory in a sterile universal container, swabs are not suitable for diagnostic purposes.

The pus is inspected for the presence of sulphur granules and then a suitable portion is mixed with sterile water in a universal container or test tube with screw-on lid and the container shaken. It is allowed to stand and the sulphur granules sink to the bottom and are easily seen. They are collected in a pasteur pipette. One granule is placed in the middle of a slide and crushed with another slide, the slides being applied to each other in the form of a cross. After separation of the two films and fixation by heat, one film is stained by Gram's method and the other by a modified Ziehl-Neelsen technique. **Microscopy.** The felted branching structure is seen with coccal and bacillary bodies. The Gram reaction is usually but not always positive. The Ziehl-Neelsen stain shows the organism to be non-acid fast.

Culture. The sulphur granules are washed in sterile saline to separate them from the pus cells and are then inoculated into 1 per cent glucose semi-solid agar which is rolled between the hands to give a uniform distribution of the granules and then incubated aerobically at 37°C. Other granules are put into broth which is incubated aerobically at 37°C. Others are inoculated on to blood agar plates which are incubated aerobically and anaerobically.

In the shake culture the maximal growth occurs 10–20 mm below the surface. The broth culture shows the presence of white granules and the anaerobic blood agar culture shows the characteristic colonies. Incubation should be continued for 14 days at least.

Microscopy of the colonies shows Gram-positive diphtheroid-like bacilli with some branching. From a human case these findings are sufficient for a diagnosis of actinomycosis. In practice it is not easy to isolate the organism if sulphur granules are not found in the specimen.

ACTINOMYCES BOVIS

On microscopy *Actino. bovis* shows a similar morphology to that of *Actino. israelii,* but clubs are more obvious. In culture the colonies of *Actino. bovis* are smoother and softer in consistency that those of *Actino. israelii* and do not adhere to the medium. *Actino. bovis* produces acid from starch. It shows no serological relationship with *Actino. israelii* or *Actino baudetii.*

ACTINOMYCES BAUDETII

Clubs absorb basic stains and not acid stains; colonies grow slowly; no serological relationship with *Actino. israelii* or *Actino. bovis.*

NOCARDIA

Nocardia is a genus of aerobic organisms, some of which are acid-fast and some chromogenic. There are more than 40 species in the genus but the majority are saprophytic.

NOCARDIA ASTEROIDES

Morphology and staining. In pus the organism appears as a branched filament 1 μm thick, occasionally with deeply staining bodies at the ends. In culture it appears as bacillary forms and branched forms.

The filaments are Gram-positive; they are acid-fast by the modified Ziehl-Neelsen method.

Cultural characters. Aerobic conditions required; no growth anaerobically or micro-aerophilically; optimum temperature 37°C; growth on ordinary nutrient media.

1. AGAR PLATE. Whitish umbonate friable colonies, later yellow and later still, pink; colony becomes star-shaped with irregular edge.

2. SERUM BROTH. Waxy pellicle in 48 h with small round fluffy masses in bottom of tube, no turbidity.

Biochemical reactions. Acid from glucose and glycerol; non-haemolytic; pink pigmentation of colony on blood agar.

Animal pathogenicity. Causes death in rabbits and guinea-pigs in 5–30 days; lungs, liver and spleen contain small white nodules; abscesses may develop, which contain branching forms of the organism.

LABORATORY DIAGNOSIS

The specimen may be empyema fluid or pus from a secondary brain abscess. The specimen should be collected in a sterile universal container; swabs are not suitable.

Microscopy. A Gram-stained film and a modified Ziehl-Neelsen stained film is prepared from the pus. The nocardia is Gram-positive and acid-fast and appears as long branched threads, some with deeply staining bodies at the ends.

Culture. Aerobic and anaerobic cultures are made on nutrient agar and blood agar, and in serum broth, and are incubated at 37°C. Growth occurs only in aerobic cultures on solid medium and the characteristic colonies appear which become pigmented on further incubation. The serum broth shows pellicle formation and fluffy deposit.

Animal inoculation of the colonies will give rise to the typical fatal illness.

NOCARDIA MADURAE

One of the causal agents of mycetoma, or madura foot, a disease not found in Great Britain but travellers to semi-tropical and tropical countries may return with it.

Morphology and staining. In tissue lesions and pus, granules are seen usually pale yellow in colour. Microscopical examination of a crushed granule reveals a mycelium or felted mass of branching filaments, 0·4–0·6 μm thick; fragmented and ovoid forms are also present. Microscopical examination of a culture shows long filaments and branched forms in young growths and fragmented forms and ovoid bodies in older ones. Staining is uniformly Gram-positive and non-acid fast.

Cultural characters. Aerobic growth only; no growth in anaerobic conditions. Optimum temperature 37°C.

1. NUTRIENT AGAR. Small round white convex colonies which at 14 days are 1–3 mm in diameter; become yellow and eventually pink; very adherent to medium and horny in consistence; rosette-like in appearance.

2. BROTH. Deposit of small puff balls; no turbidity; no pellicle formation.

Biochemical reactions. No action on sugars.

Animal pathogenicity. In rabbits, guinea-pigs, cats and mice, a local nodule appears after subcutaneous injection; lasts about a month and then disappears.

LABORATORY DIAGNOSIS

Specimen is pus from a sinus of the foot. It should be inspected for yellow granules which are separated by shaking with sterile water. Granules are stained by Gram's method and a modified Ziehl-Neelsen procedure. A Gram-positive mycelium with branched filaments is seen. Non-acid-fast by the Ziehl-Neelsen procedure.

Granules are cultured aerobically and anaerobically at 37°C on nutrient agar and in broth for at least 14 days. The organism grows only aerobically and the typical horny rosette colonies are seen on the nutrient agar. The broth culture shows a poor growth of small puff balls with a clear supernatant. Microscopy of the colonies shows the typical morphology and staining reaction.

FURTHER READING

PORTER, I. A. (1953) Actinomycosis in Scotland. *British Medical Journal*, **2**, 1084.

SULLIVAN, H. R. & GOLDSWORTHY, N. E. (1940) Comparative study of anaerobic stains of *Actinomyces* from clinically normal mouths and from actinomycotic lesions. *Journal of Pathology and Bacteriology*, **51**, 253.

27. Neisseria

The genus *Neisseria* contains two pathogenic species, *Neisseria meningitidis* (the meningococcus), the casual organism of an acute purulent meningitis, and *N. gonorrhoeae* (the gonococcus), that causes gonorrhoea, a sexually transmitted infection of the genito-urinary tract; in addition there are several commensal species, e.g. *N. catarrhalis*, some of which are potentially pathogenic. Although the two pathogenic members are morphologically and culturally very similar, they are described here separately.

NEISSERIA MENINGITIDIS

Morphology and staining. Oval Gram-negative diplococci with flattened or concave opposing edges and the long axes parallel: about 0·8 μm in diameter: typically seen in large numbers inside polymorphonuclear pus cells: films from cultures show more rounded cocci and some pleomorphism with irregular staining: although capsules are not ordinarily evident, the 'capsule-swelling' phenomenon is elicited when exudates or young cultures are mixed with specific antiserum: non-motile, non-sporing.

Cultural characters. Aerobe, but primary cultures grow better in an atmosphere containing 5–10 per cent CO_2: optimum temperature 35°–36°C (range 25°–42°C): growth on nutrient agar (pH 7·0–7·4) is enhanced by addition of blood or serum: after 24 h incubation on serum agar colonies are small, greyish, transparent, smooth disks—1–2 mm in diameter. After 48 h colonies larger, with opaque raised centre and thin transparent margins which may be crenated: no haemolysis on blood agar.

Sensitivity to physical and chemical agents. Killed at 55°C in 5 min: dies quickly at room temperature, but cultures may be maintained in sealed tubes of serum agar or Dorset egg medium at 37°C for several weeks: sensitive to sulphonamides and many other antimicrobial drugs but sulphonamide-resistant strains are now common in North America.

Biochemical reactions. Ferments glucose and maltose, but not lactose, sucrose or inulin: use peptone-water serum agar slopes in screw-capped bijou containers: oxidase reaction quickly positive when the reagent is flooded on to mixed cultures on heated blood-agar.

Antigenic characters. Four main serogroups, A, B, C, D plus some recently recognized groups, e.g. Y and Z.

Group A meningococcus is the main infecting type in countries where cerebrospinal meningitis frequently occurs in epidemics, e.g. Central Africa, but has been supplanted by groups B and C in outbreaks among military personnel and in civilian communities in North America.

Laboratory Diagnosis

Cerebrospinal fluid from suspected cases must be *urgently* submitted to the laboratory: cell-counts are done and smears of centrifuged deposit stained with methylene blue and Gram's method (with neutral red counterstain): Gram-negative diplococci are seen filling a limited proportion of the pus cells: many are extra-cellular: if scanty, diplococci may be seen more easily in MB stained smears. Culture centrifuged deposit on blood or serum agar or heated blood agar and incubate in 5–10 per cent CO_2: if organisms scanty or absent in direct smears, add glucose broth to deposit, incubate for 18 h and subculture.

A positive precipitin reaction may be sought by layering CSF on to specific antiserum in a capillary tube: a retrospective diagnosis may be attempted by testing paired sera for complement-fixing antibodies: after preliminary identification of culture, fermentation reactions may be used to confirm diagnosis.

Blood culture should be done in cases of meningitis and suspected meningococcal septicaemia with frequent subcultures up to seven days.

NEISSERIA GONORRHOEAE

Morphology and staining. Identical with *N. meningitidis*: extra-cellular as well as intracellular diplococci seen in smears of pus: pleomorphism in films of older cultures.

Cultural characters. Aerobe: addition of 5–10 per cent CO_2 essential for primary culture: optimum temperature 35°–36°C (range 30°–39°C): growth requirements similar to meningococcus: heated blood-agar or agar containing fresh sterile serum recommended: selective media, e.g. Thayer and Martin's medium (1966) or that recommended in PHLS monograph series No. 1 (1972), are needed for culture of specimens with mixed flora, e.g. cervical or high vaginal swabs from chronic infections and symptomless carriers: for rectal swabs, trimethoprim (8 μg/cm) should be added to inhibit growth of *Proteus* (Seth, 1970).

Kellogg *et al.* (1968) have shown that gonococci may be divided into four biotypes (1–4) related to colonial appearance on their special colonial type (CT) medium, auto-agglutinability and virulence as tested by intraurethral inoculation in human volunteers: types 1 and 2 produce small, glistening, convex, dark brown colonies, auto-agglutinable and virulent: types 3 and 4 produce larger, flatter, unpigmented colonies, not autoagglutinable and non-virulent.

Sensitivity to physical and chemical agents. Killed by heat at 55°C for 5 min, dies quickly under natural environmental conditions, but may remain viable in pus on linen or other fabrics for 2–3 days: cultures tend to die within a few days unless subcultured and kept at 37°C: sensitive to penicillin and other antimicrobial drugs, but penicillin-resistant strains sometimes occur, particularly among those infected in cities or abroad (MRC Report, 1961).

Biochemical reactions. In the same sugar containing media and containers as for meningococcus, *N. gonorrhoeae* ferments glucose, but not maltose, lactose or sucrose: oxidase reaction quickly positive.

Antigenic characters. Antigenically heterogeneous: shares certain somatic antigens with meningococci: not used in diagnosis.

Laboratory Diagnosis

Smears of discharge are thinly spread, fixed gently by heat and stained by Gram's method with neutral red or Sandiford's counterstain: in acute untreated cases, typical Gram-negative intracellular diplococci filling a limited proportion of the pus cells are commonly seen, but may be scanty and pleomorphic and occurring only extracellularly in chronic or treated cases: (fresh, wet preparations of vaginal discharge should be examined for trichomonas). Presumptive positive Gram-stained smears must be confirmed by culture, particularly in cases that may involve legal proceedings.

IMMUNOFLUORESCENCE. The fluorescent antibody technique (FA) for the identification of *N. gonorrhoeae* in smears of genital secretions is being used in some laboratories for on-the-spot diagnosis of gonorrhoea. The technique is especially useful for the diagnosis of the infection in women who may be symptomless carriers of the disease. The method of Somerville as modified by Thin (1970) is recommended. It is advisable to use a high quality fluorescence microscope (e.g. Zeiss) with an optical system designed to give the maximum intensity of light, since otherwise gonococci do not fluoresce brightly.

Smears from the urethra, cervix and rectum are stained with specific antiserum to *N. gonorrhoeae* prepared in rabbits and conjugated with fluorescein isothiocyanate (Difco Laboratories). In order to inhibit the fluorescence of antigenically related neisseriae and the non-specific fluorescence of *Staphylococcus aureus* and other bacteria, the conjugate is diluted before use with an equal volume of normal human serum. The bright non-specific fluorescence of leucocytes which previously caused difficulty by preventing the recognition of intracellular gonococci is counteracted by the use of naphthalein black* (added to the human serum used as the diluent in a concentration of 3 mg/ml of serum) as a counterstain. Gonococci appear as double rings of fluorescence—solid staining of the cells is unusual: they are easily recognized by an experienced viewer even when they are scanty.

The 'immediate' test can be completed within 30 min. Although it has to be confirmed by laboratory culture, on-the-spot diagnosis may be of considerable help to the clinician and

---

* Naphthalein black. TS for electrophoresis (Amidoschwarz), supplied by Messrs G. T. Gurr.

compares favourably with either Gram-stained smears or laboratory culture.

A 'delayed' technique whereby smears taken from culture media after 24 h incubation are examined in the same way, may give a somewhat higher yield of positive results than the immediate test and the results are easier to read (Thin, Williams and Nicol, 1971).

Material for culture must either be inoculated on appropriate media *immediately in the clinic* or *within 1–2 h if sent to the laboratory*: otherwise, specimens on charcoal-impregnated swabs should be placed in Stuart's transport medium in which gonococci will remain viable for 24 h or longer at room temperature. After incubation in 5–10 per cent CO_2 for 1–2 days suspicious colonies are picked for fermentation tests: plates with mixed growth should be submitted to the oxidase test: colonies seen to be developing a purplish colour within 1–2 min may be picked for subculture but the reagent is quickly lethal: or a colony is picked and applied to a piece of filter paper moistened with the oxidase reagent. A positive reaction in deep purple colour, appears almost immediately. After subculture of some suspicious colonies the remainder of the culture plate should be tested for the oxidase reaction.

To determine the MIC in penicillin sensitivity tests subcultures are made on enriched media containing doubling dilutions of penicillin from 1·0 to 0·004 $\mu g/cm$ with the Oxford staphylococcus or a reference gonococcus strain as control organisms: alternatively, disks containing 0·03, 0·25 and 1·0 unit of benzyl penicillin may be used and the zone of inhibition converted to an MIC value from a standard curve. Strains with MIC of 0·5 to 1 unit/ml are regarded as highly resistant (see Chap. 8 and PHLS monograph series No. 1, 1972).

With disks containing 1 unit of penicillin, a zone diameter of 28–26 mm indicates strain sensitivity to 0·1 unit/ml penicillin, 25–24 mm indicates strain sensitivity to 0·2 unit/ml penicillin, 20–18 mm indicates strain sensitivity to 0·4 unit/ml penicillin and 17–15 mm indicates strain sensitivity to 0·5 unit/ml penicillin. Strains giving diameters of less than 15 mm are comparatively rare.

The complement fixation test, using a suspension of recently isolated strains of gonococci as antigen, gives variable results and is most likely to be positive in persistent infections in the female and in gonococcal complications such as salpingitis and arthritis. The specificity of the test increases with increasing positivity of the reaction but both false positive and false negative results are not infrequent. Cross reactions occur with sera from patients with meningococcal antibodies and may also be found in cases of chronic bronchitis and bronchiectasis.

COMMENSAL NEISSERIAE

These organisms occur on various mucous surfaces of the body and are regularly found in the muccous secretions of the throat, nose and mouth; and less frequently, on the genital mucosae. When inflammatory or other pathological conditions affect these mucous membranes, Gram-negative diplococci may constitute a prominent feature of the bacterial flora, and may possibly act as secondary infecting agents in such conditions.

There is some uncertainty regarding the biological classification of this group of organisms, and the taxonomic significance to be attached to colony characters, pigmentation and fermentation of different carbohydrates

Table 27.1 Fermentation reactions of neisseria group

	Glucose	Maltose	Lactose	Sucrose
Meningococcus	+	+	—	—
Gonococcus	+	—	—	—
N. catarrhalis and N. flavescens	—	—	—	—
N. pharyngis (N. flava and related types)	+	+	—	d
N. mucosa	+	—	(+)	—

+ = acid; d = variation in reaction among different types; (+) = delayed reaction is doubtful. Two sub-groups may be recognized: (1) characterized by complete absence of fermentative properties, e.g. *N. catarrhalis* and *N. flavescens*; and (2) possessing such properties, e.g. *N. flava* and related types sometimes combined with *N. sicca* and *N. perflava* as *N. pharyngis* (Cowan and Steel, 1966) and *N. mucosa* (see Table 27.1).

Neisseria Catarrhalis

Morphology and staining. Practically identical with the meningococcus. In some strains the cocci are relatively large.

Cultural characters. Grows on ordinary media without serum and at room temperature; the colonies may be larger than those of the meningococcus, especially when fully grown, and are thicker and more opaque. The colony characters, however, may vary considerably, and both 'smooth' and 'rough' forms are observed: no fermentative properties. Cultures tend to be auto-agglutinable.

Neisseria flavescens

This organism has been described as the causative pathogen in a group of cases of meningitis in America. It resembles the meningococcus in morphology, but on blood agar produces golden-yellow colonies. It does not ferment carbohydrates. It may be biologically related to *N. flava*.

Neisseria Flava and Related Types

The morphology of these organisms is like that of *N. catarrhalis* and they grow on ordinary media at room temperature. Cultures develop, after 48 hours, greenish-yellow or greenish-grey colours. Young colonies may simulate those of the meningococcus.

Biochemical reactions vary according to the type.

Neisseria sicca

Resembles *N. catarrhalis*, but its colonies are markedly dry, tough and adherent to the medium. This organism may not be a separate species but a 'rough' variant of some other member of the group.

Neisseria mucosa

Differs from the other members of the group in being definitely capsulate and producing mucoid colonies. This type may represent a variant of one of the other members of the group. Strains corresponding to it have been reported in cases of meningitis.

VEILLONELLA

Members of this genus are present as commensals in natural cavities of man and animals, particularly the mouth and alimentary tract: apparently not primarily pathogenic but has been isolated from cases of appendicitis, pyorrhoea and pulmonary lesions, and is potentially pathogenic.

They are minute Gram-negative cocci about 0.3 μm in diameter and occurring in masses. Culturally anaerobic and grow best at 37°C. The type of species is *Veill. parvula*, whose distinctive characters are: the formation of hydrogen, carbon dioxide, hydrogen sulphide and indole from polypeptides, the fermentation of glucose and certain other sugars, haemolytic action, and the reduction of nitrate to nitrate.

REFERENCES

Cowan, S. T. & Steel, K. J. (1966) *Manual for the Identification of Medical Bacteria*, 2nd edn. Cambridge University Press.

PHLS Report (1972) *Laboratory Diagnosis of Venereal Disease*. A. E. Wilkinson, C. E. D. Taylor, D. A. McSwiggan, G. C. Turner, J. A. Ryecroft, G. H. Lowe. Public Health Laboratory Service: Monograph Series, No. 1.

Kellogg, D. S. *et al.* (1968) *Neisseria gonorrhoeae*: Colonial variation and pathogenicity during 35 months *in vitro*. *Journal of Bacteriology*, **96**, 596.

MRC Report (1961) Resistance of gonococci to penicillin: report of a working party to the Medical Research Council. *Lancet*, **ii.** 226.

Seth, A. (1970) The use of trimethoprim to prevent overgrowth by Proteus in the cultivation of *N. gonorrhoea*. *British Journal of Venereal Diseases*, **46**, 207.

Thayer, J. D. & Martin, J. E. (1966) Improved medium selective for cultivation of *N. gonorrhoeae* and *N. meningitidis*. *Public Health Report*, **81**, 559.

Thin, R. H. T. (1970) Immunofluorescent methods for diagnosis of gonorrhoea in women. *British Journal of Venereal Diseases*, **46**, 27.

Thin, R. H. T., Williams, I. A. & Nicol, C. S. (1971) Direct and delayed methods of immunofluorescent diagnosis of gonorrhoea in women. *British Journal of Venereal Diseases*, **47**, 27.

28. The Enterobacteriaceae: Salmonella

ENTEROBACTERIACEAE

Definition of the family. The Enterobacteriaceae are Gram-negative bacilli that are either motile with peritrichous flagella or non-motile, grow both aerobically and anaerobically on simple laboratory media and on MacConkey's bile-salt-lactose medium, are oxidase-negative and, with few exceptions, catalase-positive, and reduce nitrates to nitrites. They ferment glucose in peptone water with the production of either acid or acid and gas, and they break down glucose and other carbohydrates both fermentatively under anaerobic conditions and oxidatively under aerobic conditions, e.g. in the Hugh and Leifson test.

Other families of Gram-negative bacilli, from which the Enterobacteriaceae must be distinguished, are the Brucellaceae (parvo-bacteria), most species of which are non-motile, small-celled, exacting in nutritional requirements and lacking in fermentative ability, the Achromobacteraceae (*Acinetobacter*, non-motile and oxidase-negative; *Alcaligenes*, motile and oxidase-positive) which are non-fermentative, the Pseudomonadaceae, which have polar flagella, are oxidase-positive, and react only oxidatively with carbohydrates, and the Bacteroidaceae which are obligatory anaerobes (Table 28.1). Oxidase-positive organisms otherwise resembling Enterobacteriaceae are ascribed to a genus, *Aeromonas*, unallocated to any family.

Genera of Enterobacteriaceae. Over the years there have been a number of confusing alterations in the nomenclature of the genera that constitute the family Enterobacteriaceae. The genera recognized by Cowan and Steel (1965) are: *Citrobacter* (including the Ballerup-Bethesda group), *Enterobacter* (syn. *Cloaca*), *Escherichia* (including the Alkalescens-Dispar group), *Hafnia*, *Klebsiella*, *Proteus*, *Providencia*, *Salmonella* (including the Arizona group), *Serratia* and *Shigella*. These genera are differentiated by their biochemical characters (Table 28.2) and it is only within a genus that serological and other methods are employed for further subdivision.

Some members of the family of Enterobacteriaceae, e.g. *Salmonella* spp., *Shigella* spp. and enteropathogenic strains of *Escherichia coli*, are primary pathogens for man and their precise identification is important both clinically and epidemiologically. The other

Table 28.1 Differentiating characters of the main families of Gram-negative bacilli

Family	Motility*	Growth on simple and MacConkey's media	Growth in air	Oxidase reaction	Reaction with glucose†
Enterobacteriaceae	d	+	+	−	F
Brucellaceae	−	−	+	d	F or −
Achromobacteraceae	d	+	+	d	O or −
Pseudomonadaceae	+	+	+	+	O
Bacteroidaceae	−	−	−	−	F

* Flagella polar in Pseudomonadaceae, peritrichous in motile members of other families.
† Reaction with glucose in the Hugh and Leifson test:
   F = acid produced under anaerobic conditions (fermentatively).
   O = acid produced only under aerobic conditions (oxidatively).
   − = acid not produced either fermentatively or oxidatively.

+ = Most or all members positive.
− = Most or all members negative.
d = Different reactions in different genera, species or strains.

Table 28.2 Differentiating characters of the main genera of Enterobacteriaceae and some exceptional species

Genus	Acid from lactose	Gas from glucose	Motility	Urease	Citrate utilized*	Voges-Proskauer	Growth in KCN
Escherichia	+	+	+	–	–	–	–
Shigella	–	–	–	–	–	–	–
Citrobacter	+	+	+	d	+	–	+
Salmonella	–	+	+	–	+	–	–
Enterobacter	+	+	+	d	+	+	+
Hafnia	–	+	+	–	+	d	+
Klebsiella	+	+	–	+	+	+	+
Serratia	d	d	+	–	+	+	+
Proteus	–	+	+	+	d	–	+
Providencia	–	+	+	–	+	–	+

* Citrate utilization tested in Koser's or Simmons's medium.
  + = Most or all strains positive.
  – = Most or all strains negative.
  d = Some strains positive. Some negative.

Notable exceptions:
  Alkalescens-Dispar organisms are like *Escherichia,* but non-lactose fermenting, non-gas-producing and non-motile.
  Ballerup-Bethesda organisms are like *Citrobacter,* but non-lactose fermenting.
  Salmonella arizonae: most strains are lactose-fermenting and some are gelatin liquefying.
  Salmonella typhi is non-gas-producing and non-citrate utilizing.
  Klebsiella rhinoscleromatis is negative in all reactions tabled except that with KCN.
  Klebsiella ozaenae is late-lactose-fermenting and Voges-Proskauer negative; some strains are negative in the gas, citrate or urease tests.

enterobacteria are essentially commensals or saprophytes, but some, e.g. *Esch. coli*, are also common pathogens in the urinary tract, in wounds and in organs associated with the gut, e.g. appendix and gall-bladder, and most enterobacteria occasionally act as opportunistic pathogens in individuals with defective defences. Commensal and saprophytic enterobacteria may, therefore, be isolated from clinical specimens, but their precise identification, apart from the determination of their antibiotic sensitivities, has little clinical significance, although it may sometimes assist in tracing the sources of outbreaks of infection among patients in hospital.

The vernacular term 'coliform bacilli' is commonly used to refer to organisms resembling *Escherichia coli,* but there is no general agreement on the definition and membership of the coliform group. Some authors use the term as being synonymous with the Enterobacteriaceae, others confine its use to the lactose-fermenting enterobacteria (i.e. most species of *Escherichia, Klebsiella, Citrobacter* and *Enterobacter*) and still others use it, as generally in this book, for the enterobacteria that are urinary-tract, wound and opportunistic pathogens (e.g. *Escherichia, Klebsiella* and *Proteus*). *Pseudomonas pyocyanea* (*Ps. aeruginosa*), which is not an enterobacterium, is sometimes regarded as a 'coliform bacillus' in this last sense.

Lactose fermentation. Reactions with lactose are of great practical importance for the primary isolation of enterobacteria from clinical specimens. The specimen, e.g. faeces, is usually plated on a lactose-containing medium, such as MacConkey's medium or deoxycholate citrate agar (DCA), on which the colonies of lactose-fermenting bacteria are pink and those of non-lactose-fermenting bacteria are pale. This procedure makes possible an immediate presumptive distinction between colonies of the true intestinal pathogens, salmonellae and shigellae, which do not ferment lactose, and colonies of the common intestinal commensals, escherichiae and klebsiellae, which do ferment it. The identity of the pale colonies as salmonellae or shigellae must, however, be confirmed by further tests, because some commensal and saprophytic enterobacteria are non-lactose-fermenting, e.g. all *Proteus* and *Providencia* species and the Ballerup-Bethesda, Alkalescens-Dispar and Hafnia groups of organisms (Table 28.2).

The term 'paracolon bacillus' was frequently used in the past to describe non-lactose-fermenting coliform bacilli that did not belong to the well-defined, non-lactose-fermenting genera, *Salmonella*, *Shigella* and *Proteus*. These bacteria, however, are now regarded as being non-lactose-fermenting variants of organisms in genera that are characteristically lactose-fermenting, e.g. organisms of the Alkalescens-Dispar group as non-lactose-fermenting (and non-motile and anaerogenic) variants of *Escherichia*, organisms of the Ballerup-Bethesda group as non-lactose-fermenting variants of *Citrobacter* and organisms of the Hafnia group as non-lactose-fermenting variants of *Enterobacter*. Because their full identification is often difficult and because they are not important pathogens, many clinical bacteriologists do not identify paracolon bacilli further than to exclude the possibility that they are salmonella, shigella, proteus or pseudomonas.

Other Gram-negative bacilli isolated from clinical material are morphologically, and sometimes culturally, similar to the enterobacteria although they do not belong to any genus in the family Enterobacteriaceae. They are distinguished by their non-conformation with the criteria defining the family and they include genera such as *Acinetobacter* (including 'Bacterium anitratum'), *Alcaligenes* and *Pseudomonas*. They may be observed initially as pale colonies growing on MacConkey's medium.

Identification of genus and species. The effort necessary to identify a Gram-negative bacillus that grows readily on ordinary agar varies. Although some genera, e.g. *Proteus*, may be easy to recognize, others are particularly difficult. However, for the important intestinal pathogens, *Salmonella*, *Shigella* and the entero-pathogenic strains of *Escherichia coli*, clear-cut methods are available and full identification is essential.

Only a minority of laboratories are able to maintain stocks of all the media required to perform the full range of biochemical tests. Not only are some of the media difficult to prepare but the quality of each batch must be tested with organisms known to give both positive and negative results. Even if a diagnostic laboratory has the facilities to identify all the coliform organisms that may be isolated from clinical specimens, such detailed information is generally not of great value.

SALMONELLA

BIOLOGICAL CHARACTERS

Definition of genus Salmonella. Enterobacteria (fermentative, facultatively anaerobic, oxidase-negative Gram-negative rods) that generally are motile, aerogenic, non-lactose-fermenting, urease-negative, citrate-utilizing, Voges-Proskauer-negative and KCN-negative (KCN-sensitive).

Morphology and staining. Gram-negative bacilli, 2–4 μm × 0·6 μm, non-acid-fast, non-sporing and non-capsulate. Most serotypes ('species') are motile with peritrichous flagella, but *S. gallinarum* and *S. pullorum* are non-motile and non-motile variants (OH → O variation) of other serotypes are occasionally found. Most strains of most serotypes form type-1 (mannose-sensitive, haemagglutinating) fimbriae; *S. gallinarum*, *S. pullorum* and a few strains of other serotypes form type-2 (non-haemagglutinating) fimbriae, and most *S. paratyphi A* strains are non-fimbriate (Duguid, Anderson and Campbell, 1966).

Culture. Aerobic and facultatively anaerobic. Grow on simple laboratory media in temperature range 15°–41°C, optimally at 37°C. Many strains are prototrophic, i.e. capable of growing on a glucose-ammonium minimal medium such as that of Davis and Mingioli, but some strains are auxotrophic and require enrichment of the medium with one or more amino acids or vitamins, e.g. most *S. typhi* strains require tryptophan (Stokes and Bayne, 1958).

1. NUTRIENT AGAR AND BLOOD AGAR.

Colonies of most strains are moderately large (e.g. 2–3 mm in diameter), grey-white, moist, circular disks with a smooth convex surface and entire edge. Their size and degree of opacity varies with the serotype, e.g. those of *S. paratyphi A*, *S. abortus-ovis*, *S. pullorum*, *S. sendai* and *S. typhi-suis* are relatively small. 'Rough', non-virulent variants (S → R variation) form opaque granular colonies with an irregular surface and indented edge: R variants arise spontaneously by mutation and are commonest in platings of old laboratory strains maintained by repeated subculture. Many strains of *S. paratyphi B* and a few of some other serotypes form large mucoid colonies, or colonies surrounded by a thick mucoid 'slime wall', when plates are left at room temperature for a few days after incubation for 24 hours at 37°C. The mucoid character is due to the formation of loose extracellular polysaccharide slime. Only a few strains show capsules visible in a wet India ink film.

2. DIFFERENTIAL AND SELECTIVE SOLID MEDIA.

These media are valuable for the isolation of salmonellae from faeces and other materials contaminated with many bacteria of other kinds. They include:

(i) *MacConkey's bile-salt lactose agar medium.* After 18–24 hours at 37°C the colonies are pale yellow or nearly colourless, 1–3 mm in diameter, and easily distinguished from the pink-red colonies of lactose-fermenting coliform bacilli, which also grow well on this *unselective* differential (indicator) medium.

(ii) *Brilliant green MacConkey agar.* The addition of 0·004 per cent brilliant green, which is inhibitory to *Escherichia coli* and other commensal enterobacteria likely to outnumber the salmonellae in faeces, makes MacConkey's medium selective for salmonellae except *S. typhi.*

(iii) *Leifson's deoxycholate-citrate agar* (*DCA*). The colonies of salmonellae on DCA are similar to or slightly smaller in size than those on MacConkey's medium. They are pale, nearly colourless, smooth, shiny and translucent. Sometimes they have a black centre and sometimes they are surrounded by a zone of cleared medium. They are easily distinguished from the opaque pink colonies of lactose-fermenting coliform bacilli, which are largely inhibited on this *selective* differential medium.

(iv) *Wilson and Blair's brilliant-green bismuth sulphite agar* (*BSA*). This medium is particularly valuable for the isolation of *S. typhi*. Cultures should be examined after 24 hours, then again after 48 hours. Closely packed colonies about 1 mm in diameter may take up the dye from the medium and appear green or pale brown. Larger, discrete colonies have a black centre and a clear translucent edge. All salmonellae, including *S. typhi*, may produce hydrogen sulphide which causes the colony to be surrounded by a metallic sheen. The medium is highly selective for salmonellae, being inhibitory to coliforms and shigellae.

3. PEPTONE WATER AND NUTRIENT BROTH.

Abundant growth with uniform turbidity. A surface pellicle generally forms on prolonged incubation. 'Rough' (R) variants, which have a hydrophobic surface and are liable to autoagglutinate in saline solutions, produce a granular deposit and sometimes a thick pellicle.

4. ENRICHMENT MEDIA.

These are liquid media used to assist the isolation of salmonellae from faeces, sewage, foodstuffs and other materials containing a mixed bacterial flora. The material is inoculated into the enrichment medium and during incubation any salmonellae grow rapidly while *Escherichia coli* and most other bacteria are inhibited. The enriched culture is plated on MacConkey's or DCA medium, usually after 24 hours. Proteus, which is often present in faeces and sewage, is often able to grow in the enrichment medium and its pale colonies in the platings must be distinguished from those of salmonellae. Good enrichment media include:

(i) *Tetrathionate broth*, with or without brilliant green which increases its selectivity for most salmonellae but makes it rather too inhibitory for *S. typhi* and shigellae.

(ii) *Selenite F broth.* Perhaps the most used enrichment medium for materials that may yield either salmonellae or shigellae.

(iii) *Strontium chloride broth.* This medium was found by Iveson and Mackay-Scollay (1969) to be superior to selenite F broth for the isolation of a wide range of salmonellae from faeces and sewage. *Strontium selenite broth* was superior for the recovery of *S. typhi*.

Biochemical reactions. Although most species and strains conform with the pattern of reactions shown for *Salmonella* in Table 28.2, the decision that an organism is not a salmonella should not be based on the result of only a single test. Some strains show exceptional reactions in particular tests and it is necessary to consider the general pattern of the reactions in a group of tests.

1. FERMENTATION TESTS. Carbohydrates are generally fermented with the production of acid and gas. *S. typhi*, *S. gallinarum* and rare anaerogenic variants of other serotypes (e.g. *S. newport*) form only acid. Typically, glucose, mannitol, arabinose, maltose, dulcitol and sorbitol are fermented, but not lactose, sucrose, salicin or adonitol; the ONPG test is negative. Among exceptional strains, *S. cholerae-suis* and some strains of *S. typhi* do not ferment arabinose, whereas *S. cholerae-suis*, *S. pullorum*, most strains of *S. typhi* and some strains of *S. paratyphi A*, *S. paratyphi B*, *S. panama* and *S. worthington* do not ferment dulcitol.

2. DECARBOXYLASE TESTS. Salmonellae decarboxylate the amino acids, lysine, ornithine and arginine, but do not decarboxylate glutamic acid. *S. typhi* is exceptional in lacking ornithine decarboxylase.

'3. OTHER BIOCHEMICAL TESTS. Most salmonellae react as follows. Indole not produced. Methyl-red positive. Voges-Proskauer negative. Citrate utilized (except by *S. typhi* and *S. paratyphi A*). Malonate not utilized. Gluconate not utilized. Urease not produced. Phenylalanine deaminase not produced. H_2S produced in ferrous chloride-gelatin medium. KCN medium, no growth. Gelatin not liquefied.

Subgenera of Salmonella. A minority of serotypes gives biochemical reactions different from those just described as typical. Kauffmann (1969) has divided the genus *Salmonella* into four subgenera (Table 28.3); subgenus I, which contains the great majority of serotypes, including all those that commonly cause disease in man and mammals, gives the typical reactions, and the other subgenera give atypical reactions.

Table 28.3

	Subgenus			
	I	II	III	IV
Dulcitol	+	+	−	−
Lactose	−	−	+	−
Salicin	−	−	−	+
Malonate	−	+	+	−
KCN	−	−	−	+
Gelatin	−	+	+	+

Within each subgenus, a few strains give exceptional reactions, e.g. gelatin is liquefied by *S. abortus-bovis*, *S. azteca*, *S. schleissheim* and *S. texas* in subgenus I.

Arizona group. This group of organisms was originally named *Salmonella arizonae*. It is classified as subgenus III of *Salmonella* by Kauffmann (1969), though some authors give it the status of a separate genus, *Arizona*. The arizonae have been found mainly in reptiles and birds, but also occasionally in human patients with diarrhoea or septicaemia.

Arizona organisms exhibit important biochemical differences from typical salmonellae. Most strains ferment lactose promptly and others ferment it after several days' incubation. The ONPG test is positive, dulcitol is not fermented, malonate is usually utilized and gelatin is commonly liquefied after 7–10 days at 22°C.

Like the salmonellae, the arizonae are divided into numerous serogroups and serotypes by differences in their O and H antigens, many of which are closely similar to particular salmonella antigens though designated with different numbers (Edwards and Ewing, 1972; Kauffmann, 1969).

Antigenic structure of salmonellae. The genus *Salmonella* is subdivided in the Kauffmann-White classification into more than 1000 serotypes containing different combinations of antigens. The identification of serotypes depends on detection of the O (somatic) and H (flagellar) antigens by means of agglutination tests with specific antisera. Many different serotypes have one or more of their O or H antigens in common and their distinctive antigens have to be demonstrated in tests with 'single-factor' antisera which have been absorbed with heterologous organisms to free them from antibodies to the shared antigens. Salmonella antigens are also found in some members of other genera; the frequent sharing of O and H antigens with arizonae has already been mentioned and salmonella O-antigens are also found in some strains of *Escherichia*, *Shigella*, *Citrobacter* and *Proteus*.

O-ANTIGENS. These somatic antigens represent the side-chains of repeating sugar units projecting from the outer lipopolysaccharide layer of the bacterial cell wall. They are hydrophilic and enable the bacteria to form stable, homogeneous suspensions in saline solution. Over 60 different O-antigens have been recognized and they are designated by arabic numerals. The O-antigens are heat-stable, being unaffected by heating at 100°C for 2·5 hours, and alcohol-stable, withstanding treatment with 96 per cent ethanol at 37°C for 4 hours. The former procedure destroys flagellar and fimbrial antigens, while the latter detaches the flagella. Either method can be used to prepare bacterial suspensions susceptible to agglutination by O-antibodies but insusceptible to agglutination by H-antibodies. The O-antigens are unaffected by suspending the bacteria in 0·2 per cent formaldehyde, but if flagella are present, their fixation by the formaldehyde renders the bacteria inagglutinable by O-antibodies. As will be discussed later, the O-antigens are liable to be changed in character by the processes of *form variation* and *lysogenic conversion*, and to be lost from the bacteria in '*S → R*' *mutation*.

H-ANTIGENS. These antigens, which represent determinant groups on the flagellar protein, are heat-labile and alcohol-labile, but are well preserved in 0·04–0·2 per cent formaldehyde. Heating at temperatures above 60°C detaches the flagella from the bacteria and detachment of all flagella is achieved by heating at 100°C for 30 minutes. The deflagellated bacteria are inagglutinable by H-antibodies but the detached flagella remain immunogenic, so that suspensions of bacilli to be used for the production of O-antisera should be freed from detached flagella by centrifugation and washing or by inactivation by heating at 100°C for 2·5 hours.

In many salmonellae the production of flagellar antigens is diphasic, each strain varying spontaneously and reversibly between two phases with different sets of H-antigens. In *phase 1* (the 'specific' phase) the different antigens are designated by small letters, but because about 70 such antigens have been identified the letters a to z are insufficient and the more recently discovered antigens are designated z_1, z_2, z_3, etc. In *phase 2* (the 'group' phase) the antigens first discovered were given arabic numerals (not implying any relationship with the similarly numbered O-antigens), but later, certain phase-1 antigens, especially e, n, x and z, were found to be present in the phase 2 of some strains. Phase 2 is termed the 'group', or 'non-specific' phase because numerous serotypes share the same antigens in this phase. The identification of serotypes, therefore, largely depends on the antigens in the specific phase (phase 1).

A given culture of a diphasic salmonella may consist almost entirely of bacteria in one or other phase; e.g. a colony, or a first subculture from a colony, is likely to be mainly in one phase because it consists wholly of the recent progeny of a single cell. Alternatively, a culture may contain numerous bacteria in each phase, e.g. when a culture in one phase is subcultured serially by mass inoculation, variants into the other phase multiply until they comprise a substantial, equilibriating proportion of the population (Stocker, 1949).

Because the identification of a salmonella always requires the identification of the antigens of phase 1 and sometimes also the identification of those of phase 2, it is often necessary to obtain a culture in the alternate phase of the isolate under test. This may be done by selective cultivation of the isolate in semi-solid agar containing monophasic antiserum, e.g. by the modified Craigie tube method described later.

Flagella and flagellar antigens may be lost by a rare spontaneous mutation (*OH → O variation*). This mutation is usually irreversible, but it is sometimes possible to select motile and flagellated back-mutants by stab culture in semi-solid agar in a plate or Craigie (1931) tube; the non-motile forms remain at the site of inoculation while the motile mutants swarm away from it and so may be picked up at a distance for subculture. One or two passes by this method can also yield richly flagellated variants from strains that are poorly flagellated by their genotype. The abundance of flagella varies with the conditions of culture as well as with genotype; it is maximal in young (6 hour) broth cultures and minimal in older (24 hour) cultures on thin dry agar plates.

Kauffmann-White classification. This scheme, first developed in 1934, classifies the salmonellae into different *O-groups*, each of which contains a number of serotypes possessing a common O-antigen not found in other O-groups. The O-groups first defined were designated by capital letters A to Z and those discovered later by the number (51 to 64) of the characteristic O-antigen. Group A, for example, is characterized by O-antigen 2, group B by O-antigen 4, and group D by O-antigen 9. Some groups are divided into subgroups whose members are distinguished by a second O-antigen, e.g. group C_1 is characterized by O-antigens 6 and 7, and group C_2 by O-antigens 6 and 8. Groups A to E contain nearly all the salmonellae that are important pathogens in man and animals.

Within each O-group the different serotypes

Table 28.4   Antigens of some representatives of the genus *Salmonella* (Kauffmann-White classification)

O-group	Serotype ('species')	O-antigens* (and Vi)	H-antigens Phase 1	H-antigens Phase 2
A	S. paratyphi A	1, **2**, 12	a	–
	S. paratyphi A var. durazzo	**2**, 12	a	–
B	S. paratyphi B	1, **4**, 5, 12	b	1, 2
	S. paratyphi B var. odense	1, **4**, 12	b	1, 2
	S. java	1, **4**, 5, 12	b	(1, 2)
	S. limete	1, **4**, 12, 27	b	1, 5
	S. typhimurium	1, **4**, 5, 12	i	1, 2
	S. typhimurium var. copenhagen	1, **4**, 12	i	1, 2
	S. agama	**4**, 12	i	1, 6
	S. abortus-equi	**4**, 12	–	e, n, x
	S. abortus-ovis	**4**, 12	c	1, 6
	S. agona	**4**, 12	f, g, s	–
	S. brandenburg	**4**, 12	l, v	e, n, z_{15}
	S. bredeney	1, **4**, 12, 27	l, v	1, 7
	S. derby	1, **4**, 5, 12	f, g	–
	S. heidelberg	1, **4**, 5, 12	r	1, 2
	S. saint-paul	1, **4**, 5, 12	e, h	1, 2
	S. salinatis	**4**, 12	d, e, h	d, e, n, z_{15}
	S. stanley	**4**, 5, 12	d	1, 2
C_1	S. paratyphi C	**6, 7**, Vi	c	1, 5
	S. cholerae-suis	**6, 7**	c	1, 5
	S. cholerae-suis var. kunzendorf	**6, 7**	(c)	1, 5
	S. decatur	**6, 7**	c	1, 5
	S. typhi-suis	**6, 7**	c	1, 5
	S. bareilly	**6, 7**	y	1, 5
	S. infantis	**6, 7**	r	1, 5
	S. menston	**6, 7**	g, s, t	–
	S. montevideo	**6, 7**	g, m, s	–
	S. oranienburg	**6, 7**	m, t	–
	S. thompson	**6, 7**	k	1, 5
C_2	S. bovis-morbificans	**6, 8**	r	1, 5
	S. newport	**6, 8**	e, h	1, 2

* Numbers in bold type indicate the antigens characterizing the O-group.
Numbers in brackets are antigens that are rarely expressed.

Table 28.4—*continued*

O-group	Serotype ('species')	O-antigens* (and Vi)	H-antigens Phase 1	H-antigens Phase 2
D	*S. typhi*	**9**, 12, Vi	d	—
	S. ndolo	**9**, 12	d	1, 5
	S. dublin	1, **9**, 12	g, p	—
	S. enteritidis	1, **9**, 12	g, m	—
	S. gallinarum	1, **9**, 12	—	—
	S. pullorum	(1), **9**, 12	—	—
	S. panama	1, **9**, 12	l, v	1, 5
	S. miami	1, **9**, 12	a	1, 5
	S. sendai	1, **9**, 12	a	1, 5
E_1	*S. anatum*	**3, 10**	e, h	1, 6
	S. give	**3, 10**	l, v	1, 7
	S. london	**3, 10**	l, v	1, 6
	S. meleagridis	**3, 10**	e, h	l, w
E_2	*S. cambridge*	**3, 15**	e, h	l, w
	S. newington	**3, 15**	e, h	1, 6
E_3	*S. minneapolis*	(3), (15), **34**	e, h	1, 6
E_4	*S. senftenberg*	1, **3, 19**	g, s, t	—
	S. simsbury	1, **3, 19**	—	z_{27}
F	*S. aberdeen*	**11**	i	1, 2
G	*S. cubana*	1, **13**, 23	z_{29}	—
	S. poona	**13**, 22	z	1, 6
H	*S. heves*	**6, 14**, 24	d	1, 5
	S. onderstepoort	1, **6, 14**, 25	e, h	1, 5
I	*S. brazil*	**16**	a	1, 5
	S. hvittingfoss	**16**	b	e, n, x
Others	*S. kirkee*	**17**	b	1, 2
	S. adelaide	**35**	f, g	—
	S. locarno	**57**	z_{29}	z_{42}

* Numbers in bold type indicate the antigens characterizing the O-group.
 Numbers in brackets are antigens that are rarely expressed.

are distinguished by their particular H-antigen or combination of H-antigens. The antigenic formulae of some representative salmonellae are shown in Table 28.4, which includes the serotypes most virulent in man, those commonest in Britain and those most likely to be confused with the virulent and common serotypes. A full table of serotypes is given by Edwards and Ewing (1972) and Kauffmann (1969). It should be noted that although O-antigens 6 and 12 are shown in Table 28.4 as single entities, antigen 6 is a complex of two

factors, 6_1 and 6_2, and antigen 12 is a complex of three factors 12_1, 12_2 and 12_3; the proportions of these different factors may vary from strain to strain.

Differentiation of antigenically similar strains. As may be seen from examples in Table 28.4, not all the named serotypes have a unique antigenic structure. Thus, *S. paratyphi B*, a cause of enteric fever in man, has the same antigens as *S. java*, an animal parasite of lesser virulence for man, in whom it causes gastroenteritis but not enteric fever. *S. paratyphi C*, possesses the same O and H antigens as *S. cholerae-suis*, *S. decatur* and *S. typhi-suis*. *S. sendai*, a rare cause of enteric fever, possesses the same antigens as the less virulent *S. miami*, and *S. gallinarum* possesses the same antigens as *S. pullorum*.

The serotypes that share the same antigenic formula are distinguished by biochemical tests. *S. parathyphi B* forms mucoid colonies on prolonged incubation and does not ferment *d*-tartrate, whereas *S. java* is non-mucoid and does ferment *d*-tartrate. *S. paratyphi C* ferments *d*-tartrate and trehalose within 2 days, but not Stern's glycerol; *S. cholerae-suis* ferments *d*-tartrate but not trehalose or Stern's glycerol; *S. decatur* ferments all three substrates and *S. typhi-suis* only trehalose. *S. sendai*, which is non-fimbriate and grows poorly on conventional media, ferments arabinose but not Stern's glycerol, whereas *S. miami* grows vigorously and ferments Stern's glycerol but not arabinose. *S. gallinarum* is anaerogenic and ferments *d*-tartrate and dulcitol, whilst *S. pullorum* forms gas from glucose but fails to ferment *d*-tartrate or dulcitol.

Other surface antigens. Although the serotype of an enterobacterium is defined mainly by its O and H antigens, there may be other important antigens at the surface of the bacterial cell which can determine agglutination with homologous antibodies. These include the capsular, or K antigens of the varieties L, A, B, M and Vi (see Kauffmann, 1969), fimbrial antigens (Gillies and Duguid, 1958; Duguid and Campbell, 1969), the alpha antigen of Stamp and Stone (1944) and the beta antigen of Mushin (1949). Such antigens may cause difficulties in the serological identification of bacteria either by masking the O-antigen so that the bacilli are inagglutinable by O-antibodies or by causing non-specific cross-reactions due to their presence in otherwise unrelated organisms.

VI ANTIGEN. Almost all recently isolated strains of *S. typhi* form Vi antigen as a covering layer outside their cell wall. This antigen is an acidic polysaccharide. When fully developed, it renders the bacteria agglutinable by Vi antibody and inagglutinable by O-antibody. It was originally designated Vi because its presence appeared to determine virulence for

mice, probably by protecting the bacteria from phagocytosis and the bactericidal action of serum. Antigens identical with or closely related to the Vi antigen of *S. typhi* have been found in *S. paratyphi C* and some strains of *Escherichia* and *Citrobacter* (Ballerup-Bethesda group).

The amount of Vi antigen in different strains of *S. typhi* varies considerably. It is usually greatest in freshly isolated strains and Vi-rich strains (V forms) produce more opaque colonies than strains lacking Vi antigen (W forms). Vi-rich strains maintained by subculture on conventional media are rapidly replaced by spontaneously originating Vi-deficient mutants ($V \rightarrow W$ variation).

The Vi antigen is heat-labile. It can be removed from the bacteria by heating a suspension at 100°C for 1 hour and separating the bacteria by centrifugation from the Vi-containing fluid. The heated bacteria are inagglutinable by Vi-antibody but agglutinable by O-antibody. Even without heating, Vi antigen gradually separates from the bacteria in a saline suspension. Tests for Vi antigen are therefore best done with a bacterial suspension freshly made from an agar culture grown from a V-form colony.

M-ANTIGEN. This extracellular polysaccharide antigen is produced by those strains of *S. paratyphi B* and other serotypes that form mucoid or 'slime wall' colonies when cultures are held for several days at room temperature after incubation for 1 day at 37°C. It resembles Vi antigen in preventing agglutination by O-antibodies. Its antigenic specificity, which differs from that of the Vi antigen, is the same in the different salmonella serotypes that form it and resembles that of the capsular antigen of *Klebsiella* type 13. Heating at 100°C for 2·5 hours removes the M antigen and renders the bacteria agglutinable by O-antiserum. A motile non-mucoid mutant can sometimes be selected by serial passage through semi-solid agar ($M \rightarrow N$ variation).

FIMBRIAL ANTIGENS. Type-1 fimbriae, which are formed by most strains of salmonellae, bear antigens that determine agglutination by sera containing anti-fimbrial antibodies (Duguid and Campbell, 1969). The bacteria vary reversibly between a fimbriate phase, which predominates in 24–48 hour broth cultures, and a non-fimbriate phase which predominates in young (6 hour) broth cultures and 24-hour agar plate cultures (*fimbrial phase variation*). A common antigen is present in the fimbriae of the different salmonella serotypes and some arizona and citrobacter strains, but there is no sharing of antigens with fimbriate strains of *Escherichia*, *Shigella*, *Klebsiella* and *Enterobacter*.

The sharing of fimbrial antigens between different serotypes of salmonellae gives rise to confusing cross-reactions if tests are done with bacteria from fimbriate-phase cultures and sera containing fimbrial antibodies. Such cross-reactions are best avoided by the use of non-fimbriate-phase cultures for the preparation of agglutinable bacterial suspensions, e.g. broth cultures grown for 6 hours, glucose-broth cultures grown for 12 hours or thin agar-plate cultures grown for 24 hours.

Like the flagellar antigens, the fimbrial antigens are preserved in bacteria held in 0·1 or 0·2 per cent formaldehyde; they are detached from the bacteria by heating at 100°C for 30 min and are inactivated by heating at higher temperatures or for longer periods. Agglutination by fimbrial antibodies is best tested with formaldehyde-killed bacteria from a 48-hour broth culture. Fimbrial antiserum is prepared by injecting such fimbriate bacteria into rabbits and it may be absorbed free from O and H antibodies with non-fimbriate bacteria grown in glucose broth or on agar plates ('pure fimbrial antiserum').

R-ANTIGENS. In S → R mutation the O-antigens are lost and new 'R' antigens are revealed at the bacterial surface. The R bacteria form rough colonies and are auto-agglutinable in saline, sensitive to killing by complement and non-virulent. They tend to outgrow the parental S bacteria during serial culture in the laboratory. The S → R mutation involves the loss of an enzyme required for the formation of one of the links in either the polysaccharide core or the side chains of the cell-wall lipopolysaccharide, leading to an absence of the side chains. The exposed incomplete (R_I) or complete (R_{II}) core polysaccharides constitute the R-antigens. These antigens are the same in the R variants from different salmonella serotypes, though they differ from the R-antigens of other genera of Enterobacteriaceae.

Because they lack O-antigens and are auto-agglutinable in saline, R bacteria are unsuitable for serological tests. R cultures can be recognized by the rapid agglutination caused when a drop of dense bacterial suspension is mixed with a drop of 0·2 per cent acriflavine or trypaflavine in 0·85 per cent NaCl. This test will demonstrate 'roughness' before it is indicated either by colonial morphology or inability to form a uniform suspension in saline.

Antigenic variations. The mutations V → W (Vi-antigen loss), M → N (M-antigen loss), S → R (O-antigen loss) and OH → O (H-antigen loss) and the reversible phase variations of flagellar antigens (phase 1 ⇌ phase 2) and fimbrial antigens (fimbriate ⇌ non-fimbriate) have been described above.

Form variation is a spontaneous, reversible variation in the amount of one of the O-antigens, e.g. factor 1, 6_1, 12_2, 22, 23, 24 or 25; different amounts of the antigen are found in different colonies in a plating from a culture.

Other changes in O-antigens take place by *lysogenic conversion*. Thus, in *S. typhimurium* and other members of O-groups A, B, D, G, R and T, the formation of O-antigen 1 is dependent on the genome of a temperate A-type phage, such as P22 (Boyd and Bidwell, 1957); strains gain or lose O-antigen 1 when they are lysogenized or de-lysogenized with the phage. By a similar process, *S. anatum* (0-3,10; H-e,h:1,6) forms O-antigens 3 and 15 and so comes to resemble *S. newington* (3,15; e,h:1,6) when it is lysogenized with phage epsilon[15] derived from *S. newington*; it forms O-antigens 3, 15 and 34 when it is further lysogenized with phage epsilon[34] derived from a group-E_4 serotype such as *S. minneapolis*. Other phage-dependent O-antigens are 14 in group C and 27 in group B.

Viability. Salmonellae are readily killed by moist heat, e.g. in 1 hour at 55°C or 15 minutes at 60°C, and most strong disinfectants. Laboratory cultures survive for several months or years. Cultures on slopes of Dorset's egg kept tightly capped to prevent drying and stored at room temperature in the dark usually remain viable for at least 10–20 years. *S. typhi* and other salmonellae gradually die in contaminated moist natural environments outside the body, but some bacilli may survive for over 4 weeks in, for example, sewage-polluted water or moist soil. They die more quickly when dried, *S. typhi* often within a few hours, so that spread is less likely to take place by dust or dry contaminated objects than by water or moist foodstuffs. Many salmonellae, however, may survive for fairly long periods when dried in foodstuffs, e.g. in dried egg, milk or coconut, and infections have been carried in such products from one country to another.

Antibiotic sensitivity. Most strains are sensitive to chloramphenicol (MIC 2 μg/ml), ampicillin (MIC 2 μg/ml), streptomycin (MIC 8 μg/ml), tetracycline (MIC 1 μg/ml), cotrimoxazole and some other antibiotics. Chloramphenicol is considered to be the most effective agent for the treatment of typhoid fever. Some strains, however, are highly resistant to certain of these antibiotics as a result of mutation or the acquisition of a transmissible resistance plasmid. In some countries, Mexico for instance, there have been outbreaks of typhoid fever due to infections with strains of *S. typhi* resistant to chloramphenicol. It is necessary, therefore, to test the antibiotic sensitivities of any salmonella isolated from enteric fever or other septicaemic illness.

In recent years the selective pressure of a widespread prophylactic use of antibiotics in domestic animals has greatly increased the prevalence of resistant strains of the animal salmonellae that commonly cause food-poisoning infections in man. Salmonella food-poisoning uncomplicated by septicaemia should not be treated with antibiotics, for there is evidence that such treatment by its effect on the normal intestinal flora may paradoxically prolong the excretion of salmonellae and fail to give any clinical benefit. It is, however, useful to determine the sensitivities of food-poisoning strains so that prompt effective treatment may be given to the rare cases that become septicaemic.

LABORATORY DIAGNOSIS OF INFECTIONS

Laboratory diagnosis of salmonella infections depends mainly on the isolation and identification of the causal salmonella from a specimen of blood, faeces, urine or vomit. Testing the patient's serum for salmonella antibodies is useful only in the diagnosis of enteric fever (Widal reaction) and the significance of the results of this test is often doubtful. For the diagnosis of pyrexial illnesses, physicians should be advised to submit blood cultures to the laboratory and not to rely on the fallible serological tests. If a blood culture cannot be submitted, the bacteriologist may culture the clot taken from a blood specimen submitted for serology.

Isolation of a salmonella by blood culture is proof that the patient has a salmonella septicaemia. Isolation from the faeces is of less certain significance; in illnesses resembling enteric fever or gastroenteritis such an isolation strongly suggests that salmonella infection is the cause, but since salmonellae may be present in the faeces of carriers it does not amount to proof of a causal role.

The clinical value of identifying the serotype of a salmonella isolate lies in distinguishing the serotypes that cause enteric fever in man, namely *S. typhi*, *S. paratyphi A*, *S. paratyphi B* and *S. sendai*, from the other serotypes, which in man rarely cause septicaemic infections, though commonly causing gastroenteritis (food-poisoning). The value of identifying the serotype of a 'non-enteric-fever' salmonella is mainly epidemiological; knowledge of the serotype helps to define the sources and vehicles of infection in outbreaks of food-poisoning.

Isolation. The methods of isolating salmonellae from clinical specimens are summarized in Table 28.5. The specimen, or a preliminary enrichment culture grown in a selective liquid medium, is plated out on a solid differential medium on which salmonella-like colonies may be recognized by a characteristic appearance, e.g. by their pale colour on MacConkey's medium or black colour on Wilson and Blair's medium. These suspect colonies are picked and grown as pure subcultures which are then identified by further tests. It is essential to obtain *pure* subcultures for the identifying tests. Each subculture should be grown from a *single*, well separated colony that is homogeneous in appearance. If, for any cause,

Table 28.5   Methods for the isolation of salmonellae

Specimen	Treatment of specimen	Method of and media for inoculation	Subsequent procedure
Faeces	If delay in transit, use buffered glycerol saline or Stuart's transport medium	Plate out on MacConkey DCA BSA	Examine for suspect colonies on MacConkey and DCA after 24 hours,
	If faeces solid emulsify in broth	Put heavy inoculum into	BSA after 24 and 48 hours
Urine	Centrifuge and use deposit	selenite broth, tetrathionate broth	Incubate for 24 hours; subculture on to MacConkey, DCA or BSA, incubate and examine for suspect colonies
Vomit	Centrifuge if possible: use deposit		
Bile			
Pus			
Blood culture	See Chapter 6	—	Subculture at 48 hours and again at 7–10 days on to BA and MacConkey
Clotted blood	Remove serum for Widal reaction. Lyse clot with streptokinase, add bile-salt broth	—	
	See Chapter 6		Examine for suspect colonies
Sewage	Use Moore's swab Express fluid from swab	Dilute expressed fluid 1 in 10, add 0·1 ml to 10 ml selenite and tetrathionate broths	Incubate and subculture on to MacConkey, DCA and BSA after 24, 48 and 72 hours
			Examine solid media for suspect colonies after incubation
Solid food	Powder or homogenize: use pestle and mortar, electric blender or cut into fragments	Add approximately 25 g to 150 ml selenite and tetrathionate broths	
Liquid food		Mix with equal volumes of double strength selenite and tetrathionate broths	

BA   = Blood agar.
DCA = Deoxycholate citrate agar.
BSA = Wilson and Blair's bismuth-sulphite agar.

The surface of solid media must be sufficiently dry before inoculation otherwise a confluent growth may result. Individual colonies should be visible on at least a quarter of the plate.

e.g. crowding of colonies, there is a doubt about the purity of the colony picked, it is essential to plate it on MacConkey's agar and grow a subculture from a well-separated colony on this secondary plate for examination in the identifying tests.

In many laboratories, blood cultures are subcultured only on to non-selective blood agar, on which salmonella colonies lack distinctive features. It is imperative, therefore, that all Gram-negative bacilli isolated from blood are fully identified.

Identification. The suspect culture is first subjected to a series of biochemical tests and if the results are consistent with its being a salmonella the serotype is determined by agglutination tests. It is unwise to make the serological tests on bacteria harvested from colonies on a selective medium, because these bacteria often form unstable or mixed suspensions. Agar or broth subcultures should be used. If there is great urgency, a suspect colony can be subcultured on to a moist agar slope and slide agglutination tests attempted after 4 hours.

BIOCHEMICAL TESTS. Pick a suspect colony that is well separated from other colonies on the plate and subculture it in nutrient broth for 4 hours. Inoculate drops of this young broth culture into sugar peptone waters (e.g. lactose, glucose, sucrose, mannitol and dulcitol), ONPG broth, urea medium, peptone water (for motility and indole tests) and an agar slope (for serological tests); also plate it on MacConkey's agar to establish that it is pure. When many cultures have to be examined, labour can be saved by testing the biochemical reactions in composite media, e.g. Gillies's modification of Kohn's two-tube media (Chap. 5).

Read the tests after overnight incubation and if the results are consistent with the culture being a salmonella, proceed with slide agglutination tests. If not, discard the culture. If the initial biochemical tests suggest that the culture is a salmonella, but the serological tests fail to confirm that this is so, carry out a full range of biochemical tests for identification of the genus. If the results are still consistent with the culture being a salmonella, send the culture to a Reference Laboratory where antisera are available for identification of rare salmonella serotypes.

SEROLOGICAL TESTS. The growth on the agar slope is tested by slide agglutination against salmonella polyvalent O, polyvalent H (specific and non-specific) and Vi sera. If results are positive, further slide tests are done with single-factor sera to determine the O and H antigens. Preferably, quantitative tube agglutination tests should also be done, in particular to demonstrate the specific-phase H-antigens by agglutination to the serum's titre.

Source of antisera. Diagnostic antisera can be prepared in the laboratory by immunizing rabbits with the appropriate antigens, but agglutinins to cross-reacting antigens must be removed by absorption and the method is not only tedious but also requires considerable expertise. It is usual, therefore, to employ commercially prepared antisera. The choice of sera to be held in the laboratory will vary with the type of specimens received, but the following sera would be suitable for a large hospital or public health laboratory.

O-antisera:
Polyvalent-O, groups A–G
2-O, group A
4-O, group B
6,7-O group C_1
8-O, group C_2
9-O, group D
3,10,15,19-O, group E
11-O, group F
13,22-O, group G

Vi antiserum.

H-antisera:
Polyvalent-H, specific and non-specific
Polyvalent-H, non-specific, factors
  1,2,5,6,7
a-H (*S. paratyphi A*–H)
b-H (*S. paratyphi B*–H specific)
c-H (*S. paratyphi C*–H specific)
d-H (*S. typhi*–H)
e,h-H (*S. newport*–H specific)
f,g-H (*S. derby*–H)
g,m-H (*S. enteritidis*–H)
i-H (*S. typhimurium*–H specific)
k-H (*S. thompson*–H specific)
l,v-H (*S. london*–H specific)
m,t-H (*S. oranienburg*–H)
r-H (*S. bovis-morbificans*–H specific)

'Rapid diagnostic sera' for determination of common specific H-antigens except factor i:

Rapid diagnostic 1-H (factors b,d,E,r)
Rapid diagnostic 2-H (factors b,E,k,L)
Rapid diagnostic 3-H (factors d,E,G,k)
E = polyvalent for eh, enx, etc.
G = polyvalent for gm, gp, etc.
L = polyvalent for lv, lw, etc.

Antigens for production of antisera. O-antigens should consist of agar-grown bacteria heated at 100°C for 2·5 hours, separated by centrifugation, treated with 96 per cent ethanol for 4 hours at 37°C, centrifuged and resuspended in saline. H-antigens should consist of bacteria from a young (6 hour) broth culture grown from a colony of the required phase and killed by the addition of formaldehyde to 0·2 per cent concentration.

Slide agglutination tests. METHOD 1. Place a drop of saline solution (0·85 per cent NaCl) on a carefully cleaned microscope slide. With an inoculating wire emulsify in the drop a speck of live culture from a moist agar slope culture to produce a distinct and uniform turbidity. Add a small (e.g. $\frac{1}{5}$th to $\frac{1}{10}$th volume) drop of undiluted serum to the suspension with a wire loop and mix by tilting the slide backwards and forwards for 30–60 seconds while viewing under a good light against a dark background with the naked eye. Distinct clumping within this period is a positive result.

METHOD 2. Place a drop of diluted (e.g. 1 in 5 or 1 in 10) antiserum and a drop of saline in separate positions on a slide and emulsify in each a speck of agar culture. Mix by tilting backwards and forwards for 30 seconds. Clumping in the serum without clumping in the saline (i.e. no autoagglutination) is a positive result. Unabsorbed H-sera must be diluted 1 in 50 or 1 in 100 to obviate reactions due to their content of O-antibodies.

For safety, the used slides should at once be placed in disinfectant and left overnight before being handled again or discarded.

Determination of O-group. Provided there is no autoagglutination in saline, the results of slide agglutination tests are generally sufficient to determine the O-group of a culture. If agglutination occurs only with Vi serum, a saline suspension of the culture should be heated at 100°C for 1 hour to remove the Vi antigen and the bacteria should be separated by centrifugation, resuspended in fresh saline and then tested with polyvalent O, 6,7-O (group C_1) and 9-O (group D) antisera. Occasionally a rough (R variant) Vi-containing strain of *S. typhi* is encountered and O-antigens cannot be demonstrated; the specific H-antigen of this or other R strains may be identified by a tube agglutination test with a formaldehyde-killed broth culture.

Determination of serotype. The serotype of a culture of known O-group is determined by identification of its H-antigens. This can usually be done by slide agglutination tests on bacteria from a moist agar slope culture, but some strains are not sufficiently richly flagellated in such cultures for clear results. After finding that the culture is agglutinated by polyvalent H (specific and non-specific) serum, test it against the polyvalent H (non-specific) serum. If it is not agglutinated, assume that it is in the specific phase and attempt to determine the phase-1 antigens by making further tests with single-factor H sera or the three 'rapid diagnostic sera'. If the culture is agglutinated by the polyvalent H (non-specific) serum, proceed to secure a specific-phase culture before attempting tests with the specific-phase sera. This may be done by the Craigie tube method with non-specific-phase antiserum (see below).

For reliable identification the positive results obtained in the slide agglutination tests with H sera should be confirmed by tube agglutination tests with a formaldehyde-killed broth culture to ensure that agglutination takes place at or beyond the stated diagnostic titre of the serum.

Tube agglutination tests. Antigens are prepared as follows:

1. H-ANTIGENS. Inoculate bacteria from a single colony of the required H phase into broth and incubate for 6 hours. View a drop of the culture in a wet film to confirm that all bacteria are motile and therefore sufficiently flagellated for the tests. Kill the culture by adding formaldehyde to a concentration of 0·2 per cent and incubating for several hours at 37°C. If the broth culture is found to be poorly motile, select a highly motile variant by

passing subcultures once or twice through semi-solid agar in a Craigie tube (without antiserum) or by stab-culturing in a plate of semi-solid agar and subculturing from the periphery of the swarm.

2. O-ANTIGENS. Suspend the bacteria from an agar culture in saline and heat at 100°C to remove flagella (and fimbriae). Centrifuge to separate the bacteria from the detached flagella (and fimbriae) and resuspend in saline. Alternatively, remove the flagella by mixing a dense saline suspension of the bacteria with an equal volume of 96 per cent ethanol and incubating at 37°C for 20 hours; before use, dilute in saline to a suitable density.

3. VI-ANTIGEN. Prepare a fresh suspension of live bacteria from an opaque (Vi-rich) colony just before testing.

Before use, adjust the antigens to a density of about 2×10^8 bacteria per ml by comparison with an opacity standard.

Carry out the tests in small tubes containing 0·4 ml of the mixture of bacterial suspension and diluted serum. Prepare doubling dilutions of the diagnostic serum in saline, starting at 1 in 10 for O and Vi agglutinations and at 1 in 50 for H agglutination. Add equal volumes of bacterial suspension (0·2 ml) to the diluted serum (0·2 ml) in each tube and to a control tube containing only saline. Incubate H agglutinations for 2 hours at 50°C or 4 hours at 37°C. Incubate O agglutinations for 20 hours at 50°C or 6 hours at 37°C followed by refrigeration overnight. Incubate Vi agglutinations for 2 hours at 37°C and refrigerate overnight. Use a waterbath for the incubation. Read the results by viewing the tubes under good light against a dark background with the aid of a ×2 magnifying lens. If necessary, rotate the tubes with a careful twisting movement to swirl up granules from the deposit, but do not shake. The titre of the serum is read as the greatest dilution giving agglutination; e.g. if the limiting dilution is 1 in 200, the titre is 200.

Craigie tube method for changing H phase. The procedure is performed in tubes or bottles containing 5–10 ml semi-solid nutrient agar (0·2–0·4 per cent agar, according to quality) and a small inner tube open at both ends with the upper end projecting well above the agar. Melt the medium, cool to 50°C and add 0·5 ml

of a 1 in 5 dilution of non-specific-phase H serum to one tube and 1 ml of it to another. (The serum is previously sterilized by filtration.) After the medium has solidified, inoculate the non-specific-phase culture with a straight wire into the agar *inside* the inner tube. Incubate at 37°C and take material for subculture from the agar *outside* the inner tube after the shortest period, e.g. 8–16 hours, required for swarming. Specific-phase variants can swarm freely from the inner tube but the parental, non-specific-phase bacteria are immobilized at the site of inoculation by the non-specific-phase H-antibodies. Prepare the subcultures on agar slopes and in nutrient broth, and confirm the change of phase by demonstrating absence of agglutination with polyvalent H (non-specific) serum. Then use the subculture for identification of the specific-phase H antigens.

The method can also be used to change the specific to the non-specific phase. For this purpose, add homologous specific-phase H antiserum to the semi-solid agar.

Serological diagnosis by the Widal reaction. Tests for the presence of salmonella antibodies in the patient's serum may be of value in the diagnosis of enteric fever, but are of little help in that of salmonella food-poisoning. The patient's serum is tested by tube agglutination for its titres of antibodies against H, O and Vi suspensions of the enteric fever organisms likely to be encountered, e.g. *S. typhi* and *S. paratyphi B* in Britain. The suspensions may be prepared from suitable stock laboratory cultures in the manner described above for tube agglutination tests, but commercially prepared suspensions are nowadays generally used.

METHOD. Separately test the patient's serum in a series of dilutions against each of the different salmonella suspensions. For each series use seven small (3 × 0·5 in) test tubes, six for six serum dilutions and the seventh for a non-serum control. Place 0·4 ml saline (0·85 per cent NaCl) in each of tubes 2 to 7. Make up a 1 in 15 dilution of the patient's serum in saline and with a fresh graduated pipette add 0·4 ml of the diluted serum to each of tubes 1 and 2. Tube 2 will then contain 0·8 ml of serum diluted 1 in 30. Mix the fluid in tube 2 by pipetting up and down several times, then transfer 0·4 ml to tube 3. Repeat the process to tube 6, from which discard 0·4 ml. Each tube then contains 0·4 ml fluid, tubes 1 to 6 containing serum dilutions of 15, 30, 60, 120, 240 and 480, and tube 7 only saline. With a fresh pipette, now add 0·4 ml bacterial suspension to each tube, starting at tube 7 and working backwards to tube 1. The serum dilutions in tubes 1 to 6 are now 30 to 960. Transfer the mixtures with a capillary pipette to narrow agglutination tubes, starting at tube 7 and working backwards to tube 1. Incubate H agglutinations for 2 hours at 37°C and read after standing on the bench for half an hour. Incubate O agglutinations for 4 hours at 37°C and read after refrigeration at 4°C overnight. The large flakes of H agglutination are easily visible with the naked eye, but a magnifying lens should be used to detect the small granules of O agglutination.

Test Vi agglutination in doubling serum dilutions from 1 in 10 to 1 in 640 in 3 × 0·5 in test tubes. Incubate for 2 hours at 37°C and read with a lens after standing at room temperature overnight. In the control, the bacteria will be sedimented to form a small, compact deposit. If agglutination has occurred a granular deposit is scattered over the foot of the tube.

INTERPRETATION. The *titre* of the patient's serum for each salmonella suspension is read as the highest dilution of serum giving visible agglutination, e.g. if this dilution is 1 in 240, the titre is 240. A positive reaction is first detected about the seventh to the tenth day of the illness in enteric fever, so that a negative result at an early stage is inconclusive. The strength of the reaction for the infecting serotype increases progressively to a maximum about the end of the third week and the demonstration of such a *rising titre* between tests made in the first and third weeks is highly significant. Positive results in single tests by no means always indicate the presence of enteric fever and in interpreting them the following points should be borne in mind. (1) The serum of some normal (uninfected) persons agglutinates salmonella suspensions at dilutions up to about 1 in 50, so that titres cannot be taken as significant unless they are greater than about 100. (2) Persons who have received TAB vaccine may show high titres of antibodies to each of the salmonellae, and only if a marked rise of titre to one serotype is observed can the result be regarded as diagnostically significant. H-agglutinins tend to persist for many months after vaccination but O-agglutinins tend to disappear sooner, e.g. within 6 months. (3) For determining the type of infection, the H reaction is more reliable than the O reaction because the different salmonellae have some O-antigens in common. (4) Non-specific antigens, such as fimbrial antigens, may be present in test suspensions and then give false-positive results by reacting with an agglutinin in the serum of some uninfected individuals. (5) The Widal reaction is positive in many healthy carriers. A negative reaction does not exclude the carrier state, but a positive reaction, particularly a Vi titre of 10 or higher, is said to be helpful for the recognition of a carrier.

The serum of a patient convalescent from salmonella food-poisoning will often agglutinate a suspension of the causal serotype and the finding may enable a *retrospective* diagnosis to be made in cases from which a salmonella was not isolated.

Bacteriophage typing. Strains within a particular salmonella serotype may be differentiated into a number of *phage-types* by their patterns of susceptibility to lysis by a series of phages with different specificities. The determination of the phage-type of strains isolated from different patients, carriers or other sources is valuable in the epidemiological study of infections, because it helps to define groups of persons who have been infected with the same strain from the same source. Serotypes that can be subdivided by phage-typing include *S. typhi*, *S. paratyphi A*, *S. paratyphi B*, *S. typhimurium* and *S. enteritidis*. Thus, about 80 different phage-types of *S. typhi* and 190 phage-types of *S. typhimurium* are distinguished.

The typing of *S. typhi* is done by determining the sensitivity of the culture to a series of variants of a single phage, Vi-phage II, which have been adapted to the different types of typhoid bacillus. The specific phage-sensitivity, and thus the phage-type, of the bacillus is determined partly by its content of particular 'type-determining' symbiotic phages and partly by other heritable traits. In other serotypes the phage-typing is done with sets of unrelated O-phages collected from a variety of sources.

The techniques of phage-typing are complicated and it is usual for cultures for typing to be sent to a reference laboratory (Anderson and Williams, 1956; Anderson, 1964).

Biotyping. Strains within a particular serotype may be differentiated into biotypes by their different fermentation reaction with selected substrates. In *S. typhimurium*, for example, 21 biotypes are distinguished by their patterns of reactions with nine substrates in a scheme originally developed by Kristensen, Bojlén and Faarup (1937). Strains of the same phage-type may be subdivided into different biotypes, so that the combination of biotyping with phage-typing gives a finer discrimination between strains than does either method alone (Alfredsson, Barker, Old and Duguid, 1972, give references). In *S. typhi*, different biotypes are distinguished by reactions with arabinose, dulcitol and xylose.

REFERENCES

ALFREDSSON, G. A., BARKER, RUTH M., OLD, D. C. & DUGUID, J. P. (1972) Use of tartaric acid isomers and citric acid in the biotyping of *Salmonella typhimurium*. *Journal of Hygiene, Cambridge*, **70,** 651.

ANDERSON, E. S. (1964) The phage typing of salmonellae other than *S. typhi*. In *The World Problem of Salmonellosis*, edited by E. van Oye, p. 89. Monographiae Biologicae, volume 13, Uitgeverij Dr W. Junk: Den Hoag.

ANDERSON, E. S. & WILLIAMS, R. E. O. (1956) Bacteriophage typing of enteric pathogens and staphylococci and its use in epidemiology. *Journal of Clinical Pathology*, **9,** 94.

ASSOCIATION OF CLINICAL PATHOLOGISTS (1967) Broadsheet 58: October 1967. *The isolation and identification of salmonellae*. (From Publishing Manager, *Journal of Clinical Pathology*, BMA House, Tavistock Square, London WC1.)

BOYD, J. S. K. & BIDWELL, D. E. (1957) The type A phages of *Salmonella typhimurium*: Identification by a standardised cross-immunity test. *Journal of General Microbiology*, **16,** 217.

COWAN, S. T. & STEEL, K. J. (1965) *Manual for the identification of medical bacteria*. Cambridge University Press.

CRAIGIE, J. (1931) Studies on the serological reactions of the flagella of *B. typhosus*. *Journal of Immunology*, **21,** 417.

DUGUID, J. P., ANDERSON, E. S. & CAMPBELL, I. (1966) Fimbriae and adhesive properties in salmonellae. *Journal of Pathology and Bacteriology*, **92,** 107.

DUGUID, J. P. & CAMPBELL, I. (1969) Antigens of the type-1 fimbriae of salmonellae and other enterobacteria. *Journal of Medical Microbiology*, **2,** 535.

EDWARDS, P. R. & EWING, W. H. (1972) *Identification of Enterobacteriaceae* 3rd edition, *Burgess Publishing Company*, Minneapolis.

GILLIES, R. R. & DUGUID, J. P. (1958) The fimbrial antigens of *Shigella flexneri*. *Journal of Hygiene, Cambridge*, **56,** 303.

IVESON, J. B. & MACKAY-SCOLLAY, E. M. (1969) Strontium chloride and strontium selenite enrichment broth media in the isolation of *Salmonella*. *Journal of Hygiene, Cambridge*, **67,** 457.

KAUFFMANN, F. (1969) *The Bacteriology of Enterobacteriaceae*, 2nd edition. Copenhagen: Munksgaard.

KRISTENSEN, M., BOJLÉN, K. & FAARUP, C. (1937) Bakteriologisk-Epidemiologiske Erfaringer om Infektioner med Gastroenteritisbaciller af Paratyphusgruppen. *Bibliotek for Laeger, Copenhagen*, **129,** 310.

MUSHIN, R. (1949) A new antigenic relationship among faecal bacilli due to a common β antigen. *Journal of Hygiene, Cambridge*, **47,** 227.

STAMP, LORD & STONE, D. M. (1944) An agglutinogen common to certain strains of lactose and non-lactose-fermenting coliform bacilli. *Journal of Hygiene, Cambridge*, **43,** 266.

STOCKER, B. A. D. (1949) Measurements of rate of mutation of flagellar antigenic phase in *Salmonella typhimurium*. *Journal of Hygiene, Cambridge*, **47,** 398.

STOKES, J. L. & BAYNE, H. G. (1958) Growth-factor-dependent strains of salmonellae. *Journal of Bacteriology*, **76,** 417.

29. Shigella

BIOLOGICAL CHARACTERS

Definition of the genus Shigella. Enterobacteria (fermentative, facultatively anaerobic, oxidase-negative Gram-negative rods) that are non-lactose-fermenting, non-motile, mostly anaerogenic, urease-negative, non-citrate-utilizing and KCN-sensitive.

Morphology and staining. Like salmonellae, they are non-sporing non-capsulate Gram-negative rods, 2–$4 \mu m \times 0.6 \mu m$, but unlike most salmonellae, they are non-motile and non-flagellate. Fimbriae (type-1) are found only in *Shigella flexneri*, though not in serotype 6 and some strains in other serotypes (Duguid and Gillies, 1957).

Culture. Aerobic and facultatively anaerobic. Optimal growth temperature is 37°C; *Shigella sonnei* grows well even at 10°C and 45°C. Grow well on conventional media, but none can grow on a simple glucose-ammonium salts medium without supplementation with nicotinic acid; some strains also require other growth factors.

1. NUTRIENT AGAR AND BLOOD AGAR. Smooth, greyish or colourless, translucent colonies, often 2–3 mm in diameter, resembling those of salmonellae. Those of *Sh. sonnei* are slightly larger and more opaque than those of other shigellae. *Sh. sonnei* has two antigenic phases. Phase-1 colonies, which predominate in primary platings, are like the colonies of other shigellae. Phase-2 colonies, which arise by irreversible variation from phase 1 and are seen in early subcultures from primary isolates, are larger and less opaque and have an irregular, matt surface and a crenated edge. This variation probably corresponds to $S \rightarrow R$ variation in salmonellae.

2. MACCONKEY'S AGAR. Colonies are pale and yellowish (non-lactose-fermenting) and resemble those of salmonellae. Colonies of *Sh. sonnei*, a late fermenter of lactose, become pink when incubation is prolonged beyond 24 hours.

3. DEOXYCHOLATE CITRATE AGAR. DCA is an excellent selective plating medium for the isolation of shigellae from faeces. Colonies are pale and similar to, though usually slightly smaller, e.g. 1–1.5 mm in diameter, and more translucent than those of salmonellae. They do not form a black centre. On prolonged incubation, those of *Sh. sonnei* form pink papillae.

4. WILSON AND BLAIR'S BRILLIANT GREEN BISMUTH SULPHITE MEDIUM. Shigellae do not grow on this medium.

5. PEPTONE WATER AND NUTRIENT BROTH. Good growth with uniform turbidity on incubation overnight at 37°C. Some strains, especially fimbriate ones, form a surface pellicle on longer incubation.

6. SELENITE F BROTH. This medium will grow and enrich *Sh. sonnei* and *Sh. flexneri* serotype 6, but is inhibitory to other shigellae. Tetrathionate broth and brilliant green media are inhibitory and unsuitable for enrichment cultures.

Biochemical reactions. The shigellae are divided into four groups, or species, by their biochemical reactions and antigenic structure (Table 29.1). The groups A, B, C and D correspond to the species *Sh. dysenteriae*, *Sh. flexneri*, *Sh. boydii* and *Sh. sonnei*.

1. FERMENTATION OF CARBOHYDRATES. Most strains attack sugars with the production of acid but not gas, though some strains in two serotypes, *Sh. flexneri* serotype 6 (Newcastle and Manchester varieties) and *Sh. boydii* serotype 14, form gas. Glucose is fermented by all strains.

Lactose is not fermented within 24 hours by any strain nor on longer incubation by the majority. Most strains of *Sh. sonnei*, however, ferment lactose after several days and some strains of *Sh. dysenteriae* type 1 also produce acid on prolonged incubation.

The ONPG test is usually negative, but positive reactions may be given by strains of *Sh. dysenteriae* (especially type 1), *Sh. boydii* (regularly by type-5 strains) and *Sh. sonnei*.

Table 29.1 Biochemical reactions of *Shigella* species and serotypes

Group	Species, serotype and variety	Fermentation reactions						Indole production	Catalase reaction	Lysine decarboxylase	Ornithine decarboxylase
		Gas from glucose	Lactose	Mannitol	Dulcitol	Xylose	Sucrose				
	Sh. dysenteriae,										
A	1 (Sh. shigae)	–	–(e)	–	–	–	–	–	–	–	–
	2 (Sh. schmitzii)	–	–	–	–	–	–	+	+	–	–
	3 –10	–	–	–	–(e)	–	–	d	+	–	–
	Sh. flexneri,										
B	1–5, X and Y	–	–	+(e)	–	–(e)	–(e)	d	+(e)	–	–
	6, variety 88	+	–	+	d	–	–(e)	–	+	–	–
	6, variety Newcastle	+	–	–	(+)	–	–(e)	–	+	–	–
	6, variety Manchester	+	–	+	(+)	–	–(e)	–	+	–	–
	Sh. boydii										
C	1–15	–(e)	–	+	d	d	–	d	+	–	–
D	*Sh. sonnei*	–	(+)	+	–	d	(+)	–	+	–	+

+ = Positive reaction (sugars fermented in 24 hours).
– = Negative reaction.
(+) = Late and irregularly positive reaction (2—8 days).
d = Some strains positive, others negative.
(e) = See text for exceptions.

Mannitol reactions are important because they distinguish group-A strains, which do not ferment mannitol, from groups B, C and D, most strains of which do ferment it. There are, however, some mannitol-negative strains in nearly all serotypes, e.g. the Newcastle variety of *Sh. flexneri* serotype 6 and the biotype 'Sh. rabaulensis' of *Sh. flexneri* serotype 4a.

Dulcitol is not fermented by the majority of shigellae, but the Newcastle and Manchester varieties of *Sh. flexneri* serotype 6 and strains of *Sh. dysenteriae* serotype 5 and *Sh. boydii* serotypes 2, 3, 4, 6 and 10 are dulcitol fermenters.

Sucrose is not fermented except by *Sh. sonnei* and some strains of *Sh. flexneri* when incubation is prolonged for several days. Xylose is not fermented except by the mannitol-negative biotype of *Sh. flexneri* type 4a and some strains of *Sh. boydii* and *Sh. sonnei*. Salicin is not fermented except by rare strains of *Sh. sonnei*. Adonitol and inositol are not fermented.

2. INDOLE PRODUCTION. *Sh. dysenteriae* serotype 1, *Sh. flexneri* serotype 6 and *Sh. sonnei* are always indole-negative. Strains of other serotypes differ in their reactions.

3. CATALASE TEST. The general finding that enterobacteria produce catalase has important exceptions in *Sh. dysenteriae* serotype 1 and a few strains of *Sh. flexneri* (mostly in serotype 4a) which are catalase-negative.

4. DECARBOXYLASE TESTS. Members of groups A, B and C fail to decarboxylate lysine and ornithine. *Sh. sonnei* decarboxylates ornithine but not lysine.

5. OTHER BIOCHEMICAL TESTS. Urease negative. Methyl red positive. Voges-Proskauer negative. Citrate not utilized. KCN broth negative. Gluconate not utilized. Malonate not utilized. Phenylalanine deaminase negative. Gelatin not liquefied. H_2S not produced.

Antigenic structure. Shigellae are differentiated by their somatic (O) antigens into serotypes identified by agglutination tests with absorbed specific antisera (Edwards and Ewing, 1972; Kauffmann, 1969). Some serotypes may be identified by agglutination with unabsorbed sera, but absorbed sera must be used for other serotypes between which minor antigens are shared.

GROUP A. *Sh. dysenteriae* contains ten serotypes, each characterized by a different type antigen. Serotypes 1 and 2 are the organisms formerly called *Sh. shigae* and *Sh. schmitzii*. Serotype 2 shares a minor antigen with serotype 10.

GROUP B. For more than 50 years *Sh. flexneri* was known to have a complex antigenic structure. This structure was elucidated by Boyd in the decade 1930–40 (see Wilson and Miles, 1964). A simplified antigenic scheme for the six serotypes and two variants is set out in Table 29.2. Serotypes 1–6 are characterized by their possession of different specific *type antigens*, designated I–VI. They share other, *group antigens* from a series designated 1–8. The serotypes 1–4 are each divided into subserotypes by the nature of their group antigens. Variants X and Y have lost their type antigens and are distinguished by their different group antigens.

The O-antigens of *Sh. flexneri* represent the structure of the O-specific side chains of repeating sugar units of the cell-wall lipopolysaccharide. The type antigens reflect the nature of the linkages of secondary α-glucosyl side-chains, which differ among the serotypes, and

Table 29.2 Antigens of *Shigella flexneri* serotypes

Serotype	Subserotype	Type antigen	Group antigens*
1	1a	I	1, 2, 4
	1b	I	1, 2, 4, 6
2	2a	II	1, 3, 4
	2b	II	1, 7, 8
3	3a	III	1, 6, 7, 8
	3b	III	1, 3, 4, 6, 7, 8
	3c	III	1, 6
4	4a	IV	1, 3, 4
	4b	IV	1, 3, 4, 6
5	...	V	1, 7, 8
6	...	VI	1, 2, 4
X variant	...	—	1, 7, 8
Y variant	...	—	1, 3, 4

* Not all group antigens are listed.

the group antigens reflect common sequences in the primary side-chains (Simmons, 1971). The type antigens are determined by specific prophages and the serotype of a strain may be changed by lysogenization. The group antigens appear to be determined by genes on the bacterial chromosome.

Although serotype-6 strains are classified as *Sh. flexneri* because they share group antigens with other *Sh. flexneri* serotypes, they show differences that would justify their classification in a separate genus; their cell-wall lipopoly-saccharide has a very different basal (core) structure from that common to the other serotypes of *Sh. flexneri* (Simmons, 1971) and their gas-producing property and lack of fimbriae are also distinctive.

GROUP C. Fifteen different serotypes of *Sh. boydii* are recognized. Sharing of antigenic components among serotypes 1, 4 and 11, between serotypes 10 and 11 and between serotypes 9 and 13 makes the use of absorbed sera necessary for their identification.

GROUP D. *Sh. sonnei* is antigenically homogeneous, but the phase-2 (R) variant is antigenically different from the phase-1 (S) form.

CROSS-REACTIONS BETWEEN GROUPS. There are close relationships between the O-antigens of many shigella serotypes and those of serotypes in other *Shigella* species and certain serotypes of *Escherichia coli* and the Alkalescens-Dispar group of organisms. For example, the O-antigen of *Sh. dysenteriae* serotype 1 is related to the O-antigens of *Esch. coli* O-group 1 and A-D group 1; that of *Sh. dysenteriae* serotype 2 to those of *Sh. boydii* serotype 15 and *Esch. coli* O112a, O112c; those of *Sh. flexneri* serotypes 2, 3 and 4 to that of *Esch. coli* O13; that of *Sh. flexneri* serotype 6 to those of *Sh. boydii* serotype 5, *Esch. coli* O19a and A-D group 2; those of *Sh. boydii* serotypes 1 and 4 to that of A-D group 1 (also Boyd 1 to *Esch. coli* O2 and Boyd 4 to *Esch. coli* O53); and that of *Sh. boydii* serotype 6 to that of *Sh. sonnei* phase 2 (R). The O-antigen of *Sh. sonnei* phase 1 (S) is unrelated to the O-antigens of other enterobacteria, including *Esch. coli* O-groups 1-145, but is identical with that of a polar-flagellated oxidase-positive Gram-negative rod previously designated 'paracolon C27' and now classified as *Plesiomonas*

shigelloides. The relationships of some shigellae, particularly of *Sh. boydii* serotypes, with Alkalescens-Dispar organisms are of particular importance because the latter organisms resemble shigellae in being non-motile, anaerogenic and, in many strains, non-lactose-fermenting; tests with carefully absorbed sera are necessary for the identification of these shigellae.

K-ANTIGENS. Some strains in many shigella serotypes are inagglutinable by homologous O-antisera because they possess a K-antigen, which may or may not be visible as a capsule and which covers their O-antigen. The K-antigen in each O-serotype appears to be specific for that serotype and different from those in other serotypes; exceptions are the related K-antigens of *Sh. boydii* serotypes 10 and 11. In cases where the same O-antigen is present in a shigella serotype and an *Esch. coli* O-group, the K-antigens of the organisms are also similar. Like the B variety of K-antigen in *Esch. coli,* the K-antigens of shigellae are heat-labile and the cultures possessing them can be rendered agglutinable by O-antisera by heating at 100°C for 1 hour.

FIMBRIAL ANTIGENS. Fimbriate strains in the different serotypes of *Sh. flexneri* form identical fimbrial antigens (Gillies and Duguid, 1958). Richly fimbriated cultures obtained by prolonged or serial culture in broth, e.g. 3 passages at 37°C for 48-hour periods, are agglutinable by antisera raised to fimbriate cultures of any serotype. Minor antigens are shared between the fimbriae of *Sh. flexneri* and those of *Escherichia coli* and *Klebsiella aerogenes*, but there is no sharing with salmonella fimbriae. Antibodies to the shared coliflexneri fimbrial antigens are present in the sera of many persons and some unimmunized rabbits. Fimbriae may be removed from the bacteria by heating at 100°C for 30 minutes and washing by centrifugation, but misleading cross-agglutination reactions are best avoided by using only agar-grown non-fimbriate-phase cultures for the preparation of agglutinable bacterial suspensions and immunizing antigens.

Viability. Cultures retain their viability well, e.g. for many years on Dorset's egg. All types are killed by moist heat at 55°C in 1 hour and fairly readily by strong disinfectants, e.g. by

1 per cent phenol in 15 min. The bacilli tend to die within a few hours in faeces allowed to become acid due to the growth of commensal bacteria, but can survive for some days in faeces kept non-acid in buffered glycerol solution or preserved at 4°C. They mostly die within a few hours if dried, but under some circumstances survive for several (e.g. 5–20) days, for example in faeces dried on cloth, or on soiled lavatory seats and other fomites, in cool, damp, dark conditions. *Sh. sonnei* is more resistant and survives better in the environment than the other species of *Shigella*, a difference that may explain why Sonne dysentery has not been as readily controlled by improvements in community hygiene as the other types of bacillary dysentery.

Antibiotic sensitivity. Different strains of a serotype differ in their sensitivity to sulphonamide, chloramphenicol, tetracycline, streptomycin, neomycin and other antibiotics, and some show multiple resistance due to the acquisition of a transmissible resistance plasmid. Therapy with antibiotics tends to prolong the excretion of shigellae and is best avoided except in severe illnesses, when it should be based on the results of an antibiotic sensitivity test made on a culture isolated from the patient.

LABORATORY DIAGNOSIS OF SHIGELLA DYSENTERY

Shigellae are rarely present in the body other than in the intestine and the laboratory diagnosis of bacillary dysentery can be made only by the isolation of a shigella from the faeces. A positive finding in a case of diarrhoeal illness is practically diagnostic of shigella dysentery. Shigellae may, however, be present in the faeces of chronic carriers and so may occasionally be found in the faeces of a patient with diarrhoea due to a cause other than shigellosis, but mistakes due to such a coincidence are likely to be rare.

Determination of the serotype of an isolate is necessary to confirm its identity as a shigella and has a further, epidemiological value in defining groups of patients infected with the same serotype from a common source. Phagetyping or colicine typing of strains within a serotype defines even more precisely the similarities and differences between strains from different sources.

Specimens. The specimens submitted to the laboratory are commonly faeces or rectal swabs, rarely vomit. Faeces is preferable to a rectal swab because a rectal swab is unlikely to give a positive culture unless it is moist and visibly soiled with faeces. If the specimen of faeces cannot be transported to the laboratory under cool conditions within a few hours, it should be placed in buffered glycerol saline (Chap. 5) to prevent the shigellae being overgrown and killed by acid-forming commensal bacteria. Rectal swabs may be transported in Stuart's transport medium.

Microscopic examination. Gram-stained films are not used because shigellae are indistinguishable from the commensal Gram-negative bacilli invariably present in faeces. A wet film of a saline suspension of faeces from severe bacillary dysentery is likely to show numerous erythrocytes (blood) and polymorphs (pus) and some macrophages. Care should be taken not to mistake the macrophages for the vegetative forms of *Entamoeba histolytica*, which have relatively smaller nuclei and are usually motile in warm fresh specimens.

Isolation by culture. The specimens are cultured by the methods described for salmonellae in Chapter 28. Identical selective and enrichment media are used, because the usual request is for a search for all intestinal pathogens. It should be noted, however, that whilst MacConkey's agar, deoxycholate citrate agar and selenite F broth are generally selective for shigellae, brilliant-green bismuth sulphite agar and tetrathionate broth are inhibitory to shigellae and useful only for the isolation of salmonellae.

'Pale' (colourless or pale yellow) colonies on MacConkey's agar or DCA after not more than 24 hours' incubation are selected for further investigation. If the colonies emulsify smoothly in saline, slide agglutination tests with shigella antisera may be attempted directly and, if these tests are positive, a *provisional report* may be issued pending the growth of subcultures and the confirmation of their identity by biochemical tests.

The colonies from the selective media may,

however, be sticky and give suspensions un-suitable for slide agglutination tests. It is always necessary, therefore, to subculture single colonies of each suspect colonial form into nutrient broth and on to nutrient agar and to use the subcultures as inocula for biochemical tests. The subculture used for this purpose should also be tested for purity by plating on MacConkey's agar. If the plating shows a mixture of organisms, a pale colony should be picked from it and used to inoculate a fresh set of biochemical tests.

Biochemical tests. Tests for motility and bio-chemical reactions are used primarily to indicate that the isolate is a shigella and secondarily to suggest the species of shigella. These tests are carried out as described for suspect salmonellae in Chapter 28. Motility may be assessed either by microscopical examination of a wet film of a young (6 hour) growth in peptone water or by naked-eye observation of a stab culture in semi-solid agar, e.g. 'tube 2' of Kohn's composite test media. Isolates with the biochemical characters of one of the shigella groups must be further examined by serological agglutination tests.

Serological identification. Shigella serotypes are identified by slide and tube agglutination tests with specific O-antisera. The typing sera should be purchased for commercial sources because laborious absorptions are required to make sera sufficiently specific (Edwards and Ewing, 1972). The set of antisera held should comprise at least those for *Sh. dysenteriae* serotype 1, *Sh. dysenteriae* serotype 2, *Sh. flexneri* (polyvalent for serotypes 1–6 and variants X and Y), *Sh. boydii* (polyvalent for serotypes 1–15) and *Sh. sonnei* (phases 1 and 2). Additional sera for other *Sh. dysenteriae* sero-types and monovalent sera for the different *Sh. flexneri* and *Sh. boydii* types should be kept if the laboratory examines many faecal speci-mens.

Slide-agglutination tests will suffice for typing if the results are clear cut. If there is any doubt about the results of the slide test, tube-agglutination tests should be done. Tube tests should also be done if the biochemical reactions of the isolate are atypical or if the slide tests indicate an uncommon serotype.

The antigen for tube-agglutination tests

should be prepared by suspending the growth from a nutrient agar slope or plate either in saline containing 0·2 per cent formaldehyde or in mercuric iodide solution (HgI_2 0·1 g, KI 0·4 g, NaCl 0·45 g, 40 per cent formaldehyde 0·2 ml and distilled water to 100 ml; store at room temperature). Broth cultures should not be used because, when grown in broth, *Sh. flexneri* may form fimbrial antigens which interfere with the test. A suspension containing about 3×10^9 bacteria/ml is suitable for slide tests and it should be diluted 1 in 10 in saline for tube tests (3×10^8/ml).

If a shigella-like culture proves to be in-agglutinable by the available O-antisera, the presence of a K-antigen should be suspected. A saline suspension of the bacteria should be heated at 100°C for 0·5 to 1 hour to remove any K-antigen and after centrifugation and re-suspension in fresh formaldehyde-saline the bacteria should be tested again with the O-antisera. If results are still negative, the suspect culture should be submitted to a Reference Laboratory for fuller investigation.

If a culture shows some autoagglutination in saline, i.e. is 'rough', it may be tested in 0·1 per cent formaldehyde in distilled water or first be subcultured at 22–30°C when it may be obtained in a 'smooth' form

Bacteria that may be confused with shigellae. Gram-negative bacilli of several other genera share many biochemical reactions with the shigellae and some share antigens with parti-cular shigella serotypes. These bacteria may be mistaken for shigellae, particularly because some strains of shigella differ in one or more of their biochemical reactions from the pattern typical of their serotype.

1. *Salmonella*. Anaerogenic and non-motile strains of salmonellae may be mistaken for shigellae if only a limited range of biochemical tests is carried out. The tests of most value for the differention of such salmonellae from shigellae are those for citrate utilization, H_2S production, decarboxylation of lysine and ornithine, and agglutination with polyvalent salmonella O and H sera.

2. *Alkalescens-Dispar group*. These non-motile anaerogenic non-lactose-fermenting members of the genus *Escherichia* may mimic shigellae in the initial biochemical tests and some

strains share antigens with particular shigella serotypes. They can be differentiated in tests of bacteria heated at 100°C for 0·5 to 1 hour with absorbed type-specific sera for the different shigella and Alkalescens-Dispar serotypes. Some A-D strains are distinguished by their decarboxylation of lysine.

3. *Hafnia*. Hafnia organisms are non-lactose-fermenting bacilli that otherwise resemble organisms in the genus *Enterobacter*. They are distinguished from shigellae by their motility and their positive gluconate, malonate, ornithine-decarboxylase and citrate-utilization reactions. Some hafnia strains share O-antigens with certain shigella serotypes, e.g. *Sh. flexneri* type 4a, and *Sh. boydii* type 11.

4. *Providencia*. These non-lactose-fermenting organisms are distinguished from shigellae by their motility and their ability to deaminate phenylalanine.

5. *Plesiomonas shigelloides*. This Gram-negative bacillus, which shares antigens with *Sh. sonnei* phase 1 and resembles it in being anaerogenic and non-lactose-fermenting, is distinguished by its motility, positive oxidase reaction, positive indole reaction and failure to ferment mannitol.

Tests for shigella antibody in patient's serum. Antibody production is irregular in bacillary dysentery and tests for it have no part to play in the diagnosis of the disease.

Typing of strains for epidemiological purposes. Within groups A, B and C the determination of serotype has an epidemiological value and subdivision of the serotype is rarely attempted. The subdivision of *Sh. flexneri* by the method of phage-typing distinguishes a number of different phage-types within each serotype and a total of 123 phage-types have been identified by Milch, Laszlo, Slopek and Mulczyk (1968). *Sh. sonnei* consists of only a single serotype and it is in this species that there is the greatest requirement for subdivision by some other typing method. Phage-typing has been attempted in *Sh. sonnei*, but instability of type and the predominance of strains of one phage-type did not encourage its use (Tee, 1955); the method has, however, been found useful and reliable over a long period in Sweden where up to 21 out of about 100 recognized phage-types were distinguished in a single year (Kallings,

Lindberg and Sjöberg, 1968). In most centres, however, the method of colicine typing is used for the subdivision of *Sh. sonnei* strains because the method is simpler than that of phage-typing and the typing characters are more stable.

COLICINE TYPING OF SH. SONNEI. The majority of strains of *Sh. sonnei* are colicinogenic and different strains produce colicines active against different susceptible 'indicator' strains of *Sh. sonnei* and other enterobacteria. The ability of a strain to produce a particular colicine is a fairly stable character and strains are therefore typed by identifying the colicines they produce by a test of their ability to inhibit the growth of a set of selected indicator strains. The sensitivity of *Sh. sonnei* strains to colicines is a less stable character, so that a system of typing based on observations of the sensitivity of the strains to standard colicines is unsatisfactory.

The method of typing *Sh. sonnei* by observation of colicine production recommended by Gillies (1964) is based on that of Abbott and Shannon (1958).

Indicator strains. Fifteen strains are usually used, e.g. *Sh. sonnei* strains 2, 56, 17, 2M, 38, 56/56, 56/98, R1, R6; *Sh. schmitzii* M19; *Sh. sonnei* 2/7, 2/64, 2/15, R5; *Escherichia coli* strain Row. These are the indicator strains no. 1–15, respectively, as used by Gillies and Brown (1966) and in the scheme shown in Table 29.3. They may be obtained from Dr R. R. Gillies, Bacteriology Department, University of Edinburgh Medical School, Teviot Place, Edinburgh.

Medium. Tryptone soya (TS) agar (Oxoid) is reconstituted according to the manufacturer's instructions and horse blood is added to give a final concentration of 2·5 per cent (v/v). It is poured in Petri dishes in a layer about 3–4 mm thick.

Method. The strain to be typed is inoculated as a single streak across the diameter of a TS agar plate and the plate is incubated at 35°C (*not* 37°C) for 24 hours. The growth is removed with the edge of a glass slide and 2–3 ml CHCl₃ is put into the lid of the plate and the medium-containing dish, medium side downwards, is placed on top of it. After exposure to the chloroform vapour for a period of 10–15 min,

Table 29.3   Inhibition patterns given by seventeen colicine-type strains of *Shigella sonnei* against fifteen indicator strains

Indicator strain	Inhibition caused by producer strain of colicine type:																
	1a	1b	2	3	3a	4	5	6	7	8	9	10	11	12	13	14	15
1	+	+	−	+	+	+	+	−	−	+	+	+	−	+	−	+	+
2	+	+	+	+	+	+	+	+	−	−	+	+	−	+	+	+	−
3	+	+	+	+	+	+	+	−	+	+	+	+	−	−	+	+	+
4	−	−	−	−	−	v	v	−	−	−	−	−	−	−	−	v	+
5	−	−	−	+	+	+	+	−	−	+	v	+	−	+	−	+	+
6	+	+	−	+	+	−	+	+	−	−	+	+	−	+	+	+	−
7	+	+	−	+	+	−	+	+	−	−	+	+	−	+	+	+	−
8	−	−	−	+	+	+	+	−	−	+	+	+	−	+	−	+	+
9	−	+	+	+	+	+	+	+	−	−	+	+	−	+	+	+	−
10	+	+	−	+	−	−	+	−	−	−	−	+	−	−	−	−	−
11	−	−	−	+	+	+	+	−	−	−	−	−	−	−	−	+	+
12	−	−	−	+	+	+	+	−	−	−	−	−	−	−	−	−	−
13	−	−	−	+	+	+	+	−	−	+	+	+	−	+	−	+	+
14	−	−	−	+	+	−	−	−	−	−	−	−	−	−	−	−	+
15	+	+	+	+	+	+	+	+	−	+	+	+	+	+	+	+	+

+ = Indicator strain inhibited by colicine-type strain;
− = indicator strain not inhibited;
v = variable reaction.

sufficient for the killing of all bacteria, the chloroform is decanted and the plate exposed to air for a further 10–15 min. The indicator strains, which have been grown overnight in nutrient broth, are inoculated on to the plate in parallel streaks at right angles to the line of the original growth. The plate is then incubated at 37°C for 8–12 hours and observed for any inhibition of the streak-growths of the indicator strains.

Interpretation of results. More than 17 colicine-types of *Sh. sonnei* are distinguished according to the different combinations of the indicator strains inhibited by their colicines (Table 29.3).

REFERENCES

ABBOTT, J. D. & SHANNON, R. (1958) A method of typing *Shigella sonnei* using colicine production as a marker. *Journal of Clinical Pathology*, **11**, 71.

ASSOCIATION OF CLINICAL PATHOLOGISTS. Broadsheet 60: January 1968. *Identification of shigella.* (From Publishing Manager, *Journal of Clinical Pathology*, BMA House, Tavistock Square, London WC1.)

DUGUID, J. P. & GILLIES, R. R. (1957) Fimbriae and adhesive properties in dysentery bacilli. *Journal of Pathology and Bacteriology*, **74**, 397.

EDWARDS, P. R. & EWING, W. H. (1972) *Identification of Enterobacteriaceae*, 3rd edition. Minneapolis: Burgess Publishing Co.

GILLIES, R. R. (1964) Colicine production as an epidemiological marker of *Shigella sonnei*. *Journal of Hygiene, Cambridge*, **62**, 1.

GILLIES, R. R. & BROWN, D. O. (1966) A new colicine type (type 15) of *Shigella sonnei*. *Journal of Hygiene, Cambridge*, **64**, 305.

GILLIES, R. R. & DUGUID, J. P. (1958) The fimbrial antigens of *Shigella flexneri*. *Journal of Hygiene, Cambridge*, **56**, 303.

KALLINGS, L. O., LINDBERG, A. A. & SJÖBERG, L. (1968) Phage typing of *Shigella sonnei*. *Archivum Immunologiae et Therapiae Experimentalis*, **16**, 250.

KAUFFMANN, F. (1969) *The Bacteriology of the Enterobacteriaceae*, 2nd edition. Copenhagen: Munksgaard.

MILCH, H., LASZLO, G., SLOPEK, S. & MULCZYK, M. (1968) Lysotypes of *Shigella flexneri*. *Archivum Immunologiae et Therapiae Experimentalis*, **16**, 265.

SIMMONS, D. A. R. (1971) Immunochemistry of *Shigella flexneri* O-antigens: a study of structural and genetic aspects of the biosynthesis of cell-surface antigens. *Bacteriological Reviews*, **35**, 117.

TEE, G. H. (1955) Bacteriophage typing of *Shigella sonnei* and its limitations in epidemiological investigations. *Journal of Hygiene, Cambridge*, **53**, 54.

WILSON, G. S. & MILES, A. A. (1964) *Principles of Bacteriology and Immunity*, 5th edition, page 855. London: Arnold.

30. Escherichia, Klebsiella, Proteus and other Enterobacteria

The genera of Enterobacteriaceae remaining to be described comprise *Escherichia*, *Klebsiella*, *Enterobacter* (syn. *Cloaca*) *Hafnia*, *Serratia*, *Citrobacter*, *Proteus* and *Providencia*.

Morphology and staining. The bacteria of these eight genera are alike in being Gram-negative bacilli, 2–4 μm $\times$ 0·6 μm, and non-sporing, but show differences in the presence or absence of motility (always due to peritrichous flagella), fimbriae and capsules.

Cultural characters. Members of most genera form 'coliform-type' colonies on simple solid media, i.e. circular, 1–3 mm in diameter, low convex, smooth surfaced, colourless to grey and translucent. On MacConkey's agar the colonies may be *pink*, indicating that the organism ferments lactose rapidly, or *pale* (yellow-grey), indicating that it either does not ferment lactose or gives 'late' fermentation only after several days' incubation. Some species, however, give characteristic appearances, e.g. the large mucoid colonies of klebsiellae and the swarming colonies of proteus on non-inhibitory media.

Biochemical characters. Differences in biochemical activities provide the main means of differentiating the genera and species. Table 30.1 shows some of the most useful discriminating biochemical reactions along with the properties of motility and capsulation. It should be considered in conjunction with the descriptions of the most constant differential features in the text below (see also Cowan and Steel, 1965, pp. 78 and 79). The results of the different tests are not given equal importance in the identification of a particular genus or species. Although equal weight is given to all characters in classification by the Adansonian principle, it is legitimate and, indeed, essential for diagnostic purposes to put different weightings on different characters (Cowan, 1965). Thus, less weight should be given to a highly variable than to a more constant character. The representation of results by the notation ' + ', ' − ' and 'd' in Table 30.1 is not sufficiently precise to indicate the amount of weighting to be given to a reaction, but the proper weighting can be assessed when the proportion of strains in the species that give a positive result is known. This information is available and enables identification to be done by the statistical expression of the results of a selected range of tests. Such an assessment may be done with the aid of a computer, as in certain reference laboratories (e.g. Computer Laboratory, Central Public Health Laboratory, Colindale Avenue, London). Commercially prepared 'kits' of tests embodying this principle can now be purchased and used in any laboratory; they enable a range of biochemical tests to be carried out simply and are issued with instructions on how the results should be interpreted (e.g. api system, API, Philpot House, Rayleigh, Essex; Encise system, Roche Products Ltd, Diagnostics Department, 15 Manchester Square, London).

Antigenic structure. Although much is known of the antigenic composition of the various genera (Edwards and Ewing, 1972; Kauffmann, 1969), this information is not generally used in ordinary diagnostic medical bacteriology. Where, however, it has a special value, e.g. in the identification of the enteropathogenic strains of *Escherichia coli*, the necessary antisera are available from commercial sources.

ESCHERICHIA COLI

The genus *Escherichia* was formerly subdivided into a number of species by differences in sugar fermentation reactions, but nowadays only one species, *Escherichia coli*, is recognized and it is subdivided into biotypes and serotypes. The characters of *Escherichia* that distinguish it from other enterobacteria are that it is motile, forms gas from glucose, ferments lactose, produces indole, gives a positive methyl-red reaction and a negative Voges-Proskauer reaction and does not utilize citrate, grow in KCN, decompose urea or liquefy gelatin (Table 30.1). Some strains differ from the typical in one or two of these

Table 30.1 Reactions of *Escherichia coli* and some other enterobacteria

Reaction	Escherichia coli	A–D Group	Klebsiella aerogenes	Klebsiella pneumoniae	Klebsiella edwardsii	Klebsiella atlantae	Klebsiella ozaenae	Klebsiella rhinoscleromatis	Enterobacter cloacae	Enterobacter aerogenes	Enterobacter liquefaciens	Hafnia alvei	Serratia marcescens	Citrobacter	Proteus vulgaris	Proteus mirabilis	Proteus morganii	Proteus rettgeri	Providencia
Motility	+	–	–	–	–	–	–	–	+	+	+*	+*	+	+	+	+	+	+	+
Capsule	–	–	+	+	+	+	+	+	–	–	–	–	d	–	–	–	–	–	–
Glucose (gas)	+	–	+	+	–	–	d	–	+	+	+*	+*	d	d	+	+	+	–	d
Lactose (acid)	+	d	+	+	(+)	(+)	(+)	–	+	+	d	+	(±)	d	–	–	–	–	–
ONPG	+	d	+	+	+	+	+	+	+	+	+	+	+	d	–	–	–	–	(+)
Sucrose (acid)	d	d	+	+	+	+	d	+	+	+	+	d	+	d	+	(+)	–	d	–
Salicin (acid)	d	d	+	+	+	+	+	+	+	+	+	d	+	d	+	(±)	–	d	d
Adonitol (acid)	–	–	d	–	–	–	+	+	d	+	+	–	d	–	–	–	–	+	–
Dulcitol (acid)	d	d	–	d	d	d	–	–	d	d	d	–	–	d	–	–	–	–	d
Inositol (acid)	–	–	+	–	+	+	+	+	d	–	–	+	d	d	+	–	–	–	d
Mannitol (acid)	+	+	+	+	+	+	+	+	+	+	+	+	+	+	+	+	–	+	+
Indole	+	+	–	–	+	+	–	+	–	–	–	–	–	+	+	–	+	+	+
Methyl Red	+	+	+	+	+	+	+	+	–	–	d*	+*	–	d	+	d	+	+	+
Voges-Proskauer	–	–	+	+	+	+	–	–	+	+	+	+*	+	d	d	d	–	–	–
Citrate	–	–	+	+	+	+	+	+	+	+	+	–*	+	+	–	+	–	+	+
Gelatin	–	–	–	–	–	–	–	–	–	–	+	+	+	–	+	+	–	–	–
Phenylalanine	–	–	–	–	–	–	–	–	(+)	d	–	–	–	–	+	+	+	+	+
Urease	–	–	+	+	+	+	d	+	d	d	d	d	+	d	+	+	+	+	–
Hydrogen sulphide	–	–	–	–	–	–	–	–	–	–	–	–	–	–	+	+	–	–	–
KCN	–	–	+	d	+	+	+	–	+	+	+	+	+	+	+	+	+	+	+
Gluconate	–	–	+	d	+	+	+	+	+	+	+	d	d	–	–	–	–	–	–
Malonate	–	+	+	+	+	+	+	+	d	d	d	+	d	d	–	–	–	–	–
Lysine decarboxylase	+	+	+	+	+	+	–	+	–	+	+	+	+	–	–	–	–	–	–
Ornithine decarboxylase	d	d	+	–	–	–	d	–	+	+	+	+	+	d	–	+	+	–	–

+   = Result positive with at least 80% of strains.
–   = Result negative with at least 80% of strains.
d   = Different result in different strains.
(+) = Delayed positive result (e.g. 2–8 days).
... = Results not given.
* tests done at 25°–30°C.

characters, e.g. motility, gas formation, lactose fermentation or non-utilization of citrate, but are nevertheless accepted as *Esch. coli* (Sojka, 1965).

Morphology. Gram-negative non-sporing bacilli. Most strains (about 80 per cent) are motile, though motility is often feeble on primary isolation, and most strains (again about 80 per cent) are fimbriate. The fimbriae are type 1, i.e. haemagglutinating and mannose-sensitive, and are found both in motile and non-motile strains (Duguid, Smith, Dempster and Edmunds, 1955). (About 30 per cent of strains possess a mannose-resistant somatic haemagglutinin either in addition to or in the absence of a fimbrial haemagglutinin; Duguid, 1964). A few strains are capsulate and many others form abundant loose slime when grown on sugar-containing medium at 15°–20°C (Duguid, 1951, 1964).

Cultural characters. Since most strains ferment lactose rapidly, the colonies on MacConkey's medium, which are smooth, glossy and translucent, are rose-pink in colour. Growth is either impaired or totally inhibited on deoxycholate citrate agar; any colonies that do grow are small, pink and opaque. On blood agar the colonies of some strains are surrounded by zones of haemolysis. Most strains are prototrophic and grow on simple synthetic media such as a glucose-ammonium-salts agar without supplementation with amino acids or vitamins. *Esch. coli* is uninhibited by bile salt in MacConkey's medium, but is inhibited by the citrate in Leifson's DCA medium and by sodium selenite, sodium tetrathionate, brilliant green and other substances used in media selective for salmonellae and shigellae. It is also inhibited by 7 per cent NaCl in salt media used for isolation of staphylococci.

Biochemical reactions. Carbohydrates are attacked fermentatively, with the production of acid and gas; a few strains are anaerogenic, producing acid but not gas. Traditionally, the prompt fermentation of lactose (within 24 hours, and usually within 8 hours) was a character essential for the identification of a strain as *Esch. coli*, but it is now accepted that the species includes some late-lactose-fermenting or lactose-negative strains. Other substrates with which different biotypes of *Esch. coli*

react differently include raffinose, rhamnose, sorbose, sucrose, xylose, adonitol, dulcitol, glycerol, sorbitol, salicin, arginine, glutamic acid and ornithine (see Sojka, 1965).

For classifying enterobacteria isolated from drinking-water supplies, bacteriologists commonly use the so-called 'IMViC' reactions; thus the faecal coliform bacillus, *Esch. coli*, is distinguished from klebsiellae, enterobacters and other coliforms derived from soil and vegetation by the pattern of reactions: indole positive, methyl-red positive, Voges-Proskauer negative and citrate-utilization negative. It is also distinguished from the other coliforms by its ability to form gas from lactose in tests incubated at 44°C (Eijkman test).

Antigenic structure. Three kinds of surface antigens demonstrable in agglutination tests are observed for the serotyping of *Esch. coli*: the O (somatic), K (capsular) and H (flagellar) antigens. Fimbrial antigens also take part in the agglutination reactions of bacilli that are phenotypically in the fimbriate-phase; they are widely shared between strains of different serotypes, so that misleading cross-reactions may be obtained unless serotyping tests are done with bacilli from non-fimbriate-phase cultures (e.g. agar-grown cultures) or bacilli defimbriated by heating at 100°C for 1 hour (Gillies and Duguid, 1958).

In the Kauffmann - Knipschildt - Vahlne scheme for the serological classification of strains of *Esch. coli* the primary subdivision is made according to the specific character of the lipopolysaccharide O-antigen of the cell wall. A different 'O-group' of strains is defined by the presence of each different O-antigen. The original scheme (Kauffmann, 1947) included 25 O-group and O-antigens, but over 140 such groups and antigens have now been described (Sojka, 1965; Kauffmann, 1969; Edwards and Ewing, 1972). The O-groups are subdivided into serotypes according to the K and H antigens present. At least 91 different K-antigens and 49 different H-antigens are known. The serotype of a strain is defined by its full antigenic formula, i.e. its O, K and H antigens, e.g. *Esch. coli* 055:K59:H6.

The term K-antigen is used to include three kinds of antigens that lie outside the cell wall and the O-antigen; these are the L, A and B types of K-antigen. The A type of K-antigen is associated with the presence of a typical capsule visible in wet India ink films on bacteria from ordinary cultures; alternatively, the capsule may be seen by its 'swelling' with the homologous K-antiserum in a wet film. Strains with L or B antigens generally show capsules only if grown on sugar-containing medium at 15°–20°C. The properties of these three kinds of antigen differ also in the way they are affected by heat and treatment with chemicals. A knowledge of their differential susceptibilities is necessary for the preparation of pure antisera to the individual antigenic components and details are given by Edwards and Ewing (1972) Sojka (1965) and Kauffmann (1969). An important feature is that the ability of the L and B antigens to mask agglutination by the appropriate O-antiserum is nullified by heating at 100°C for 1 hour, whereas removal of the A-antigen requires autoclaving at 121°C for 2·5 hours.

Originally the K-antigens of the L and A types were numbered consecutively but the B-antigens were numbered in a separate series. Subsequently the B-antigens were renumbered so that they could be included in the same series as the other K-antigens and both their old and new numbers are often shown in the designation of a strain's serotype, e.g. *Esch. coli* O55:K59(B5):H6. It should be noted that with few exceptions any one strain can possess only one of the three kinds of K-antigen, i.e. L, A *or* B.

Recent studies of the immunoelectrophoretic patterns of water (60°C) extracts of the O and K antigens of *Esch. coli* strains in all known O-groups suggest that only a minority of strains have a polysaccharide K-antigen separate from the O-antigen, that most B-antigen-containing strains lack such an independent K-antigen and that some B-antigens may represent labile material corresponding to part of the O-antigen (Ørskov, Ørskov, Jann and Jann, 1971; Ørskov and Ørskov, 1972). These authors have proposed that the antigenic formula should omit the K-antigen designation in cases where an independent K-antigen has not been demonstrated; e.g. serotypes O55:K59(B5):H6 and O111:K60(B4):H2 should instead be given as O55:H6 and O111:H2. They found that nearly

all the strains possessing an independent K-antigen were strains that possessed L-type antigens and belonged to serotypes frequently found in the normal intestine and in extra-intestinal disease such as septicaemia and urinary infections, e.g. O1:K51, O2:K56, O3: K2, O4:K3, O5:K4, O6:K2, O7:K7, O11:K10, O25:K19, O75:K?. (These K-antigens are acidic thermostable polysaccharides that appear to inhibit host defence mechanisms such as phagocytosis and complement.) The O-antigens of the commonly encountered O-groups were predominantly kathodic (non-acid) in migration but those of some groups, including the groups associated with 'dysentery-like' disease (O112ac, O124, O28 and O136) were wholly anodic (acidic). Most of the enteropathogenic serotypes associated with infantile gastroenteritis (e.g. O26, O55, O86, O111, O119, O127, O128 and O142) had wholly kathodic (non-acidic) O-antigens and no independent K-antigens.

Viability. *Esch. coli* is generally similar to other enterobacteria in its susceptibility to inimical agents and conditions, though it is slightly more resistant to heat, to some chemicals and to drying than are the salmonellae and shigellae. It is killed by moist heat at 60°C usually within 30 min, though occasionally some bacteria may survive pasteurization in milk at 62°–63°C for 30 min. It can remain alive in water for several weeks or months, though it does not appear to grow in natural waters·outside the body. It can survive for several days when dried on clothing or in dust, and pathogenic serotypes have been found to be viable and numerous in floor dust, in air and on clothing, napkins and ward equipment in hospitals containing infants with gastroenteritis (Rogers, 1951; Hutchinson, 1957).

Antibiotic sensitivity. *Esch. coli* is similar to many other enterobacteria in its susceptibility to antibiotics and different strains differ markedly in the degree of their sensitivity to several of the drugs commonly used to treat coliform infections. Strains from the faeces of healthy persons or from infections, e.g. in the urinary tract, in patients outside hospitals are commonly sensitive to readily attainable concentrations of sulphonamides, ampicillin (minimum inhibitory concentration about 8 μg/ml), tetracycline (1 μg/ml), chloramphenicol (4 μg/ml), streptomycin (4 μg/ml), kanamycin (2 μg/ml) and polymyxin (0·25 μg/ml). All strains are resistant to the concentrations of benzylpenicillin and phenoxymethyl penicillin that are attainable in the blood and tissues, but many are sensitive to concentrations readily attainable in the urine after oral or parenteral administration (e.g. 32–64 μg/ml). All strains are highly resistant to methicillin, cloxacillin, erythromycin, fucidin and vancomycin.

Strains of *Esch. coli* can acquire high-level resistance to some of the antibiotics (e.g. streptomycin) to which most strains are sensitive by spontaneous genetic mutation and an infecting strain sometimes undergoes such a change during the treatment of a patient. Strains may also acquire resistance to one or several antibiotics by the receipt of a transmissible plasmid from another, already resistant bacterium. Strains with resistance that is dependent on mutated chromosomal genes or on transmissible plasmids are commonly present in hospital patients receiving antibiotics, e.g. in urological wards, where they commonly cause cross-infections.

LABORATORY DIAGNOSIS OF INFANTILE GASTROENTERITIS DUE TO ESCHERICHIA COLI

Esch. coli in the healthy intestine. *Esch. coli* strains predominate among the aerobic commensal organisms present in the healthy gut. Strains of any O-group may be present as commensals, though some groups, e.g. O1, O2, O4, O6, O7, O18 and O75 appear to occur more commonly than others. Many serotypes may be present in an individual's intestine at any one time but over a period the types change; some types ('residents') persist over relatively long periods of time, e.g. many months, whereas others ('transients') persist for only a few days or weeks (Sears, Brownlee and Uchiyama, 1950). A strain of a new serotype deliberately swallowed in large numbers rarely becomes established as a resident. The intestinal commensal strains commonly act as pathogens in the urinary tract (cystitis, pyelitis, pyelonephritis), appendix abscess, peritonitis, cholecystitis, septic wounds and bedsores, but do not act as primary pathogens in the intestine and are not known to cause gastroenteritis.

Enteropathogenic serotypes of Esch. coli. Certain serotypes of *Esch. coli*, the 'enteropathogenic types', have a primary pathogenicity in the intestine and cause gastroenteritis, mainly in infants. Most outbreaks take place in infants under 18 months, though many cases are in children up to 5 years old and some infections cause diarrhoea in adults. The two serotypes, *alpha* (Bray, 1945) and *beta* (Smith, 1949), first shown to be the cause of outbreaks of infantile diarrhoea were later typed as O111:K58(B4) and O55:K59(B5). The biotypes Dyspepsikoli A IV and Dyspepsikoli A I which were identified as causes of infantile gastroenteritis by Adam (1927) were also later typed as O111:K58 and O55:K59 respectively. Further serotypes have since been found in cases and outbreaks of infection, e.g. in O-groups 26, 44, 86, 112, 114, 119, 124, 125, 126, 127, 128, 142 and 158 (Rowe, Gross, Lindop and Baird, 1974). Not all strains in these enteropathogenic serotypes are able to cause gastroenteritis. In a nursery studied by McDonald and Charter (1956), for example, waves of intestinal colonization of the infants with strains of O-groups 26, 111, 125 and 126 caused no illness. The particular strains that cause gastroenteritis are distinguished from others in the same serotype by their ability to form an enterotoxin demonstrable by the production of fluid secretion and distension in ligated loops of intestine in rabbits; most strains of the same serotypes found in symptomless excreters do not form enterotoxin (Taylor, Wilkins and Payne, 1961; Smith and Halls, 1967; Sack, Gorbach, Banwell, Jacobs, Chatterjee and Mitra, 1971). The power to produce enterotoxin can be acquired by a nontoxigenic strain by the receipt of a plasmid transmitted on conjugation from a toxigenic strain (Smith and Halls, 1968).

Demonstration of enteropathogenic Esch. coli in faeces. It is usual to examine faeces for the presence of enteropathogenic *Esch. coli* when a patient with diarrhoea is under 5 years old; these specimens should also be examined for salmonellae and shigellae, as in the case of older patients. There is no selective medium that will grow only the enteropathogenic strains of *Esch. coli*, so that unselective media have to be used for culture of the faeces. The method, however, is commonly successful because during acute infections the enteropathogenic strain is very numerous and is usually the predominant organism in the faeces.

Inoculate the faeces lightly both on a blood agar plate and a plate of MacConkey's medium and incubate for 18–24 hours. Test separately at least ten coliform-type colonies for serotype. (Note that the colonies of enteropathogenic strains do not differ in appearance from the colonies of other strains of *Esch. coli* and that an enteropathogenic strain sometimes grows on blood agar when it does not grow on MacConkey's agar.) First identify the K-antigen by testing a portion of the colony (live bacteria) directly by slide agglutination and then identify the O-antigen by slide and tube tests with bacteria heated at 100°C for 1 hour. H-antigen identification is generally not done except in reference laboratories.

It should be noted that the usual procedure of identifying enteropathogenic strains by the demonstration of their serotype is subject to the limitations that not all strains in the recognized 'enteropathogenic' serotypes produce enterotoxin and that some strains in supposedly 'non-enteropathogenic' serotypes may do so. In a study of *Esch. coli* strains isolated from the faeces of 29 children with diarrhoea not yielding salmonella or shigella, Gorbach and Khurana (1972) found that 24 of the children yielded *Esch. coli* strains forming enterotoxin demonstrable by intragastric inoculation in infant rabbits, but that only 9 of the 29 children yielded strains of 'enteropathogenic' serotypes and only 6 of these 9 strains formed enterotoxin.

Diagnostic sera. Laboratories should maintain a stock of polyvalent antisera. Two or three 'pools', commercially available, contain combinations of antisera to the individual enteropathogenic serotypes. Laboratories examining large numbers of faecal samples from children should keep also the monovalent antisera, e.g. those for serotypes O26:K60(B6), O44:K74(L), O55:K59(B5), O86:K61(B7), O111:K58(B4), O112:K66(B11), O114:K90(B), O119:K69 (B14), O124:K72(B17), O125:K70(B15), O126: K71(B16), O127:K63(B8), O128:K67(B12), O142:K86(B). It should be noted that the K-antigens possessed by enteropathogenic strains are almost all of the B type and that the diagnostic sera contain agglutinins both to the K-antigens and to the O-antigens.

Slide agglutination test. Test the colonies from the blood agar plate rather than those from the MacConkey plate because the latter may give misleading reactions. Emulsify a portion of the colony in a drop of physiological saline solution on a slide, add a drop of polyvalent antiserum and tilt back and forwards for up to 1 min. If a colony gives strongly positive agglutination with one of the pools of polyvalent serum, inoculate a further portion of it on to a nutrient agar slant and incubate to grow a culture for testing with monovalent sera; grow such slope cultures from at least three colonies. Prepare a heavy suspension of bacteria from each slope culture in saline and perform slide agglutination tests with monovalent OK sera to identify the K-antigen. Then heat the bacterial suspension at 100°C for 1 hour, cool and repeat the slide agglutination test with the OK sera to identify the O-antigen.

Tube agglutination test. Finally confirm the O-group by making a tube agglutination test with the heated bacterial suspension and the indicated serum, which should be titrated in appropriate serial dilutions, e.g. 1 in 200 to 1 in 6400. The tests should be read after incubation for 18 hours at 50°C or after incubation for 4 hours at 37°C and refrigeration overnight at 4°C.

Biochemical tests. If there is any doubt about the identity of the subcultures as *Esch. coli*, they should be examined in the appropriate biochemical tests. Tests with adonitol, dulcitol, sorbitol, salicin and other substrates may be done to distinguish different biotypes within a single enteropathogenic serotype.

Demonstration of O-antibodies. The antibody response to clinical or subclinical infection with enteropathogenic strains may often be detected by an indirect haemagglutination test in which the patient's serum is reacted with red blood cells on to which O-antigen prepared from bacteria of known O-group has been adsorbed (Neter, Bertram and Arbesman, 1952).

LABORATORY DIAGNOSIS OF URINARY-TRACT INFECTIONS DUE TO ESCHERICHIA COLI

The fresh or refrigerated specimen of urine is inoculated on to plates of blood agar and MacConkey agar with a standard loop or by some other method that will enable an approximate viable count to be made. If coliform-type colonies are found in numbers suggesting a significant bacteriuria ($>10^5$ per ml) a colony is identified as *Esch. coli* and tested for sensitivity to antibiotics suitable for therapy of urinary-tract infection, e.g. ampicillin, tetracycline, nalidixic acid, nitrofurantoin, a sulphonamide, cotrimoxazole and a cephalosporin.

Serotyping of *Esch. coli* from the urinary tract is done only in special circumstances, e.g. in epidemiological studies of cross-infection in a urological or gynaecological hospital or in the prospective investigation of patients with chronic infection in whom it is wished to distinguish reinfection with a new strain from relapsing infection with the strain formerly present. The serogroups most commonly responsible for urinary-tract infections are O1, O2, O4, O6, O7, O9, O11, O18, O39 and O75 (Grüneberg and Bettelheim, 1969). Commercially prepared antisera are available for these groups.

As an alternative to serotyping, colicine typing may be employed in epidemiological studies (McGeachie and McCormick, 1967).

Demonstration of O-antibodies. The demonstration in a bacterial (Widal-type) agglutination test that the serum of a patient contains a significant (e.g. >64) or rising titre of O-antibodies to the strain of *Esch. coli* isolated from the urine is considered to be evidence of involvement of the kidney in a urinary-tract infection (Brumfitt and Percival, 1964).

ALKALESCENS-DISPAR (A-D) ORGANISMS

The A-D group of organisms includes non-motile anaerogenic enterobacteria that ferment lactose late (B. dispar) or not at all (B. alkalescens), but otherwise resemble *Esch. coli* in their biochemical reactions. Many members of the group have the same O and K antigens as typical strains of *Esch. coli* and they are now classified in this species. In their biochemical reactions they are easy to confuse with *Shigella* (see Chap. 29). They resemble *Esch. coli* in occurring in the intestine in healthy persons and in some cases of urinary-tract infection.

KLEBSIELLA

The genus *Klebsiella* is a group of coliform bacteria which has given rise to many problems in classification. The scheme adopted in this book is that proposed by Cowan, Steel, Shaw and Duguid (1960) which excludes motile and gelatin-liquefying forms. The characters that distinguish *Klebsiella* from other enterobacteria are that all klebsiella strains are non-motile, do not liquefy gelatin and do not produce ornithine decarboxylase or phenylalanine deaminase and that most strains are capsulate, produce gas from glucose, ferment lactose, adonitol and inositol, do not produce indole but give positive reactions in the Voges-Proskauer, citrate, urease and KCN tests.

The majority of strains isolated from vegetation, soil, water and faeces form a biochemically homogeneous group, *Klebsiella aerogenes*, which traditionally has been recognized as being lactose-fermenting and having the IMViC reactions: indole negative, methyl-red negative, Voges-Proskauer positive and citrate positive. Motile enterobacteria with similar reactions, many of which liquefy gelatin, are now placed in the genus *Enterobacter* (syn. *Cloaca*). Klebsiellae isolated from the healthy or diseased respiratory tract are more heterogeneous in their reactions. Some give reactions identical with those of *K. aerogenes* and others show several differences. The species other than *K. aerogenes* recognized by Cowan *et al.* are *K. pneumoniae, K. ozaenae, K. rhinoscleromatis, K. edwardsii* var. *edwardsii* and *K. edwardsii* var. *atlantae*; for convenience, the last two of these species are named in this book *K. edwardsii* and *K. atlantae* respectively. The distinguishing reactions of these species are shown in Table 30.1.

Morphology. Gram-negative non-sporing non-motile bacilli which tend to be short and thick, e.g. 1–2 μm × 0·8 μm. Virtually all freshly isolated strains form a well-defined polysaccharide capsule which is readily visible in wet India ink films or by its 'swelling' reaction in films with homologous antiserum; the capsule is largest in cultures on sugar-containing media, especially those with a high ratio of sugar to other nutrients. Some of what appears to be the same extracellular polysaccharide is secreted from the bacteria as a loose, soluble slime, and it is the accumulation of the loose slime that gives colonies their large 'mucoid' form (Duguid, 1951; Wilkinson, Duguid and Edmunds, 1954). The power to form capsules and slime is generally well preserved in laboratory cultures, but non-capsulate non-slime-forming mutants appear from time to time and can be recognized by the smaller, non-mucoid appearance of their colonies. Rarely, a non-capsulate but still slime-forming mutant is produced and such a mutant forms mucoid colonies.

Fimbriae of one or more of three types, 1, 3 and 6, are present in a majority of strains (Duguid, 1959; Thornley and Horne, 1962; Duguid, 1968, Table 1). Most strains of *K. aerogenes* produce both type-1 fimbriae (mannose-sensitive, haemagglutinating, about 7 nm in width) and type-3 fimbriae (mannose-resistant, haemagglutinating only with tannic-acid-treated erythrocytes, about 5 nm in width), though in different phases of their growth they may form only the one type or the other or neither. A few strains of *K. aerogenes* form only type-1 fimbriae and a few form only type 3. *K. pneumoniae* forms only type-1 fimbriae, whereas *K. edwardsii*, *K. atlantae*, *K. rhinoscleromatis* and *K. ozaenae* are non-fimbriate with the exception of a few *K. ozaenae* strains which form the non-haem-agglutinating type-6 fimbriae (Duguid, 1968).

Cultural characters. Grow well on ordinary nutrient media and on glucose-ammonium-salts agar unsupplemented with growth factors. Temperature range for growth is 12°–43°C, optimum 37°C. Colonies are large, raised, moist and viscid, i.e. 'mucoid'; the degree of mucoidness depends on the amount of loose slime produced and this depends on the amount of carbohydrate in the culture medium as well as varying from strain to strain. The colonies of non-capsulate non-slime-forming mutants resemble those of other non-capsulate coliform bacteria. Most strains ferment lactose and

their colonies on MacConkey's medium are pink, though this colour may not be clearly apparent in very mucoid colonies.

Biochemical reactions. The reactions of the different species of *Klebsiella* are shown in Table 30.1. All species fail to liquefy gelatine and none produces ornithine decarboxylase or phenylalanine deaminase. Most species hydrolyse urea but do so much more slowly than *Proteus* species. *K. aerogenes* is the most active fermenter among the klebsiellae and it produces acid and gas from the widest range of carbohydrates; its IMViC reactions are indole negative, methyl-red negative, Voges-Proskauer positive and citrate positive. *K. pneumoniae*, all strains of which appear to ferment dulcitol and belong to capsule serotype 3, differs from *K. aerogenes* in being methyl-red positive, Voges-Proskauer negative and KCN negative. *K. edwardsii* and *K. atlantae*, which form large capsules and very mucoid colonies even on media not containing added sugar, differ from *K. aerogenes* in usually giving only delayed fermentation of lactose, a positive methyl-red reaction and a negative malonate reaction; *K. edwardsii* is anaerogenic. *K. ozaenae* is also a late fermenter of lactose; it is methyl-red positive, Voges-Proskauer negative, gluconate negative and malonate negative. *K. rhinoscleromatis* is the least active biochemically; it is anaerogenic, fails to ferment lactose, is methyl-red positive, Voges-Proskauer negative, citrate negative but malonate positive.

Antigenic structure. O and R somatic (cell wall) antigens have been recognized in smooth and rough variant strains of klebsiellae. Five different O-antigens have been distinguished, four of which, O1, O3, O4 and O5, are related to *Esch. coli* O-antigens 19b, 9, 20 and 8 respectively. These O-antigens occur in different combinations with K-antigens in different strains (see Table 37, Kauffmann, 1969). The O-antigens are masked by the K-antigens in capsulate strains and because the K-antigens are heat-stable at 100°C for 2·5 hours, the O-antigens are identifiable only in non-capsulate mutants. Because of this difficulty in demonstrating them, they are not observed in ordinary typing studies.

K-antigens. The klebsiellae are differentiated into 72 capsule serotypes by the identification of their K-antigens (no. 1–72), which is usually done by the microscopical demonstration of capsule 'swelling' in wet films with capsular antiserum (Edwards and Ewing, 1972). A loopful of a freshly prepared *dilute* suspension of bacteria is mixed on a slide with a loopful of undiluted antiserum or antiserum appropriate diluted to obviate cross-reactions. A coverslip is applied and the preparation is observed with the ×100 oil-immersion objective for the appearance of a refractile margin to the capsule, which in the absence of homologous antibody remains invisible. A positive reaction is usually observed within a minute or so. Loose slime dissolved in the bacterial suspension competes for capsular antibody and interferes with the reaction, so that the amount of loose slime present should be minimized by the use of a young (4–6 hour) broth culture or of bacteria washed free from slime by centrifugation. Pooled and monovalent capsular antisera are available commercially. Slide and tube agglutination tests and precipitation tests may also be used to determine the K-antigen of a strain, but the O-antigens may participate in these reactions and K-antisera absorbed free from O-antibodies are required for such tests.

The six species of *Klebsiella* determined by biochemical reactions were found by Cowan *et al.* to contain strains of different capsular serotypes as follows: *K. aerogenes*, all 72 serotypes; *K. pneumoniae*, type 3; *K. edwardsii*, types 1 and 2; *K. atlantae*, type 1; *K. rhinoscleromatis*, type 3; *K. ozaenae*, types 3, 4, 5 and 6.

M-antigen. This term has sometimes been used for the loose-slime polysaccharide antigen that can be demonstrated in bacteria-free culture supernates by precipitation with capsular antiserum. It appears to have the same chemical composition and antigenic specificity as the K-antigen of the same strain (Edwards and Fife, 1952; Wilkinson, Duguid and Edmunds, 1954).

ENTEROBACTER (CLOACA) AND HAFNIA

These are motile organisms that otherwise resemble *K. aerogenes* in many of their bio-chemical characters. Enterobacter strains are mostly fimbriate (type-1 fimbriae) and slime-forming; they generally do not show defined capsules in wet India ink films, but K-antigens often render them O-inagglutinable. They have the same IMViC reactions as *K. aerogenes*, but differ from that species in producing ornithine decarbocylase, in generally failing to form urease and in commonly liquefying gelatin (Table 30.1).

Three species of *Enterobacter* are recognized: *Ent. cloacae* (Cloaca A), which always liquefies gelatin, but only slowly (after 7 days at 22°C), and fails to produce gas in glycerol and inositol, *Ent. aerogenes* (Cloaca B); which commonly fails to liquefy gelatin even slowly, and *Ent. liquefaciens* (Cloaca C), which liquefies gelatin rapidly (within 2 days), but fails to form gas from carbohydrates unless incubated at temperatures lower than 37°C, e.g. at 25°–30°C.

The independent status of the genus *Hafnia*, with its type species *Hafnia alvei*, is in doubt. These organisms are probably best regarded as being non-lactose-fermenting members of the genus *Enterobacter*, i.e. as *Ent. hafnia*. They resemble *Ent. liquefaciens* in having a low optimum temperature for growth and they give regular, characteristic results in motility and biochemical tests only when incubated at 25°–30°C. They do not liquefy gelatin. Some strains of hafnia form type-1 fimbriae and many strains have an O-antigen related to those of *Salmonella basel* ($58:1,z_{13},z_{28}:1,5$) and *Shigella flexneri* serotype 4a (Sedlák and Kertészová, 1968). Many strains possess the thermolabile surface alpha-antigen of Stamp and Stone (Emslie-Smith, 1961) and since many rabbit sera have a high natural titre of alpha-agglutinins, agglutination tests with live hafnia bacteria commonly give false-positive reactions.

Enterobacter and hafnia organisms are saprophytes found in water, soil and vegetation, but sometimes also in human faeces.

SERRATIA

Members of the genus *Serratia* are motile enterobacteria which resemble *Enterobacter* organisms in their biochemical reactions but are distinguished from them by the production of a non-diffusible red pigment. The only well characterized species is *Serratia marcescens*. The serratias are free-living saprophytes in soil and water, but occasionally act as opportunistic pathogens, causing a variety of infections in man.

Serr. marcescens is a small Gram-negative coccobacillus, $0.7–1.5 \mu m \times 0.7 \mu m$, with peritrichous flagella and fimbriae (types 1 and 3); it may form a capsule on sugar-containing medium.

Most strains form a red pigment, prodigiosin, which is insoluble in water and does not diffuse away from the colonies on agar medium; these, therefore, are pink or red. The optimum temperature for growth is 30°–37°C, but pigmentation may be poor at such temperatures and may be strong only in cultures grown at lower temperatures, e.g. 15°–20°C. The pigment is formed only in cultures grown aerobically and in some strains it may be inapparent in cultures grown on ordinary media. Non-pigmented variant strains commonly originate by mutation in laboratory cultures and occasionally are isolated from clinical specimens. They are closely similar in their characters to *Ent. liquefaciens*.

The IMViC reactions are indole negative, methyl-red negative, Voges-Proskauer positive and citrate positive. All strains liquefy gelatin rapidly, produce ornithine decarboxylase, are gluconate positive and are urease negative. Colonies on MacConkey's agar are usually pink but many strains fail to ferment lactose. Little or no gas is formed in the fermentation of sugars.

CITROBACTER

Members of the genus *Citrobacter* are motile enterobacteria that resemble salmonellae in their IMViC reactions (indole usually negative, methyl-red positive, Voges-Proskauer negative, citrate positive), but differ from salmonellae by being KCN positive and lysine decarboxylase negative.

The type species, *Citrobacter freundii*, is a rapid fermenter of lactose. It corresponds to the organisms known to water bacteriologists as 'intermediate coliform bacilli' and formerly it was called '*Escherichia freundii*'. It is distinguished from *Esch. coli* by being citrate positive, KCN positive, hydrogen sulphide positive and lysine decarboxylase negative (Table 30.1).

Late-lactose-fermenting and non-lactose-fermenting members of the genus *Citrobacter* constitute the Bethesda-Ballerup group. Because they form pale colonies on MacConkey's and DCA media and share somatic antigens with salmonellae, they may be mistaken for salmonellae when they are encountered in cultures of faeces. They are distinguished, however, by their negative lysine decarboxylase and positive KCN reactions. Certain strains possess a K-antigen closely related to the Vi antigen of *S. typhi* and *S. paratyphi C* (see Chap. 28), but they are saprophytes and lack the pathogenicity of salmonellae.

PROTEUS

The genus *Proteus* consists of highly motile ('swarming') enterobacteria that are urease positive, phenylalanine deaminase positive and KCN positive. Four species are recognized, *Proteus vulgaris*, *Pr. mirabilis*, *Pr. morganii* and *Pr. rettgeri*. By far the commonest species encountered in clinical bacteriology is *Pr. mirabilis*. This and the other species of *Proteus* are free-living saprophytes in soil, vegetation, water and sewage, and are found in the intestine in many healthy persons. They occur also in infections of the urinary tract, wounds and other sites.

Morphology. Non-capsulate Gram-negative rods varying in length from short coccobacilli to long filaments; filamentous cells are common in young swarming cultures on agar media. Most strains are highly motile and richly flagellated, but non-flagellate non-motile variant strains are encountered. All four species are fimbriate (type-4 fimbriae; Hoeniger, 1965; Duguid, 1968).

Cultural characters. Proteus organisms are usually first recognized by their fishy smell and their swarming appearance when grown on non-inhibitory solid media such as nutrient agar and blood agar. *Pr. morganii* differs from the other species of *Proteus* by failing to swarm on the conventional agar media, though it does swarm on 'soft' agar media with a reduced content of agar-agar. Swarming appears as a thin, colourless, transparent film extending from the margins of a young colony and spreading in several waves demarcated by a raised margin until most or all of the surface of the culture plate is covered. Colonies of other organisms on the plate are covered and contaminated by the film of proteus growth, which sometimes is so thin that its presence may at first be overlooked. The fishy smell draws attention to the likelihood that proteus is present and if the apparently clean surface of the medium is stroked lightly with an inoculating loop, material from the inapparent film of growth will be seen to accumulate on it.

When the presence of proteus in a clinical specimen makes it difficult to isolate in pure culture another organism such as *Strept. pyogenes* or *Staph. aureus*, the specimen should be plated on a medium that inhibits swarming, e.g. blood agar containing two to three times the usual concentration of agar-agar. Swarming is inhibited and compact 'pale' (non-lactose-fermenting) colonies are formed on MacConkey's medium and deoxycholate citrate agar. It is simple, therefore, to separate from proteus the other enterobacteria that grow on these bile-salt media.

Dienes phenomenon. When two identical proteus cultures are inoculated at different points on the same plate of non-inhibitory medium the resulting swarms of growth coalesce without signs of demarcation. When, however, two different strains of a *Proteus* species are inoculated, the spreading films of growth fail to coalesce and remain separated by a narrow, easily visible furrow. The observation of this appearance, the 'Dienes phenomenon', has been used to determine the identity or non-identity of strains in epidemiological studies (Skirrow, 1969).

Biochemical reactions. Two tests serve to distinguish *Proteus* species from other enterobacteria: (1) the demonstration of its ability to hydrolyse urea rapidly (within a few hours) and (2) the demonstration of its ability oxidatively to deaminate phenylalanine to phenylpyruvic acid. Proteus shares the latter property with species of *Providencia*. Reactions differentiating the four species of *Proteus* are shown in Table 30.1. In fermenting glucose and other carbohydrates all species except *Pr. rettgeri*

usually produce gas. *Pr. vulgaris* is alone in fermenting maltose, only *Pr. mirabilis* fails to form indole and only *Pr. rettgeri* ferments mannitol.

Antigenic structure. Strains of *Pr. vulgaris* and *Pr. mirabilis* have been classified by their O-antigens into 49 O-groups and the groups subdivided according to different H-antigens into a larger number of serotypes (see Kauffmann, 1969, Table 40). Similarly, 57 serotypes of *Pr. morganii* and 45 serotypes of *Pr. rettgeri* have been described.

Certain types of proteus are agglutinated by the serum of patients with typhus fever. This reaction, the Weil-Felix reaction, is used as a diagnostic test. The strain employed, *Proteus* X19 has the biochemical reactions of *Pr. vulgaris*. The Weil-Felix reaction is dependent on a close relationship between the specific O-antigen of *Proteus* X19 and a somatic antigen in *Rickettsia prowazekii*, the causative organism of typhus fever.

Another proteus type designated XK (biochemically *Pr. mirabilis*) is agglutinated by the serum of patients with 'scrub typhus', an infection due to *Rickettsia tsutsugamushi*. A diagnostic agglutination test similar to the Weil-Felix test is based on this antigenic relationship.

PROVIDENCIA

Members of the genus *Providencia* are motile, non-lactose-fermenting Gram-negative bacilli which resemble *Proteus* in their ability to deaminate phenylalanine but differ from *Proteus* by failing to hydrolyse urea. They do not swarm on ordinary agar media but can swarm on soft agar media containing half the usual concentration of agar-agar. They occur in some infections of the urinary tract and are found in the faeces in some cases of diarrhoea, but their role in the causation of diarrhoeal disease is doubtful.

Two biotypes and many serotypes are recognized. The biotypes are regarded by some authors as distinct species. *Providencia alcalifaciens* (Providence I, Providence A) produces gas from glucose and acidifies adonitol but not inositol. *Providencia stuartii* (Providence II, Providence B) is anaerogenic and acidifies inositol but not adonitol.

REFERENCES

ADAM, A. (1927) Dyspepsiekoli. Zur Frage der backteriellen Aetiologie der sogenannten alimentaren Intoxikation. *Jahresbericht Kinderheilkunde Berlin (1927–31)*, **116**, 8.

BRAY, J. (1945) Isolation of antigenically homogeneous strains of *Bact. coli neapolitanum* from summer diarrhoea of infants. *Journal of Pathology and Bacteriology*, **57**, 239.

BRUMFITT, W. & PERCIVAL, A. (1964) Pathogenesis and laboratory diagnosis of non-tuberculous urinary tract infection: A review. *Journal of Clinical Pathology*, **17**, 482.

COWAN, S. T. (1965) Principles and practice of bacterial taxonomy—a forward look. *Journal of General Microbiology*, **39**, 143.

COWAN, S. T., STEEL, K. J., SHAW, C. & DUGUID, J. P. (1960) A classification of the klebsiella group. *Journal of General Microbiology*, **23**, 601.

COWAN, S. T. & STEEL, K. J. (1965) *Manual for the identification of medical bacteria.* Cambridge: University Press.

DUGUID, J. P. (1951) The demonstration of bacterial capsules and slime. *Journal of Pathology and Bacteriology*, **63**, 673.

DUGUID, J. P. (1959) Fimbriae and adhesive properties in klebsiella strains. *Journal of General Microbiology*, **21**, 271.

DUGUID, J. P. (1964) Functional anatomy of *Escherichia coli* with special reference to enteropathogenic *E. coli*. *Revista Latinoamericano de Microbiologia*, **7**, Supls 13–14.

DUGUID, J. P. (1968) The function of bacterial fimbriae. *Archivum Immunologiae et Therapiae Experimentalis*, **16**, 173.

DUGUID, J. P., SMITH, I. W., DEMPSTER, G. & EDMUNDS, P. N. (1955) Non-flagellar filamentous appendages ('fimbriae') and haemagglutinating activity in *Bacterium coli*. *Journal of Pathology and Bacteriology*, **70**, 335.

EDWARDS, P. R. & FIFE, M. A. (1952) Capsule types of klebsiella. *Journal of Infectious Diseases*, **91**, 92.

EDWARDS, P. R. & EWING, W. H. (1972) *Identification of Enterobacteriaceae*, 3rd edition. Minneapolis: Burgess Publishing Company.

EMSLIE-SMITH, A. H. (1961) *Hafnia alvei* strains possessing the alpha antigen of Stamp and Stone. *Journal of Pathology and Bacteriology*, **81**, 534.

GILLIES, R. R. & DUGUID, J. P. (1958) The fimbrial antigens of *Shigella flexneri*. *Journal of Hygiene, Cambridge*, **56**, 303.

GORBACH, S. L. & KHURANA, C. M. (1972) Toxigenic *Escherichia coli*: a cause of infantile diarrhoea in Chicago. *New England Journal of Medicine*, **287**, 791.

GRÜNEBERG, R. N. & BETTELHEIM, K. A. (1969) Geographical variation in serological types of urinary *Escherichia coli*. *Journal of Medical Microbiology*, **2**, 219.

HOENIGER, J. F. M. (1965) Development of flagella by *Proteus mirabilis*. *Journal of General Microbiology*, **40**, 29.

HUTCHINSON, R. I. (1957) *Escherichia coli* (O-types 111, 55 and 26) and their association with infantile diarrhoea: A five-year study. *Journal of Hygiene, Cambridge*, **55**, 27.

KAUFFMANN, F. (1947) The serology of the Coli-Group. *Journal of Immunology*, **57**, 71.

KAUFFMANN, F. (1969) *The Bacteriology of Enterobacteriaceae*, 2nd edition. Copenhagen: Munksgaard.

MCDONALD, J. C. & CHARTER, R. E. (1956) *Escherichia coli* serotypes in a nursery. *Proceedings of the Royal Society of Medicine*, **49**, 85.

MCGEACHIE, J. & MCCORMICK, W. (1967) Importance of potency in typing by colicine production. *Journal of Clinical Pathology*, **20**, 887.

NETER, E., BERTRAM, L. F. & ARBESMAN, C. E. (1952) Demonstration of *Escherichia coli* O55 and O111 antigens by means of a haemagglutination test. *Proceedings of the Society for Experimental Biology and Medicine, New York*, **79**, 255.

ØRSKOV, F., ØRSKOV, I., JANN, B. & JANN, K. (1971) Immunoelectrophoretic patterns of extracts from all *Escherichia coli* O and K antigen test strains, correlation with pathogenicity. *Acta pathologica microbiologica scandinavica*, Section B, **79**, 142.

ØRSKOV, F. & ØRSKOV, I. (1972) Immunoelectrophoretic patterns of extracts from *Escherichia coli* O antigen test strains O1 to O157, examinations in homologous OK sera. *Acta pathologica microbiologica scandinavica*, Section B, **80**, 905.

ROGERS, K. B. (1951) The spread of infantile gastro-enteritis in a cubicled ward. *Journal of Hygiene, London*, **49**, 140.

ROWE, B., GROSS, R. J., LINDOP, R. & BAIRD, R. B. (1974) A new *E. coli* O group O158 associated with an outbreak of infantile enteritis. *Journal of Clinical Pathology*, **27**, 832.

SACK, R. B., GORBACH, S. L., BANWELL, J. G., JACOBS, B., CHATTERJEE, B. D. & MITRA, R. C. (1971) Enterotoxigenic *Escherichia coli* isolated from patients with severe cholera-like disease. *Journal of Infectious Diseases*, **23**, 378.

SEDLÁK, J. & KERTÉSZOVÁ, V. (1968) On the taxonomy of the genus *Hafnia*. *Archivum Immunologie et Therapiae Experimentalis*, **16**, 243.

SEARS, H. J., BROWNLEE, I. & UCHIYAMA, J. K. (1950) Persistence of individual strains of *Escherichia coli* in the intestinal tract of man. *Journal of Bacteriology*, **59**, 293.

SKIRRÓW, M. B. (1969) The Dienes (mutual inhibition) test in the investigation of proteus infections. *Journal of Medical Microbiology*, **2**, 471.

SMITH, J. (1949) The association of certain types (α and β) of *Bact. coli* with infantile gastro-enteritis. *Journal of Hygiene, Cambridge*, **47**, 221.

SMITH, H. W. & HALLS, S. (1967) Studies on *Escherichia coli* enterotoxin. *Journal of Pathology and Bacteriology*, **93**, 531.

SMITH, H. W. & HALLS, S. (1968) The transmissible nature of the genetic factor in *Escherichia coli* that controls enterotoxin production. *Journal of General Microbiology*, **52**, 319.

SOJKA, W. J. (1965) *Escherichia coli in domestic animals and poultry.* Commonwealth Agricultural Bureaux, Farnham Royal, Bucks, England.

TAYLOR, J., WILKINS, M. P. & PAYNE, J. M. (1961) Relation of rabbit gut reaction to enteropathogenic *Escherichia coli*. *British Journal of Experimental Pathology*, **42**, 43.

THORNLEY, M. J. & HORNE, R. W. (1962) Electron microscope observations on the structure of fimbriae, with particular reference to klebsiella strains, by the use of the negative staining technique. *Journal of General Microbiology*, **28**, 51.

WILKINSON, J. F., DUGUID, J. P. & EDMUNDS, P. N. (1954) The distribution of polysaccharide production in aerobacter and escherichia strains and its relation to antigenic character. *Journal of General Microbiology*, **11**, 59.

31. Vibrio: Spirillum

The genus *Vibrio* belongs to the family Spirillaceae and consists of various species, pathogenic, commensal and saprophytic, which may be differentiated from two closely related genera, *Aeromonas* and *Plesiomonas*; it has been suggested that these three genera could be grouped in a new family, the Vibrionaceae. Besides the classical *Vibrio cholerae* and its El Tor biotype, currently responsible for the seventh pandemic of cholera, other vibrios may be associated with diarrhoeal diseases; in particular, pathogenic strains of *V. parahaemolyticus* cause a form of food-poisoning first noted in Japan but since reported from other areas (see footnote, p. 442).

Morphology and staining. Gram-negative, slender bacilli, usually, in young cultures, curved like a comma, with rounded or pointed ends (approximately $2 \cdot 0 \times 0 \cdot 5$ μm); actively motile with one long polar flagellum; in liquid media vibrios often occur in pairs or short chains giving an S or spiral appearance; elongated undivided spirals may also occur; pleomorphic or involution forms (globular, clubbed, etc.) common in older cultures; vibrio appearance less obvious after frequent subculture; non-sporing, non-capsulate.

Cultural characters. Aerobe; optimum temperature 37°C (range 16°–40°C); grows well and quickly on ordinary media, but is inhibited by acid reaction; optimum pH 8·0–8·2; after 12–18 h, colonies are translucent glistening disks 1–2 mm diameter, with bluish colour in transmitted light; colonial variants are more opaque, mucoid or rugose with dry wrinkled surface; colonies on MacConkey's agar are at first colourless then pinkish red, then dark red; grows quickly in alkaline peptone water (pH 8·4) with surface pellicle and uniform turbidity; funnel-shaped liquefaction in gelatin-stab culture; serum not usually liquefied; grows on numerous selective and enrichment media which are particularly useful for isolation of cholera vibrios from the stools of convalescent cases and carriers and from foodstuffs.

Sensitivity to physical and chemical agents. Killed by heat at 56°C in 30 min; dies out quickly in the environment and in sewage-polluted waters; may survive in clean alkaline stagnant water or sea water for 1–2 weeks; limited period of survival (several days) on fruit, vegetables, fish, cooked foods; the El Tor vibrio is more resistant than the classical cholera vibrio (see Barua, 1970). Each biotype is sensitive to a wide range of antimicrobial drugs, e.g. tetracyclines, chloramphenical, furazolidone, sulphonamides; the El Tor vibrio is resistant to the polymyxin group and this forms one useful taxonomic marker.

Biochemical reactions. Ferments glucose, sucrose, mannose, maltose (acid, no gas) but not lactose, dulcitol or arabinose. Heiberg's classification of vibrios into six groups is related to the fermentation of mannose, sucrose, and arabinose; a strain falling into Heiberg's group I with a positive cholera-red reaction and negative Voges-Proskauer reaction is probably a true *V. cholerae*; a positive *cholera red reaction*, the reddish-pink colour which develops immediately after adding a few drops of pure

Table 31.1 Biochemical reactions which help to differentiate *Vibrio* from *Aeromonas* and *Plesiomonas*

Genus	Gas in glucose	Decarboxylases:		Acid from Mannitol
		lysine	arginine	
Vibrio	−	+	−	+
Aeromonas	d usually +	−	+	+
Plesiomonas	−	+	+	−

d = Different reactions in different strains.

440

sulphuric acid to a 24-hour peptone-water culture, indicates the production of indole and nitrites. A Gram-negative motile, mono-flagellate rod growing in air which ferments glucose to produce acid only and is catalase and oxidase positive may be more precisely identified by the reactions listed in Table 31·1.

Biological activities. Cholera vibrios produce a classical toxin; it is an exotoxin or 'entero-toxin' which stimulates a persistant and excessive secretion of isotonic fluid by the intestinal mucosal cells (Field, 1971). A similar, probably identical, exotoxin is produced in peptone water cultures of *V. cholerae* and also *V. cholerae* El Tor which causes increased tissue permeability when injected intradermally in rabbits. Classical cholera vibrios do not produce a soluble haemolysin whereas many of the El Tor strains do so; the latter also haemagglutinate chicken and sheep red-blood cells, are resistant to polymyxin 5 (50 units) and resist lysis by cholera group IV phage at routine test dilution; differentiation of the two biotypes depends on a combination of these tests.

Antigenic characters. The two cholera vibrio biotypes may be distinguished from other vibrios by a distinctive O (somatic) antigen; they may be further subdivided into two main serotypes, called Inaba and Ogawa, which are differentiated by the surface prominence of either of the subsidiary O antigens; an intermediate type, Hikojima, seems to exhibit both these subsidiary antigens; S → R variation in the cholera vibrio is associated with the loss of the O antigen. Vibrios isolated from faeces or polluted waters which do not have the basic cholera O antigen have been called non-agglutinatory vibrios or NAG: they may be associated with other diarrhoeal diseases; vibrios with different O antigens may possess the same H (flagellar) antigen as the cholera vibrios. Variation from the Ogawa to the Inaba serotype is sometimes noted in the individual excretor or the convalescent patient or during the course of a localized outbreak of disease due to the Ogawa serotype (Sakazaki and Tamura, 1971).

Animal pathogenicity. A number of models for the production of a cholera-like syndrome have been developed in recent years, e.g. outpouring of fluid into isolated intestinal loops after local inoculation (rabbit, guinea-pig, rat, chicken); oral or intestinal inoculation of baby rabbits (10–14 days) followed by acute diarrhoea and death; oral infection in mongrel dogs after neutralization of stomach acid with resultant cholera syndrome; mice can be infected by intraperitoneal injection.

Laboratory Diagnosis

Faecal specimens from early acute cases, preferably collected by rubber catheter (No. 24–26) into a sterile container, or on a rectal swab, should be placed directly on bile salt agar or nutrient agar since vibrios are present in enormous numbers (10^7–10^9 per ml); collection from a bedpan should be avoided because of the risk of contamination or the presence of disinfectant. In examination of specimens from convalescent cases or suspected carriers, moistened rectal swabs are most convenient and should be cultured on both enrichment and selective media; alkaline peptone water (pH 8·4) to which may be added 0·1–0·2 per cent Teepol to inhibit spore-bearing contaminants is incubated for 6–8 h, then subcultured on a plate of selective medium and into a second peptone water tube. If there is likely to be delay of 12–24 h in rectal swabs reaching the laboratory, the specimen should be added to a transport medium, e.g. alkaline taurocholate tellurite broth (pH 9·0); larger faecal specimens (1–3 ml) may be added to 10 ml sea water or to Venkatraman-Ramakrishnan fluid. In urgent cases, dark field microscopy of fresh diarrhoeal specimens or of young peptone water cultures combined with an immobilization test with specific antisera will give positive results in 90 per cent of acute cases; or stereoscopic examination with oblique transmitted light of a culture after 4–5 h incubation on a non-selective medium may be used to pick out bluish-grey vibrio colonies but diagnosis must be confirmed by slide-agglutination with group O antiserum.

In the use of selective culture media, of which there are many, the laboratory worker should become thoroughly acquainted with at least one reliable medium; those most commonly used are TCBS medium and MONSUR's medium (gelatin taurocholate tellurite agar), both of highly alkaline reaction (pH 8·5); on each medium the vibrios have characteristic colonial appearances. Classical vibrios may grow more freely on either Monsur's or on Aronson's medium which some workers still prefer; TCBS agar is more inhibitory and is therefore better suited to the isolation of El Tor strains. It was developed from a medium intended for the recovery of *V. parahaemolyticus* from sea foods and suspected victims of sea-food poisoning. The cautious worker, faced with the investigation of gastro-enteritis of uncertain exotic origin, might well prefer to use at least two of the many types of selective media available for the isolation of pathogenic vibrios.

Colonies should be picked for slide agglutination with group O and monospecific antisera, testing 5–10 colonies or a sweep if first results are negative; colonies taken from TCBS agar may not emulsify properly and should be re-examined after subculture on salt-free nutrient agar; further identification, including biotypes, requires fermentation tests (mannose, sucrose, arabinose) VP test, haemolytic test (Sakazaki *et al.*, 1971), haemagglutination of chicken or sheep cells, resistance to 50 unit polymyxin and resistance to group IV cholera phage at routine test dilution. In endemic areas, periodic checks should be made for sensitivity to tetracycline and other commonly used antimicrobial drugs.

Retrospective diagnosis may be made serologically by testing paired sera (1–3 days and 7–10 days) for agglutinins or vibriocidal antibodies (Holmgren *et al.*, 1971).

For fuller details of laboratory diagnosis of cholera cases and carriers, see Barua (1970).

VIBRIO PARAHAEMOLYTICUS*

This vibrio has been incriminated as a frequent cause of food-poisoning, particularly in Japan and the Far East, but also in S.E. Asia, Australia and U.S.A. It is a halophilic, Gram-negative marine vibrio and has been isolated from shellfish and other fish in many countries with warm coastal waters. The clinical infection is characterized by the sudden onset of acute gastro-enteritis with an incubation period of 10–20 h (range 2–40 h) and lasts for only a

few days: vibrios are expected in large numbers in the stools during the illness but decrease rapidly with clinical recovery (Peffers *et al.*, 1973).

Morphology. Similar to *V. cholerae* and other vibrios.

Cultural characters. After overnight incubation on selective culture media, e.g. TCBS, large (3–4 mm) smooth, dome-shaped colonies with opaque centre and green colour: films show pleomorphic Gram-negative bacilli: actively motile from fluid culture: halophilic (growth on 6–9 per cent salt agar): non-sporing, non-capsulate: sensitive to same vibriocidal drugs as the cholera vibrio.

Biochemical reactions. Acid but no gas in glucose oxidation-fermentation test: no other sugar fermentation reactions: oxidase+: catalase+: indole+: VP−: urease−: lysine and ornithine decarboxylase+: arginine dehydrolase−.

Antigenic characters. Numerous serotypes based on O and K antigens (Sakazaki, personal communication).

Laboratory Diagnosis

Procedures for isolation and identification similar to those for the cholera vibrios except for serological tests.

Other Vibrios

Certain species of vibrios have been described in association with diseases of animals, e.g. *V. fetus*, *V. jejuni*, *V. coli* and *V. metchnikovi*; some are now classified in the genus *Campylobacter*. They rarely cause human disease. Other saprophytic vibrios have been recovered from water, cheese, fish, and other foods. Brief descriptions of some of the animal pathogenic vibrios are given in Cruickshank (1965).

SPIRILLUM MINUS

A causative organism of rat bite fever in man. Morphologically, Gram-negative spiral organism usually 2–5 μm but up to 10 μm in length with regular short coils each about 1 μm across; very actively motile with darting movements (but no undulations like spirochaetes) due to

---

* This vibrio and *V. alginolyticus* have been re-allocated to a new genus, *Beneckea* (Baumann, Baumann and Mandal, 1971).

terminal flagella, varying in number from 1–7 at each pole; motility and flagella best demonstrated by dark-field microscopy. Stained by Romanowsky stains (e.g. Leishman) and also by ordinary aniline dyes; *Spirillum minus* has not been grown on artificial culture media. Guinea-pigs, white rats and mice can be infected experimentally.

Laboratory Diagnosis

Spirilla may be demonstrated in local lesion, affected regional lymph nodes (by aspiration) and sometimes in the blood, either by direct microscopic examination or after inoculation of the infective material into a susceptible animal; in guinea-pigs a progressive disease with septicaemia and finally death occurs; in inoculated mice, there is no clinical disease, but spirilla may be demonstrable in the blood after 5–14 days; sensitive *in vivo* to tetracyclines and penicillin.

REFERENCES

BARUA, D. (1970) Principles and practice of cholera control. *Public Health Paper No.* 40, p. 47. Geneva: World Health Organization.*

BAUMANN, P., BAUMANN, L. & MANDAL, M. (1971) *Taxonomy of marine bacteria*, the genus *Beneckea, Journal of Bacteriology*, **107**, 268.

CRUICKSHANK, R. (1965) *Medical Microbiology*, 11th edn., pp. 269–270. Edinburgh: Livingstone.

FIELD, M. (1971) Intestinal secretion: effect of cyclic AMP and its rôle in cholera. *New England Journal of Medicine*, **284**, No. 20, 1137.

HOLMGREN, J., SVENNERHOLM, A. M., OUCHTERLONY, O. (1971) Quantitation of vibriocidal antibodies using agar plaque techniques. *Acta Pathologica Microbiologica Scandinavica, Sect. B*, **79**, No. 5, 708.

PEFFERS, A. S. R., BAILEY, J., BARROW, G. I. & HOBBS, B. C. (1973) *Vibrio parahaemolyticus:* gastro-enteritis and international air travel. *Lancet*, **i**, 143.

SAKAZAKI, R. & TAMURA, K. (1971) Somatic antigen variation in *Vibrio cholerae. Japanese Journal of Medical Science and Biology*, **24**, No. 2, 93.

SAKAZAKI, R., TAMURA, K. & MURASE, M. (1971) Determination of the haemolytic activity of *Vibrio cholerae. Japanese Journal of Medical Science and Biology*, **24**, No. 2, 83.

*This W.H.O. report also describes classification and characteristics of vibrios, including survival in the environment and on food, water, etc.; phage-typing; pathogenesis; clinical features and treatment of cholera.

32. Pseudomonas: Loefflerella

PSEUDOMONAS

Members of this large genus, which contains over 140 species, are widely distributed in nature as saprophytes and plant pathogens. Only a few species, among which *Pseudomonas pyocyanea (Ps. aeruginosa)* is pre-eminent, cause disease in man. *Ps. pyocyanea* flourishes in warm moist situations in the human environment, including sink and bath drains, respirator humidifiers and disinfectant solutions, can be found in the faeces of up to 40 per cent of hospital patients, and is a common cause of hospital-acquired infections. Derangement of local or general defence mechanisms often precedes infection; for this reason the species is often isolated from infected burns, bed-sores, surgical wounds, the middle ear, and the urinary tract. Deep infections, e.g. of the lung, or septicaemia can occur in patients whose immunological defence has been upset by disease or immunosuppressive drugs, and may be fatal. The organism has often been transferred from inanimate sources to susceptible human tissues in contaminated disinfectant solutions. A few other species of *Pseudomonas* occasionally cause infection in man.

All pseudomonads are aerobic Gram-negative rods, motile with polar flagella (mono- or multi-trichous); oxidase-positive and catalase-positive. Typically the breakdown of carbohydrates is oxidative. Many species produce water-soluble pigments.

PSEUDOMONAS PYOCYANEA

Morphology and staining. Gram-negative non-sporing rods, motile with (usually) one polar flagellum. Fimbriae may be present. Some strains, notably from respiratory tract infection in children with fibrocystic disease, produce large amounts of extracellular polysaccharide slime.

Cultural characters. Most strains are strict aerobes. The growth range is 5–42°C, optimum 37°C. *Ps. pyocyanea*, but few other *Pseudo-*

monas species, will grow in serial subculture at 42°C.

1. NUTRIENT BROTH. Uniform turbidity and surface pellicle.
2. NUTRIENT AGAR. After 24 h at 37°C colonies are large, low-convex, rough and often oval with the long axis in the line of the inoculating streak. Cultures have a distinctive musty smell, and the surface of confluent growth often shows an iridescent sheen in reflected light. Most strains produce pigments which colour the colonies (slightly) and the surrounding medium (often intensely) blue-green (pyocyanin), yellow-green (fluorescin) or dark brown (pyorubrin). Colonies of slime-producing strains are large, smooth and mucoid.
3. MacCONKEY'S AGAR. Colonies have much the same appearance as on nutrient agar. They are 'pale', i.e. non-lactose-fermenting.
4. GELATIN STAB. At 20°C there is liquefaction from the surface and pigmentation mainly in the liquefied medium.
5. PIGMENT-ENHANCING MEDIA (King, Ward and Raney, 1954). Used to ensure recognition of weakly pigment-producing strains.

(a) *Medium A (for pyocyanin)*. Dissolve, by heating, peptone 20 g, glycerol 10 g, K_2SO_4 10 g and $MgCl_2$ 1·4 g, in water 1 litre; adjust to pH 7·2; add 20 g agar and dissolve by autoclaving at 115°C for 10 min; filter; sterilize by autoclaving at 115°C for 10 min. Incubate cultures at 37°C for 24 to 96 h.

(b) *Medium B (for fluorescin)*. Proteose peptone 20 g, glycerol 10 g, K_2HPO_4 1·5 g, $MgSO_4.7H_2O$ 1·5 g, water 1 litre; prepare as for Medium A. Incubate cultures at 37°C for 24 h and then at 22°C or room temperature for 72 h.

Identification of pigments. Pyocyanin is blue-green and non-fluorescent; it is formed in peptone media, and is soluble in both chloroform and water. Fluorescin is yellow-green and fluorescent; it is formed only in the presence of phosphate and is soluble in water but not in chloroform. The production of pyocyanin is demonstrated by shaking several millilitres of $CHCl_3$ with a broth culture or disintegrated agar culture; on standing, pyocyanin (but not fluorescin) will appear in the $CHCl_3$ once the phases have separated out.

Biochemical reactions. Tests that may be used to characterize *Ps. pyocyanea* are shown in Table 32.1 (Snell, 1973). Indole and H_2S are not produced; the Vosges-Proskauer and methyl-red reactions are negative.

Pyocine typing. Observations of pyocine production are made to characterize strains for epidemiological purposes; serotyping and phage-typing are less reliable. In the method of Gillies and Govan (1966) and Govan and Gillies (1969) the strain to be typed is streaked as a 1 cm wide band across the centre of tryptone soya agar medium (Oxoid) containing 5 per cent horse blood in a *glass* petri dish, and the culture is incubated for 14 h at 32°C. Visible growth is then scraped off with a slide and the growth remaining is killed by exposure for 15 min to 3–5 ml $CHCl_3$ poured into the lid of the dish. Excess $CHCl_3$ is decanted and traces of vapour are removed by exposing the plate to the air for a few minutes. Eight or more 'indicator' strains of *Ps. pyocyanea* are then applied in marked positions as streaks placed at right angles to the original inoculum, and the plate is re-incubated at 37°C for 8–18 h. The patterns of inhibition which are produced allow recognition of 37 stable pyocine types and of up to 8 subtypes within the common pyocine type 1.

Antibiotic sensitivity. *Ps. pyocyanea* is naturally resistant to many antibiotics. Those most likely to be effective against it clinically and *in vitro* are gentamicin, polymyxin and carbenicillin. Very large doses (up to 30 g daily) of the last are necessary in severe infections. The size of inhibition zones produced by gentamicin in surface disk diffusion tests is inversely related to the magnesium content of the medium (Garrod and Waterworth, 1969). Some strains are sensitive to streptomycin and kanamycin.

Multiple resistance can be turned to advantage in the laboratory by using a strain of *Ps. pyocyanea* with a low MIC for gentamicin to assay serum levels of this drug in the presence of other antibiotics to which the species is usually resistant.

Disinfectant resistance. The ability of *Ps. pyocyanea* to withstand and even flourish in the use-dilutions of common hospital disinfectants (hypochlorites are a noteworthy exception) has resulted in many and sometimes tragic outbreaks of hospital infection (for references, see Snell, 1973 and Lowbury, 1968) and is a major influence on hospital disinfectant policies. This resistance may also be used to advantage in the laboratory by incorporating disinfectants, e.g. 0·03 to 1 per cent cetrimide, in nutrient agar or broth, which then become selective for *Ps. pyocyanea*. On 'improved' cetrimide agar (Brown and Lowbury, 1965) colonies of *Ps. pyocyanea* show brilliant yellow fluorescence.

Laboratory diagnosis. Isolation of *Ps. pyocyanea* in surveys of carriers or environmental sources or from mixed cultures is best attempted with selective cetrimide broth or cetrimide agar in addition to blood agar and MacConkey agar. *Ps. pyocyanea* can be rapidly and presumptively identified by its characteristic colony morphology on solid media and its pellicle formation in broth; by green pigmentation on nutrient or MacConkey agar or the media of King *et al.* (1954); by its distinctive musty smell, its characteristic antibiotic sensitivity pattern, its production of oxidase, and its ability to grow in serial subcultures at 42°C. Further tests, to confirm identity, are listed in Table 32.1

Strains identified as *Ps. pyocyanea* may be stored for later pyocine typing on slants of nutrient agar or Dorset's egg medium.

PSEUDOMONAS PSEUDOMALLEI

This organism, which is also known as *Malleomyces pseudomallei, Loefflerella pseudomallei* and *Loefflerella whitmori*, is the causal agent of melioidosis, a disease of rodents. Man is seldom infected, and then only as an end-host, either by eating food contaminated with infected rodent excreta, or by direct contact with infected animals. Virtually all human cases contract infection in South East Asia or the northern tip of South America. Clinically the human disease, which is difficult to treat and often fatal, may be a chronic indolent infection resembling glanders, with the formation of

Table 32.1 Reactions of *Pseudomonas* spp. and some other non-fermenting Gram-negative bacteria (after Snell, 1973)

Species	Growth on MacConkey, 1 day	Urease activity, 5 days	Motility at 22°C, 1 day	O/F test, 10 days	Oxidase (Kovacs), 1 day	ONPG, 2 days	Growth in KCN broth, 2 days	Gelatin liquefied, 5 days	Malonate utilized, 1 day	Arginine desmidase, 5 days	Maltose ASS, 10 days	Ethanol ASS, 10 days	Tween 80 hydrolysis, 5 days
Ps. pyocyanea	+	+	+	Ox.	+	-	+	+ (d)	+ (d)	+	-	+	+
Ps. cepacia	+	+	+	Ox.	+	+	-	+	-	-	+	+	+
Ps. maltophilia	+	-	+	Alk.	+	-	+	+	+	-	+	-	-
Ps. putida	+	-	d	Ox.	+	-	-	-	- (d)	+	-	-	-
Ps. fluorescens	+	d	+	Ox.	+	-	d	+	-	+	-	-	-
Ps. pseudomallei	+	d	+	Ox.	+	-	+	+	- (d)	+	+	d	+
L. mallei	-	d	-	Ox.	d	-	-	d	-	+	d	-	...
Alcaligenes odorans	+	-	+	Alk.	+	-	+	d	-	-	-	+	-
Moraxella	d	- (d)	-	Alk./-	+	-	-	- (d)	-	-	-	-	d
Acinetobacter anitratus	+	+ (d)	-	Ox.	-	-	+ (d)	- (d)	+	-	- (d)	+ (d)	+
Flavobacterium	+	-	-	Ox.	+	+	-	+	-	- (d)	+ (d)	+	d
Chromobacterium lividum	d	d	+	Ox.	+	d	-	+	d	-	+	-	-

Methods: Arginine desmidase after Thornley (1960). Maltose and ethanol utilization in ammonium salt sugars (ASS) of Smith, Gordon and Clark (see Cowan and Steel, 1965, p. 109). Tween 80 hydrolysis after Sierra (1957). Other tests by methods of Cowan and Steel (1965).

Results: + = positive; − = negative; d = different reactions (+ or −) in different strains; + (d) = most strains positive; − (d) = most strains negative; Ox. = oxidative production of acid; Alk. = alkaline reaction; ... = undetermined.

caseous nodules round embolic foci and multiple abscess formation in the skin, bone and internal organs, or it may present as a fulminant septicaemia.

On nutrient agar *Ps. pseudomallei* produces unusual and distinctive rough, dry, coherent colonies (Lapage, Hill and Reeve, 1968). Biochemically *Ps. pseudomallei* broadly resembles other pseudomonads, but it does not produce a definite pigment on nutrient agar and its cultures do not fluoresce on medium B of King *et al.* (1954). Like *Ps. pyocyanea* it grows well at 41–42°C. Tests for differentiation are shown in Table 32.1.

OTHER PSEUDOMONAS SPECIES

Pseudomonas cepacia. Also known as 'Eugonic Oxidizer −1', *Pseudomonas multivorans*, and *Pseudomonas kingii*. This species was originally isolated as a plant pathogen causing soft rot in onions, but is being isolated with increasing frequency from human infections, and has caused a distinctive form of 'trench foot' in troops training in swamps (Taplin, Bassett and Mertz, 1971). The species is resistant to an even wider range of antibiotics than *Ps. pyocyanea*; most strains are resistant to polymyxin and a few to gentamicin.

Pseudomonas maltophilia and *Pseudomonas putida* have also been isolated from human infections. The former fails to metabolize glucose in the Hugh and Leifson test but will metabolize maltose oxidatively. These species may be identified by the tests shown in Table 32.1.

Pseudomonas fluorescens is generally regarded as non-pathogenic for man; its chief importance lies in the need to distinguish it from *Ps. pyocyanea.*

LOEFFLERELLA

LOEFFLERELLA MALLEI

This organism, which is also known as *Malleomyces mallei* and *Pfeifferella mallei*, causes glanders in the horse, a disease characterized by the formation of nasal abscesses and cutaneous and lymphatic nodules ('farcy buds') or abscesses. Human disease may take the form of an acute fulminant febrile illness or a chronic indolent infection producing abscesses in the respiratory tract or skin. It is not common and almost totally restricted to persons handling horses in those countries, principally in Asia and South America, from which the disease has not yet been eradicated. Human laboratory-acquired infection is a hazard: few organisms are so dangerous to work with as this.

In its morphology and biochemical characters *L. mallei* closely resembles *Ps. pseudomallei* (see Table 32.1) but shows a number of negative differences: it is non-motile, has a narrower range of carbon and energy sources, does not grow on MacConkey's medium, and is variable in oxidase and gelatinase production. It has been suggested by Redfearn, Palleroni and Stanier (1966) that the two species shared a common ancestor, and that the negative differences of *L. mallei* are the result of functional and structural loss-adaptation to a strictly parasitic mode of existence.

Guinea-pigs are susceptible to experimental inoculation. Intraperitoneal injection of small amounts of a pure culture causes in 2 to 3 days testicular swelling due to bacillary invasion of the tunica vaginalis, which increases up to the tenth day. This 'Straus reaction' may be followed by death of the animal.

OTHER NON-FERMENTING GRAM-NEGATIVE BACILLI

In recent years there have been increasing numbers of isolations, from clinical specimens, of Gram-negative non-fermenting bacilli that are primarily either free-living saprophytes or harmless commensals, but which occasionally act as secondary or opportunistic pathogens in human disease processes. The significance of their presence in particular patients is often uncertain, namely whether they are harmless contaminants or harmful pathogens, though where large numbers are present their content of endotoxin is likely to have an injurious effect.

Growing attention is being paid to their identification and a detailed account of their differentiation by biochemical tests is given by Snell (1973). Table 32.1 shows the reactions of some of the species described.

REFERENCES AND FURTHER READING

BROWN, V. I. & LOWBURY, E. J. L. (1965) Use of an improved cetrimide agar medium and other culture methods for *Pseudomonas aeruginosa*. *Journal of Clinical Pathology*, **18**, 752.

COWAN, S. T. & STEEL, K. J. (1965) *Manual for the Identification of Medical Bacteria*. Cambridge: Cambridge University Press.

GARROD, L. P. & WATERWORTH, P. M. (1969) Effect of medium composition on the apparent sensitivity of *Pseudomonas aeruginosa* to gentamicin. *Journal of Clinical Pathology*, **22**, 534.

GILLIES, R. R. & GOVAN, J. R. W. (1966) Typing of *Pseudomonas pyocyanea* by pyocine production. *Journal of Pathology and Bacteriology*, **91**, 339.

GOVAN, J. R. W. & GILLIES, R. R. (1969) Further studies in the pyocine typing of *Pseudomonas pyocyanea*. *Journal of Medical Microbiology*, **2**, 17.

KING, E. O., WARD, M. K. & RANEY, D. E. (1954) Two simple media for the demonstration of pyocyanin and fluorescin. *Journal of Laboratory and Clinical Medicine*, **44**, 301.

LAPAGE, S. P., HILL, L. R. & REEVE, JEANNE D. (1968) *Pseudomonas stutzeri* in pathological material. *Journal of Medical Microbiology*, **1**, 195.

LOWBURY, E. J. L. (1968) *Pseudomonas aeruginosa*. In *Recent Advances in Clinical Pathology*, Series 5. Edited by S. C. Dyke. London: Churchill.

REDFEARN, M. S., PALLERONI, N. J. & STANIER, R. Y. (1966) A comparative study of *Pseudomonas pseudomallei* and *Bacillus mallei*. *Journal of General Microbiology*, **43**, 293.

SIERRA, G. (1957) A simple method for the detection of lipolytic activity of micro-organisms and some observations on the influence of the contact between cells and fatty substrates. *Antonie van Leeuwenhoek*, **23**, 15.

SNELL, J. J. S. (1973) The distribution and identification of non-fermenting bacteria. PHLS Monograph Series No. 4. London: HMSO.

TAPLIN, D., BASSETT, D. C. J. & MERTZ, PATRICIA (1971) Foot lesions associated with *Pseudomonas cepacia*. *Lancet*, **2**, 568.

THORNLEY, M. J. (1960) The differentiation of *Pseudomonas* from other Gram-negative bacteria on the basis of arginine metabolisms. *Journal of Applied Bacteriology*, **23**, 37.

33. Anthrax Bacillus

Large straight Gram-positive rods occurring in chains which grow aerobically and form heat-resistant spores are members of the genus *Bacillus*. Most species are Gram-positive. The spores are ubiquitous and are extremely common in dust so that a large proportion of the bacteria which contaminate cultures belong to this group. These organisms exist as saprophytes in soil, water, air and on vegetation, e.g. *Bacillus cereus* and *Bacillus subtilis*. *Bacillus anthracis*, the causative organism of anthrax, is the only pathogen of the group, though very occasionally species such as *B. subtilis* have been isolated from the tissues in terminal disease (agonal infection). *B. cereus* has been incriminated as a cause of food-poisoning.

Anthrax is primarily an infectious disease of domestic herbivores; in them it occurs usually as a fulminating septicaemia. Man contracts the disease sporadically by coming into contact with infected animals or contaminated animal products. Anthrax is uncommon in the United Kingdom and North America but is relatively common in many other parts of the world.

BACILLUS ANTHRACIS

Morphology. Rods 4–8 μm × 1–1·5 μm. Square-ended or ends recurved; arranged in chains in culture; occurs singly or in pairs in animal's blood. Spores central, oval and non-bulging; not formed in animal tissues. Non-motile. Capsule formed in animal body, on serum media and in bicarbonate media in excess of CO_2.

Staining reactions. Gram-positive, especially in tissues. Blue bacillus with purple granular surround when stained by polychrome methylene blue (McFadyean); purple bacillus with red capsule by Giemsa. Non-acid-fast. Spores not stained without mordant.

Cultural characters. Aerobic and facultative anaerobe; growth temperature range 12°–45°C; grows on all ordinary media. Aerobic condi-tions necessary for sporulation; optimum temperature for sporulation 25°–30°C. Germination of spores occurs under aerobic conditions.

On agar plate greyish, granular, circular disks (3 mm diameter after 24 h at 37°C); wavy margin, 'medusa-head' appearance; colony is one continuous convoluted thread of bacilli in chain formation; it is sticky and a projection is left in air when touched with loop; difficult to emulsify and gives a 'sheen' on spreading. On agar slope, thick greyish, opaque sticky growth with irregular edges; ground glass appearance. Slight haemolysis round colony on blood agar.

On broth growth develops as silky strands; usually pellicle formation occurs. In gelatin stab growth along wire puncture with lateral spikes longest near surface; 'inverted fir tree'; liquefaction late and starts at surface: partial liquefaction of coagulated serum.

Biochemical reactions. In glucose, sucrose, maltose, trehalose and dextrin acid but no gas production; nitrate reduced to nitrite.

Viability. Vegetative cells destroyed at 60°C for 30 min; spores usually destroyed at 100°C (boiling) for 10 min; may resist 140°C for 1 h; spores destroyed by 0·1 per cent mercuric chloride in 30 min and by 4 per cent potassium permanganate in 15 min. Spore germination and growth of most strains *in vitro* inhibited by penicillin (0·1 μg/ml), streptomycin (0·5–2 μg/ml), tetracyclines (0·1–0·5 μg/ml), erythromycin (1 μg/ml), chloramphenicol (2·5–10 μg/ml), and sulphonamides.

Antigenic structure. Three distinct antigenic components are described: an anthrax toxin complex, a capsular polypeptide (D-glutamic acid) and a somatic polysaccharide.

Pathogenicity. Man, cattle, sheep, goats, pigs and camels naturally affected. Experimental mice, guinea-pigs, rabbits, hamsters and monkeys all susceptible to infection: Infection usually septicaemic with marked splenic enlargement in most animals naturally or experimentally infected.

Laboratory Diagnosis

All procedures connected with the handling of *Bacillus anthracis* should be carried out with the greatest of care in a safety cabinet.

Malignant pustule. The best specimen is fluid from an unbroken vesicle round the lesion. Films made from exudate stained by Gram's method and Giemsa's stain; the finding of bacilli morphologically like *B. anthracis* suggestive; very few pus cells seen in the preparations unless pyogenic organisms are present.

Note that the usual heat fixation and staining of microscopic preparations from cultures of the anthrax bacillus may not affect the viability of the spores, and laboratory infection from handling such materials has been recorded. All stained smears should be autoclaved after examination.

Cultures are made on blood agar and nutrient agar plates and in broth. The cultures are best stored in a closed container that can be autoclaved after use. The container should be clearly labelled '*B. anthracis*'.

After overnight incubation on solid media typical medusa-head colonies seen if *B. anthracis* present; little or no haemolysis on the blood agar.

Broth culture. A pellicle with a deposit which stirs up in a silky-like whirl if the tube is shaken gently.

Films made from the media are stained by Gram's method, characteristically a long tangled Gram +ve chain of bacilli, several showing central spores.

In all cases the identity of the suspected organism must be confirmed by subcutaneous inoculation of a guinea-pig or mouse with the suspected culture. A small dose of culture is sufficient to produce a lethal effect in 24–48 h. The occurrence of the bacilli in the heart blood and in the spleen in considerable numbers, and the other post-mortem appearances described below, are diagnostic.

Diagnosis of anthrax in domestic animals (post-mortem). The usual form of post-mortem examination is not made, since it is essential to prevent any distribution of sporing bacilli from the carcase. In the body sporulation does not take place, but spores are readily formed when the bacilli are exposed to air under most conditions. Films of blood taken from a superficial vein in the ear are prepared, and stained by Gram's method and by McFadyean's methylene-blue method (see above). Characteristic bacilli (without spores) in the blood giving the methylene-blue reaction are diagnostic. If necessary, the organism can be cultivated and identified by the procedure described above, a specimen of blood from the ear being used for the investigation.

Isolation of Bacillus anthracis from heavily contaminated materials. The methods used are culture and animal inoculation of a 'wash' made from the material. The material (e.g. hair, hide, tissue, bone meal) is liable to be heavily contaminated with other organisms and a portion of about 25 g in 100 ml sterile water is shaken up and allowed to stand with occasional shaking for 3 h. The supernatant

Table 33.1 Various types of media used for isolation of *B. anthracis*

Author	Agar	Additions (per ml)	Method of inoculation
Pearce and Powell, 1951	2% peptone	40 μg haemin 60 μg lysozyme	Spread plate
Morris, 1955	2% peptone	20 units polymyxin 100 μg propamidine	Spread plate
Green and Jamieson, 1958	Yeastrel + 0·5% peptone	None	Pour plate
Gillissen and Scholz, 1961	Synthetic	100 μg polymyxin	Spread plate + layer 24 h later
Knisely, 1966	Heart infusion agar	30 units polymyxin 40 μg lysozyme 300 μg EDTA 40 μg thallous acetate	Spread plate

EDTA = ethylene-diamine-tetra-acetic acid

fluid is heated at 70°C for 10 min to destroy all non-spored bacteria.

The 'wash' can be cultured aerobically on a variety of culture media from simple agar media to complex media containing antibiotics (Table 33.1). The media are used as spread or pour plates depending on their constituents.

Any colonies which require further investigation are stabbed into the inner tube of a Craigie tube and incubated overnight at 37°C. Colonies of *B. anthracis* appear as a fine feathery growth along the length of the stab. Most other members of the genus *Bacillus* are motile and therefore migrate down the inner tube and appear on the surface outside the inner tube. Non-motile members grow only on the surface of the agar in the inner tube.

Final identification of the organisms isolated *B. anthracis* must be made by the subcutaneous inoculation of a small amount of culture into a mouse or guinea-pig. A very small inoculum of a pure culture, 0·1 ml of a 1 in 100 dilution of an overnight broth culture (approximately 100 bacilli) will kill a mouse in 24–48 h.

For direct isolation by animal inoculation centrifuge 50 ml (or more) of the heat-treated 'wash' described above at 3000 rev/min for 15 min. Discard the supernatant and inoculate the residue intramuscularly into a guinea-pig which has been passively immunized 24 h previously with *Cl. welchii* antitoxin 1000 units, *Cl. septicum* antitoxin 500 units, *Cl. oedematiens* antitoxin 1000 units and tetanus antitoxin 1000 units. For a mouse one-third of the dose of antitoxin for a guinea-pig is used. Death due to anthrax occurs in 2–3 days.

The post-mortem examination should be carried out with care to avoid spread of the spores of the bacilli. The examination should be carried out with the animal laid on its back and pegged out on aluminium foil which can be wrapped round the animal at the end of the examination and the whole package incinerated. Characteristic appearances are: gelatinous oedema at the site of inoculation and petechial haemorrhages spread widely over the peritoneal surface; the black blood clots slowly when shed; smears made from the heart blood and spleen stained by McFadyean's method (see above) and Giemsa's stain show (1) *McFadyean*

—large number of blue bacilli and purplish granular material. (2) *Giemsa*—bacilli purple and capsules red with red granular material round bacilli.

Death may occur within 24 h of infection from gas-gangrene, usually due to *Cl. septicum* or *Cl. bifermentans*. Aerobic cultures made from the blood, spleen or local site of injection may yield a few colonies of *B. anthracis* after overnight incubation. A smear of the spleen may show one or two capsulate bacilli by McFadyean's method or Giemsa among a number of other non-capsulate bacilli—some of which contain spores, i.e. are *Clostridia*.

A rapid method of identification is the immunofluorescent method of Cherry and Freeman (1959) applied to a culture of *B. anthracis* grown on a bicarbonate medium.

Serological Diagnosis

It is not always possible to isolate *B. anthracis* from patients who clinically are suffering from cutaneous anthrax. There are two possible methods for demonstrating antibodies to the anthrax toxin, the gel diffusion test described by Thorne and Belton (1957) and the *in vivo* neutralization test in the rabbit described by Darlow *et al.* (1956). Reference should be made to these papers for the details of the tests.

Antibodies are rarely found in uncomplicated cases of cutaneous anthrax but these uncomplicated cases tend to develop antibodies after a single subsequent dose of anthrax vaccine, instead of after three doses as in individuals with no past history of exposure of anthrax (Darlow and Pride, 1969).

Precipitin test for demonstration of anthrax infection. This test was first used by Ascoli for the recognition of anthrax infection in organs and tissues from suspected carcasses, and may be applicable even in the case of putrefied material. It depends on the occurrence of a specific precipitin in the serum of an immunized animal. Immune sera vary in their precipitin content, and for the test a serum with known precipitating properties must be selected. An extract of the tissue is made in slightly acidified saline with heat. The fluid is cooled and then filtered through paper. 0·5 ml of the serum is placed in a narrow tube and the filtrate is carefully run on to the top. The development within 15 min of a white ring of precipitate at the junction of the two fluids denotes a positive result.

OTHER SPECIES OF GENUS BACILLUS

These organisms are saprophytes and comprise a large number of different species. Their classification is complicated and for detailed differential features of the various species, reference can be made to Bergey (1957).

The general characters of the commoner species encountered in diagnostic laboratory work may be summarized as follows:

Morphology and staining. Certain large-cell species resemble *B. anthracis*, e.g. *B. cereus* and *B. megaterium*. Others are shorter, thinner with rounded ends, e.g. *B. subtilis*. All these species are Gram-positive, but there are others which are Gram-variable, e.g. *B. stearothermophilus*, *B. polymyxa*.

The spore varies in position in the bacillus and also may cause swelling of the sporangium.

Cultural characters. The optimum temperature is between 30° and 37°C but some are themophilic, with optimum temperature at 55°C, e.g. *B. stearothermophilus*; aerobes but, usually,

also facultative anaerobes; abundant growth occurs on all the ordinary culture media. The appearance of the growth varies considerably among different species.

B. subtilis produces a white, glistening adherent, somewhat membranous growth, which tends to spread; rather similar growths are seen among other species.

Table 33.2 shows some of the differential features of species of *Bacillus*. *B. anthracis* is included as being the important pathogen for man, which must be distinguished from the others.

McGaughey and Chu (1948) have shown that of the group of aerobic sporing bacilli only *B. mycoides*, *B. cereus*, and to a less extent, *B. anthracis*, are capable of splitting the lecithin of egg-yolk incorporated in a culture medium. This reaction, which is due to an enzyme, phospholipinase, separates them quite sharply from *B. subtilis* and other members of the group. *B. cereus* is commonly found in heat-treated milk and it may be identified by culture on an egg-yolk-agar plate.

The various species are usually non-pathogenic on inoculation into laboratory animals. *B. cereus*, however, may be pathogenic to mice and guinea-pigs but does not give the appear-

Table 33.2 Some differential features of species of *Bacillus*

	Motility	Capsule	Spore	Pathogenicity for mouse	Optimum temperature °C	Egg yolk reaction
(a) Large celled 2–8 × 1–2 μm						
B. anthracis	−	+	C	High	35	Weak
B. cereus	+	−	C	Low	30	+
B. cereus var mycoides	+	−	C	None	30	+
B. megaterium	+	±	C	None	35	−
(b) Small celled 1·5–5 × 0·5–0·8 μm						
B. subtilis	+	−	C	None	37	−
B. subtilis var globigii (B. globigii)	+	−	C	None	37	−
B. pumilis	+	−	C	None	37	−
xB. polymyxa	+	−	C or ST	None	35	−
xB. stearothermophilus	+	−	T	None	55	−

Spore C = central; T = terminal; ST = subterminal.

    x = Gram variable, sporangia swollen by oval spores.

Egg yolk reaction: + = wide zone of turbidity spreading beyond colony; Weak = narrow zone of turbidity just wider than colony; − = no turbidity.

ances associated with *B. anthracis*, i.e. no evidence of capsulated bacilli in blood or tissues.

REFERENCES AND FURTHER READING

BERGEY (1957) *Manual of Determinative Bacteriology* (7th edn.). Baltimore: Williams and Williams Company.

CHERRY, W. B. & FREEMAN, E. M. (1959) Staining bacterial smears with fluorescent antibody. V. The rapid identification of *Bacillus anthracis* in culture and in human and marine tissue. *Zeitschrift für Bakteriologie*, **175**, 582.

DARLOW, H. M., BELTON, F. C. & HENDERSON, D. W. (1956) The use of anthrax antigen to immunize man and monkey. *Lancet*, **ii,** 476.

DARLOW, H. M. & PRIDE, N. B. (1969) Serological diagnosis of anthrax. *Lancet*, **ii,** 430.

GILLISSEN, G. & SCHOLTZ, H. G. (1961) Die Selektion von Milzbrandbazillen aus Flussigkerten mit Storker Verunreinigung durch *E. coli*. *Zeitschrift für Bakteriologie*, **182,** 232.

GREEN, D. M. & JAMIESON, W. M. (1958) Anthrax and bone meal fertilizer. *Lancet*, **ii,** 153.

KNISELEY, R. F. (1966) Selective medium for *Bacillus anthracis*. *Journal of Bacteriology*, **92,** 784.

McGAUGHEY, C. A. & CHU, H. P. (1948) The egg-yolk reactions of aerobic sporing bacilli. *Journal of General Microbiology*, **2,** 334.

MORRIS, E. J. (1955) A selective medium for *Bacillus anthracis*. *Journal of General Microbiology*, **13,** 456.

PEARCE, T. W. & POWELL, E. O. (1951) A selective medium for *Bacillus anthracis*. *Journal of General Microbiology*, **5,** 387.

THORNE, C. B. & BELTON, F. C. (1957) An agar diffusion method for titrating *Bacillus anthracis* immunizing antigen and its application to a study of antigen production. *Journal of General Microbiology*, **17,** 55.

34. Brucella

Brucellosis is essentially an infection of animals, mainly domestic animals, caused by organisms of the genus *Brucella*. There are three main species. *Br. melitensis* which infects sheep and goats, *Br. abortus* which infects cattle and *Br. suis*, the cause of brucellosis of swine. Human infections occur through contact with infected animals or their discharges or through consumption of infected milk or milk products. Infection is readily acquired by inhalation of infected dust in a cow-shed.

Morphology and staining. Round or oval coccobacilli, about 0·4 μm in diameter, but definite bacillary forms, 1–2 μ may also be seen. They occur singly, in pairs, or short chains: Gram-negative, non-motile, non-capsulate, non-sporing.

Cultural character. Aerobic, but *Br. abortus* requires an atmosphere containing 5–10 per cent CO_2 when first isolated from blood or tissues: *Br. melitensis* and *Br. suis* do not require additional CO_2. Optimum temperature 37°C. Growth is best on medium enriched with serum. On solid medium the colonies appear as small smooth transparent disks about 1 mm in diameter increasing to 2–3 mm. They are slow to develop and may not appear for several days.

Viability. Killed at 60°C in 10 min: hence killed in milk by pasteurization: moderately sensitive to acid and die out within a few days in fresh cheese undergoing lactic acid fermentation. They may survive for a number of days in butter made from infected milk: very sensitive to direct sunlight, but if unexposed may persist in dust or soil for two to three months and in dead foetal material for longer periods: susceptible to sulphonamides, streptomycin, the tetracyclines, chloramphenicol, ampicillin, but not to penicillin.

Biochemical reactions. Although carbohydrates are utilized, brucellae produce insufficient acid or gas to be demonstrable by the ordinary methods.

Animal pathogenicity. Laboratory animals may be experimentally infected, the guinea-pig being the most susceptible to small inocula. The infection is not usually progressive and the guinea-pig normally recovers spontaneously although infection by *Br. melitensis* may be fatal. If the animal is killed after six to eight weeks the lymph nodes in the region of the site of inoculation are usually swollen, the spleen is greatly enlarged and necrotic areas are seen in the liver and spleen from which the organisms may be cultured. Agglutinating antibodies are detectable in the serum.

Differential Biological Tests

The three main species *Br. abortus*, *Br. melitensis* and *Br. suis* differ in certain characters which form the basis for their classification. These are (1) CO_2 requirement; (2) production of H_2S; (3) sensitivity to certain dyes; (4) urease activity.

1. CO_2 requirement. When cultivation is attempted directly from the animal body, *Br. abortus* requires an atmosphere containing 5–10 per cent CO_2. Screw-capped bottles should be only loosely closed. After continued culture *Br. abortus* will grow aerobically; *Br. melitensis* will grow and may even benefit from the CO_2 atmosphere, but *Br. suis* may be inhibited by it.

2. Production of H_2S. *Br. abortus* and most strains of *Br. suis* form H_2S, the latter more markedly and for a longer period. A strip of lead acetate paper is inserted into a tube containing a glucose serum agar slope culture and held in place with the cotton-wool stopper. The paper is examined daily and renewed as soon as it becomes blackened. *Br. melitensis* and certain strains of *Br. suis* found only in Denmark do not produce H_2S.

3. Inhibition by dyes. Characteristically the three main types of brucella are differentiated by means of media containing 1 in 25 000 basic fuchsin and 1 in 50 000 thionin respectively. *Br. melitensis* is not inhibited to any extent by either dye, *Br. abortus* is typically inhibited by thionin, not by fuchsin, whereas *Br. suis* is inhibited by fuchsin but not by thionin (Table 34.1). Methyl violet, 1 in 50000, and pyronin, 1 in 100000 give results similar to those with basic fuchsin. Biotypes of the three species with characteristics that differ from the normal also exist (see below).

These dye-sensitivity tests may be carried out either by:

(a) Cruickshank's method which is useful in laboratories where only occasional strains are examined. Sterilized strips of filter paper (6 by 0·5 cm) are impregnated with the dye solutions, dried and stored for future use: the following concentrations have been found satisfactory: thionin 1 in 600, basic fuchsin 1 in 200. The strips are placed in parallel on the surface of a plate of solid medium (e.g. glucose serum agar) and then covered by pouring the same medium (melted) over them to form an additional layer. Stroke inoculations from cultures of the strains to be tested are made at right angles to the strips. After incubation in 5–10 per cent CO_2 for two to three days the results are determined as follows: if the organism resists the dye it grows across the strip; if sensitive, growth is inhibited for some distance (up to 10 mm) from the strip.

(b) Huddleson's method recommended by the FAO/WHO Brucellosis Centre, Weybridge, England. Useful for frequent examinations or research purposes.

Each dye is added to glucose serum agar at 50°C to give a final concentration in each case as follows: basic fuchsin 1 in 25000; thionin 1 in 50000; methyl violet 1 in 50000; pyronin 1 in 100000. The two latter dyes may be useful but are not normally used. Stock solutions (1 per cent in distilled water) of the dyes are relatively stable and may be stored for long periods, but the dilutions employed should be freshly prepared each time the medium is made and added after sterilization of the medium.

Each dye-agar mixture is poured into a Petri dish and allowed to solidify. Suspensions of the unknown strains and of known strains of the three species to act as control are grown first on glucose serum

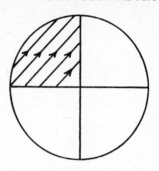

FIG. 34.1

agar without dyes and should be in the smooth phase. Suspensions of each are then prepared in a concentration of about 3×10^9 organisms per ml and are inoculated on to a quarter of each plate, five strokes being made, commencing from the edge and working inwards without recharging the loop so that the smallest inoculum is made nearest the centre (see Fig. 34.1). If five inocula of different sizes are used there is less likelihood of unsatisfactory results due to too large or too small an inoculum. The plates are incubated for five days in an atmosphere of 10 per cent CO_2.

Urease activity. One ml of a buffered 5 per cent urea solution (pH 4·0) containing phenol red as an indicator is inoculated with a loopful of a 48-h culture of the unknown strain grown on a solid medium. The tubes are incubated at 37°C in a waterbath and readings made after 15 min, 30 min, 1 h and hourly thereafter until a pink colour develops indicating a positive result. In general *Br. abortus* requires 2 h or more for the pink colour to develop whereas *Br. suis* gives a positive result in 15–30 min. *Br. melitensis* gives variable results sometimes resembling *Br. abortus* and sometimes *Br. suis* (Table 34.1).

Antigenic Analysis

Agglutination by monospecific sera. *Br. melitensis*, *Br. abortus* and *Br. suis* show a close antigenic relationship and direct agglutination tests with unabsorbed antisera fail to distinguish them. Agglutinin-absorption tests, however, elicit a difference between *Br. meliten-*

Table 34.1 Biological tests for the differentiation of brucella types.

	CO₂ require-ment	H₂S production (days)					Growth in presence of			Urease activity demonstrable within (min)	Serological Monospecific serum	
		1	2	3	4	5	Basic fuchsin 1 in 25 000	Thionin 1 in 50 000	Methyl violet 1 in 50 000		Abortus	melitensis
Br. melitensis	−	− (or slight)					+	+	+	variable	−	+
Br. abortus	+	+	+	++	+	−	+	−	+	120 or more	+	−
Br. suis (American strains)	−	++	++	++	+	+	−	+	−	15–30	+	−

Danish strains of *Br. suis* are similar to the American strains but do not produce H₂S

sis on the one hand and *Br. abortus* and *Br. suis* on the other; the latter two cannot be distinguished serologically. The difference in antigenic constitution is quantitative rather than qualitative. The three species possess two similar antigenic constituents A and M, though in different proportions, one constituent (M) being dominant in *Br. melitensis* and the other (A) dominant in *Br. abortus* and *Br. suis*.

To identify an unknown brucella strain, a suspension of organisms is prepared and diluted to a density corresponding to tube 4 of Brown's Opacity Tubes. The suspension is tested for agglutination by monospecific sera available commercially. Strains of *Br. abortus* and *Br. suis* are agglutinated to titre by mono-specific A antiserum and *Br. melitensis* by M antiserum only.

Biotypes of Brucella

Strains of brucella which differ in some of their characteristics from the normal species pattern may be identified as biotypes of one or other of the three main species by means of oxidative metabolic, phage-susceptibility and other tests. The rates of oxygen uptake by brucella cultures on eight amino-acids and four carbohydrate substrates have been determined and shown to form a different pattern for each of the three species. By this means strains may be identified as belonging not only to one or other of the three species but also to biotypes within the species. There are three types of *Br. melitensis*, at least nine of *Br. abortus* and four of *Br. suis*, type 1 in each case being the normal (prototype) of the species.

The *phage-susceptibility test* is performed with a standard reference phage, known as Tbilisi (Tb), at two dilutions, RTD (Routine test dilution) and 10 000 × RTD (these phage preparations may be obtained from the Central Veterinary Laboratory, Weybridge, Surrey, England). Since the oxidative metabolic tests are highly specialized and time consuming, it is recommended that atypical brucella strains should first be identified as far as possible using the conventional tests and phage-typing, and should then be sent to an active brucellosis centre for final identification. A table showing the main characters of the various biotypes of

Brucella and their reactions to four of the metabolic tests is given in the WHO fourth report on brucellosis (1964) and is reproduced here in a modified form (Table 34.2).

On the basis of the results of these differential tests it is thought that a number of brucella types that were regarded and named as additional species may, in fact, be biotypes of one or other of the three main species. They include two types that have given rise to human brucellosis, viz., *Br. rangiferi tarandi*, an organism that infects reindeer in U.S.S.R., Canada and Alaska, and which is known to cause brucellosis in Eskimos who handle the meat of those animals, and *Br. canis*, isolated from cases of canine abortion of beagles, which has given rise to infection in laboratory staff working with the strains.

Variation

Whilst typical, virulent brucellae produce colonies that are smooth and transparent, growth on laboratory media may result in mutation to a rough type of colony with corresponding loss of virulence; mucoid colonies may also appear. The organisms also change antigenically so that they are no longer agglutinated readily by homologous sera. Variation may also take place *in vivo*. The level of dissociation of a strain of brucella can be determined by inoculating a glucose serum agar plate with one smooth colony (determined by microscopic examination). After 72 h incubation at 37°C, a loopful of culture is emulsified in a drop of physiological saline on a slide and a drop of acriflavine solution (1 in 1000) is added. If the organism is still smooth the suspension remains smooth and homogeneous: if rough variants have developed, flocculation occurs and if a mucoid mutant has emerged a mucoid reaction takes place. The acriflavine solution should be kept in a brown flask to prevent its deterioration.

LABORATORY DIAGNOSIS

Blood Culture in Brucella Infections

Blood cultures should be carried out repeatedly on all suspected cases, but they are not likely to be positive in more than 30–50 per cent of cases. *Br. melitensis* and *Br. suis* are more readily isolated from blood cultures than *Br. abortus*. It is not necessary to limit the tests to the febrile phase. At least 10 ml blood should be withdrawn as the organisms may be relatively scanty. Blood cultures should be carried out in duplicate in glucose serum broth, one of each pair being incubated in an atmosphere of 10 per cent CO_2. Subcultures on to solid medium are made every few days and characteristic colonies looked for. The blood cultures should be retained for as long as six weeks before they are discarded as negative.

Castaneda's method of blood culture. This method may be more successful and obviates the need for frequent subcultures with the accompanying risk of laboratory infection. Three per cent melted glucose serum agar is allowed to solidify on one of the narrow sides of a 120 ml flat rectangular bottle (medical flat) with a perforated screw cap. 20 ml sterile glucose serum broth are added. The bottle is closed and the cap protected with a viscap during storage. Five ml of patient's blood are added to the broth by inserting the syringe needle through the perforation in the screw cap and the mixture is allowed to flow over the agar. CO_2 is introduced into the bottle aseptically by a needle inserted through the perforation in the cap to give approximately 10 per cent concentration. The bottle is incubated in the upright position and the agar surface is examined daily for colonies; if no colonies are seen in 48 h the blood broth is allowed to flow gently over the agar by suitably tilting the bottle which is again incubated in the upright position. If brucellae are present in the blood, colonies can usually be observed within a week.

Urine culture. In *Br. melitensis* infections the organisms may sometimes be isolated by culturing the urine.

Serological Tests

Because blood culture is often negative the laboratory diagnosis of human brucellosis has to rely mainly on serological tests, the results of which vary with the clinical form and stage of infection: (a) standard agglutination test

Table 34.2 Differential characters of the three species of the genus *Brucella* and their biotypes.

Species	Type	CO_2 requirement	H_2S production	Thionin a	Thionin b	Thionin c	Basic fuchsin d	Basic fuchsin e	Urease	Aggl. A	Aggl. M	Phage Tb* at RTD†	Glutamic acid	Ornithine	Ribose	Lysine
Br. melitensis	1	−	−	−	+	+	+	+	+ or ±	−	+	−	+	−	−	−
	2	−	−	−	+	+	+	+	+ or ±	+	−	−	+	−	−	−
	3	−	−	−	+	+	+	+	+ or ±	+	+	−	+	−	+	−
Br. abortus	1	+(−)	+	−	−	+	+	+	±	+	−	+	+	−	+	−
	2	+	+	−	−	−	+	−	±	+	−	+	+	−	+	−
	3	−(+)	+	−	−	+	+	+	±	+	−	+	+	−	+	−
	4	+(−)	+	−	+	+	+	+	±	−	+	+	+	−	+	−
	5	−	−	−	+	+	+	+	±	−	+	+	+	−	+	−
	6	−	−	−	+	+	+	+	±	+	+	+	+	−	+	−
	7	+	− or +	−	+	+	+	+	±	+	+	+	+	−	+	−
	8	+	+	−	+	+	+	+	±	−	+	+	+	−	+	−
	9	− or +	+	−	+	+	+	+	±	−	+	+	+	−	+	−
Br. suis	1	−	++	+	+	+	−	−	++	+	−	−	−	+	+	+
	2	−	−	−	+	+	−	−	++	+	−	−	+	+	+	−
	3	−	−	+	+	+	+	+	++	+	−	−	+	+	+	+

± = weak reaction

Br. abortus, type 5 = British melitensis
Br. suis, type 2 = Danish suis
* Tb = Tbilisi
† RTD = Routine test dilution

a = 1 in 25 000
b = 1 in 50 000
c = 1 in 100 000
d = 1 in 50 000
e = 1 in 100 000

(SAT); (b) mercaptoethanol test (agglutination in the presence of 2-mercaptoethanol); (c) antihuman-globulin (Coombs) test for non-agglutinating antibodies; (d) complement-fixation test (for a detailed description of these tests as applied to the diagnosis of human brucellosis see Kerr *et al.*, 1968).

(a) A positive agglutination reaction may be detected 7–10 days after infection has occurred. Serum dilutions from 1 in 10 to 1 in 1280 or more in 0·05 ml volumes of phenol saline should be tested against an equal volume of carefully standardized antigens, e.g. 'Wellcome' *Br. abortus* 'agglutinable concentrated suspension' diluted 1 in 15, or any other *Br. abortus* suspension diluted to the same packed cell concentration (the agglutinating titre of a serum varies with the density of the cell suspension used as antigen). In order to avoid false-negative readings due to prozones that may occur in the later stages of the acute phase it is advisable to include dilutions of over 1 in 1000 in the series. The tubes are kept at 37°C for 2 days and are read in indirect light in a viewing box or a darkened room. Reactions of partial or complete clearing and deposit of cells are reported as positive. The degree of clearing is an indication of the strength of the reaction and may be reported as + + (complete), + (partial) and tr (trace) reactions. Precisely the same techniques should always be followed in the laboratory in order that successive tests may be strictly comparable.

The titre of the serum should be recorded as the highest serum dilution to give partial or complete agglutination.

(b) The mercaptoethanol test determines the type of immunoglobulin responsible for the agglutination in the standard agglutination test. In the acute stage of the infection agglutination may be associated with both IgM and IgG immunoglobulins. After recovery the antibody levels fall gradually but low-titre agglutination due mainly to residual amounts of IgM antibody may continue for many months or even years. The agglutination activity of IgM is destroyed by 2-mercaptoethanol and therefore agglutination in this test is indicative of the continuing presence of IgG and the likelihood of continuing infection. The test is carried out simultaneously with and in the same manner as the standard agglutination test except that the normal saline used as diluent contains 0·05 M-2-mercaptoethanol (MW 78: obtainable from Koch-Light Laboratories). A stock solution of 0·2 M in phosphate-buffered saline is prepared initially and stored at 4°C in an opaque bottle. It is further diluted to 0·05 M with normal saline for use as the diluent in the test. The solutions should be prepared in the fume cupboard and should not be inhaled.

(c) Antihuman-globulin test. The disease, if not effectively treated, may progress from the acute to the chronic form. The organisms are then localized intracellularly. The IgM antibodies decrease and IgG antibodies, although still present at high levels, lose their ability to agglutinate readily. The agglutination titre falls to a low level and may finally be absent even when the patient is still ill. The complete absence of agglutination therefore does not rule out the possibility of infection. Non-agglutinating antibodies may be detected by the antihuman-globulin (Coombs') test as follows: an agglutination test is set up using as antigen a *Br. abortus* suspension that is more concentrated than that used in the standard agglutination test, e.g. Wellcome concentrated suspension diluted 1 in 6. The same range of serum dilutions is prepared as for the standard agglutination test. The tubes are incubated at 37°C for 24 h: any tubes showing agglutination are recorded and not proceeded with further. At this stage the titre is less than that of the routine agglutination test because of the more concentrated antigen. Tubes not showing agglutination are centrifuged at 2000 rev/min for 15 minutes and the supernatant is discarded. The deposit is thoroughly washed by resuspension in physiological saline; a pasteur pipette is used to draw the suspension up and down at least ten times. This process of centrifugation and resuspension is repeated three times in order to remove all traces of human protein. After the final washing the cells are resuspended in 0·45 ml saline and to each tube 0·05 ml of suitably diluted antihuman-globulin (AHG Wellcome) is added and mixed in by shaking. The final dilution of AHG in each tube is that recommended by the manufacturers, e.g. if a final dilution of 1 in 160 is recommended, the antihuman-globulin is first diluted 1 in 16 and 0·05 ml of this dilution is added to each tube to give a final dilution of 1 in 160. The tubes are kept at 37°C for a further 24 h and examined for agglutination which, if present, is due to the antihuman-globulin reacting with the nonagglutinating antibody fixed to the bacterial cells.

(d) Complement-fixation test. As long as infection continues, IgG antibodies remain in the serum; although they may no longer be capable of agglutination they are detected by their continuing ability to fix complement. The test is set up in a WHO plastic plate using a four-volume technique with veronal buffer as a diluent. The patient's serum dilutions commence at 1 in 4. *Br. abortus* suspension as used in the standard agglutination test is used as antigen and should be diluted to an optimum concentration shown by titration not to be anticomplementary. A 2 per cent sensitized sheep red cell suspension constitutes the haemolytic system. The long-fixation technique at 4°C is recommended with 1·5 haemolytic units of complement determined by titration in the presence of antigen and normal serum (pooled negative serum).

Interpretation of Serological Findings

It should be noted that sera from a proportion of the normal population contain antibodies in low dilutions due either to a latent or past infection. The percentage is higher in rural than in urban areas. In latent infections the complement-fixation test is likely to be positive whereas in past infections it is negative. Agglutinins for brucellae may be present in the serum of persons who have been immunized against cholera. After recovery from brucellosis the antibody level falls slowly sometimes taking many months to reach low levels. (Kerr *et al.* (1968).)

Reference to Table 34.3 may help in interpreting the results of the three main diagnostic tests.

Intradermal Brucellosis Test

The intradermal injection of 0·1 ml killed suspension of brucellae or of purified extracts, e.g. brucellin, elicits a delayed tuberculin-like allergic reaction of erythema and induration in persons who have been infected. The test should be used with caution since a violent local reaction with generalized symptoms may occur in persons who are still actively infected, or who are hypersensitive as a result of frequent exposure to the organism, e.g. veterinary surgeons, abattoir workers or dairy farmers. A positive intradermal test should be interpreted as merely indicating a state of hypersensitivity in the individual. It has no other diagnostic significance. The levels of existing brucella antibodies tend to rise shortly after the test dose has been introduced (Report, 1972).

Laboratory Diagnosis in Animals

The agglutination test on the serum of supposedly infected animals using standardized

Table 34.3

Type of brucellosis	Agglutination test	Complement-fixation test	Antihuman-globulin test
Acute	positive	positive	. . .
Chronic	weak or negative	positive	positive
Past infection	weak or negative	negative	weak or negative

brucella suspensions has been used in diagnosis. Results in which 50 per cent agglutination occurs in dilutions of 1 in 40 or over are generally regarded as evidence of infection.

The *milk ring test* (MRT) is a very sensitive means of detecting agglutinins in milk samples (see Chapter 11). Since a positive reaction may occur in the milk of cows vaccinated in adult life with the avirulent strain of *Br. abortus* S19, the significance of a positive reaction should be further tested either by culturing the organism directly from the cream or by inoculating guinea-pigs with cream and with the deposit after centrifuging the milk. A convenient confirmatory test is the whey-agglutination test which is rarely affected by vaccination of cattle prior to breeding age (see Chapter 11).

REFERENCES

KERR, W. R., McCAUGHEY, W. J., COGHLAN, JOYCE D., PAYNE, D. J. H., QUAIFE, R. A., ROBERTSON, L. & FARRELL, I. D. (1968) Techniques and interpretations in the serological diagnosis of brucellosis in man. *Journal of Medical Microbiology*, **1**, 181.

REPORT (1972) Appraisal of brucellin skin test. Report of working party to the director of the public health laboratory service. *Lancet*, **i**, 676.

WORLD HEALTH ORGANIZATION, EXPERT COMMITTEE ON BRUCELLOSIS (1964) *World Health Organization Technical Report Series*, No. 289.

35. Yersinia, Pasteurella, Francisella

These three groups of organisms were previously classified together within the genus *Pasteurella*, but some of the species are now considered to be so closely related and to have sufficient distinctive characteristics to warrant their inclusion in a separate genus, viz. '*Yersinia*'. Thus the plague bacillus, previously known as *Pasteurella pestis,* and the causative organism of pseudotuberculosis of guinea-pigs and other animals (*Pasteurella pseudotuberculosis*) are now referred to as *Yersinia pestis* and *Yersinia pseudotuberculosis* respectively and grouped with *Yersinia enterocolitica*, an organism that in recent years has been recognized as a cause of enteritis and mesenteric lymphadenitis in man. The genus *Pasteurella* is now restricted to a number of animal pathogens notably *Pasteurella multocida* (*Past. septica*), the cause of septicaemic diseases in a variety of animal species. It is of medical importance because it is transmissible to man through contact with infected animals especially through animal bites. The bacillus of tularaemia of animals and man now forms a new genus *Francisella* and is known as *Francisella tularensis*.

All of these species are small Gram-negative bacilli, some of which show extreme variations in size and shape (involution forms) that are particularly marked in older cultures. When stained with methylene blue, bipolar staining is a characteristic feature. The main distinguishing features of the four species that are of medical importance are shown in Table 35.1.

YERSINIA PESTIS (PASTEURELLA PESTIS, THE PLAGUE BACILLUS)

Morphology. Characteristic morphology is seen best in films made directly from tissues or exudate; short, oval bacillus with rounded ends (cocco-bacillus) about 1·5 μm by 0·7 μm, singly or in pairs. On culture, especially in old cultures, pleomorphism is marked, e.g. enlarged, elongated or irregular cells, some of which may be pear-shaped or globular and suggestive of yeast cells. Involution in culture can be hastened by the addition of 3 per cent NaCl and this phenomenon may be used as a means of identification. In fluid culture the bacilli tend to form chains: capsulate, non-motile, non-sporing.

Staining. Gram-negative; in smears from the tissues, stained with methylene blue, the bacilli show characteristic bipolar staining, but in culture the bipolar staining is less obvious and involution forms stain only faintly.

Capsules. In exudates from lesions *Y. pestis* exhibits typical capsules; less obvious in culture although capsules may be seen in

Table 35.1 Criteria for differential diagnosis of yersinia, pasteurella and francisella infections.

	Growth on routine nutrient medium	Growth on bile-salt medium	Motility at 22°C	Motility at 37°C	Acid (no gas) from Maltose	Acid (no gas) from Sucrose	Indole	Urease	Oxidase	Catalase
Y. pestis	+	+	−	−	+	−	−	−	−	+
Y. pseudotuberculosis	+	+	+	−	+	−	−	+	−	+
Y. enterocolitica	+	+	+	−	+	+ (late)	−	+	−	+
P. multocida	+	−	−	−	−	+	+	−	+ or −	+
P. pneumotropica	+	−	−	−	+	+	+	+	+	+
P. haemolytica	+	+ or −	−	−	−	+	−	−	+	+ or −
P. ureae	+	−	−	−	−	+	−	+	+	+
F. tularensis	−	.	−	−	.	.	.	.	.	.

cultures grown at 37°C rather than at the optimum temperature of 27°C.

Cultural requirements. Aerobe and facultative anaerobe: temperature range 14°C to 37°C; optimum temperature for primary culture is 27°C: somewhat sensitive to free oxygen and growth may not develop aerobically if the inoculum is small; this inhibition may be avoided by the addition to the medium of blood or sodium sulphite, or by excluding air. Colonies on blood agar are at first very small, transparent, white circular discs, 1 mm or less in diameter but later enlarging to 3 or 4 mm and becoming opaque. In older cultures the mixture of opaque and transparent colonies gives the appearance of a mixed growth.

In broth, growth results in a granular deposit at the bottom and on the sides of the tube. If the inoculum is added to a flask of broth and a drop of oil then allowed to float on the surface, a characteristic growth develops, consisting of 'stalactites' hanging down into the liquid medium from the oil drop. Unlike some of the other members of the group *Y. pestis* grows on MacConkey's bile salt medium.

Sensitivity to physical and chemical agents. Killed at 55°C for 15 min and by 0·5 per cent phenol within the same time: very susceptible to natural drying, but laboratory cultures remain viable for months if kept moist and at a low temperature. The risk of laboratory infection from pathological material or cultures is considerable.

Drug sensitivity. *Y. pestis* is sensitive to tetracycline, the drug of choice for bubonic and pneumonic plague; sensitive to sulphonamides which, however, are not effective for the treatment of pneumonic plague; sensitive to streptomycin, but the use of this drug alone is not recommended since the large doses necessary to control the disease may give rise to severe intoxication; resistant to penicillin.

Biochemical reactions. Poor growth in peptone water and sugar fermentation reactions may take up to two weeks to be complete. The various biochemical reactions are as shown in Table 35.1.

Antigenic structure. Virulent and avirulent strains of *Y. pestis* are antigenically homogeneous; a close antigenic relationship exists with *Y. pseudotuberculosis* so that cross reactions take place in agglutination tests. Two main antigenic complexes are concerned with virulence and immunogenicity, one somatic and heat-stable, the other capsular and heat-labile. The capsular antigen is important for efficient vaccine production since it contains the protective fraction F1 obtained as a non-toxic capsular component from saline extracts of acetone-dried cultures. The conditions that determine immunogenicity vary according to the species of animal used to test it. Fraction F1 also contributes to the virulence of the capsulated organisms because of its anti-phagocytic activity. Two other antigens known as V and W also contribute to the organisms' resistance to phagocytosis. For development of killed vaccine that may be effective against plague in man see Keppie, Cocking Witt and Smith (1960).

Laboratory Diagnosis

The diagnosis of plague is confirmed by demonstrating *Y. pestis* in fluid from buboes in the case of bubonic plague or in the sputum in pneumonic plague. In septicaemic plague the bacilli may be demonstrated in blood films and isolated by blood culture or from the spleen at post-mortem examination.

Bubonic plague. The bubo is punctured with a hypodermic syringe and exudate withdrawn. This is used for (a) preparing films to be stained with Gram's stain and methylene blue; (b) culturing on blood agar from which single colonies are picked for further identification tests; and (c) inoculating laboratory animals, viz. guinea-pigs or white rats. In the films characteristic Gram-negative bacilli which show bipolar staining with methylene blue are highly suggestive of plague bacilli. Identification of pure cultures from single colonies is carried out by (1) demonstrating the ability of the organism to grow on MacConkey's bile salt agar; (2) biochemical reactions as shown in Table 35.1; (3) the production of involution forms on 3 per cent salt agar; (4) chain formation in broth culture; and (5) stalactite growth from oil drops in fluid culture medium.

Pneumonic plague. Films are made from the sputum, stained by Gram's stain and methylene blue and examined microscopically for the characteristic bipolar stained bacilli. For identification the organisms should be isolated in pure culture, as with material from bubonic plague.

For animal inoculation with sputum in which other virulent microorganisms may be present, successful infection can be most readily effected by applying the material to the nasal mucosa or to a shaved area of skin. The plague bacillus has been successfully recovered from contaminated sources by the use of a simple selective medium devised by Kniseley, Swaney and Friedlander (1964).

Post-mortem examination. There may be racial prejudices against obtaining material for laboratory examination *post-mortem*. If excision of buboes, liver, spleen, bone marrow or lung tissue is not allowed, specimens of tissue may be obtained by needle puncture.

Animal pathogenicity. Necropsy carried out on a rat found dying of plague or on guinea-pigs or white rats that have died as a result of inoculation reveals a marked local inflammatory condition at the site of infection with necrosis and oedema; the regional lymph nodes are enlarged; the spleen is enlarged and congested and may show greyish white patches in the tissue. The characteristic cocco-bacilli are seen in large numbers in films made from local lesions, lymph nodes, spleen-pulp and heart-blood.

Diagnosis of plague in wild rats. It is important to differentiate plague from infection due to *P. pseudotuberculosis*. In plague, necropsy reveals the following features: enlargement of the lymphatic nodes with periglandular inflammation and oedema that is most frequent in cervical lymph nodes due to the tendency for the flea to attack the rat's neck region; pleural effusion; enlargement of the spleen which may show small white areas in the pulp; liver congested and mottled; congestion and haemorrhages under the skin and in internal organs.

Films and cultures made from heart-blood, lymph nodes and spleen are examined for characteristic appearances and differential biochemical tests.

Material from lesions in dead rats should be inoculated on to the nasal mucosa of guinea-pigs or white rats as for sputum (see above).

YERSINIA PSEUDOTUBERCULOSIS

This is the causative organism of pseudotuberculosis of animals and birds. It causes human infection that sometimes results in a severe septicaemic typhoid-like illness with a high fatality rate. More commonly it gives rise to acute mesenteric lymphadenitis simulating acute or subacute appendicitis sometimes with erythema nodosum: this milder infection usually clears up spontaneously.

Morphology and staining. A small, oval, Gram-negative bacillus similar to *Y. pestis*; slightly acid-fast; differs from *Y. pestis* in being motile at 22°C, readily demonstrated in Craigie tubes, one of which is incubated at 22°C and another at 37°C.

Cultural characteristics. Aerobe and facultative anaerobe. Grows on ordinary nutrient medium and on MacConkey's medium.

Biochemical reactions. These are shown in Table 35.1. It differs from the plague bacillus in its ability to produce urease.

Antigenic structure. There are 5 serological types (types 1–5) based on highly specific thermostable somatic antigens and thermolabile flagellar antigens (present only in cultures grown at 22°C). There is a common *rough* somatic antigen shared by all five types and with *Y. pestis*. More than 90 per cent of *Y. pseudotuberculosis* infections in man are caused by type 1 (Mair, 1969). An antigenic relationship exists between types II and IV and certain salmonellae of groups B and D respectively.

Laboratory Diagnosis

The diagnosis is confirmed by isolating the organism from the mesenteric lymph nodes and by demonstrating antibodies in the patient's serum during the acute phase of the illness. This may be done by slide-agglutination confirmed by tube agglutination tests using live, smooth suspensions of the five serotypes of *Y. pseudotuberculosis* grown at 22°C. Antibodies usually disappear fairly rapidly.

The organism is sensitive to certain bacteriophages and this provides a useful means of identification. A drop of bacteriophage is added to one of two tubes of peptone water culture of *Y. pseudotuberculosis* and incubated at 37°C. The tube containing the bacteriophage shows complete clearing after 24 hours. The *Y. pseudotuberculosis* bacteriophages are also specific for *Y. pestis*.

An intradermal test similar to the tuberculin or brucellin tests is positive in infections due to all types of *Y. pseudotuberculosis*. The reaction may persist for many years after the infection has cleared.

For full details of methods of diagnosis see Mair (1969).

PASTEURELLA MULTOCIDA
(P. SEPTICA)

Pasteurella multocida produces haemorrhagic septicaemia in various animals and is the cause of septic wounds following trauma from animal bites, operation, cranial fracture, etc.

Morphology and staining. Small, oval, Gram-negative cocco-bacilli: exhibits bipolar staining in films made directly from blood and tissues stained with methylene blue: capsulated: non-motile.

Cultural characteristics. Aerobe and facultative anaerobe: with rare exceptions does not grow on MacConkey's medium.

Drug-sensitivity. Sensitive to penicillin, ery-thromycin, sulphonamides, tetracycline and streptomycin. In cases of osteomyelitis following animal bites drug treatment must be continued for at least eight weeks.

Biochemical reactions. P. multocida differs from other members of the group in certain cultural and biochemical details (Table 35.1). Sugars are fermented without gas production.

Antigenic structure. The species is not antigenically homogeneous. Serological methods have revealed a certain degree of grouping (Coghlan, 1958). Five types have been determined by cross-protection tests (Hudson, 1959).

Laboratory Diagnosis

The diagnosis is confirmed by culturing the organism on blood agar from swabs of dog or cat bite wounds, from cerebrospinal fluid in cases of meningitis and from secretions in suppurative conditions of the respiratory system. Identification is made by cultural and biochemical tests (Table 35.1).

Other Organisms of Pasteurella Genus

Strains of Pasteurella which differ from *P. multocida* in certain biochemical features have been named *P. pneumotropica*, occasionally isolated from animal bites, and *P. haemolytica* and *P. ureae* (Jones, 1962) sometimes isolated from chronic respiratory tract infections, although their pathogenicity has not been established. For their distinguishing characteristics see Table 35.1. *P. pneumotropica* may be classified as a variant of *P. multocida* as *P. ureae* may be a variant of *P. haemolytica* (Winton and Mair, 1969).

FRANCISELLA TULARENSIS
(PASTEURELLA TULARENSIS)

F. tularensis is the cause of tularaemia, a plague-like disease of rodents and other small mammals, transmissible to man as a typical zoonosis, through either direct or indirect contact with infected animals or the improper handling of laboratory cultures. Human infections may produce a variety of clinical manifestations, mild or severe. In Europe water-borne and airborne infections tend to produce an influenza-like type of illness but in American outbreaks there is usually ulceroglandular, oculoglandular, pulmonary or typhoidal manifestations.

Morphology. Small cocco-bacillus which on first isolation does not exceed 0·7 μm by 0·2 μm, but on artificial media may appear as a moderately sized bacillus 1·5 μm by 0·5 μm with a marked tendency to pleomorphism; capsulate, non-motile and non-sporing. In infected animals occurs within cells of the spleen and liver where it probably multiplies.

Staining. Stains well with methylene-blue: Gram-negative: dilute carbol-fuchsin should be used as a counter-stain but smears from post-mortem specimens may require gentle heating to allow penetration of the stain.

Cultural requirements. Strict aerobe. Fresh isolates cannot be cultivated on ordinary laboratory media but require a complex medium containing blood or tissue extracts and cystine (see Chap. 5). Minute droplet-like colonies develop in 48–72 h at 37°C. Growth in liquid cultures may be obtained using casein hydrolysate with added thiamine and cystine.

Sensitivity. Easily killed by heat at 56–58°C in 10 min. May remain viable in cultures kept at 10°C for many years and in humid soil and water for 30 and 90 days respectively (Zidon, 1964).

Drug sensitivity. Sensitive to tetracycline which is the drug of choice and should be used in high dosage for a prolonged period; sensitive to streptomycin. Severe infection may require the use of chloramphenicol.

Laboratory Diagnosis

Human infections are usually diagnosed by inoculating laboratory guinea-pigs and mice with exudates from the glands and ulcers and subsequent isolation of *F. tularensis* from the liver and spleen of the infected animals *post-mortem*, on glucose cystine blood agar. Slide agglutination tests on animal blood and fluorescent antibody test on spleen imprints may also be carried out. Patient's serum may be tested for specific antibodies by slide and tube agglutination, haemagglutination, complement fixation and antihuman globulin (Coombs) tests using antigens prepared from suspensions of *F. tularensis* grown on solid medium (Haug and Pearson, 1972). It should

be noted that the serum of cases of brucellosis may contain agglutinins for *F. tularensis*.

REFERENCES

Coghlan, Joyce D. (1958) Isolation of *Pasteurella multocida* from human peritoneal pus and a study of the relationship to other strains of the same species. *Journal of Pathology and Bacteriology*, **76**, 45.

Haug, R. H. & Pearson, A. D. (1972) Human infections with *Francisella tularensis* in Norway. Development of a serological screening test. *Acta pathologica et microbiologica scandinavica, Section B*, **80**, 273–280.

Hudson, J. R. (1959) In *Infectious Diseases of Animals; Diseases Due to Bacteria*, p. 413, edited by A. W. Stableforth and I. A. Galloway. London: Butterworth.

Jones, D. M. (1962) A Pasteurella-like organism from the human respiratory tract. *Journal of Pathology and Bacteriology*, **83**, 143.

Keppie, J., Cocking, E. C., Witt, K. & Smith, H. (1960) The chemical basis of the virulence of *Pasteurella pestis*. III An immunogenic product obtained from *Pasteurella pestis* that protects both guinea-pigs and mice. *British Journal of Experimental Pathology*, **41**, 577.

Kniseley, R. F., Swaney, L. M. & Friedlander, H. (1964) Selective media for the isolation of *Pasteurella pestis*. *Journal of Bacteriology*, **88**, 491.

Mair, N. S. (1969) The laboratory diagnosis of infections with *Pasteurella pseudotuberculosis*. In *Recent Advances in Clinical Pathology*, 4th edn., Chap. 3.

Winton, F. W. & Mair, N. S. (1969) *Pasteurella pneumotropica* isolated from a dog-bite wound. *Microbios.*, **2**, 155.

Zidon, J. (1966) Tularaemia. In *Zoonoses*, Chap. 5, p. 74, edited by J. van der Hoeden. Amsterdam: Elsevier.

36. Bacteroides: Streptobacillus: Donovania

THE GRAM-NEGATIVE NON-SPORING ANAEROBIC BACILLI

With the exception of the debated *Bacteroides corrodens* sub-group, organisms of the *Bacteroides-Fusiformis* group are strict anaerobes. In their anaerobic requirements, they are generally more exacting than *Clostridium welchii* or *Cl. bifermentans*, and less exacting than *Cl. tetani*.

Morphology. They are typically Gram-negative rod-shaped bacilli, but they may be very short or very long and they also vary markedly in width. Often they are wider towards the centre of the bacillus and the fusiform appearance may be thin and delicate or broad and coarse with a tendency to stain less intensely in the central area. Pleomorphism in this group is common and it varies in degree from moderate to extreme. The organisms may occur singly, in pairs or in chains; filamentous forms often show subdivisions as seen in septate fungi, but the filaments are usually finer than fungal hyphae.

All of the bacteroides organisms are non-sporing. Some produce strangely swollen spherical bodies that may resemble sporing forms. Some are motile, but most are non-motile.

Nutritional requirements. The nutritional requirements of this heterogeneous group vary. Most of the species of medical interest grow better on enriched media such as freshly poured or pre-reduced blood agar. Even with such favourable media, development of visible colonies of some strains may require 48 h. Some have special requirements for haemin and vitamin K (menadione, 5 μg per ml). The presence of 10 per cent CO_2 in the anaerobic atmosphere often markedly enhances growth.

Colonial appearance is variable, depending on the species and the medium, from tiny ·pin-point translucent colonies to large grey circular or irregular colonies at 24–48 h.

Biochemical reactions. They may ferment various sugars such as glucose and sucrose, sometimes producing gas. Some are proteolytic, some produce indole and some produce hydrogen sulphide. *B. necrophorus* produces a lipase and, on egg-yolk agar, its colonies develop a 'pearly layer'. Some strains produce a heparinase.

Identification of genera and species. There is confusion at present regarding the taxonomy of the Gram-negative anaerobic bacilli. Not only are the characters of the different groups apparently variable, but the reproducibility of various laboratory tests is compromised by difficulties of culture and problems of purification of strains. Technical problems associated with sugar fermentation tests are well recognized in this context (see Rutter, 1970). When variable results occur commonly, it is difficult to use a taxonomic key based on clear positives and negatives. Accordingly, a provisional approach to the identification of various species is indicated in Table 36.1, and some of the common characters of these species are listed here.

Bacteroides fragilis (Bacillus fragilis, Fusiformis fragilis)

This is a delicate moderately pleomorphic non-motile Gram-negative rod, 2–3 μm by 0·4–0·8 μm. It grows well on freshly poured blood agar incubated anaerobically with 10 per cent CO_2 to produce at 24 h small (1 mm) greyish to greyish-white translucent, non-haemolytic smooth circular convex colonies. *B. fragilis* is saccharolytic but not proteolytic. Some strains produce a deconjugase that releases free bile acid from bile salt.

Bacteroides necrophorus (Bacteroides funduliformis, Actinomyces necrophorus, Sphaerophorus necrophorus, Fusobacterium necrophorum)

This fairly large non-motile Gram-negative anaerobe often occurs as a long rod with a central unstained bar, but highly pleomorphic

Table 36.1   A provisional approach to the identification of Gram-negative anaerobic bacilli. (Bacteroides spp.).

PRIMARY TESTS	Observed result with the test species*				
Growth strictly anaerobic	+	+	+	–	+
Colonies α or β-haemolytic on blood agar	–	+	+	–	–
Pearly layer on egg-yolk agar	–	+	– (+)	–	–
Oxidase	–	–	–	+	–
Catalase	–	–	–	–	–
Penicillin sensitivity (1-2-unit disk)	R	S	S	S	S
Rifampicin sensitivity‡ (10–15 μg disk)	S	S/R	S	S	S
Gelatinase activity	–	–	+	–	–
Hydrolysis of aesculin	+	–	–	–	+
Sugar fermentations: (Glucose, Lactose, Sucrose, Maltose)	GLSM	–	GSM (–)	–	GLSM

SECONDARY TESTS	PRESUMPTIVE SPECIES				
	B. fragilis	B. necrophorus	B. melanino-genicus	B. corrodens	F. fusiforme
Black pigment produced†	–	–	+	–	–
Pitting growth on agar media	–	–	–	+ (–)	–
Indole production	–	+	+	–	– (+)
H₂S production	+	+	+	–	– (+)
Lysine decarboxylase	...	...	...	+	...

* – = negative result, + = positive, symbol in brackets = variation recorded, ... = observation not recorded.
† see p. 470.
‡ Gram-negative anaerobic bacilli resistant to rifampicin are classified as *Sphaerophorus* species by Sutter and Finegold (1971); see p. 470.

forms range from short bacteria to long filaments. 'Ghost cells' that stain feebly may be seen. The microorganism grows a little more slowly on anaerobic blood agar with 10 per cent CO_2 than *B. fragilis*. At 48 h however, its colonies are well developed (2–3 mm) irregularly circular, high convex or papillate, greyish or yellowish opaque at the centre with granular translucence peripherally, producing a greenish α-haemolytic effect or, at times, a frankly β-haemolytic appearance. *B. necrophorus* is non-saccharolytic and non-proteolytic. It produces a lipase and its colonies on egg-yolk media have an associated 'pearly layer'.

Fusobacterium fusilforme (Bacteroides fusiformis, Bacillus fusiformis, Fusiformis fusiforme, F. plauti-vincentii, Leptotrichia buccalis)

This is a large non-motile Gram-negative bacillus, typically stout spindle-shaped or cigar-shaped with a less deeply stained central area; may occur in highly pleomorphic forms; filamentous forms are common.

This anaerobe grows on blood agar anaerobically with 10 per cent CO_2 to produce in 48 h small circular convex colonies, later becoming irregular, sometimes with zones of doubtful haemolysis. *F. fusiforme* is saccharolytic but non-proteolytic.

Bacteroides melaninogenicus (Ristella melaninogenica, Fusiformis melaninogenicum)

This anaerobe occurs as a small non-motile Gram-negative bacillus, or diplobacillus, sometimes with filamentous forms. Growth on fresh blood agar under strictly anaerobic conditions with 10 per cent CO_2 produces small circular convex colonies (about 1 mm) that later develop a black pigment derived from haem. This organism appears to grow more readily in mixed culture.

It is saccharolytic and proteolytic and it produces indole and hydrogen sulphide.

Bacteroides corrodens

This small fairly regular Gram-negative organism produces occasional filamentous forms. It is non-motile. An occasional fimbria-like process has been observed in electron micrographs.

Many strains are capable of aerobic growth on enriched media, but growth is generally better under anaerobic conditions and some strains are clearly anaerobes (see below). Growth is enhanced by carbon dioxide.

Colonies on blood agar at 24 h are small (0·2–0·5 mm) greyish translucent non-haemolytic dots burrowing into the agar and producing a corroded appearance. Not all strains produce this pitting effect and it is not unique for B. corrodens. Older colonies develop up to 3 mm in diameter.

The B. corrodens group is non-proteolytic and appears to be non-saccharolytic. It is oxidase-positive and decarboxylases (for lysine and ornithine) may be produced. The group's aerotolerance and resistance to lincomycin sets it apart from other bacteroides-like organisms: recent papers by Hill, Snell and Lapage (1970) and Jackson et al. (1971) should be consulted for further details of this group's characteristics and classification. It now seems that aerotolerant strains originally classified as B. corrodens should be included in Eikenella and should not be regarded as Bacteroides-like organisms (see Lancet, 1973).

A Note on Classification

Although the above descriptions take account of the significant contributions of Finegold and Sutter in this field, the classification evolved by these workers is not incorporated here and various species recognized by them are not included; the Sphaerophorus group certainly merits the attention of clinical microbiologists. The reader is referred to recent papers by Finegold, Sugihara and Sutter (1971) and by Sutter and Finegold, (1971) for details of their classification and laboratory procedures. Alternatively, special procedures are described and detailed criteria for identification are listed in a manual on clinical methods in anaerobic bacteriology published by Cato et al. (1970) from the Virginia Polytechnic Institute, Blacksburg, U.S.A.

A Note on Pigment Production by Bacteroides-like Organisms

In a recent study of chromogenesis in Bacteroides spp., Tracy (1969) noted that black 'pigments' could be produced by B. fragilis, B. necrophorus and B. melaninogenicus when given a source of cysteine and ferrous sulphate. The black material produced was colloidal ferrous sulphide and this is unrelated to the true pigment produced by B. melaninogenicus on media containing blood (Duerden, to be published).

THE LABORATORY DIAGNOSIS OF INFECTIONS DUE TO BACTEROIDES-LIKE ORGANISMS

The general procedures outlined for the isolation and identification of anaerobes are recommended, but the following special points should be noted. It must be stressed that the medical microbiologist is obliged to make a reasonably accurate identification with reasonable speed; the procedures described here take account of this.

Microscopy. Bacteroides-like organisms in a Gram-stained smear may be missed if a careful examination is not made. The organisms may be mistaken for coliform bacteria, which are generally less pleomorphic and more robust in appearance and in staining, or for Haemophilus species, which they may resemble

Table 36.2 Commonly observed antibiotic sensitivity patterns of some Gram-negative anaerobic bacilli.

Antibiotic (and amount in disk)	Sensitivity (S) or resistance (R) of the test species				
	Bacteroides fragilis	B. necrophorus F. fusiforme	B. melanino-genicus	B. corrodens·	Sphaerophorus varius, S. mortiferus S. ridiculosus
Penicillin (2 units)	R	S	S	S	S
Erythromycin (60 µg)	S	S	S	S	R
Neomycin (1000 µg)	R	S	S	S	S
Kanamycin (1000 µg)	R	S	R	S	S
Colistin (10 µg)	R	S	S(R)	S	S
Rifampicin (15 µg)	S	S	S	S	R
Lincomycin* (2 µg)	R*	S	S	R	S

* Note that a disk of low potency is used to demonstrate these patterns for lincomycin; this is of use for laboratory identification, but it does not relate to clinical use.

closely. Failure to recover a Gram-negative bacillus that has been observed in significant numbers in a smear suggests that a *Bacteroides* organism or a demanding *Haemophilus* species may be involved.

Culture. Prompt submission of an adequate specimen and meticulous anaerobic procedure in cultivation are essential. Manipulation in an anaerobic cabinet is not obligatory; the important factors include the provision of freshly prepared or pre-reduced media, the prompt and careful seeding of these media and their incubation in a reliably anaerobic atmosphere with 10 per cent of carbon dioxide present.

Recommended media for primary cultures are: (1) freshly prepared horse blood agar with and without neomycin 70–100 µg per ml; (2) egg-yolk agar or neomycin egg-yolk agar; and (3) cooked-meat broth, pre-steamed for 30 min at 100°C and cooled promptly to 37°C before seeding. Incubate all media in an anaerobic jar using a standardized procedure or a Gaspak system (Becton Dickinson Ltd.). Vancomycin 7·5µg per ml may be added to neomycin blood agar for the isolation of Gram-negative anaerobes, and kanamycin 100 µg per ml may have some advantages over neomycin as a selective agent (Finegold *et al.*, 1971).

Antibiotic sensitivities. The patterns of susceptibility of commonly encountered members of the bacteroides-fusiformis group are indicated in Table 36.2. These may vary to some extent, but multiple resistance transfer has not yet been observed in this group.

REFERENCES

CATO, E. P., CUMMINS, C. S., HOLDEMAN, L. V., JOHNSON, J. L., MOORE, W. E. C., SMIBERT, R. M. & SMITH, L. D (1970) *Outline in Clinical Methods in Anaerobic Bacteriology.* Virginia Polytechnic Institute Anaerobe Laboratory (Publishers): Blacksburg, U.S.A.

FINEGOLD, S. M., SUGIHARA, P. T. & SUTTER, V. L. (1971) Use of selective media for isolation of anaerobes from humans. In *Isolation of Anaerobes,* The Society for Applied Bacteriology Technical Series No. 5, pp. 99–108, edited by D. A. Shapton and R. G. Board, Academic Press: London and New York.

HILL, L. R., SNELL, J. J. S. & LAPAGE, S. P. (1970) Identification and characterisation of *Bacteroides corrodens. Journal of Medical Microbiology,* **3,** 483.

JACKSON, F. L., GOODMAN, Y. E., BEL, F. R., WONG, P. C. & WHITEHOUSE, R. L. S. (1971) Taxonomic status of facultative and strictly anaerobic 'corroding bacilli' that have been classified as *Bacteroides corrodens. Journal of Medical Microbiology,* **4,** 171.

LANCET (1973) Editorial. HB-1 Bacteria become *Eikenella. Lancet,* **i,** 1227.

RUTTER, J. M. (1970) A study of the carbohydrate fermentation reactions of *Clostridium oedematiens (Cl. novyi). Journal of Medical Microbiology,* **3,** 283.

SUTTER, V. L. & FINEGOLD, S. M. (1971) Antibiotic disc susceptibility tests for rapid presumptive identification of Gram-negative anaerobic bacilli. *Applied Microbiology,* **21,** 13.

TRACY, O. (1969) Pigment production in bacteroides. *Journal of Medical Microbiology,* **2,** 309.

37. Clostridium I

THE GAS GANGRENE GROUP: FOOD POISONING

The genus *Clostridium* is comprised of anaerobic or microaerophilic large, straight or slightly curved Gram-positive spore-bearing rods, 3–8 μm × 0·6–1 μm with slightly rounded ends. Gram-variable and Gram-negative forms are often seen and pleomorphic forms are common. Most species of this genus are saprophytes that normally grow in soil, water and decomposing plant and animal matter, playing an important part in the process of putrefaction. Some, e.g. *Clostridium welchii* and *Cl. sporogenes*, are commensal inhabitants of the animal and human intestine, and just before or immediately after death of their host, rapidly invade the blood and tissues and play a major part, along with aerobic bacteria such as *Proteus*, in putrefying and decomposing the corpse. A few species are opportunistic pathogens and can produce disease; these include *Cl. welchii*, *Cl. septicum* and *Cl. oedematiens*, the causes of gas gangrene and other infections; *Cl. tetani*, the cause of tetanus; and *Cl. botulinum*, the cause of botulism. With only a few exceptions, the bacteria producing powerful exotoxins belong to this genus. *Cl. welchii* is otherwise known as *Cl perfringens*; and *Cl. oedematiens* as *Cl. novyi*. The commonly encountered species can be roughly grouped in descending order of their tolerance of oxygen as follows:

1. *Cl. histolyticum*, *Cl. tertium* and *Cl. carnis* are able to grow in the presence of trace amounts of air, and some strains may grow in air.
2. *Cl. welchii* type A, can grow in trace amounts of air if a young culture is seeded on to a good fresh medium. This is not recommended for routine practice and growth may be poor or absent.
3. *Cl. septicum* and organisms of the *Cl. bifermentans—Cl. sordellii* group are not regarded as particularly exacting anaerobes.
4. *Cl. sporogenes* is a strict anaerobe.
5. *Cl. oedematiens* type A and *Cl. tetani* are very strict anaerobes.
6. *Cl. oedematiens* type D is an exceedingly strict anaerobe.

The above grading may be challenged as the successful growth of any anaerobe is also dependent upon the provision of a suitable nutrient medium and may be markedly influenced by the gaseous atmosphere.

For the routine surface culture of anaerobes of medical importance, freshly poured blood agar incorporating a good base is recommended and carbon dioxide 10 per cent should be present in the anaerobic atmosphere (Watt, 1973). Details of anaerobic culture procedures are given in Chapter 6.

All clostridia produce spores but vary markedly in their readiness to do so. The shape of the spore and its position in the bacillus is of significance in classification. *Clostridium welchii* (*Cl. perfringens*) and the type species *Cl. butyricum* produce capsules. Almost all members of the genus are motile, but *Cl. welchii* is not. Some motile species do not show active motility under the relatively aerobic conditions of the usual wet-film preparations. These may be examined in tissue fluid preparations following animal inoculation. A semi-solid nutrient-agar medium for the demonstration of motility is recommended. Stab cultures in this medium, freshly prepared with 1 per cent glucose added to enhance anaerobiosis, should be examined frequently before excessive gas production invalidates the test. A non-motile species (e.g. *Cl. welchii*) may show lateral spikes of growth along 'faults' extending from the stab line, but the appearance is not likely to be confused with the diffuse growth of a truly motile species. The active motility of species such as *Cl. septicum* and *Cl. sporogenes* may be of advantage or of distinct disadvantage in the isolation of pure cultures on solid media. This is discussed on p. 480.

The *saccharolytic clostridia* grow rapidly and vigorously in carbohydrate media with the production of acid and abundant gas. Saccharolytic species ferment glucose and may, in addition, be usefully examined for fermentation of lactose, maltose, sucrose and salicin. In routine sugar fermentation tests a small iron nail may be included in each tube. The nail should not project above the level of the fluid medium. The indicator dyes in such tests become reduced and may be irreversibly decolourized so that it is advisable to add a little fresh indicator to the tests when recording the results or to check their final reaction by spot tests on a tile with bromothymol blue indicator. When grown in cooked-meat broth, saccharolytic clostridia rapidly produce acid and gas but do not digest the meat; the cultures may have a slightly sour smell and the meat is often reddened. Gas production is not necessarily indicative of sugar fermentation, as proteolysis may be accompanied by evolution of gas bubbles.

The *proteolytic clostridia* digest protein and liquefy gelatin and coagulated serum. Cultures in meat medium cause blackening of the meat, decomposing it and reducing it in volume with the formation of foul-smelling products.

Cl. welchii, Cl. septicum, Cl. tertium and *Cl. fallax* are predominantly saccharolytic; *Cl. sporogenes* and *Cl. histolyticum* are actively proteolytic, and *Cl. tetani* is slightly proteolytic.

Morphological and biochemical variations within strains of the same species, and within subcultures of the same strain, render identification of the clostridia difficult. Whenever possible, the identity of a toxigenic species should be confirmed by specific toxin neutralization tests, although it should be borne in mind that non-toxigenic strains of toxin-producing species occur.

Strains may be preserved by freeze-drying or by storage in various media. Cooked-meat broth containing chalk and minced cooked egg-white is a useful preservation medium. Germination of spores is sporadic, especially following heat-resistance tests, and this is considered to be partly due to fatty acids in the sub-culture medium. The inhibitory effect may be reduced by incorporating soluble starch or serum in the medium when subcultures are made from preservation media or from heat-resistance tests.

Table 37.1   The major lethal toxins and minor lethal or non-lethal factors produced by the various types of *Clostridium welchii* (after Brooks, Sterne and Warrack, 1957).

Type	Occurrence	Major lethal toxins				Minor lethal or non-lethal factors							
		α	β	ε	ι	γ	δ	η	θ	κ	λ	μ	ν
A	Gas gangrene Puerperal infection Septicaemia	+++	-	-	-	-	-	(+)	+-	+-	-	+-	+-
	Food-poisoning	+++	-	-	-	-	-	-	(+)	+-	-	+-	++
B	Lamb dysentery	+++	+++	++	-	++	(+)	-	++	-	+++	+++	++
C	'Struck' in sheep	+++	+++	-	-	++	+++	-	+++	+++	-	-	+-
	Enteritis in other animals	+++	+++	-	-	?	-	-	+++	+++	-	-	+-
	Enteritis necroticans in man	+++	++	-	-	++	-	-	-	-	-	-	+++
D	Enterotoxaemia of sheep and pulpy kidney disease	+++	-	+++	-	-	-	-	++	++	++	+-	+-
E	Doubtful pathogen of sheep and cattle	+++	-	-	+++	-	-	-	++	++	++	(+)	+-

+++ = produced by all strains.   ++ = produced by most strains.   +- = produced by some strains.
(+) = produced by very few strains.   +++ = large amounts.

CLOSTRIDIUM WELCHII
(*Cl. perfringens*)

Five types (A to E) are distinguished by the different combinations of major lethal toxins that they produce (Table 37.1). The classical *Cl. welchii* of *gas gangrene* belongs to type A.
Morphology and staining. A relatively large Gram-positive bacillus, about 4–6 μm by 1 μm, with stubby ends, occurring singly or in pairs, and often capsulate when seen in the tissues. In sugar media the bacilli are shorter, whereas in protein media they tend to become filamentous. They are non-motile. Spores are formed, but only in the absence of fermentable carbohydrates and abundantly only on special media such as Ellner medium. They are typically oval, subterminal and not bulging, but many bizarre forms are seen. Sporulation in Ellner medium is very variable, even when different cultures of the same strain of *Cl. welchii* are studied (Cash and Collee, 1962).
Cultural characters. Anaerobe, but may be grown under microaerophilic conditions. Optimum temperature range 37–45°C. Grows best on carbohydrate-containing media, e.g. glucose agar or glucose-blood agar.

Surface colonies are large, round, smooth, regular, convex and slightly opaque disks. Other types of colonies occur, including one having a raised opaque centre and a flat transparent border that is radially striated. Rough flat colonies with an irregular edge resembling a vine-leaf may also be seen. On horse-blood agar the colonies are usually surrounded by a variable zone of complete haemolysis; a wider zone of incomplete haemolysis may occasionally develop.

A variant occasionally produces very mucoid broth cultures and tenacious colonies on blood agar.
Biochemical reactions. *Cl. welchii* is actively saccharolytic and ferments, with gas production, glucose, lactose, sucrose, maltose, starch and, in the case of some strains, salicin, glycerol and inulin. Mannitol and dulcitol are not fermented.

In litmus milk medium, the organism produces acid and gas. The acid clots the milk and the gas breaks up the clot, resulting in the 'stormy clot' reaction that is produced by almost all strains of *Cl. welchii* but is not specific for this organism. The culture has a sour, butyric-acid odour.

Gelatin is liquefied. Coagulated serum is usually not liquefied. In cooked-meat medium the meat is reddened and no digestion occurs. Hydrogen sulphide is produced. The organism produces an active phospholipase-C (lecithinase), which causes a typical effect on egg-yolk media.
Viability. *Cl. welchii* spores generally resist routinely used antiseptics and disinfectants with the exception of formaldehyde and glutaraldehyde. The spores of classical type A strains of *Cl. welchii* do not survive boiling for more than a few minutes, whereas the spores of typical food-poisoning strains and certain type C strains are markedly heat-resistant.
Toxins. The five types of *Cl. welchii* can be differentiated on the basis of their production of the four major lethal toxins. Type A strains produce alpha toxin; type B strains typically produce alpha, beta and epsilon toxins; type C strains produce alpha and beta toxins; type D strains produce alpha and epsilon toxins; and type E strains produce alpha and iota toxins (Table 37.1).
Alpha toxin. Produced by all types of *Cl. welchii* but notably by type A strains, the alpha toxin is lethal for laboratory animals and necrotizing on intradermal inoculation. The toxin is a Ca^{2+} or Mg^{2+}—dependent phospholipase (lecithinase-C) and is formally defined as E.C. 3.1.4.3.: phosphatidylcholine choline phosphohydrolase. In the presence of free Ca or Mg ions it produces opalescence in serum or egg-yolk preparations by splitting lipoprotein complexes. The reaction can be inhibited by specific antitoxin.

The enzyme attacks phospholipid constituents of the red blood cells of various animals, and the alpha toxin is thereby haemolytic for the red cells of most species with the exception of the horse and the goat. The clear zones of haemolysis typically seen around colonies of classical type A strains of *Cl. welchii* grown on horse blood agar are produced by the theta toxin and not by the alpha toxin. With the red cells of the sheep in particular the alpha toxin provides an example of a 'hot-cold' lysin.

Alpha toxin activity may thus be assayed by several methods, including turbidity tests with egg-yolk emulsion (lecitho-vitellin, LV) or human serum as indicator, and sheep red cell lysis tests incorporating antisera to other haemolytic toxins that may be produced by *Cl. welchii*.

Nagler's reaction. Several clostridia produce phospholipase enzymes that give rise to opalescence in both human serum and egg-yolk media. The reaction produced by *Cl. welchii* is specifically neutralized by *Cl. welchii* alpha antitoxin (but the serologically related lecithinase of *Cl. bifermentans* is also inhibited).

For the rapid detection of *Cl. welchii* in direct plate culture, a plate of good quality digest agar containing 5 per cent of egg yolk is prepared and dried. On one half of the plate (which is appropriately marked) two or three drops of standard *Cl. welchii* antitoxin are spread and allowed to dry. The plate is then seeded with the test organism or with the exudate under investigation and then incubated anaerobically at 37°C. On the section containing no antitoxin, *Cl. welchii* colonies show a surrounding zone of opacity, i.e. the Nagler reaction, whereas colonies of the organism on the remainder of the plate show no change. The incorporation of neomycin sulphate inhibits aerobic sporing organisms and coliform organisms (Lowbury and Lilly, 1955). The complex medium of Willis and Hobbs (1959) also incorporates lactose and neutral red to indicate lactose-fermenting organisms and milk as an indicator of proteolysis. As results of culture on Willis and Hobbs' medium can be variable and are occasionally confusing, a simpler selective medium such as that of Lowbury and Lilly is preferred and a concentration of neomycin of 70 μg per ml is recommended for general use.

Beta toxin. Types B and C produce this lethal necrotizing toxin. Intradermal inoculation in the guinea-pig produces a purple-tinged necrotic area which is almost circular in the case of type C filtrates, but with type B filtrates is more extensive and irregular in shape due to the associated hyaluronidase produced by type B strains.

Epsilon toxin. This is produced by type B and D strains as a prototoxin. It is lethal and necrotizing and its activity is largely dependent upon the presence of an activating proteolytic enzyme and an alkaline environment. Filtrates may be trypsinized before assay.

Iota toxin is produced by type E strains. It is lethal and necrotizing and is formed as a prototoxin that is activated by proteolytic enzymes.

Theta toxin is lethal and cytolytic; it is an oxygen-labile haemolysin related to streptolysin-O and may be produced by all types of *Cl. welchii*, but not by typical food-poisoning strains or by strains associated with enteritis necroticans in man. It lyses the red cells of the horse, ox, sheep and rabbit, but is virtually inactive against mouse erythrocytes. Many animal sera inhibit theta toxin, and tissue lipids and cholesterol inactivate it. It is adsorbed on to meat particles so that strains assayed for theta production must be grown in medium free of meat particles. Culture supernatants (unfiltered, as the toxin is oxygen-sensitive) are then titrated for haemolytic activity against horse red cells in the presence of alpha antitoxin and under reducing conditions.

Gamma toxin is a minor lethal toxin.

Delta toxin is lethal. It is haemolytic for the red cells of sheep, goats, pigs and cattle.

Eta toxin is a minor lethal toxin.

Kappa toxin is a collagenase. It attacks native collagen, hide powder and gelatin.

Lambda toxin is a proteinase and gelatinase. It decomposes hide powder but not native collagen.

Mu toxin is a hyaluronidase.

Nu toxin is a deoxyribonuclease.

Cl. welchii also produces (1) enzymes that destroy blood-group substances, (2) a neuraminidase, (3) a diffusible or soluble haemagglutinin, and (4) an enterotoxin.

Toxin-antitoxin neutralization tests for the typing of Cl. welchii. Antitoxin to the types of *Cl. welchii* commonly encountered in disease will neutralize the major lethal antigens of these types as follows:

Type A antitoxin neutralizes only the homologous toxin.

Type B antitoxin neutralizes the toxins of types A, B, C and D.

Type C antitoxin neutralizes the toxins of types A and C.

Type D antitoxin neutralizes the toxins of types A and D.

The neutralization tests may be performed by intracutaneous or intravenous challenge of guinea-pigs or mice respectively, with mixtures of toxin and antitoxin. Epsilon and iota toxins do not occur in fully active form in cultures and these prototoxins require to be activated by trypsinization of samples of the culture filtrates prior to neutralization tests. A combination of *in vivo* and *in vitro* tests has been recommended for the routine typing of *Cl. welchii* (Oakley and Warrack, 1953).

Intracutaneous Serum Neutralization Tests in Guinea-pigs and Mice

The following procedure has been developed at the Wellcome Research Laboratories, Beckenham, England, and is recommended:

Aliquots (0·5 ml) of bacteria-free filtrate from a 5-h cooked-meat broth culture are made up to 0·8 ml quantities by adding nutrient broth and 0·1 ml volumes of specific antisera as indicated below (see Table 37.2). A similar set of mixtures is prepared after activation of any epsilon and iota prototoxins and destruction of any beta toxin present, by treatment of the crude filtrate with 0·005 per cent (w/v) crystalline trypsin for 1 h at 37°C. The filtrate-antitoxin mixtures are held at room temperature for 30 min, and 0·2 ml of each is then injected into the skin of a depilated albino guinea-pig. Reactions are read at 24 and 48 h. Death of the guinea-pig is occasionally due to excess epsilon toxin and this necessitates repetition with filtrate diluted (1 in 5 or 1 in 10) with broth. The alpha toxin produces a spreading yellowish necrotic lesion on intracutaneous injection. The beta toxin produces a purplish necrotic lesion. Epsilon toxin causes a whitish necrotic lesion with occasional patches of small purplish haemorrhages, and iota toxin produces a circular area of purplish white necrosis vaguely outlined with purple.

Table 37.2   Toxin-antitoxin mixtures employed in neutralization tests for the typing of *Clostridium welchii*[1]

Substance tested	Mixture number	Type-specific antiserum added (0·1 ml volumes)	Sterile broth added (ml)	Reactions with *Cl. welchii* type				
				A	B	C	D	E
Untreated filtrate	1	–	0·3	+	+	+	+	+
	2	A	0·2	–	+	+	–*	(±)
	3	A & C	0·1	–	–*	–	–*	(±)
	4	A, C & D	–	–	–	–	–	(±)
	5	–	0·3	(±)	+	–*	+	+
Trypsin-treated filtrate	6	A	0·2	–	+	–*	+	+
	7	A & D	0·1	–	–*	–*	–	+
	8	A, C & D	–	–	–	–	–	+
	(9†	A & E	0·1	–	+	–*	+	–)
		Toxins identified		alpha	beta and epsilon	beta	epsilon	iota

† Often omitted as iota toxin seldom encountered
– = no reaction (intracutaneous test); survival (intravenous test)
+ = necrotic lesion (intracutaneous test); death (intravenous test)
(±) = variable result
–* = nearly always negative either because epsilon is in inactive prototoxin form, or beta toxin is destroyed by trypsin
[1] Table amended and reproduced by courtesy of Wellcome Research Laboratories.

Two 0·3 ml volumes of each mixture prepared as for the intracutaneous tests are injected intravenously into pairs of mice which are subsequently observed for three days. The presence or absence of the major lethal antigens is indicated by death or survival of the appropriate mice.

Animal pathogenicity. Virulence for guinea-pigs can be demonstrated by subcutaneous or intramuscular injection of 0·5–1 ml of a 24-h culture in cooked-meat broth into the thigh. A control animal can be protected by an injection of 300–500 units of *Cl. welchii* antitoxin given 24 h before challenge. In the test animal, a spreading inflammatory oedema develops with gelatinous exudate and gas production in the tissue planes; the affected muscles become pink, sodden and necrotic and virtually liquefy at the site of the injection. The products of growth in a young culture increase the organism's aggressiveness. Washed organisms are practically non-pathogenic. An equal volume of a sterile 5 per cent solution of calcium chloride mixed with the inoculum just before injection increases the pathogenicity of a strain.

Occurrence. *Cl. welchii* occurs normally in numbers of about 10^4 per gram wet weight of faeces in the large intestine of healthy man and animals. It occurs in the air and soil and may gain access to wounds from the patient's skin (as a result of faecal soiling), or as a result of accidental or surgical release of intestinal contents. It may occur in uterine infections, e.g. in septic abortion, and occasionally a *Cl. welchii* bacteriaemia occurs.

Cl. welchii is therefore a common environmental contaminant and, because of its capacity for rapid growth in cooked-meat broth, it may be present in misleadingly large numbers on secondary plate cultures seeded from primary broth cultures. When it is truly involved in a clostridial myositis (gas gangrene), *Cl. welchii* is usually capsulate and can generally be recovered in large numbers on primary plates.

Table 37.3   The soluble antigens of the *Clostridium oedematiens* group (after Oakley and Warrack, 1959).

Designation	Biological activity	Biochemical activity	Presence in filtrates of *Cl. oedematiens* type			
			A	B	C	D
Alpha	necrotizing, lethal cytotoxin		++	+++	–	–
Beta	haemolytic, necrotizing, lethal	phospho-lipase	–	+	–	++
Gamma	haemolytic, necrotizing	phospho-lipase	+	–	–	–
Delta	oxygen-labile haemolysin		+	–	–	–
Epsilon	production of pearly layer in egg-yolk media	lipase	+	–	–	–
Zeta	haemolytic		–	+	–	–
Theta	production of opalescence in egg-yolk media	lipase*	–	tr	–	+

– = none
tr = trace present
+, ++, +++ = increasing amounts
* see Rutter and Collee (1969).

CLOSTRIDIUM OEDEMATIENS
(CLOSTRIDIUM NOVYI)

This Gram-positive bacillus is large and only moderately pleomorphic. It possesses peritrichous flagella but its motility is not active and is inhibited in the presence of oxygen. Its spores are oval and central or sub-terminal. Four types of *Cl. oedematiens* A, B, C, D, are differentiated on the basis of the toxins or 'soluble antigens' that they produce (Table 37.3, and see Rutter and Collee, 1969). Type A strains and occasionally type B strains may be associated with a severe form of gas-gangrene in man.

Type A strains are very strictly anaerobic. Type B and type C strains are even more exacting, and type D strains are among the most exacting of the strict anaerobes that can be cultured as a routine on solid media. All types may be grown satisfactorily in freshly made cooked-meat broth, but special solid media are required for reliable surface growth of types B, C and D. Types B, C and D are not typically associated with human disease. The following observations relate to type A strains which will grow on simple solid media if the atmosphere is strictly anaerobic. Surface colonies are raised, opaque, sometimes dome-shaped and circular in very young cultures but often flattened, large and irregular in older cultures. The colonies tend to fuse and form a spreading, sometimes swarming, growth. Tracks produced by motile daughter colonies may be seen. Discrete colonies show two zones of haemolysis on horse blood agar: there is a narrow inner zone of complete haemolysis and an outer zone of partial lysis. This pattern is not seen with a spreading growth. On blood agar, growth is more abundant and is also enhanced by 10 per cent CO_2.

On egg-yolk media, the organism's gamma toxin produces a zone of opacity due to its phospholipase (lecithinase) activity and this can be inhibited by specific antitoxin. In addition, the epsilon toxin (a lipase) produces a pearly layer effect that is more restricted and overlies the colonies.

Changes produced in litmus milk medium are slight and indefinite.

Culture of types B, C and D on solid media. The cysteine-dithiothreitol system of Moore (1968) incorporated in blood agar by Watt (1972) is recommended for the reliable culture of these difficult anaerobes (p. 124). A much less effective but useful and inexpensive alternative is to sprinkle sterile iron filings on a freshly poured blood agar plate just after inoculating the organisms; the plate must be promptly incubated anaerobically. Colonies develop initially around the iron filings (Collee, Rutter and Watt, 1971).

Biochemical reactions. Cl. oedematiens type A is saccharolytic and mildly proteolytic. It ferments glucose, maltose and dextrin with gas production and glycerol with or without gas production. Fermentation of mannose is variable, and various sugars including lactose, sucrose, fructose and salicin are not fermented (Table 37.4).

Gelatin is liquefied, but milk agar, coagulated serum and cooked meat are not digested.

Table 37.4 The carbohydrate fermentation reactions of the *Clostridium oedematiens* group (from Rutter, 1970).

Cl. oedematiens type	Fermentation test result* with						
	dextrin	glucose	glycerol	inositol	fructose	maltose	mannose
A	+	+	+ or ⊥	−	−	+	v
B	−	+	v	+	+ or ⊥	+	+
C	−	+	−	−	⊥	−	+
D	−	+	−	+	+ or ⊥	−	+

* + = positive, ⊥ = doubtful positive, − = negative result, v = variable result.
(All types produced *negative results* with: dulcitol, galactose, lactose, mannitol, salicin, sorbitol, sucrose and xylose.)

Hydrogen sulphide is produced: nitrates and nitrites are reduced. Type A strains do not produce indole or reduce sulphite (Rutter, 1970)

Serology. All types seem to share at least one common O antigen and this is of practical value in the application of a direct immuno-fluorescence procedure for the prompt identification of *Cl. oedematiens* (Chap. 1). The soluble antigens are listed in Table 37.3.

Animal pathogenicity. An intramuscular injection of 0·2–1 ml of an actively growing culture of *Cl. oedematiens* type A in cooked-meat broth into the thigh muscles of a guinea-pig may cause overwhelming gas gangrene with minimum gas production, but massive oedema. With some strains, there may be difficulty in initiating the infection and the procedure outlined at p. 476 should be followed.

CLOSTRIDIUM SEPTICUM

Morphology and staining. Moderately large Gram-positive bacillus with rounded ends, about 3–10 μm by 0·6–1 μm; pleomorphic. Short forms, swollen 'citron bodies' and long curved filaments occur. Degenerate Gram-negative forms are common. Actively motile with peritrichous flagella. Spores are readily formed and are oval, central or subterminal and distend the bacillus.

Cultural characters. Obligatory anaerobe but less strict than *Cl. tetani.* Optimum temperature 37°C. Grows on ordinary media, but glucose promotes growth. Grows well on blood agar to produce irregular transparent colonies, later becoming greyish and opaque with fairly coarse projecting radiations; often produces confluent spreading growth. Colonies on horse blood agar show a narrow zone of haemolysis.

Biochemical reactions. Ferments various sugars including glucose, lactose, maltose, salicin, but not mannitol and usually not sucrose. Slight acid production in litmus milk medium may cause slow clotting. Liquefies gelatin but not coagulated serum; no proteolytic effect on milk agar. The meat in cooked-meat broth is reddened but not digested. Hydrogen sulphide is produced but not indole. Nitrates are reduced to nitrites. Sulphites are reduced.

Cl. septicum does not produce a phospholipase (lecithinase) or a lipase; colonies on egg-yolk agar show no visible effect.

Antigenic characters. Six groups can be distinguished on the basis of two somatic antigens (1, 2) and five H-antigens (a–e). There is marked cross-relationship with *Cl. chauvoei,* which shares a common spore antigen with *Cl. septicum* (Moussa, 1959).

Accordingly, there are good reasons to consider *Cl. septicum* and *Cl. chauvoei* as different types within the same species. However, most *Cl. chauvoei* strains have a specific O antigen (3) and this is exploited in the use of a direct immunofluorescence procedure for the prompt identification of these two species by ultraviolet microscopy (see p. 492).

Soluble antigens. The alpha toxin of *Cl. septicum* is a lethal haemolytic necrotizing substance. The beta toxin is a deoxyribonuclease. The gamma toxin is a hyaluronidase, and the delta toxin an oxygen-labile haemolysin (see Table 37.5). A fibrinolysin is produced and the organism also produces a haemagglutinin and a neuraminidase.

Animal pathogenicity. Intramuscular injection of cultures into guinea-pigs produces gas gangrene. The organisms invade the blood and the animal dies within a day or two. Smears from the liver show long, filamentous forms and also citron bodies.

Table 37.5   The named toxins of *Clostridium septicum.*

Product	Biological activity
Alpha toxin	Lethal, haemolytic and dermonecrotic; an oxygen-stable haemolysin
Beta toxin	Deoxyribonuclease; a leucocidin
Gamma toxin	Hyaluronidase; a spreading factor
Delta toxin	Haemolytic and dermonecrotic; an oxygen-labile haemolysin

Laboratory Diagnosis

The microscopical appearances, cultural characteristics and the results of pathogenicity tests in guinea-pigs allow initial identification. Differentiation from *Cl. chauvoei* may present difficulties and is discussed below and on p. 492.

CLOSTRIDIUM CHAUVOEI
(CLOSTRIDIUM FESERI)

Morphology. Resembles closely *Cl. septicum*. Individual organisms tend to occur singly or in pairs, and not in long filaments. 'Citron bodies' may be seen in the tissues. The bacilli are motile, with numerous peritrichous flagella. Spores are usually central or subterminal in position, elliptical in shape, and are broader than the bacillus.

Cultural characters. Strict anaerobe; optimum temperature 37°C, but grows at room temperature. Grows poorly on ordinary medium and a blood or minced meat medium is preferable. Liver infusion aids growth.

Cl. chauvoei ferments glucose, lactose, sucrose, maltose, but not mannitol or inulin, and usually not salicin.

Antigenic characters. A somatic antigen is common to all strains.

Flagellar antigens distinguish two groups. Cross-reactions with *Cl. septicum* occur as there is a common spore antigen.

Culture-filtrates are lethal, necrotizing and haemolytic; they also contain a deoxyribonuclease, a hyaluronidase, and an oxygen-labile haemolysin. The organism is pathogenic for guinea-pigs and mice; death occurs 24–36 h after inoculation.

Laboratory Diagnosis

In the differentiation of *Cl. septicum* and *Cl. chauvoei*, stress has been laid on the morphological elements seen in infected guinea-pigs; *Cl. chauvoei* exhibits 'citron' and club-shaped forms, but no elongated filaments are observed on the peritoneal surface of the liver of inoculated animals, as in the case of *Cl. septicum*. *Cl. chauvoei* ferments sucrose but usually not salicin; *Cl. septicum* ferments salicin but usually not sucrose. The two organisms, how-ever, are closely related. Specific antisera have now been conjugated to different fluorescent dyes at the Wellcome Research Laboratories. Direct microscopic examination of tissue smears stained by these conjugates and illuminated by ultraviolet light allows prompt differentiation between *Cl. septicum* and *Cl. chauvoei* infections (Batty and Walker, 1963).

CLOSTRIDIUM BIFERMENTANS AND
CLOSTRIDIUM SORDELLII

Cl. bifermentans and *Cl. sordellii* are closely related species; the former is non-pathogenic whereas some strains of the latter are pathogenic.

Morphology. Short stubby Gram-positive bacilli with rounded ends, often occurring in chains and often showing large oval central spores that do not typically bulge but seem to make the whole organism look bigger. Chains of these sporing forms in Gram smears or in wet films under the phase-contrast microscope look like necklaces set with bright beads.

The organisms grow readily and are relatively non-exacting anaerobes. Growth on blood agar is abundant and may be spreading. Discrete colonies may be greyish-white convex roughly circular with irregularly crenated edges. More irregular colonies are common. Colonies on blood agar are often but not always haemolytic.

The name *bifermentans* refers to the ability to decompose both sugars and proteins, and the *sordellii* group shares this double activity with variations: *Cl. bifermentans* ferments glucose, maltose, mannose, sorbitol and salicin, whereas *Cl. sordellii* ferments glucose and maltose, but not the other sugars noted above. Neither ferments lactose or sucrose (cf. *Cl. welchii*). Both groups are strongly proteolytic; they liquefy gelatin and decompose milk protein, coagulated serum and cooked meat. *Cl. bifermentans* does not decompose urea, whereas *Cl. sordellii* produces an active urease. Both produce indole and hydrogen sulphide, and both groups produce a phospholipase (lecithinase) that is serologically related to the alpha toxin of *Cl. welchii* and is partially neutralized by *Cl. welchii* antitoxin on egg-yolk agar plates.

Pathogenic strains of *Cl. sordellii* produce a lethal necrotizing toxin and are occasionally associated with wound infections in man. Experimental inoculation of 0·5–1·0 ml of an actively growing cooked-meat broth culture of such a strain into the thigh of a guinea-pig produces a rapidly lethal oedematous myositis.

CLOSTRIDIUM HISTOLYTICUM

This organism is a long slender Gram-positive rod. It is not a strict anaerobe and can be cultured aerobically. It is proteolytic but non-saccharolytic. In meat medium, digestion occurs with the formation of white, crystalline masses consisting of tyrosine. When cultures are injected into animals, in-vivo digestion of the tissues results. This organism is pathogenic to experimental animals and produces a lethal necrotizing exotoxin, an active collagenase, a proteinase, an elastase, an oxygen-labile haemolysin, and various other biologically active products. It may be associated with gas gangrene in man.

CLOSTRIDIUM TERTIUM

This slender rod is also a non-exacting anaerobe and will grow suboptimally under aerobic conditions. It is weakly motile. The spores are terminal and, when fully developed, oval in shape. The organism is actively saccharolytic. In milk, acid is formed with gas production and slow clotting. Meat is reddened, but not digested. Neither gelatin nor coagulated serum is liquefied. Its pathogenicity is doubtful, but when present in wounds it may give rise to gas production. No exotoxin is produced.

CLOSTRIDIUM FALLAX

This organism resembles *Cl. welchii* in some respects, and has sometimes been mistaken for it (hence the name 'fallax': Latin deceitful). It is, however, more slender. The spores are usually subterminal. In milk, the organism produces clotting and gas formation, but these changes take place slowly (as compared with *Cl. welchii*). It is saccharolytic. It does not liquefy either gelatin or coagulated serum. A relatively weak exotoxin is formed, and when freshly isolated the organism is pathogenic on experimental inoculation in animals.

CLOSTRIDIUM SPOROGENES

This Gram-positive motile bacillus is very widely distributed and is generally regarded as a harmless saprophyte. It is usually longer and more slender than *Cl. welchii*. It forms oval central or subterminal spores which may be highly resistant so that the organism is frequently encountered in mixed cultures in the laboratory, even after preliminary heating of these cultures to select heat-resistant pathogens. Its spores may survive boiling for periods of 15 min up to 6 h.

Cultural characters. *Cl. sporogenes* grows well on simple media, provided that anaerobic conditions are maintained. It is a relatively strict anaerobe. Surface colonies may present a 'medusa-head' appearance (cf. *B. anthracis*) if the plate is dry. Young colonies may be small, circular, raised and slightly opaque; they soon produce outgrowths and the spreading margin of the colony becomes irregular with coarse feathery projections. On horse-blood agar the colonies may appear to be haemolytic, but this is not caused by a true haemolysin: they are usually irregular and transparent with some central greyish opacity where the colonies are raised. Shake colonies show as 'woolly' balls of growth. A stab culture develops, like that of *Cl. tetani*, with lateral spikes.

The organism decomposes protein, producing amino-acids, ammonia, hydrogen sulphide, etc. and cultures have an exceedingly putrid odour.

In milk media, the casein is precipitated and digested.

In meat medium, the meat is blackened and digested. Gelatin and coagulated serum are liquefied.

Acid and gas are produced from some sugars, including glucose and maltose. Lactose and sucrose are not fermented.

Occurrence. *Cl. sporogenes* is a ubiquitous saprophyte and also occurs in the intestine of man and animals. It is frequently isolated from wound exudates in association with accepted

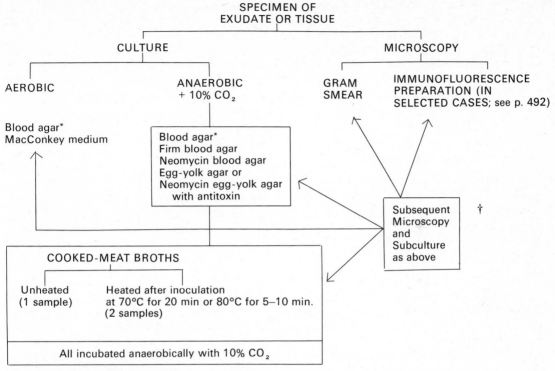

* Possibly with primary disk-sensitivity tests, etc.
† Special procedures such as spore stain, phase-contrast microscopy, motility tests, biochemical tests, etc. may be used for final identification.

FIG. 37.1. A guide to the initial steps that may be taken in the isolation and preliminary identification of anaerobic pathogens.

Table 37.6 Some differential characters of clostridia of medical interest.

Species	Saccharolytic activity	Fermentation of lactose	Gelatinase Activity (1–5 days)	Marked proteolytic activity (48 h)	Phospho-lipase (Nagler) effect	Lipase (pearly layer) effect	Production of indole
Cl. welchii type A	+++	+†	+	−	+	−	−
Cl. septicum	+++	+	+	−	−	−	−
Cl. oedematiens type A	++	−	+	−	+	+	−
Cl. tertium	+++	+	−	−	−	−	−
Cl. fallax	+++	+	−	−	−	−	−
Cl. bifermentans	++	−	+	+	+	−	+
Cl. sordellii	++	−	+	+	+	−	+
Cl. histolyticum	−	−	+	+	−	−	−
Cl. sporogenes	++	−	+	+	+	+	−
Cl. botulinum	++	−	{+‡ −	{+‡ −	+	+	−
Cl. tetani	−	−	+	−	−	−	+

− = no activity, ++ = active against a limited range,   +++ = active against a wide range of sugars (e.g. glucose, maltose, lactose, sucrose); † + in this and subsequent columns denotes a positive result;
‡ *Cl. botulinum* types A, B and F are proteolytic (See Chap. 38, p. 4)

pathogens. While its presence may accelerate anaerobic infection by enhancing local conditions, it is not regarded as a pathogen in its own right: it presumably participates in secondary proteolysis.

In pure culture it is virtually non-pathogenic to laboratory animals.

LABORATORY DIAGNOSIS OF GAS GANGRENE

The bacteriological diagnosis of gas gangrene is usually combined with a general bacteriological examination of the infected wound with which this condition is associated (see Fig. 37.1). It is convenient here to give special reference to the recognition of the clostridia (see Table 37.6, but see also references to *Bacteroides* infections, Chap 36).

Specimens of exudate should be taken from the wound, particularly from the deeper parts and from parts where the infection seems to be most pronounced. Sterile swabs rubbed over the wound surface and soaked in the exudate serve reasonably well for the purpose, but their prompt submission to the laboratory is imperative and desiccation in transit must be avoided.

Two swabs should be taken from the wound, one of which is used for film preparations, the other for culture. If there are sloughs or necrotic tissue or an adequate amount of exudate present in the wound, good samples of these should be placed in a sterile screw-capped bottle and used for microscopical examination and culture.

Microscopical examination. Films are made in the usual way and stained by Gram's method. If gas gangrene is present, Gram-positive bacilli may predominate. Thick, stubby, Gram-positive bacilli suggest the presence of *Cl. welchii, Cl. fallax* or *Cl. sordellii*; 'citron bodies', boat- or leaf-shaped pleomorphic bacilli with irregular staining may indicate *Cl. septicum*; slender bacilli with round terminal spores suggest *Cl. tetani* or *Cl. tetanomorphum*; *Cl. oedematiens* occurs as large bacilli with oval subterminal spores, but these may appear to be relatively scanty in the wound exudate, even in an active infection.

The immunofluorescence staining procedure of Batty and Walker (1963) is a most useful diagnostic aid.

Cultures. In addition to the media routinely used for the detection of aerobes, the following media should be seeded: (a) blood-agar plate to be incubated anaerobically; the surface should be well dried before inoculation to prevent colony spreading of certain anaerobes. If the agar content of a solid medium such as blood agar is increased to about 4·5 per cent, depending upon the brand of agar used and the other constituents of the medium, the spreading tendency of organisms is inhibited (see below). Although the firm agar does not prevent the growth of any species, colonies tend to be smaller and morphologically atypical. (b) Plate of Lowbury and Lilly's medium or a good nutrient agar containing egg-yolk (5 per cent, v/v) and neomycin sulphate (70–100 μg per ml). (c) Two tubes or bottles of cooked-meat medium; after inoculation, one is heated for 20 min at 70°C to kill non-sporing organisms. Alternative recommendations in this section include heating different bottles for 0–20 min at 100°C (Willis, 1972).

The anaerobic plates and tubes are incubated anaerobically with 10 per cent CO_2 and examined after 24 and 48 hours' incubation. These may yield growths of various facultative anaerobes as well as the strict anaerobes. Comparison of the aerobic and anaerobic plates affords some indication of the presence of strictly anaerobic organisms in the wound exudate, but any suspected anaerobe must later be tested in subculture to ensure that it is unable to grow under aerobic conditions. *Cl. tertium, Cl. histolyticum* and *Cl. carnis* can grow to some extent aerobically. The colony characters of suspected anaerobes on blood-agar are carefully studied with the naked eye and plate-culture microscope; films are made and stained by Gram's method. Each type of organism present must be isolated in pure culture for further examination, e.g. fermentation tests and animal inoculation. Tables 37.6 to 37.8 provide a guide to identification and list some differential characters. The lactose egg-yolk milk-agar medium developed by Willis and Hobbs is useful for the preliminary

Table 37.7 A guide to the provisional identification of clostridia of medical interest.

	Observed result with								
	Cl. welchii	1. *Cl. sordellii* 2. *Cl. bifermentans*	*Cl. oedematiens* type A	1. *Cl. sporogenes* 2. *Cl. botulinum* types A, B, F	*Cl. botulinum* types C, D, E	*Cl. histolyticum*	*Cl. tetani*	1. *Cl. septicum* 2. *Cl. tertium*	*Cl. chauvoei*
Primary tests:									
Nagler effect	+	+	+	+	+	−	−	−	−
Pearly layer effect	−	−	+	+	+	−	−	−	−
Lactose fermentation	+	−	−	−	−	−	−	+	+
Indole production	−	+	−	−	−	−	+	−	−
Gelatinase activity (1–5 days)	+	+	+	+	−	+	+	+	+
Marked proteolytic activity (48 h)	−	+	−	+	−	+	−	−	−
Confirmatory tests:									
Direct immunofluorescence microscopy	…	1. … 2. …	+	1. … 2. +	+	…	+	1. + 2. …	+
Specific neutralization of Nagler effect	+	1. ± 2. ±	+	−	−	…	…	…	…
Fermentation of sucrose	+	1. + 2. −	−	−	type E +	−	−	−	+
Production of urease	−	1. + 2. −	−	−	−	−	−	1. − 2. +	−
Microaerophilic or aerobic growth	±	−	−	−	−	+	−	−	−
Animal pathogenicity specific syndrome (antitoxic protection tests sometimes possible)	+	1. v 2. −	+	1. − 2. +	+	+	+	1. + 2. −	+

… = not done; − = negative result; + = positive result, ± = doubtful positive, v = variable.

Table 37.8 Some differential characters of clostridia.

	Morphology in culture*	Typical Colonies on blood-agar	Cooked meat medium	Milk medium	Liquefaction of coagulated serum	Fermentation of GLSMSa†	Pathogenicity to guinea-pigs and mice
Cl. tetani	Slender bacilli with round terminal spores; usually Gram-negative	Transparent, with long feathery spreading projections; usually haemolytic; often swarming	*Slight* digestion blackening and pungent odour	Unaltered	– (but may be softened)	– – – – –	+ (tetanus produced)
Cl. tetanomorphum	Resembles *Cl. tetani*; round terminal spores	Small and transparent, with irregular outline	Gas; no digestion; no putrefactive odour	Unaltered	– (but may be softened)	+ – – + –	–
Cl. welchii	Large, thick, stubby bacilli; spores usually absent	Large circular, with regular outline; haemolytic	Gas; no digestion, meat reddened	Acid, gas, rapid clotting; 'stormy-clot'	–	+ + + + – (+)	+
Cl. septicum	Pleomorphic, often short with central or subterminal spores‡	Transparent, irregular, with spreading projections; usually haemolytic; often swarming	Gas; no digestion, meat reddened	Acid, gas, slow clotting	–	+ + – + + (+) (–)	+
Cl. oedematiens type A	Large Gram-positive rods; some pleomorphism; central or sub-terminal spores (not numerous)	Translucent, convex round or irregular flat; tend to fuse and form spreading film, usually haemolytic	Gas; no digestion, meat reddened	Sometimes slow clotting	–	+ – – + –	+
Cl. histolyticum	Filamentous in old cultures or if grown aerobically; spores oval and subterminal	Irregular, round opaque, greyish-white colonies; haemolytic	Digestion of meat with evolution of H_2S; white crystals deposited late	Acid, gas; casein precipitated and digested	+	– – – – –	+

484

Table 37.8—continued

	Morphology in culture*	Typical Colonies on blood-agar	Cooked meat medium	Milk medium	Liquefaction of coagulated serum	Fermentation of GLSMSa†	Pathogenicity to guinea-pigs and mice
Cl. bifermentans¹	Usually numerous sporing forms, often in chains; spores large, oval, central	Round, crenated or irregular; greyish to white; usually haemolytic	Gas, digestion, blackening and putrefactive odour; whitish mucoid deposit	Acid, gas, digestion	+	+ − − + +	−
Cl. sordellii					+	+ − − + −	(±)
Cl. botulinum	Large, pleomorphic bacilli; oval spores, usually subterminal	Large irregular colonies with opaque raised centre; usually haemolytic	Gas, types vary in proteolytic activity (see text)	Casein precipitated and digested by some types; others produce no digestion	(±)	+ − − + −	+
Cl. sporogenes	Somewhat slender bacilli, central or subterminal spores	Usually irregular colonies with feathery projections; young colonies small, circular, opaque; pseudo-haemolytic	Gas, digestion, blackening and putrefactive odour	Acid, clot, digestion, later alkaline	+	+ − − + − (+)	−

* All these organisms are Gram-positive, but Gram-negative forms are seen in older cultures; they are all motile, with peritrichous flagella, except Cl. welchii.

† G = glucose, L = lactose, S = sucrose, M = maltose, Sa = salicin.

‡ Morphological forms seen in tissues are referred to in the text (vide supra).

+ Under fermentation signifies acid and gas production.

Single symbols in brackets signify occasional atypical reactions; double symbols in brackets signify variability in reaction among strains.

¹ For a discussion of the differentiation between Cl. bifermentans and Cl. sordellii and for full details of the biological and other characters of the various members of the clostridia, consult Clostridia of Wound Infection, A. T. Willis (1969), Butterworths, London.

485

examination of pure cultures of clostridia, but results tend to vary with different batches of this medium. It indicates lactose-fermenting colonies; phospholipase-active colonies produce a marked zone of opalescence extending beyond the colony (Nagler effect); and zones of clearing develop around proteolytic colonies. Opalescence restricted to the medium underlying a colony and associated with an overlying iridescent 'pearly-layer' indicates lipase activity.

In the cooked-meat medium both aerobes and anaerobes flourish; this growth is useful for later subculture should the plate cultures fail to yield successful isolation of organisms present in the wound. Film preparations also yield further information on the morphological types of vegetative organisms, and sporing forms that may have developed can be seen.

Additional methods. Reducing agents such as ascorbic acid (0·1 per cent), or sodium thioglycollate (0·1 per cent) or reduced iron or iron strips may be incorporated in fluid media to make them more suitable for the growth of anaerobes.

Control of Spreading Growth on Anaerobic Plates

Control of the swarming growth of unwanted organisms in plate cultures presents various problems. Pre-treatment of the proposed inoculum by differential heating may be effective, but it carries the risk of killing vegetative cells of likely non-sporing and sporing pathogens. Moreover, the spores of some pathogens are not markedly heat resistant and may be inactivated, or their prompt germination may be inhibited. The use of firm agar containing 3–4 per cent agar is recommended as a general control method, but colonial morphology is altered. Alternatively, some workers pay particular attention to drying the surface of agar plates to inhibit swarming; but the availability of nutrients for the initiation of colonial growth on a relatively dry surface may be critically impaired. An 'alcohol' plate is sometimes used; here the surface of the unseeded medium is flooded with ethanol, the excess is removed and the plate is exposed in an incubator to dry it at 37°C. The medium is then seeded in the usual manner. If the pathogen to be isolated can grow on MacConkey agar, it should be noted that *Proteus* and *Pseudomonas* species do not spread on this medium. It is sometimes possible to exclude these spreading species by exposing the seeded plate to chloroform vapour for some minutes prior to anaerobic incubation.

Specific serological control of the swarming growth of *Cl. tetani* and *Cl. septicum* was achieved by Williams and Willis (1970) and Willis and Williams (1972). When commercial tetanus antitoxin 40–60 units per ml is incorporated into the agar medium, motile strains of *Cl. tetani* grow as discrete colonies. Similarly, *Cl. septicum* did not spread on plates on which 0·2–0·5 ml of a *Cl. septicum* O antiserum prepared against the two serological groups of Moussa (1959) was spread.

CL. WELCHII FOOD-POISONING

Strains of *Cl. welchii* type A that produce non-haemolytic or feebly haemolytic colonies on horse-blood agar and having markedly heat-resistant spores, are typically associated with a mild form of food-poisoning (Vol. I, Chapter 36); however, classical type A strains producing relatively heat-sensitive spores and strains that produce spores of intermediate heat-resistance may also produce food-poisoning.

The bacteriological diagnosis of *Cl. welchii* food-poisoning usually involves the isolation of typical food-poisoning strains from faeces of patients and those at risk and from the suspected food. (1) Isolation of these strains from faeces is facilitated by their being present in spore form. A portion of faeces is carefully emulsified by coating a swab with the faecal specimen and stirring this into a tube of cooked-meat broth. The inoculated tube is then held in a steamer at 100°C for an hour, cooled and incubated overnight at 37°C. If heat-resistant *Cl. welchii* is present, a virtually pure culture will frequently be obtained by this simple procedure and pure subcultures can readily be obtained on solid media. When a pure culture of *Cl. welchii* is obtained in this way, the result is of no quantitative significance; only direct plating procedures on selective media are of value in this respect. Large particles of faeces should not be inoculated into the tube since many organisms are protected from the heat and survive to produce a very mixed culture including non-sporing organisms. (2) Isolation of typical food-poisoning strains from *food* by selective heating is rarely successful because spores of *Cl. welchii* are not normally abundant in food. The vegetative organisms are recovered by selective culture methods. Weighed samples of the suspected food should ideally be macerated and suspended in broth. Measured volumes are then pipetted on to selective media such as Lowbury and Lilly's medium, or an egg-yolk agar medium containing 70 μg of neomycin sulphate per ml, or horse-blood agar containing this concentration of neomycin. Suspected colonies are counted and further identified. Typical strains show lack of true haemolytic activity on horse-blood agar; although they produce alpha toxin which may cause zones of doubtful haemolysis, they do not produce theta toxin which is the cause of the complete β-haemolysis typical of the colonies of classical strains grown on horse-blood agar. In order to demonstrate the heat-resistance of food-poisoning strains, it is necessary to produce sporing cultures, e.g. in Ellner medium; adequate numbers of spores are produced by most strains after culture for 2–4 days in cooked-meat broth, but commercially available cooked-meat broth is usually unsuitable for this purpose. Samples of sporing culture deposits are held in cooked-meat broth at 100°C for an hour, cooled and then incubated. As some strains do not produce spores readily, this may be a laborious task. Final identification of the serological type of a typical food-poisoning strain is done by slide agglutination tests of colonies taken from blood-agar cultures and tested against a range of agglutinating antisera prepared against different food-poisoning strains (Hobbs' types).* Typical food-poisoning strains with markedly heat-resistant spores can be assigned to 24 types (1–24), and other strains that resemble classical type A organisms can be assigned to 18 types (i–xviii). Untypable strains occur quite fre-

quently.

The finding of large numbers of classical strains of β-haemolytic *Cl. welchii* in a sample of suspected food may be significant (see Vol. I, Chap. 36). For a detailed account of the isolation and enumeration of *Cl. welchii* from food and faeces, the account of Sutton, Ghosh and Hobbs (1971) should be consulted.

A sub-group of *Cl. welchii*, type C, is associated with *enteritis necroticans* in man; the strains produce markedly heat-resistant spores.

REFERENCES

BATTY, I. & WALKER, P. D. (1963) Differentiation of *Clostridium septicum* and *Clostridium chauvoei* by the use of fluorescent labelled antibodies. *Journal of Pathology and Bacteriology*, **85**, 517.

BROOKS, M. E., STERNE, M. & WARRACK, G. H. (1957) A re-assessment of the criteria used for type differentiation of *Cl. perfringens*. *Journal of Pathology and Bacteriology*, **74**, 185.

CASH, J. D. & COLLEE, J. G. (1962) Sporulation and the development of resistance in sporing cultures of *Clostridium welchii*. *Journal of Applied Bacteriology*, **25**, 225.

COLLEE, J. G., RUTTER, J. M. & WATT, B. (1971) The significantly viable particle: a study of the subculture of an exacting sporing anaerobe. *Journal of Medical Microbiology*, **4**, 271.

LOWBURY, E. J. L. & LILLY, H. A. (1955) A selective plate medium for *Cl. welchii*. *Journal of Pathology and Bacteriology*, **70**, 105.

MOORE, W. B. (1958) Solidified media suitable for the cultivation of *Clostridium novyi* type B. *Journal of General Microbiology*, **53**, 415.

MOUSSA, R. S. (1959) Antigenic formulae for *Clostridium septicum* and *Clostridium chauvoei*. *Journal of Pathology and Bacteriology*, **77**, 341.

OAKLEY, C. L. & WARRACK, G. H. (1953) Routine typing of *Cl. welchii*. *Journal of Hygiene (London)*, **51**, 102.

OAKLEY, C. L. & WARRACK, G. H. (1959) The soluble antigens of *Clostridium oedematiens* type D (*Cl. haemolyticum*). *Journal of Pathology and Bacteriology*, **78**, 543.

RUTTER, J. M. (1970) A study of the carbohydrate fermentation reactions of *Clostridium oedematiens* (*Cl. novyi*). *Journal of Medical Microbiology*, **3**, 283.

RUTTER, J. M. & COLLEE, J. G. (1969) Studies on the soluble antigens of *Clostridium oedematiens* (*Cl. novyi*). *Journal of Medical Microbiology*, **2**, 395.

SUTTON, R. G. A., GHOSH, A. C. & HOBBS, B. C. (1971) Isolation and enumeration of *Clostridium welchii* from food and faeces. In *Isolation of Anaerobes*, pp. 39–47. edited by D. A. Shapton and R. G. Board, The Society

* Dr Betty C. Hobbs, Director, Food Hygiene Laboratory, Central Public Health Laboratory, Colindale Avenue, London.

for Applied Bacteriology Technical Series 5, London and New York: Academic Press.

WATT, B. (1972) The recovery of clinically important anaerobes on solid media. *Journal of Medical Microbiology*, **5,** 211.

WATT, B. (1973) The influence of carbon dioxide on the growth of obligate and facultative anaerobes on solid media. *Journal of Medical Microbiology*, **6,** 307.

WILLIAMS, KATHLEEN & WILLIS, A. T. (1970) A method of performing surface viable counts with *Clostridium tetani*. *Journal of Medical Microbiology*, **3,** 639.

WILLIS, A. T. (1969) *Clostridia of Wound Infection*, London: Butterworths.

WILLIS, A. T. (1972) *Anaerobic Infections*. Public Health Laboratory Service Monograph Series No. 3. London: Her Majesty's Stationery Office.

WILLIS, A. T. & HOBBS, G. (1959) Some new media for the isolation and identification of clostridia. *Journal of Pathology and Bacteriology*, **77,** 511.

WILLIS, A. T. & WILLIAMS, KATHLEEN (1972) Prevention of swarming of *Clostridium septicum*. *Journal of Medical Microbiology*, **5,** 493.

38. Clostridium II

THE ORGANISMS OF TETANUS AND BOTULISM

CLOSTRIDIUM TETANI

Tetanus occurs in man and animals when a wound is infected with *Clostridium tetani* under conditions that allow the organism to multiply and produce a powerful exotoxin. Absorption of the toxin to the central nervous system leads to hyperexcitability of voluntary musculature and the disease is characterized by increased muscle tonus and exaggerated muscular responses to trivial stimuli. Trismus occurs when the muscles of the jaw are affected and, as this is quite frequently an early sign of tetanus in man, the disease is sometimes called lockjaw.

Morphology. A slender rod 2–5 μm by 0·4–0·5 μm with rounded ends; pleomorphic; filamentous forms occur; motile, with numerous long peritrichous flagella, but movement is usually sluggish. The spores, early in development, may produce an oval and subterminal enlargement. The fully developed spore is characteristically terminal and spherical, two to four times the diameter of the bacillus (drumstick). Strains vary in their tendency to produce spores. If sporing forms are scanty in normal culture media, the strain may be encouraged to produce spores by stab subculture in a tube of horse-flesh agar with 1 per cent glucose, incubated for two to three days.

Staining. Gram-positive, but Gram-negative forms usually seen, especially in broth cultures. Only the periphery of the mature spore is stained by the Gram counterstain.

Cultural characters. A strict anaerobe; temperature range 14°–43°C; optimum, 37°C; grows on ordinary nutrient media but is more readily grown in cooked-meat medium or in Fildes' peptic blood broth or on fresh blood agar.

Colonies on solid media show fine branching projections. After 48–72 hours' incubation the central part of the colony, which rarely grows more than 1 mm in diameter, becomes slightly raised and has a ground-glass appearance with a delicately filamentous periphery. A fine spreading growth may extend over the entire surface of the medium and the spreading film of growth may not be apparent on cursory examination. On blood agar, haemolysis is evident in the region of initial confluent growth and may develop below individual colonies, but frequently does not appear below the spreading growth in young cultures.

Non-motile variants may produce quite isolated colonies lacking the characteristic feathery processes.

Agar stab culture. No growth occurs on the surface; a white line of growth appears along the track of the inoculating wire but stops short of the surface; lateral spikes, which are longest in the deeper part of the tube, develop from the central growth.

Biochemical reactions. Nutrient gelatin is slowly liquefied. Coagulated serum is slowly rendered more transparent and softened but not liquefied. Litmus milk medium may show no coagulation or there may be delayed clotting. Cooked-meat medium shows slight digestion and blackening of the meat. Some gas is evolved due to breakdown of amino-acids, but no carbohydrates are fermented by typical strains of *Cl. tetani*. Cultures have an unpleasant slightly pungent odour.

Viability. The resistance of spores of *Cl. tetani* varies. Some are killed by exposure to boiling water for 5–15 min, but rarer, more resistant, strains require boiling for up to three hours before being killed. They may resist dry heat at 150°C for one hour, 5 per cent phenol or 0·1 per cent mercuric chloride for up to two weeks or more, but they are inactivated by exposure to iodine 1 per cent in watery solution or hydrogen peroxide (10 volumes) within a few hours.

Antigenic characters. Ten types are distinguishable by agglutination tests involving flagellar H antigens. Type 6 consists of non-flagellate strains. All types produce the same neurotoxin, and toxigenic and non-toxigenic strains may belong to the same type.

Toxin. The neurotoxin *tetanospasmin* develops in cooked-meat broth cultures after 5–14 days' growth at 35°C, the optimum time varying with the strain.

Tetanolysin, another product, is an oxygen-labile haemolysin.

When tetanus toxin is injected into guinea-pigs or mice, the animals die within a day or two with the typical signs of tetanus. In animals, tetanus spasms may start in the muscles related to the site of injection ('local tetanus').

Laboratory Diagnosis

Films made from the wound exudate and stained by Gram's method may show 'drum-stick' bacilli; this is suggestive evidence of the presence of *Cl. tetani*, but it is not conclusive as other organisms with terminal spores morphologically indistinguishable from *Cl. tetani* may be present. Moreover, it is often impossible to detect the tetanus bacilli in wounds by microscopic examination.

Direct plating on blood agar incubated anaerobically may reveal *Cl. tetani*, provided that spreading or abundant growth of other organisms does not mask it. The production of tetanus in mice by subcutaneous injection of an anaerobic fluid culture prepared from wound material may also be attempted, but this technique is limited by the fact that some strains of *Cl. tetani* from cases of human tetanus do not seem to produce the disease in mice. The injection, e.g. 0·2 ml of a five- to ten-day cooked-meat broth culture, is made into the tissues to the right of the base of the animal's tail. Within a day or so in a positive test there may be stiffness of the tail and the hind limbs. The right hind leg is subsequently paralysed and the tail and spine of the animal tend to curve to the right. Thereafter, more generalized muscular involvement becomes increasingly evident, and tetanic convulsions may be elicited by trivial stimuli. Control animals are each protected with a dose of tetanus antitoxin, e.g. 500 units, injected sub-cutaneously or intraperitoneally one hour prior to inoculation of the culture.

Although significant results may thus some-times be obtained with impure or mixed cultures from the wound, it is desirable that the tetanus bacillus, if possible, should be obtained in pure culture so that it can be identified by its biological characters and its specific toxicity. In Fildes' method, which exploits the tendency of *Cl. tetani* colonies to spread and extend beyond the growth of other bacteria, the material is incubated anaerobic-ally in 5 per cent peptic-blood broth for two to four days at 37°C. The culture is then heated at 65°C for 30 min to kill spreading non-sporing organisms such as *Proteus*. The condensation water of a peptic-blood agar slope is seeded from the heated culture, and the tube is incubated anaerobically. After 24–48 hours, the edge of the culture is examined with a hand lens and a growth of tetanus bacilli may be seen as a mass of very fine filaments. Sub-cultures from the marginal growth frequently yield pure cultures of *Cl. tetani*. (It is advan-tageous to keep the blood-agar tubes prior to inoculation until the surface of the medium is dry at the top.)

This method of isolation will not be success-ful if a non-motile type 6 strain is involved, and it is advisable to employ additional methods. It is also recommended, when possible, to vary the degree of preliminary heating of portions of the specimen under investigation. Thus, tissue from the wound may be ground up with sand under sterile conditions. After direct plating on blood agar for anaerobic incubation, one-quarter of this material may be extracted and used for direct animal inoculation. The remaining three-quarters is dispensed into six universal con-tainers of freshly prepared, cooked-meat medium. Two of these are heated at 80°C for 10 min, two at 70°C for 30 min and two are not heated. After several days' incubation at 37°C, subcultures from these may be made to blood agar plates, into shake cultures and into the condensation water of Fildes' peptic-blood-agar slopes as already described.

An antitoxin-controlled plate haemolysin test for the presumptive identification of *Cl. tetani* involves the use of fresh blood agar plates half-smeared with tetanus antitoxin (Lowbury and Lilly, 1958). *Cl. tetani* produces haemolysis which is inhibited by the antiserum. Although there are several objections to this technique (see Willis, 1964), the method is convenient for the provisional screening of large numbers of strains. Confirmation by mouse inoculation is recommended.

Cl. tetani may be stained specifically by the direct immunofluorescence procedure of Batty and Walker (1965) (see p. 492).

Antibiotic sensitivity. Cl. tetani is usually sensitive to penicillin and the tetracyclines.

CLOSTRIDIUM BOTULINUM

Botulism is a fatal form of food poisoning characterized by pronounced toxic effects, mainly on the parasympathetic system, that include oculomotor and pharyngeal paralyses and aphonia. It is not a common disease in this country, only four incidents having been recorded since the Loch Maree tragedy in 1922 when eight victims died after eating duck paste infected with *Cl. botulinum*. Six main types of *Cl. botulinum*, A, B, C, D, E and F are differentiated on the basis of their antigenically distinct toxins. Types A, B and E are most frequently associated with botulism in the human subject, but types C, D and F have also caused disease in man.

Morphology and staining. A sporing bacillus with rounded ends, about 4–6 μm by 0·9–1·2 μm occurring singly and in pairs. Spores are oval, sub-terminal and slightly distend the bacillus. The bacilli are motile with peritrichous flagella, and stain Gram-positively unless degenerate. The spore of toxigenic strains of *Cl. botulinum* type E bears very many (*c.* 200) tubular appendages protruding from the spore surface and enclosed by a delicate exosporium (Hodgkiss and Ordal, 1966).

Cultural characters. Strict anaerobe. Grows on ordinary media. The optimum temperature for type A strains is around 33°C. Strains of type A or type B will not grow or produce toxin at temperatures below about 10°C, whereas type E strains can grow (slowly) and produce toxin at low temperatures, e.g. 1–5°C. The lower limit of pH for growth is approximately pH 5·0–5·5, and for toxin production around pH 4·6, but many factors merit consideration (Riemann, 1969, p. 310).

Surface colonies are smooth, large, irregular, greyish, semi-transparent with a central 'nucleus' and a reticular or fimbriate border; incompletely haemolytic on horse blood agar. Rough colony forms occur. The semi-transparent colonies of toxigenic type E strains were said to revert to opaque-sporing (OS) non-toxigenic colonial mutants, but this hypothesis has been challenged (Hobbs, Roberts and Walker, 1965; Hodgkiss and Ordal, 1966).

Biochemical reactions. All types ferment glucose, fructose and maltose. Types A, B and F are proteolytic; they liquefy gelatin and coagulate serum and digest meat in cooked-meat broth, blackening it and producing a foul smell. They produce hydrogen sulphide. Types C, D and E are essentially non-proteolytic or very weakly so (Dolman, 1957); their effect on gelatin is generally recorded as negative, they do not decompose meat and they do not produce hydrogen sulphide. All types are indole-negative and catalase-negative. They all produce a phospholipase (lecithinase) and a lipase; colonies on egg-yolk agar produce zones of opacity and a pearly-layer effect. Colonies of the proteolytic types A, B and F may also show a clearing effect on egg-yolk media and this is more readily seen on simple milk agar or on the lactose egg-yolk milk agar medium of Willis and Hobbs.

Viability. Spores of some strains of *Cl. botulinum* withstand moist heat at 100°C for several hours, but are usually destroyed by moist heat at 120°C within 5 min. Spores of type E strains are generally not markedly heat-resistant; they may be inactivated by exposure to 80°C (wet heat) for 30 min.

Spores of *Cl. botulinum* also resist gamma radiation (see Grecz, 1965; Roberts and Ingram, 1965).

Antigenic characters. The different types produce immunologically different toxins that are completely neutralizable only by the appropriate antitoxin. Type C toxin has two components: C_α antitoxin neutralizes C_α and C_β toxins, whereas C_β antitoxin does not completely neutralize C_α toxin.

Differentiation between strains of types A or B and type E. Type E strains are typically associated with a marine source, but type A or B strains may also occur in a marine environment. Type E spores are often heat-sensitive; they are usually destroyed within 5 min by boiling at 100°C and do not generally resist 80°C wet heat for 30–40 min. Type E strains ferment mannose and sucrose whereas type A strains do not, and type E strains are essentially non-proteolytic.

Cl. botulinum may be stained specifically by the direct immunofluorescence procedure developed by Batty and Walker (q.v.). Commercially available labelled antisera (Wellcome) differentiate three groups:

1. the proteolytic types A, B, F;
2. the non-proteolytic types C, D; and
3. the non-proteolytic type E.

Animal pathogenicity. Laboratory animals are susceptible to experimental inoculation and feeding with cultures. Mice show paresis of the hindquarters and difficulty in breathing. The guinea-pig similarly shows difficulty in breathing, flaccid paralysis of the abdominal muscles and salivation after intraperitoneal injection; marked congestion of the internal organs, extensive thromboses and haemorrhages may be noted at necropsy.

Laboratory Diagnosis

It is occasionally possible to demonstrate the presence of toxin in the patient's blood or in post-mortem material such as blood or liver by direct inoculation into animals.

Gram-stained films of the food may first be examined for sporing bacilli. The food is then macerated in sterile salt solution and an extract cleared by centrifugation. This may be sterilized or further clarified by filtration prior to inoculation into animals. Activation of type E toxin by overnight incubation with 1 per cent trypsin is worth while. A 0·5 ml dose of the extract is injected intraperitoneally (1) into unprotected mice, and (2) into groups of mice protected with the individual commercially available type-specific antitoxins (0·5 ml). Alternatively, mixtures of 0·5 ml of extract or culture material and 0·1 ml of type-specific antitoxin may be injected subcutaneously in mice. The instructions of the supplier of the antitoxin should be followed

as the volume of antitoxin to be used depends upon its potency. If a specific botulinum toxin is involved, this may be indicated by the second group of tests; injections of test material heated for 10 min at 100°C and given without antitoxin to unprotected mice should not cause death.

Cl. botulinum may be isolated in pure culture from the food by preliminary heating of various samples at 65°–80°C for 30 min to eliminate non-sporing bacteria. Unheated samples should be processed, as spores of type E strains may be readily inactivated by heat. Cultures may then be made at 32°C (Silliker and Greenberg, 1969) under anaerobic conditions on solid media, including a selective medium such as Willis and Hobbs' medium, and in cooked-meat broth. Subsequent identification of *Cl. botulinum* involves demonstration of its biological characters and its toxigenicity. Culture filtrates may be prepared from five- to ten-day cooked-meat broth cultures and tested for toxicity by inoculation into animals as described above. The fluorescent labelled antibody procedure is a valuable diagnostic aid.

The identification of clostridia by direct staining with fluorochrome labelled antibody (see Batty and Walker, 1965). This procedure is of use for the identification of *Clostridium septicum*, *Cl. chauvoei*, *Cl. oedematiens*, *Cl. botulinum* types A, B, F, C, D and E, and *Cl. tetani*. Conjugated globulins are commercially available from Wellcome Reagents Ltd., Beckenham, England BR3 3BS.

Procedure. An air-dried smear is fixed by immersion of the slide in reagent grade anhydrous acetone for 10 min. A drop of the conjugated globulin is spread on the smear and left at room temperature for 30 min in a humid atmosphere provided by a wet filter paper in a plastic box.

The excess conjugate is quickly rinsed off the smear with phosphate-buffered saline at pH 7·6 (NaCl 8·5 g, Na_2HPO_4 1·28 g, $NaH_2PO_4.2H_2O$ 0·156 g, in 1 litre of distilled water); the smear is held in several changes of this buffer during the following 10–15 min. It is then gently blotted dry and mounted with buffered glycerol at pH 8–9 ($NaHCO_3$ 0·0715 g, Na_2CO_3 0·016 g, water to 10 ml, glycerol to 100 ml) and a glass (not plastic) coverslip.

The prepared smear should be examined with a suitable fluorescence microscope fitted with appropriate filters.

REFERENCES AND FURTHER READING

BATTY, I. & WALKER, P. D. (1965) Colonial morphology and fluorescent labelled antibody staining in the identification of species of the genus *Clostridium*. *Journal of Applied Bacteriology*, **28,** 112.

DOLMAN, C. E. (1957) Recent observations on type E botulism. *Canadian Journal of Public Health*, **48,** 187.

GRECZ, N. (1965) Biophysical aspects of clostridia. *Journal of Applied Bacteriology*, **28,** 17.

HOBBS, G., ROBERTS, T. A. & WALKER, P. D. (1965) Some observations on OS variants of *Clostridium botulinum* type E. *Journal of Applied Bacteriology*, **28,** 147.

HODGKISS, W. & ORDAL, Z. J. (1966) The morphology of the spore of some strains of *Clostridium botulinum* type E. *Journal of Bacteriology*, **91,** 2031.

LOWBURY, E. J. L. & LILLY, H. A. (1958) Contamination of operating-theatre air with *Clostridium tetani*. *British Medical Journal*, **ii,** 1334.

RIEMANN, H. (1969) Botulism—types A, B and F. In *Food-borne Infections and Intoxications*, p. 310. Edited by H. Riemann, New York and London: Academic Press.

ROBERTS, T. A. & INGRAM, M. (1965) The resistance of spores of *Clostridium botulinum* type E to heat and radiation. *Journal of Applied Bacteriology*, **28,** 125.

SILLIKER, J. H. & GREENBERG, R. A. (1969) Laboratory methods. In *Food-borne Infections and Intoxications*, pp. 455–487. Edited by H. Riemann, New York and London: Academic Press.

WILLIS, A. T. (1964) *Anaerobic Bacteriology in Clinical Medicine*, Vol. 2, p. 69. London: Butterworths.

39. Treponema: Syphilis Serology: Borrelia

TREPONEMA PALLIDUM

Syphilis is an infectious venereal disease caused by *Trep. pallidum*. Clinically the disease includes a sore on the genitalia which is followed by generalization of the infection with protean clinical manifestations.

Morphology. An exceedingly delicate, spiral filament 6–14 μm (average 10 μm) by 0·2 μm, with six to twelve coils which are comparatively small, sharp and regular. The length of the coils is about 1 μm and the depth 1–1·5 μm. The ends are pointed and tapering. The organism is feebly refractile, and in the unstained condition requires dark-ground illumination for its demonstration.

In electron micrographs *Trep. pallidum* is seen to be covered by an outer periplast which covers the whole organism. When this periplast is removed by digestion with pepsin or trypsin four fine filaments about 10 nm in diameter are seen twisted around the organism and conforming to its coils (Swain, 1955) (Fig. 39.1).

In addition to the typical form, as described, some variation in morphology may be observed: the number of coils to the unit of length may be more or less than normal, the filament may be thicker than normal in whole or part and the coils may be shallower and less regular than usual.

The spirochaete shows rotary corkscrew-like motility and also movements of flexion. The coils remain relatively rigid, but there may be some expansion and contraction. Angulation, with the organism bending almost to 90° towards its centre is highly characteristic. Its progression is relatively slow as compared with many of the motile bacteria.

The organism divides by transverse binary fission. There is good evidence for the existence of a more complicated life cycle of reproduction in the case of cultivated non-pathogenic strains of treponemes such as the Reiter spirochaete, in which a granular, filterable phase has been described. Division into four and even more fragments has also been described. Some observers have claimed that granules or bud-like structures may be split off, remaining attached by pedicles or stalks before final separation. This budded form has also been regarded as a phase in the life history of the organism, and various supposed developmental bodies differing morphologically from the normal spirochaete have been described as originating from such structures.

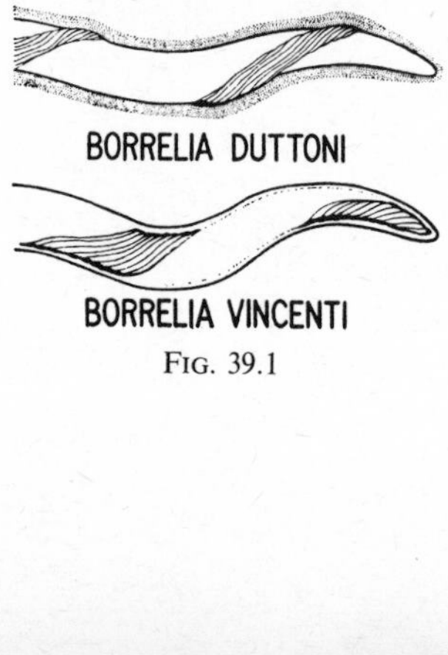

Staining. *Trep. pallidum* cannot be demonstrated by the ordinary staining methods. It can be stained by Giemsa's solution applied in a 1 in 10 dilution over a prolonged period (twenty-four hours) or in a 1 in 2 dilution for an hour, and appears faint pink in colour in contrast to the purplish colour of the coarser non-pathogenic spirochaetes. The organism may also be demonstrated by Fontana's silver or the India ink methods using the exudate from the chancre. In tissues, the spirochaetes can be stained by Levaditi's silver impregnation method.

Cultivation. It is generally agreed that pathogenic *Trep. pallidum* has not been cultivated in artificial media or in embryonated eggs or tissue cultures. The organism does grow in the testicles of experimentally inoculated rabbits and pathogenic strains can be maintained in

INTERNAL STRUCTURE OF
SPIROCHAETES

LEPTOSPIRA

TREPONEMA PALLIDUM

BORRELIA DUTTONI

BORRELIA VINCENTI

FIG. 39.1

this way (e.g. Nichol's strain). Certain other strains (e.g. Reiter's strain, not *Trep. pallidium*) can be cultured under strictly anaerobic conditions in Smith-Noguchi medium, or in digest broth enriched with serum. These latter strains, although originally isolated from syphilitic lesions, may have been contaminating saprophytes.

Viability outside the body is feeble under ordinary conditions. This spirochaete is a strict parasite; it dies rapidly in water and is very sensitive to drying. On the other hand it has been found that *Trep. pallidum* can retain its viability and virulence in necropsy material for some time at ordinary temperatures, and in serum kept in sealed capillary tubes it remains motile for several days. It is readily killed by heat (even at 41·5°C in an hour) and dies out more slowly (in two to three days) if kept at 0°–4°C. *Trep. pallidum* remains viable in tissue slices of rabbit testis for long periods at temperatures of −55° to −65°C.

Animal pathogenicity. Monkeys have been infected experimentally by inoculation of a scarified area on the eyebrows and genitals, or by implanting tissue from a syphilitic lesion under the epidermis. The anthropoid apes are the most susceptible, and lesions typical of primary and secondary syphilis may result in these animals. Rabbits can also be infected in some cases by inoculation in certain sites: inoculation into the anterior chamber of the eye produces keratitis and iritis; intratesticular injection leads to a syphilitic orchitis; and inoculation of the skin of the scrotum may set up a chancre-like sore. Metastatic lesions may succeed the primary infection.

Inoculation of mice produces no lesions, and though infection takes place it is symptomless and apparently latent.

Laboratory Diagnosis

The clinical diagnosis of syphilis is confirmed in the laboratory by finding *Trep. pallidum* in the exudates from the lesions or in the tissues and by demonstrating antibodies in the serum.

The Examination of Syphilitic Exudates

There is a serious risk of infection to the person who collects specimens from patients with primary or secondary syphilis and it is impor-

tant to wear rubber gloves and to exercise great care in handling the lesions. The sore is first cleansed carefully with a gauze swab soaked in warm normal saline and the margins are gently scraped so that superficial epithelium is abraded. Gentle pressure is applied to the base of the chancre until serum exudes from its surface; if this serum is bloodstained it should be wiped away and the process repeated until a clear fluid is obtained. Excessive numbers of red blood cells in the specimen must be avoided as they tend to obscure the spirochaetes. Wet films are now made on thin glass slides, covered with a thin coverslip and examined under the dark-ground microscope. If the examination has to be made in a laboratory at some distance some of the exudate should be taken up into several capillary tubes, both ends of which are then sealed in a flame. Do not store in the refrigerator or the incubator.

If a local antiseptic has been applied to the sore, spirochaetes may not be found until a wet dressing of gauze soaked in sterile normal saline has been applied to the sore for 24–48 h. When antisyphilitic treatment (e.g. with penicillin), has been used before the examination the likelihood of a successful microscopic diagnosis is greatly diminished.

If a primary sore is healing the microscopic examination of the exudate is often negative. At this stage, however, the spirochaetes may be found in the fluid aspirated with a syringe from enlarged inguinal lymph glands. Before acceptance of negative findings, the microscopical examination must be repeated on at least three occasions at daily intervals.

The observation of living motile spirochaetes under the *dark-ground microscope* is the most satisfactory method and in experienced hands provides a rapid and reliable diagnosis. *Trep. pallidum* is recognized by its slender spiral structure, characteristic slow movements, and angulation. It must be carefully distinguished from other spirochaetes which may be found in ulcerating sores (e.g. *Trep. calligyrum*). If no dark-ground microscope is available a wet film of the exudate mixed with India ink may be examined or Fontana's staining method can be used. A final identification of the spirochaete from a lesion as *Trep. pallidum* can be made by the use of the fluorescent antibody technique.

The necessary antiserum may be obtained from rabbits after infection with the Nichol's strain of *Trep. pallidum* and the other necessary reagents are those that are used in the FTA ABS test.

In the secondary stage of syphylis spirochaetes can be demonstrated in the serous exudate obtained from the skin eruption by scarifying and 'cupping' with test-tubes. The spirochaetes are also present in large numbers in the mucous patches in the mouth and in condylomata about the vulva and anus. Specimens from these situations, however, may contain large numbers of non-pathogenic spirochaetes which may be morphologically identical with *Trep. pallidum* so that great caution is required in reporting the observations.

OTHER TREPONEMATA

Treponema calligyrum (or *gracile*). This organism may occur in the secretions of the genitals, and morphologically resembles *Trep. pallidum*. Its differentiation from the latter is therefore of practical importance in syphilis diagnosis. It is not usually found if care has been taken to obtain serum from below the surface of the chancre. It is thicker than *Trep. pallidum* and its spirals are shallower; by the dark-ground illumination method it appears 'glistening', whereas *Trep. pallidum* is 'dead white'; it stains more readily than *Trep. pallidum* by Giemsa's method.

Treponema genitalis, which is very similar to *Trep. pallidum*, has also been described as a commensal on the genital mucosa.

Treponema microdentium. This organism flourishes in carious teeth, and may be found in the secretion between the teeth. It closely resembles *Trep. pallidum* in morphology, but is shorter (3–10 µm) and the coils are shallower. It is more easily stained by the ordinary methods than *Trep. pallidum*.

Treponema mucosum. Similar to *Trep. microdentium* in morphology, but is stated to have the property of producing a mucin-like substance.

Treponema macrodentium. Occurs in the mouth like *Trep. microdentium*. It bears some resemblance to *Trep. pallidum*, but is larger and thicker, with larger and less regular coils,

usually two to eight in number. Its motility is also more active. It is more easily stained than *Trep. pallidum* and is coloured blue by Giemsa's method.

Treponema cuniculi. Associated with an infectious disease of rabbits, which usually takes the form of a chronic local and superficial infection of the genitals. The spirochaetes can be demonstrated in the exudate from the lesions and in tissue sections. They are morphologically identical with *Trep. pallidum*.

SEROLOGICAL METHODS

Three distinct antibodies appear in the serum after a syphilitic infection. The first is known as a lipoidophil antibody 'reagin' and reacts with an antigen composed of an alcoholic extract of heart muscle to which cholesterol and lecithin have been added; it can be demonstrated either by flocculation as in the Kahn or similar tests or by complement fixation as in the Wassermann reaction. Reactions which demonstrate the presence of the 'reagin' are known as the standard tests for syphilis (STS) or as conventional tests. A second antibody reacts with a protein component found in the spirochaetal bodies of a non-pathogenic strain of *Trep. pallidum* and can be demonstrated by the Reiter Protein Complement Fixation Test (RPCFT). The third antibody reacts directly with a pathogenic strain of *Trep. pallidum* and can be demonstrated in the Treponema Pallidum Immobilization (TPI) and the Fluorescent Treponemal Antibody tests (FTA ABS).

FLOCCULATION TESTS FOR SYPHILIS

The direct mixture of syphilitic sera with antigens of the type used in the Wassermann reaction results in the appearance of a flocculent deposit which is easily seen with the hand lens and which may also be visible to the naked eye. Such reactions, however, may occur in non-syphilitic infections (e.g. tuberculosis, leprosy, malaria, hepatitis, infectious mononucleosis, etc.) and the tests may therefore react positively in many different infections. The sensitivity of the reaction may be reduced by adjusting the conditions under which the test is performed so as to render the test almost specific for syphilis; many flocculation reactions give results that are closely parallel to those of the complement-fixation technique. The value of flocculation tests lies in the simplicity of the technique employed and the fact that they can be carried out in places where complement and the reagents of the haemolytic system of the Wassermann test are not available. Ideally the tests are used as a first screening investigation and any positive sera are then subjected to a fuller investigation. Many varieties of the flocculation reaction are described and have been used as the Meinicke, Hinton, Mazzini and Kahn tests (see Cruickshank, 1972). One of the best tests employing cardiolipid antigen was devised by the Venereal Disease Research Laboratory, CDC, Atlanta and is generally known as the VDRL test.

The VDRL Flocculation Test

A rapid screening test that is simple to perform is of great value in dealing with large numbers of sera. The method described here is very satisfactory (see WHO Bulletin, 1951). The following reagents are required.

1. *Antigen*. This is an alcoholic solution of the following composition:

Cardiolipin	.	.	0·03 per cent
Lecithin	.	.	0·24 per cent
Cholesterol	.	.	0·9 per cent

It may be purchased from Messrs Wellcome Reagents Ltd.

2. *Diluent*. Buffered saline prepared as follows:

Formaldehyde, neutral reagent			
grade AR .	.	.	0·5 ml
$Na_2HPO_4, 12H_2O$.	.	.	0·093 g
KH_2PO_4	.	.	.	0·170 g
NaCl .	.	.	.	10·0 g
Distilled water	.	.	1000 ml

This solution has a pH of $6·0 \pm 0·1$.

3. *Unbuffered saline*. 0·9 per cent sodium chloride.

4. *Serum under test*. Should be clear and free of any trace of haemolysis. Inactive for 30 min at 56°C. Cerebrospinal fluid is not activated; if it is contaminated with blood it is not possible to carry out a satisfactory test.

Control sera. Pools of positive sera that react at dilutions of 1 in 4 and 1 in 8 are prepared and stored in sealed tubes in aliquots of 0·25 ml at −20°C. Similar stocks of non-reactive sera are needed.

5. *Antigen emulsion*. In a stoppered bottle place 0·4 ml of the buffered saline and add to it drop by drop from a pipette 0·5 ml of antigen. Ensure that the antigen is added during a period of approximately 6 sec and that the bottle is continuously rotated during this time. After the addition, the bottle is rotated vigorously for a further 10 sec. Now add 4·1 ml of 1·0 per cent buffered saline. Gently shake about 30 times in 10 sec and allow to stand for 5 min. The antigen is now ready and can be used during the next eight hours.

The qualitative serum test. Use $3 \times \frac{1}{2}$ in tubes. Transfer 0·5 ml inactivated serum to a tube and add to it 0·5 ml diluted antigen. Place for 10 min in a rack in the Kahn shaker and shake for 5 min. The tubes are now spun at about 2000 rev/min in a straight-headed centrifuge. After this the tubes are shaken again for exactly one minute and the test is read at once. Visible aggregation in a clear or very faintly turbid medium are read as positive. A slightly turbid appearance with a 'silken swirl' on gentle shaking is the typical negative appearance. All borderline reactions should be reported as negative. The test can be used quantitatively with serial doubling dilutions of the patient's serum, ranging from neat to 1 in 8 in weakly reactive sera to, for strongly positive sera, neat to 1 in 128. The weakest dilution giving a positive reaction is reported as the titre of the serum.

The VDRL test can be carried out more economically on slides when small quantities of the reagents are placed on 76×50 mm slides with ceramic rings using 0·016 ml and 0·01 ml droppers. Rotation is carried out by a mechanical slide rotator.

Wassermann Syphilis Reaction

This reaction depends on the 'fixation' of complement by a suspension of a phosphatide lipid (similar to lecithin and extracted from certain normal animal tissues) along with the *heated* serum of a person infected with syphilis, and constitutes an important diagnostic test. It becomes weakly positive at the second or third week after the appearance of the primary sore and by the sixth week of the disease is usually strongly positive.

For complement-fixation tests, an indicator of the presence of complement is required. The 'haemolytic system' used in these tests serves this purpose. It consists of the red corpuscles of a particular animal species 'sensitized' with the corresponding haemolytic antibody, e.g. the red cells of the ox or sheep *plus* the serum of a rabbit that has been immunized with the red cells of the species used. The immunoglobulin in the serum is thermostable. The serum is inactivated at 56°C and stored in bottles or tubes or preserved in the dry state (see above). The heated serum is nonhaemolytic by itself, but in the presence of a suitable complement brings about lysis of the homologous red corpuscles. Fixation of complement is denoted by the absence of lysis in the haemolytic system.

In its simplest form the Wassermann reaction can be represented as shown in Fig. 39.2.

It should be noted that the Wassermann test is carried out on a quantitative basis. Not only must it indicate whether the reaction is positive, but the various degrees of the reaction have also to be determined, from a strong positive ($+++$) to a weak positive ($+$) or a doubtful positive ($\pm$). Quantitative testing is most important in assessing the value of treatment or the completeness of cure.

The technical application of the reaction demands very accurate standardization of each reagent. Further, the amount of complement used in relation to the quantities of antigen and serum must be adjusted with such delicacy that the weakest reactions can be accepted as significant.

Antigen*

Fresh ox hearts are obtained from the slaughter house and are freed of fat and connective tissue. They are cut into pieces no longer than 1 cm and weighed. About 50 g of the cut muscle is pounded with sintered glass in a mortar for a minute or two. This mixture is transferred to a 2-litre flask and 9 ml absolute alcohol are added for every gram of muscle. Not more than 100 g muscle should be treated in one flask. The flask is now tightly stoppered, shaken thoroughly, and left for five days at room temperature in a dark cupboard. The flask must be shaken well every day. The mixture is now filtered through No. 1 Whatman filter paper at room temperature and is stored in the refrigerator overnight. Filter once again through Whatman No. 1 filter paper while still cold in the refrigerator. Store the filtrate in amber glass bottles away from the light in a cool place.

For use, 6 parts of the alcoholic extract are added to 4 parts of a 1 per cent solution of cholesterol and this mixture is then diluted with saline according to the optimal titre of the antigen. If, for example, the optimal titre is 320, 0·25 ml of the cholesterol antigen mixture is accurately pipetted to the bottom of a 100 ml measuring cylinder and 80 ml saline is measured into a similar cylinder. The saline is now poured *rapidly* into the measure containing the antigen and the mixture is completed by pouring from

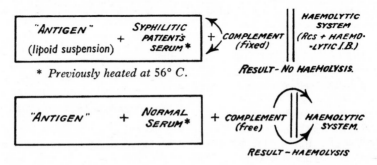

FIG. 39.2

* A suitable antigen (Maltaner Cardiolipin Antigen) is available commercially from Wellcome Reagents Ltd., London.

one cylinder to the other six times. The resultant opalescent mixture is the antigen to be used in the test; it should stand for 20 min before use and can be used throughout the working day. It should not be used after 8 h.

Human heart muscle has always been reputed to make a very sensitive Wassermann antigen but it may give non-specific results.

Before use the antigen must be tested in the following three ways: (1) it must be shown to have complement-fixing ability; (2) the anti-complementary action of the antigen must be determined by itself and also in the presence of normal serum; and (3) the antigen must be titrated by the method of optimal proportion to discover the appropriate dilution to be used in the test. With commercially prepared antigens these steps have usually been carried out by the makers who supply instructions for the use of their product in the test. Full details of the method of titration of antigens are given by Price (1950a) but the essential steps are as follows. First, the anticomplementary activity of the antigen in the presence of normal serum is determined. To accomplish this a chess-board titration is set up with a series of antigen dilutions and a series of complement dilutions. The antigen is prepared in seven doubling dilutions from 1 in 20 to 1 in 1280 and the complement in seven dilutions ranging from 1 in 10, 1 in 20 and so on to 1 in 70. Each tube also contains normal human serum and the haemolytic system (see above). When the titration is read the complement titre for each antigen dilution is recorded and from these figures the 'diagnostic doses' of complement needed in the next step is calculated by the method on page 500.

The optimal proportion titration of the antigen employs the same series of antigen dilutions that were used in determining the anti-complementary activity. They are set up in a fresh chess-board titration against a series of seven dilutions of a positive serum ranging from 1 in 10, 1 in 20 to 1 in 70. To each serum-antigen mixture the appropriate 'diagnostic dose' of complement, and (after an interval for fixation) the haemolytic system is added. The known positive serum is preferably of moderate strength with a titre of about 1 in 40. The end point of the titration is that antigen dilution which reacts with the greatest dilution of the serum. It is often necessary to read the result by interpolation and since the reactivity may be spread over a zone of antigen dilutions it is permissible to take the mid-point of the zone as an end point. As a final step this antigen dilution is taken as a working suspension and retitrated to determine the amount of it to be used in the test proper. The antigen suspension is now diluted in saline in a series of seven doubling dilutions ranging from 1 in 2 to 1 in 64. It is next set up in a chess-board titration against the positive serum diluted 1 in 2, 1 in 4 and so on to 1 in 64. The volumes of reagents used and the technical procedures are those described below.

Cardiolipin (as antigen in the syphilis serum reactions)

This substance, isolated from the phosphatide fraction of lipoidal extracts of heart muscle, has been extensively used in recent years in the Wassermann and flocculation tests for syphilis. It has been claimed that cardiolipin yields more specific results than those obtained with the unpurified lipoid preparations usually employed as antigen in these reactions. It is also supposed that the specific activity of these lipoid preparations with syphilitic sera depends on 'cardiolipin'. This substance contains phosphorus but no nitrogen; on saponification it yields fatty acids, a non-reducing carbohydrate, and phosphoric acid.

In the syphilis reactions it is used along with lecithin and cholesterol, and preparations containing an appropriate admixture of these constituents are available for diagnostic tests, e.g. the cardiolipin (Whitechapel) antigen, obtainable from Burroughs Wellcome & Co., London, which has the following composition: cardiolipin 0·3 per cent, lecithin 0·0175 per cent, and cholesterol 0·0875 per cent. The titre in which the antigen should be used is specified by the makers. This antigen is suitable for the Wassermann test, in substitution for the original antigen employed in this method.

Patient's Serum

A specimen of blood is obtained by vein puncture as for blood culture. The blood is then placed in a sterile stoppered test-tube or screw-capped bottle and allowed to coagulate. It is advisable to obtain about 5 ml of blood. The serum, which should be free from haemolysis, is pipetted off after separation and heated in a waterbath at 56°C for 30 min. Heating *eliminates the fallacy of non-specific fixation effects which may occur with normal unheated sera plus the antigen*; it also deprives the serum of its complementing property.

It is thought that the albumin fraction in unheated syphilitic serum may act as a protective colloid and that it tends to reduce precipitation in flocculation reactions. Heating the fraction eliminates this effect.

Complement

Fresh or specially preserved guinea-pig serum is used (see Chap. 11). It contains an active haemolytic complement for the red corpuscles of the ox or sheep sensitized with the homologous haemolytic antibody. When fresh serum is used, the blood is obtained 12 to 18 h before the test by severing the large vessels of the neck over a 6-in funnel, from which the blood is collected in a measuring cylinder; it is allowed to coagulate and stand overnight in the refrigerator. The complement in serum too recently withdrawn is apt to be excessively 'fixable', and in consequence is unsuitable for the Wassermann test.

If possible the pooled serum of several guinea-pigs should be used.

It should be noted that complement is unstable and deteriorates on keeping at ordinary temperatures. It is advisable throughout the experiment to keep the guinea-pig serum on ice. If storage at −30°C is available the fresh serum may be divided into small portions and kept frozen for a few weeks.

It is now a general practice to use specially preserved serum pooled from a number of animals and it is recommended that it should be absorbed with packed sheep erythrocytes (0·1 m cells/ml guinea-pig serum for 30 min at 4°C). The method for the preservation of complement is described in Chapter 11.

Titration of Complement

Price's method (1949) is recommended. A pool of six or more normal sera and another of strongly reacting positive sera are required. Prepare a series of ten dilutions of complement in saline ranging from 1 in 10, 1 in 20, and on to 1 in 100. Set out five rows of $3 \times \frac{1}{2}$ in tubes as follows:

Row 1 has 10 tubes, to which are added:
  1 volume complement at dilutions 1 in 10 to 1 in 100
  2 volumes saline.

Row 2 has 5 tubes, to which are added:
  1 volume complement dilutions at 1 in 10 to 1 in 50
  1 volume saline
  1 volume antigen diluted as in test.

Row 3 has 5 tubes, to which are added:
  1 volume complement dilutions at 1 in 10 to 1 in 50
  1 volume saline
  $\frac{1}{5}$ volume pooled normal serum
  1 volume antigen.

Row 4 has 7 tubes, to which are added:
  1 volume complement dilutions at 1 in 10 to 1 in 70
  2 volumes saline
  $\frac{1}{5}$ volume pooled positive serum.

Row 5 has 7 tubes, to which are added:
  1 volume complement dilutions at 1 in 10 to 1 in 70
  2 volumes saline
  $\frac{1}{5}$ volume normal serum.

Plastic plates of the WHO type are a convenient alternative to the $3 \times \frac{1}{2}$ tubes. The usual volume employed in the test is 0·11 ml, as in the Wyler technique, and the reagents are conveniently added by standard dropping pipettes attached to suitable separating funnels. Droppers of three different sizes are required (Donald's Method) (1) for *saline, complement* and *sensitized cells* a piece of glass tubing is drawn out, inserted into a Rawco gauge and cut squarely at a point where its outside diameter is 0·75 cm; (2) for the *antigen* suspension a dropper is cut in the same manner with an outside diameter of 0·9 cm; (3) for *undiluted human sera* the pipette dropper is inserted into the No. 56 hole in the Starrett gauge and cut as near to the surface of the gauge as possible. Pipettes (1) and (2) deliver per drop 0·11 ml of the reagents for which they are designed. Pipette (3) delivers in 1 drop 0·022 ml of inactivated human sera, i.e. $\frac{1}{5}$ the volume of that discharged by (1) and (2). It is necessary to check the pipettes for accuracy before use.

When the reagents have been added, the rack is incubated for 1 h in a 37°C bath. At the end of this period, the rack is removed from the bath and to every tube is added 1 volume of sensitized red blood cells. The rack is returned to the bath for a further 30 min and the results are then read. The last tube in the serial dilutions to show complete sparkling haemolysis is taken as the end-point.

Two amounts of complement will be needed in the test proper:

(*a*) *For the serum controls.* This dilution of complement is the highest to show complete haemolysis in row 4 or 5. *This is the serum control dose.*

(*b*) *For the diagnostic test.* This dose is calculated by taking the end-point in row 3 and multiplying it by $\frac{5}{4}$. For example, if 1 in 40 were the end-point then the complement would be used at a dilution of $\frac{1}{40} \times \frac{5}{4} = \frac{5}{160} = \frac{1}{32}$. *This is the diagnostic dose.* The 25 per cent margin of extra complement used is sufficient to cover the occasional anti-complementary activity of normal sera.

Haemolytic System

With guinea-pig complement, a haemolytic system consisting of sheep red corpuscles sensitized with the appropriate haemolytic antibody is used.

Defibrinated blood is obtained at the abattoir. The required quantity is thoroughly mixed with several volumes of normal saline and then centrifuged to separate the corpuscles, the supernatant fluid being pipetted off. This process has generally been designated 'washing' the blood corpuscles and is repeated three or four times. The centrifuged deposit of corpuscles after the final washing is suspended in normal saline to form a 6 per cent suspension. Sheep cells should not be used until one week old when they are uniformly susceptible to lysis.

STANDARDIZATION OF THE RED BLOOD SUSPENSION. Transfer exactly 1·0 ml of the suspension to a special haematocrit tube (Price and Wilkinson, 1947).* After centrifuging for

*Obtainable from Messrs R. B. Turner & Co. Ltd., London.

ten minutes at 2500 rev/min the height of the column of packed cells is read off. The standard packed cell volume required in the test is 0·05 ml and the original 6 per cent suspension is adjusted to this content by dilution by simple proportion. The following example shows the method of calculation:

6 per cent suspension packed volume = 0·057
Desired packed cell volume = 0·050
Dilution factor $\frac{0·057}{0·050}$ = 1·14

Thus, 0·14 ml saline should be added to each 1·0 ml of the original 6 per cent cell suspension.

Equal volumes of this standard suspension and saline containing 12 MHD of the haemolytic serum per unit volume are mixed, shaken vigorously, and incubated in the water-bath for 30 minutes at 37°C. Some workers prefer to ensure complete mixing by passing a current of air through the suspension during the period of incubation.

PRESERVATION OF SHEEP RED BLOOD CELLS. Sheep blood for complement fixation tests may be preserved at 4°C in an equal volume of sterile modified Alsever's solution consisting of:

Glucose . . . . 2·05 per cent
Sodium chloride . . 0·42 per cent
Trisodium citrate . . 0·8 per cent
Citric acid in distilled water 0·055 per cent

Sheep cells have been satisfactory for use for a period of six weeks after collection in this solution.

HAEMOLYTIC ANTISERUM. The following method is recommended. Rabbits receive on alternate days a series of five *intracutaneous* inoculations of whole sheep blood in the following doses: 0·5, 1·0, 2·0, 2·5 ml. These are followed on the twelfth and fifteenth days by the intravenous inoculation of 1·0 ml of a 20 per cent suspension of sheep red blood cells in normal saline to which has been added 0·01 per cent magnesium sulphate. A trial bleeding is taken from the rabbit's ear on the eighteenth day and if the haemolysin content of the serum is satisfactory (the titre should be over 10 000) the rabbit is exsanguinated and the serum is separated. If the titre is not high, further intravenous injections are given. High-titre serum is usually

Table 39.1

					Tube No.					
	1	2	3	4	5	6	7	8	9	10
Saline solution	None	ml 0·5	ml 1·0	ml 1·5	ml 2·0	ml 0·5	ml 0·5	ml 0·5	ml 0·5	ml 0·5

preserved by adding to it an equal volume of sterile glycerol.

The haemolysin titre of the serum (sometimes referred to as its minimum haemolytic dose) is estimated as follows: Set out ten tubes and add to them saline as shown in Table 39.1.

Prepare a 1 in 1000 dilution of the haemolytic serum and add 0·5 ml of it to the first five tubes of titration. Then proceed as shown in Table 39.2.

Now add to each tube 0·5 ml of a 1 in 10 dilution of complement and 0·5 ml of 3 per cent suspension of red blood cells prepared as above. Incubate for one hour at 37°C in a water-bath; the last serum dilution to show complete haemolysis is taken as the end-point. The lowest titre which is acceptable for the purpose of sensitizing red blood cells for the Wassermann reading is 1000.

Haemolytic serum for *sheep* red corpuscles (Wellcome Reagents Ltd.) may conveniently be used in preparing a haemolytic system for the test. This anti-sheep haemolytic serum is obtained from the horse. It tends to exert a pronounced agglutinating effect on the homologous corpuscles, with rapid sedimentation of the cells. It is advisable therefore to add the serum to the corpuscles just before the haemolytic system is required.

An alternative method for the preparation of a haemolytic antiserum for sheep's red blood cells is that used by Sawyer and Bourke which employs the stroma of lysed erythrocytes as the antigen and a shorter inoculation schedule thereby minimizing the shock reactions that are liable to occur with the usual immunization procedures.

Sensitized cells for the test are made by mixing equal volumes of the standard 6 per cent suspension and the haemolytic serum diluted to contain 12 MHD per unit volume. After vigorous shaking, the mixture is incubated for one hour in a 37°C water-bath.

The Wassermann Test

The method is that of Price, 1950*b*.

Small test-tubes $3 \times \frac{1}{2}$ in or WHO plates are used and the reagents are added to them either with graduated pipettes or according to Donald's dropping method.

The first step, before commencing the test, is to titrate the complement using the sensitized red blood cell suspension to be used in the test. This is necessary because even pooled preserved complement-serum may vary in activity against different specimens of red blood cells.

Table 39.2

Tube No.	Procedure	Final haemolysin dilution: 1 in
1	None	1000
2	Mix. Discard 0·5 ml	2000
3	Mix. Transfer 0·5 ml to tube 6. Discard 0·5 ml	3000
4	Mix. Transfer 0·5 ml to tube 7. Discard 1·0 ml	4000
5	Mix. Transfer 0·5 ml to tube 8. Discard 1·5 ml	5000
6	Mix. Transfer 0·5 ml to tube 9	6000
7	Mix. Transfer 0·5 ml to tube 10	8000
8	Mix. Discard 0·5 ml	10 000
9	Mix. Discard 0·5 ml	12 000
10	Mix. Discard 0·5 ml	16 000

The test proper is a screening procedure and each serum has two tubes allocated to it. The reagents are added as follows:

Tube 1. Serum control tube:

Patient's serum . . .	$\frac{1}{5}$ volume
Saline	2 volumes
Complement serum control dose	1 volume

Tube 2. Diagnostic tube:

Patient's serum . . .	$\frac{1}{5}$ volume
Saline	1 volume
Complement diagnostic dose .	1 volume
Antigen	1 volume

After adding the reagents the racks are shaken thoroughly and placed in a water-bath for 1 h at 37°C. At the end of this time the racks are placed on the bench and to each tube is added one volume of sensitized red blood cells. After shaking again, the racks are replaced in the water-bath for a further 30 min, after which the test is read.

Complete haemolysis in both tubes is read as negative reaction. No haemolysis in the diagnostic tube with complete haemolysis in the control tube is read as a positive reaction. Partial haemolysis in the serum diagnostic tube and complete haemolysis in the control tube is read as a weakly positive reaction. No result can be given if the serum control tube of any particular specimen of serum fails to show complete haemolysis. Positive and weakly positive sera are set aside to be put up for a quantitative test.

Quantitative tests. In this method doubling dilutions of the serum in saline from 1 in 5 to 1 in 160 are used. Seven tubes are required for each serum and they are set up as follows:

Tube 1. Serum control tube:

Serum diluted 1 in 5 . .	1 volume
Saline	1 volume
Serum control dose of complement	1 volume

Tubes 2–7. Diagnostic quantitative tubes:

Serum appropriate dilution (1 in 5 to 1 in 160) . .	1 volume
Complement diagnostic dose .	1 volume
Antigen	1 volume

The sensitized red blood cells are added in the same manner as in the test proper and the incubation times are the same. The end-point is taken as that tube which just fails to show sparkling haemolysis.

The results are reported in terms of the serum dilutions, e.g. 'Positive with serum diluted 1 in 30'.

Cerebrospinal fluid. In this test the procedure is closely similar to that used for serum. Neat cerebrospinal fluid is used in the test proper and one volume is added to both the diagnostic and control tubes instead of the one-fifth volume used for sera. The test is made quantitative by making doubling dilutions from neat cerebrospinal fluid and results are recorded as 'Positive, fluid diluted 1 in 2, 1 in 4' and so on.

Each batch of tests should include known positive sera of varying degrees of reactivity and a known negative serum. Controls should be set up for each of the reagents used.

There is a cold complement fixation technique (Kolmer) which is useful in other methods (see Eleventh Edition of this book, page 938).

Reiter Protein Complement Fixation Test (RPCFT)

The antigen for this test is prepared from mass cultures of the Reiter treponema, and by disrupting the washed spirochaetes by ultrasonication. The resulting emulsion is purified by dialysis against 70 per cent ammonium sulphate and the protein of the resulting precipitate is used as the complement-fixing antigen. It is used at its optimum titre (about 1 in 40) which must be checked with each batch (Foster, Nicol and Stone, 1958).

The technique is as for the Wassermann Test and the test is particularly valuable when carried out in parallel with other serum tests for syphilis.

The Reiter treponeme, which is non-pathogenic, shares a common group antigen with *Trep. pallidum* and with other treponemes. This antigen is distinct from the lipoidal antigen that detects the antibody in the conventional standard serological tests for syphilis. The Reiter antibody appears early in primary syphilis and can often be detected about 10 days after the appearance of the primary chancre. It is always present in the secondary stage when its titre is high; thereafter the titre in latency declines (see Chap. 34, Vol. I). When both the reagin and the RCPFT are positive there is a very high degree of probability of treponemal infection. If both tests are negative it is unlikely that treponemal infection has occurred. If there is a disagreement between the results of these two methods confirmation is required from other tests such as the FTA-ABS, the TPHA and TPI tests (Table 39.3).

Table 39.3

RPCFT	Reagin	Interpretation
+	+	Treponemal infection
+	−	Treponemal disease, e.g. treated cases of yaws and syphilis
−	+	Reagin tests non-specific in a proportion of cases
−	−	Treponemal infection unlikely

Absorbed Fluorescent Treponemal Antibody (FTA-ABS) Test

This is an indirect immuno-fluorescence technique for detecting antibodies in the serum that react with *Trep. pallidum*. Such an antibody may be produced as a result of the presence of commensal treponemes in the body, but most often results from infection with *Trep. pallidum* and other pathogenic treponemes. Quantitative FTA-ABS, IgG and IgM tests are valuable in assessing the significance of foetal antibodies that follow intrauterine infections (Johnston, 1972). The technique here described follows closely that of the Venereal Disease Research Laboratory, Communicable Disease Research Centre, Atlanta (1968).

1. Materials and equipment. Fluorescent microscope with alternative facilities for darkground illumination at a magnification of about × 500 and also a quartz-iodine light source and filters for fluorescence work (see Chap. 1).

2. Special thin microscope slides with ground glass ends inscribed with two circles 10 mm in diameter. They must be scrupulously clean.

3. Phosphate buffered saline pH 7·2 PBS.

4. Treponeme suspension. This is prepared from the testes of rabbits infected by the Nichol's strain of *Trep. pallidum*. A tissue suspension is prepared in phosphate buffered saline to contain 40–50 spirochaetes per high dry field of the dark field microscope objective. The coarse cellular debris is removed by centrifugation for 10 min at 1000 rev/min. When 0·1 per cent sodium azide has been added the suspension can be preserved in 1·0 ml aliquots for about six weeks at 4°–5°C. Lyophylized suspensions are available commercially (e.g. Wellcome Reagents Ltd.).

Treponemal suspensions should always be tested before use with a range of known positive and negative sera. A further necessity is to test them against a conjugate prepared against rabbit gammaglobulin to make certain that the treponemes have not been sensitized by the antibodies of their rabbit host.

5. Prepared slides are made by spreading 0·1 mm loopful of the treponeme suspension within each of the engraved circles on the special slides. Dry for 15 min then fix for at least 15 min in 10 per cent methanol in distilled water. Allow to dry. Prepared slides are used in the preliminary standardization of the reagents as well as in the test proper.

6. Fluorescein-conjugated anti-human gammaglobulin serum. It is best to use a commercial product of high quality, e.g. Wellcome Reagents Ltd. Each new conjugate has to be tested with the treponemes and known, strongly, medium, weakly and negative reactive sera. Such sera may be purchased from Difco Baltimore Laboratories, but as the routine work of the laboratory continues, sera should be selected from batches of tests as they are reported. Before testing the conjugate enough prepared slides are rinsed in two changes of PBS and then rinsed in distilled water before being allowed to dry. To each set of slides is added a series of two-fold dilutions of the conjugate in PBS ranging from 1 in 10 to 1 in 320. Another set of slides is set up in similar fashion with another conjugate of known reactivity. After incubation, for a minimum of 30 min at 37°C, the slides are rinsed as before and mounted in buffered glycerol (9 parts glycerol with one part PBS). The end-point of the titration is taken as one-half of the greatest dilution of the conjugate that gives + + + + fluorescence with a strongly positive serum, and + + fluorescence with a medium reactive serum. This is the future working dilution of the conjugate provided always that even at a dilution of 1 in 10, there is no trace of non-specific fluorescence.

Absorbing agent. This is used to remove group anti-treponemal antibodies from the serum being investigated and does not react with the antibodies specific for *Trep. pallidum*. It is an extract obtained from a dense culture of Reiter-treponemes in 10 per cent serum thioglycollate medium containing about 100 spirochaetes per dry high power field. After autoclaving for 10 min at 121°C the suspension is centrifuged and the extract is prepared and assayed by the method described by Wilkinson *et al.* (1972). The preparation is available commercially from Difco, Baltimore Laboratories.

The absorbent is used at the greatest dilution at which reactivity of a non-specific control serum is abolished; but the specific reactivity of a positive control serum should not be specifically decreased.

A simple way of preparing an absorbing agent for the removal of group antigens is by ultrasonication of the Reiter treponemes followed by centrifugation of the broken organisms and washing them with PBS in the centrifuge.

Technique of the FTA-ABS Test

1. Lay out enough prepared slides of treponemes as described above and number them. Each slide (two engraved circles) will accommodate two test sera. Allow three slides (six circles) for the test controls.

2. Set out a row of $3 \times \frac{1}{2}$ in (Wassermann Tubes) one for each of the test or control sera to be used. To each of them pipette 0·2 ml of the absorbing agent diluted to its working titre in distilled water.

3. With Pasteur pipettes graduated to deliver 0·05 ml add this volume to each inactivated serum to the individual tubes and mix thoroughly by drawing up the fluid and expelling it for at least eight times. Use a clean Pasteur pipette for each serum. The procedure is the same for test and control sera. Allow to stand at room temperature for no more than 30 min.

Controls that have no non-specific fluorescence are as follows:

   Positive $+ + + +$ serum
   Positive $+ +$ serum
   Positive $+$ serum
   Non-reactive serum
   Phosphate buffered saline alone.

4. Set out special slides that have no treponemes for controls of the individual reagents.
   (*a*) The absorbing agent plus phosphate buffered saline.
   (*b*) The non-reactive serum plus the absorbing agent.

5. Transfer one drop of the test serum-adsorbent agent mixtures as well as all controls to the circles of the numbered slides. Spread each drop over the whole area. Incubate for 30 min at 37°C in a moist chamber.

6. Rinse the slides gently in running water to remove excess serum and then rinse in PBS in Coplin jars for five minutes on two occasions. Rinse again in distilled water. Dry in air.

7. Now add one drop of the conjugate diluted to its working titre in PBS to all the circles with test and control sera and where needed to the control slides. Incubate again for 30 min at 37°C.

8. Rinse again as in step 5 and when dry mount in a drop of buffered glycerol and examine.

9. Examine firstly the control slides which must show the expected pattern of reactions.

10. Now read the test sera. Those with $+ +$, $+ + +$ and $+ + + +$ fluorescence are reported as positive. Those with weak $(+)$ fluorescence similar in degree to the $+$ control serum are reported as doubtful. Such sera and any others from patients whose clinical findings appear to conflict with a diagnosis of treponemal infection should be re-examined with all the tests available locally and if necessary referred to the reference laboratory for the TPI test. Sera giving no fluorescence or weak $\pm$ reactions are regarded as negative.

The Treponema Pallidum Immobilization (TPI) Test

This test depends on the observation of immobilization of living spirochaetes when they are incubated with syphilitic sera. Dilutions of the serum to be tested are mixed with a suspension of motile *Trep. pallidum* (Nichol's strain) which are maintained in the laboratory by the intra-testicular inoculation of rabbits.

An appropriate amount of fresh complement is added and after incubation the test is read by determining, under the dark-ground microscope, the proportion of treponemes which have been immobilized. This proportion is then compared with a similar estimate of the spirochaetes immobilized by normal and known positive control sera (Nelson and Mayer, 1949; Wilkinson and Johnston, 1959). The test is complicated to perform, expensive in animals and reagents, and is very time consuming. It is not suitable for use as a routine test and is reserved for specially selected cases.

The TPI test is generally accepted as being almost completely specific and a positive finding is a reliable indication of syphilitic infection. The sensitivity of the test, however, is not so great as that of the STS and negative findings may be obtained in untreated cases of primary and early secondary syphilis and also in congenital syphilis (Sequeira and Wilkinson, 1955; Wilkinson and Sequeira, 1955). The main value of the test is in latent and tertiary syphilis and in clarifying those problems which arise when discrepancies occur in the STS, e.g. biological false positive reactions. The TPI test remains positive for long periods even after the STS have become negative and thus it is of little value in following the effects of treatment. Since the TPI test has the highest specificity of all the tests for syphilitic antibodies it is used as a reference in assessing the value of other tests. Essentially it is reserved for the practice of the treponemal reference laboratory.

The Treponema Pallidum Haemagglutination Test (TPHA)

Passive haemagglutination of erythrocytes is a familiar and very sensitive method for the detection of many antibodies to bacterial and viral antigens. Its application to syphilis was first reported by Rathlev (1965–1967, see Vol. I) and has been greatly developed; the micromethod described by Johnston (1972) is easy to perform and offers a simple and sensitive alternative to those laboratories that are not able to carry out the more elaborate FTS-ABS and TPI tests.

The reagents for this test include formalized tanned sheep red blood cells sensitized with fragments of an ultrasonicated suspension of the Nichol's pathogenic strain of *Trep. pallidum*. Control unsensitized cells are needed, an absorbent and the test diluent. All are obtainable in kit form from the Fuji Yoki Pharmaceutical of Tokyo in Japan or through Mr A. Baker of Micro-bio Laboratories of London, England.

The TPHA test can be performed by a micro-method in U-type microtitre plates either qualtitatively or quantitatively (Johnston, 1972). The sensitivity and specificity of this test compare favourably with the TPI and FTA-ABS tests in both syphilis and yaws (Garner *et al.*, 1972).

The TPHA test has been assessed thoroughly and seems likely to assume an important place in the serological investigations of syphilis: it may replace some of the more complex tests presently being used.

BORRELIA

Borreliae are large, motile spirochaetes and their general morphology and pathogenicity was described in Chapter 34 of Volume I.

BORRELIA VINCENTII

Borrelia vincentii is generally associated with a large fusiform bacillus—*Fusobacterium fusiforme*—and large numbers of both these organisms can be found in a variety of mouth lesions and ulcerative and necrotic processes elsewhere in the body. They are constantly observed in the exudates of the pseudomembranous ulcers on the pharynx and tonsils in Vincent's angina and in the inflamed gum margins in acute ulcerative gingivitis; they are also occasionally found in the lesions of acute balanitis, lung abscess, bronchiectasis, and in chronic ulceration of the skin, especially in tropical countries.

Morphology and staining. *Borr. vincentii* is 7–18 μm long and 0·2–0·6 μm wide. There are three to eight loose, open coils varying greatly in amplitude and the organism is actively motile with coarse lashing movements. It resembles *Borr. refringens*, but is sometimes described as smaller and more delicate. The spirochaetes are Gram-negative and stain readily with dilute carbol fuchsin, methyl violet, and with Giemsa's and Leishman's stains. Under the electron microscope *Borr. vincentii* is seen to have a clear-cut wall within which some ten axial filaments are twisted spirally around the protoplasm of the body of the spirochaete.

Cultivation. *Borr. vincentii* is an obligate anaerobe. It can be cultivated in sealed tubes containing digest broth enriched with ascitic fluid; it grows abundantly in mixed primary cultures but is extremely difficult to maintain in pure culture.

Laboratory Diagnosis

Smears are made directly from the ulcerative lesions in the mouth or from swabs and are stained with dilute carbol fuchsin. A clinical diagnosis of Vincent's infection would be confirmed when very large numbers of both the spirochaetes and the typically barred fusiform bacilli are seen together with the many pus cells which indicate the presence of an active inflammatory process. Cultural procedures are not satisfactory for diagnosis of the infection but are necessary because other pathogenic organisms such as haemolytic streptococci or diphtheria bacilli may also be present.

BORRELIA RECURRENTIS (OBERMEIERI)

Morphology and staining. This organism is a spiral filament, cylindrical or flattened, with tapering ends, varying in length, as a rule, from 10 to 20 μm, and about 0·3–0·5 μm broad, with about five to seven fairly regular coils 0·9–1·7 μm in amplitude. Active motility of a rotatory or oscillating type is noted in fresh preparations. Multiplication is by transverse fission. The structure of the organism as it is seen under the electron microscope is that of a bundle of some twelve filaments twisted spirally around the spirochaetal body external to the cell wall. These filaments are similar to those seen in *Trep. pallidum* and are probably concerned in the contractile movements of the organism. They are rather easily displaced during the manipulations of staining and may resemble flagella, for which at one time they were mistaken. The whole spirochaete is covered by a layer of slime-like material to a thickness of about 0·08 μm.

This spirochaete stains readily with Romanowsky stains (e.g. Leishman's), and may exhibit uniform staining or beading. It can be stained also with carbol fuchsin, and is Gram-negative. In fresh preparations of blood it can be seen with the ordinary microscope, but dark-ground or preferably phase-contrast illumination is more suitable for its demonstration in the living state. Silver impregnation methods may also be used for demonstrating the spirochaete in films or tissues.

Cultivation. Artificial cultures were first obtained by anaerobic growth in Smith-Noguchi medium, citrated blood containing spirochaetes from an infected animal, e.g. a white rat, being used as the inoculum.

Cultures have also been obtained in the following media, but the organism does not readily adapt itself to artificial growth in the laboratory: (1) horse serum diluted with 2 parts of saline solution, and with 1 ml of broth, containing 10 per cent peptone, added to 10 ml of the diluted serum; for subcultures, a drop of rabbit blood is also added; the medium is covered with a paraffin seal; (2) 20 per cent rabbit serum with 80 per cent Hartley's broth in tubes to each of which 1 g of coagulated egg albumin is added; petroleum jelly is superimposed and the cultures are incubated at 30°C; (3) egg albumin is placed in a test-tube and coagulated by heat in the form of a slope; 5 ml of horse serum diluted 1 in 10 or rabbit serum diluted 1 in 5 are then added, the serum having previously been heated at 58°–60°C for one hour; the medium is covered with sterile petroleum jelly; before an inoculation is made, a drop of fresh rabbit or human blood is added. The spirochaetes may also be grown in the chick embryo. The inoculum is introduced into the allantoic cavity of 17–18-day embryos and on hatching large numbers of spirochaetes can be found in the chick's blood (Oag, 1940).

BORRELIA DUTTONII

This organism is morphologically similar to *Borr. obermeieri*, but represents a separate species. Granules with the staining reactions of chromatin have also been observed in the spirochaete; these apparently are separate from the spirochaete, and have been regarded as a phase in the life history of the organism. There is electron microscopical evidence that these granules contain coiled-up spirochaetes. It seems probable that they are formed under adverse physical conditions and that they represent a resting phase rather than a stage in reproduction. Such granules have been noted in the Malpighian tubules of infective ticks.

Borr. duttonii is transmitted by ticks (*Ornithodorus moubata* and other species). After taking a blood meal a tick may remain infective for as long as five years. The spirochaetes are transmitted transovarially to succeeding generations of ticks. Man is infected in most cases from contamination of the bite wound by infective excreta of the tick, but occasionally the bite itself or particularly the bite of the larva may also transfer the spirochaetes. The main mammalian reservoir of infection is small rodents but pigs, porcupines, opossums and armadillos may also harbour the spirochaetes.

Borr. duttonii is pathogenic to monkeys and certain laboratory animals (e.g. rat, mouse). It possesses a greater virulence for monkeys and other animals than *Borr. recurrentis*. Like *Borr. recurrentis*, *Borr. duttonii* is sensitive to penicillin and the tetracyclines.

Laboratory Diagnosis

During the pyrexial phases, the spirochaetes can frequently be demonstrated in the blood, but not during apyrexial intervals.

Thin or thick blood films are made as in malaria diagnosis, and stained by Leishman's method.

Some workers prefer to stain the films with dilute carbol fuchsin.

If a drop of blood is mounted on a slide under a coverslip and examined with the oil-immersion lens, the spirochaetes may be detected in the unstained condition and show active movement. A more satisfactory method of demonstrating them, however, is by dark-ground, or phase-contrast illumination.

If spirochaetes are not detectable, inoculation intraperitoneally of white mice with 1·0–2·0 ml blood drawn from a vein may reveal the infection, the organisms appearing in considerable numbers in the blood of the animals. A drop of blood from the tail of the inoculated animal is examined daily for a considerable period. An inoculum of 0·2 ml of blood into the chorio-allantoic sac of the chick embryo may also be used.

Lice taken from a case can be examined for spirochaetes by keeping them in a test-tube for a day, then placing them in drops of distilled water on slides and piercing them with a needle so that the haemocele fluid becomes mixed with the water, which is then examined microscopically by dark-ground illumination. The spirochaetes can also be demonstrated in ticks by examining stained films from the stomach contents.

REFERENCES AND FURTHER READING

D'ALESSANDRO, G. & DARDANONI, L. (1953) Isolation and purification of the protein antigen of the Reiter treponeme. *American Journal of Syphilis*, **37**, 137.

BEKKER, J. H. (1962) Limitations of the Reiter protein complement-fixation (RPCF) test. *British Journal of Venereal Diseases*, **38**, 131.

CRUICKSHANK, R. (1972) *Medical Microbiology*, 11th edn, revised reprint. Edinburgh: Livingstone.

FOSTER, W. D., NICOL, C. S. & STONE, A. H. (1958) Reiter's protein complement-fixation test. Report of a trial in 1000 unselected cases. *British Journal of Venereal Diseases*, **34**, 196.

JOHNSTON, N. A. (1972) Neonatal congenital syphilis. *British Journal of Venereal Diseases*, **48**, 464.

JOHNSTON, N. A. (1972) *Treponema pallidum* haemagglutination test for syphilis. Evaluation of a micro-method. *British Journal of Venereal Diseases*, **48**, 474.

GARNER, M. F., BACKHOUSE, J. L., DASKALOPOULOS, G. & WALSH, J. L. (1972) *British Journal of Venereal Diseases*, **48**, 470, 479.

NELSON, R. A. & MAYER, M. M. (1949) Immobilization of *Treponema pallidum in vitro* by antibody produced in syphilitic infection. *Journal of Experimental Medicine*, **89**, 369.

OAG, R. K. (1940) The comparative susceptibility of the chick embryo and the chick to infection with *Borrelia duttoni*. *Journal of Pathology and Bacteriology*, **51**, 127.

PRICE, I. N. O. (1950 a & b) Complement fixation technique; Wassermann reaction. *British Journal of Venereal Diseases*, **26**, 33, 172.

SEQUEIRA, P. J. L. & WILKINSON, A. E. (1955) Studies on the reproducibility and specificity of the treponemal immobilization test. *British Journal of Venereal Diseases*, **31**, 124.

SEQUEIRA, P. J. L. (1959) An examination of the treponemal Wassermann reaction and Reiter protein complement-fixation test. *British Journal of Venereal Diseases*, **35,** 139.

SWAIN, R. H. A. (1955) Electron microscopic studies of the morphology of pathogenic spirochaetes. *Journal of Pathology and Bacteriology*, **69,** 117.

VENEREAL DISEASES RESEARCH LABORATORY (1968) Technique for the fluorescent treponemal antibody-absorption (FTA-ABS) test. *Health Laboratory Science*, **5,** 23.

WILKINSON, A. E. & JOHNSTON, N. A. (1959) Results of parallel tests with the Reiter protein complement-fixation test, the treponemal immobilization test and the treponemal Wasserman reaction on 1046 sera. *British Journal of Venereal Diseases*, **35,** 175.

WILKINSON, A. E. & SEQUEIRA, P. J. L. (1955) Studies on the treponemal immobilization test. *British Journal of Venereal Diseases*, **31,** 143.

WILKINSON, A. E., TAYLOR, C. E. D., MCSWIGGAN, TURNER, G. C., RYCROFT, J. A. & LOWE, G. H. (1972) Laboratory diagnosis of venereal disease. *Public Health Laboratory Service Monograph Series No.* 1. London: H.M.S.O.

WORLD HEALTH ORGANISATION BULLETIN (1951) Cardiolipin antigens, **4,** 151.

40. Leptospira

The genus *Leptospira* consists of a group of spirochaetal organisms some of which cause leptospirosis in animals and secondarily in man. It includes both saprophytic and parasitic members. Only one species is recognized, viz. *Leptospira interrogans*, but there are many serotypes that are distinguished by cross-agglutination and agglutinin-absorption tests or by agglutinogenic factor analysis. There are two main groups or 'complexes', designated interrogans and biflexa, the former containing most of the pathogenic serotypes. Classically, the infection in man, a zoonosis, occurs as a haemorrhagic jaundice (Weil's disease), but a febrile anicteric syndrome is common and benign meningitis may be the most prominent feature. Serological tests have also shown that infection may occur without any obvious symptoms of disease being produced. These subclinical cases are mostly found in certain occupational groups, e.g. agricultural workers where the risk of infection is high.

Morphology. Spiral organisms, 6–20 μm in length, 0·15–0·2 μm in diameter and 0·3–0·5 μm in wavelength. The coils are very numerous and so closely set together that they are difficult to demonstrate in stained preparations though quite obvious by dark-ground illumination. In addition to these 'elementary' spirals, larger secondary coils may be seen especially in stained films. Hooked ends are a characteristic feature but are not always present. Active movement is observed in fresh preparations examined with the dark ground microscope. The movement is mainly rotary with rapid spinning around the long axis, but the organisms are also seen to glide across the fields, sometimes with a sinuous, boring movement especially in semi-solid media, with either end foremost, occasionally bending and straightening again into the characteristic rigid form.

Staining. Can be stained by aniline dyes and by silver impregnation methods of Levaditi and Fontana (q.v.) but satisfactory results are not readily achieved. Faulkner and Lillie's modification of Warthin-Starry silver impregnation technique is suitable for demonstrating leptospires in individual sections of infected tissue (Faine, 1965).

Cultivation. Liquid, semi-solid or solid media may be used. The addition of either serum or bovine albumin (fraction V) with tween (polysorbate) as in EM medium (Ellinghausen and McCulloch, 1965) is necessary. Rabbit serum is the most satisfactory serum since it contains the highest concentration of bound vitamin B_{12} which is essential for the multiplication of leptospires, but guinea-pig, cattle and sheep serum may be used provided no natural antibodies are present (serum should be tested for the presence of leptospiral antibodies before it is incorporated in the medium). Because individual animal serum may be unsuitable, it is advisable to use pooled sera from many animals (commercially produced serum is available). Liquid media are used for preparing antigenic suspensions and for serological tests: Stuart's and Korthof's and EM liquid media are recommended. Semi-solid media are prepared by adding 0·2–0·5 per cent w/v agar to any suitable liquid media. Agar appears to favour the multiplication of leptospires and semi-solid media are used for isolating strains. They have the advantage of evaporating less rapidly than liquid media and are thought to maintain the virulence of the organisms far longer since subculturing need not be done so frequently. They may also be used for the intravenous inoculation of rabbits in order to produce hyperimmune serum. Fletcher's medium and Dinger's modification of Noguchi's medium are examples of semi-solid media. Solid culture medium (Cox and Larson, 1957; Cox, 1966) contained in Petri dishes has been successfully used for the isolation of leptospires from contaminated material such as water or urine. It contains 0·8–1·3 per cent w/v agar depending on the brand: the optimum concentration must be determined by trial. The organisms produce discrete hemi-spherical colonies just below the surface of the medium.

They may be difficult to see without oblique light and a dark background. For best results the agar should be 6–8 mm deep, the Petri dishes should be sealed to prevent dehydration and incubated in a moist chamber or in polythene bags. Incubation should be continued for up to six weeks if necessary. Kirschner and Graham (1959) used solid medium in test-tubes and found it suitable for isolating strains from homogenized liver and kidney tissue and for the maintenance of strains. Growth appears as a turbidity extending downwards for 10–20 mm.

Leptospires grow best between 28°C and 32°C.

Viability. It is unlikely that the pathogenic serotypes multiply much outside the animal body although they may survive for many days if the external conditions are favourable. They require moisture for their survival and since they are particularly susceptible to acid, they seldom remain viable for long in localities where the pH of the water is less than 6·8. Salt water has a deleterious effect. They die out rapidly in acid urine, in sewage and in badly polluted water. They are susceptible to heat: 10 min at 50°C or 10 sec at 60°C kills them. They may survive for a time in infected animal tissue provided it is kept at a low temperature; thus guinea-pig liver has remained infective for up to 26 days at 4°C and for 100 days at −20°C and leptospires of the serotype *canicola* have been cultured from pigs' kidneys from a butcher's shop. They are rapidly dissolved by bile and by trypsin. The organisms in culture and in experimental animals are moderately sensitive to penicillin, streptomycin and the tetracyclines and these antibiotics may have value as therapeutic agents in man if given *early* in the infection.

Laboratory Diagnosis

Because of variability in the severity of the infection and the frequent absence of jaundice, leptospirosis should always be considered in cases of undiagnosed pyrexia when the patient is likely to have been exposed to infection either through the conditions of his work or from some other cause (see above).

When attempting a laboratory diagnosis of suspected leptospirosis, the following points should be borne in mind: (a) During the first week of illness, leptospires are present in the blood, but leptospiraemia is rare after the eighth day. (b) Leptospires may be present in the urine during the second week of the illness and continue to be excreted intermittently for 4 to 6 weeks after the onset (infrequently for longer periods). They are more readily detected during the second and third weeks than later. Since leptospires are very sensitive to acid urine and may be lysed by antibodies present in the urine, the urine should be examined immediately after being voided. (c) Antibodies may generally be detected in the blood serum towards the end of the first week (although their demonstration is occasionally delayed for longer periods) and increase in amount during the second and third weeks, after which they begin to decline. Residual amounts of agglutinating antibodies may remain for many years after an infection. It is advisable to examine a specimen of serum during the early days of the illness and at 4 to 5 day intervals thereafter in order to demonstrate a rise in titre. This is necessary to eliminate the possibility that the reaction may be due to residual antibodies. Paradoxical reactions in which the titres of heterologous antibodies may at first exceed those of the homologous ones are also clarified in this way.

EXAMINATION OF BLOOD (a) *Dark-ground Microscopy*. During the first week leptospires may be detected by dark-ground microscopic examination of untreated blood. Only a small percentage of cases of leptospiraemia are likely to be detected in this way, but the technique of differential centrifugation of Ruys (Wolff, 1954) may enhance the chances of seeing the organisms and thereby make an early diagnosis possible. This is done on a blood specimen to which a buffered anticoagulant (pH 8) has been added. (1 ml of 1 per cent solution of sodium oxalate in buffer to 10 ml blood or 1 ml of 1 per cent 'liquoid' in sterile saline to 5 ml blood. These are preferable to sodium citrate which may have a deleterious effect on leptospires). The blood is centrifuged at 500 rev/min for 15 min. A drop of plasma is examined by dark-ground microscopy (guinea-pigs may be inoculated with the sediment). If negative the plasma is centrifuged at 10 000 rev/min for 20 minutes and the sediment examined microscopically. (b) *Cultivation*. Bijou bottles containing 3 ml fluid culture medium are inoculated with 3 to 4 drops of the patient's whole blood, great care being paid to aseptic technique (leptospires will not usually grow in the presence of contaminants). Alternatively, the deposit after differential centrifugation (see above) may be re-suspended in 2·0 ml phosphate buffered saline (pH 8·1) and a few drops of it used to inoculate 4 to 6 bottles of culture medium. Daily culturing of the blood during the first few days of the infection considerably enhances the chances of isolating the organisms. (c) *Animal Inoculation*. Laboratory animals, usually guinea-pigs and hamsters, are inoculated intraperitoneally with whole blood during the first few days of the illness. Three days after inoculation and daily thereafter peritoneal fluid is withdrawn with a finely drawn-out Pasteur pipette introduced into the lower part of the abdomen while the animal is held in an upright position with stretched hind legs. As soon as leptospires are detected microscopically in the peritoneal fluid where they tend to localize during the early stages of infection, blood is withdrawn by cardiac puncture and a few drops introduced into several bottles of culture medium. Differences occur in the susceptibility of laboratory animals to the various leptospiral serotypes, thus guinea-pigs are very susceptible to serotype *icterohaemorrhagiae*, whereas the golden hamster (*Cricetus auratus*) is more susceptible than the guinea-pig to serotype *canicola*. The animals should be used when about 6 weeks old, since older animals may be more resistant. In typical cases, the inoculated animals die in 8 to 12 days with jaundice, haemorrhages in the lungs, under the serous membranes and in the muscles.

EXAMINATION OF URINE. During the second and third weeks and sometimes for longer periods leptospires may be present in the urine. They may be seen by dark-ground examination of the sediment after centrifuging a portion of the urine at 3000 rev/min for 10 minutes. Direct culture of urine is not usually successful because of contaminating organisms, but they may be demonstrated by the inoculation of two young guinea-pigs intraperitoneally with 2 ml of freshly voided urine and subsequent culture of the animals' blood (see above).

IDENTIFICATION OF NEWLY ISOLATED STRAINS. The procedure of identifying newly isolated strains may be a lengthy one and require the use of stock antigens and antisera not available in the average diagnostic laboratory. In such cases, or whenever there is doubt about the identity of a newly isolated strain, it is recommended that help should be sought from one of the WHO/FAO Leptospirosis reference laboratories. For the addresses of these laboratories see WHO Report (1967).

SEROLOGICAL DIAGNOSIS. Two methods are described below for carrying out a diagnostic serological investigation of the patient's serum.

1. *Microscopic agglutination test.* The following technique is based on the standard procedure used in laboratories throughout the world and first developed by Schuffner (see Wolff, 1954).

For the test well-grown cultures of leptospires in Korthof's or Stuart's media are used. They should be from 7 to 10 days old and uniform in suspension. Separate tests are set up against each serotype likely to be responsible for the case under investigation. Dilutions of the patient's serum are made by the dropping method either in tubes or in depressions in porcelain plates. The procedure is summarized in Table 40.1.

The mixtures are incubated at 32°C (or 37°C) for 3 hours and allowed to stand at room temperature for 1 hour before being read. Alternatively, if specimens are received late in the day the test mixtures are kept in the refrigerator (4°C) overnight and read the following morning. Place a drop from each tube on a slide and examine with a 16 mm objective using dark-ground illumination. Wolff advocates the use of water instead of immersion oil between the condenser and the slide since it gives adequate illumination and is much cleaner than oil. It is not necessary to place a cover-slip over the drop and if each drop is quickly examined consecutively a large number may be included on one slide. Agglutination appears as lightly refractile, spherical masses of living leptospires. Lysis, which was previously thought to occur, does not take place.

Table 40.1

Tube No.	(1)	(2)r	(3)	(4)	(5)	(6)
First row:						
Saline	8	9	9			drops
Serum	2	1,	1,			drops
		from (1)	from (2)			
Dilution of serum	5	50	500			
Second row:						
Culture	3	3	3	3	3	3 drops
Saline		2		2		2 drops
Serum 1 in 500					3	1 drops
Serum 1 in 50			3	1		drops
Serum 1 in 5	3	1				drops
Final dilution:	10	30	100	300	1 000	3000

2. *Agglutination test* (*Broom*). This involves essentially the same technique as the above method except that to kill the cultures add formaldehyde to give a final concentration of 0·08 per cent. The formalin should be neutralized with magnesium carbonate, since any traces of formic acid will cause non-specific agglutination. For screening purposes, a battery of pools of antigens, consisting of formolized suspensions, representing every leptospiral serogroups may be used. By this means agglutinins of all known serotypes should be detected. The serum-antigen mixtures are kept in the refrigerator overnight before being examined for agglutination. Agglutination appears as loose, irregular cotton-wool-like clumps, quite different from agglutinated living leptospires. Killed antigens are more convenient and safe for routine work and stock suspensions of various serotypes may be stored until required. Titres of agglutination are slightly lower than those attained with living cultures.

Diagnostic titres. The titre of the serum is regarded as the highest dilution in which 50 per cent or more of the leptospires are agglutinated. This is judged by the proportion of organisms free in suspension between the agglutinated clumps. Since many serotypes are related serologically (e.g. *canicola* and *icterohaemorrhagiae* have common antigens) there may be a certain amount of cross-reaction between the strains used in one test. Bearing in mind the possibility of non-specific agglutination and residual antibodies (see above) the significance of a single positive titre must remain in doubt unless and until a rising titre can be demonstrated.

A control must be included in both methods.

Other serological tests may also be employed. A rapid macroscopic-slide test has been devised by Galton *et al.* (1958) and is being used in some laboratories as a screening test. In the *erythrocyte sensitization test* (Chang and McComb, 1954), human red blood cells are treated with an ethanol extract of leptospires and are rendered agglutinable by serum antibodies. In the *sensitized erythrocyte lysis test* (Sharp, 1958), the addition of complement to this system causes the lysis of sensitized cells. Both these tests are genus specific, their main value being the rapid screening of human sera for evidence of antibodies resulting from leptospiroses of all kinds.

Complement-fixation tests are now being used for screening purposes. Previously, the antigens used were type-specific in their reaction. Sturdza and Elian (1960) reported successful results from a genus specific antigen prepared by adding sodium merthiolate in a concentration of 1 in 10 000 to an 8–10 day-old culture of the saprophytic serotype *biflexa* strain Patoc 1, and this antigen is recommended for use in laboratories where complement fixation tests are used routinely (Turner, 1968). For example, the antigen can be included in the battery of viral antigens used for screening sera from patients suffering from PUO. The complement-fixation test can be used to exclude leptospiroses as a cause of jaundice or aseptic meningitis.

EXAMINATION OF RATS AND OTHER

RODENTS FOR LEPTOSPIRAL INFECTION. Carcases of rats dead for even a few hours are unsatisfactory for examination. Whenever possible the live animal should be sent to the laboratory. It is then possible to anaesthetize the animal and to obtain blood by cardiac puncture for examination by the methods described. Indirect evidence of infection can be obtained by the agglutination test with serum since infected animals can have low titres of agglutinins or even be seronegative the kidneys should also be examined by both cultivation and animal inoculation methods.

In screening rats and other rodents for leptospiral infection satisfactory results have been obtained by inoculating culture media with small particles of kidney tissue punched out with a sterile Pasteur pipette after the surface of the kidney has been seared with a red-hot scalpel blade.

EXAMINATION OF WATER FOR PATHOGENIC LEPTOSPIRES. This can be done by immersing a shaved and scarified area of skin of a young guinea-pig in the water for an hour at 30°C. Infection takes place through the skin with the resulting characteristic condition as described above.

Pathogenic Leptospires

Over 100 different pathogenic serotypes have been identified, many of which are associated with disease in man. They tend to differ in the degree of their pathogenicity to man and animals and in their natural hosts, but the only reliable method of classifying them is on the basis of their serological differences demonstrated by agglutination and agglutinin-absorption tests.

In Great Britain serological evidence has shown that at least 7 leptospiral serogroups are represented, although only two serotypes, viz. *icterohaemorrhagiae* and *canicola* have so far been isolated from human cases of leptospirosis. It has been ascertained that field mice, voles and hedgehogs are carriers of a number of pathogenic serotypes, e.g. *sejroe*, *saxkoebing*, *bratislava* and *ballum* (Broom and Coghlan, 1958, 1960). Man may become infected indirectly from contact with contaminated vegetation or by handling animals, e.g. cattle that have become infected through grazing on fields contaminated by the urine of these small wild animals.

The following exemplify the various pathogenic serotypes which have been recognized in different parts of the world.

Icterohaemorrhagiae. This organism is one of the more virulent forms of Leptospira. It is the most frequent cause of classical Weil's disease (haemorrhagic jaundice) although milder conditions may result. It is carried by species of rats (notably *R. norvegicus*) and other rodents in all parts of the world and human cases arise under conditions where rats abound.

Canicola. This serotype is closely related antigenically to *icterohaemorrhagiae* but may be distinguished from it by serological tests. It is the cause of so-called 'canicola fever' in man and of a common infection of dogs characterized by nephritis often chronic in nature and, rather inconstantly, by a variable degree of jaundice. The leptospires are excreted in large numbers and may invade through abrasions in the skin of people whose hands become contaminated with dog urine. Other animals including pigs may become accidentally infected, and piggery workers have contracted the infection through handling infected pigs (Coghlan, Norval and Seiler, 1957).

Canicola fever in man is one of the milder forms of leptospirosis, in which meningeal symptoms predominate. Jaundice is only occasionally produced and then only in a slight degree. As with most forms of leptospirosis, renal involvement is a common feature, but the symptoms vary considerably in their intensity. The disease is rarely fatal.

Hebdomadis. This organism is responsible for 'seven-day fever' of the East, which is a non-icteric febrile illness with meningitis. It is carried by a field-mouse (*Microtus montebelloi*) and consequently, field workers are liable to the infection through contaminated with infected mouse urine.

Autumnalis. This organism has been found associated with a disease in Japan called Akiyami or harvest sickness clinically indistinguishable from 'seven-day fever'. *Autumnalis* can be distinguished from *hebdomadis* by its high infectivity to guinea-pigs, in which it produces typical haemorrhagic jaundice. It is carried by certain species of field-mice and rats. 'Fort Bragg fever', which occurred among troops in North Carolina, U.S.A., was found by serological tests to have been caused by a closely related organism.

Pomona. This organism was first isolated from cases of 'seven-day fever' among dairy farmers in North Queensland. It was later found to be the cause of 'swineherds'' disease in Switzerland. Pigs act as the reservoir hosts and usually suffer little effect; cattle are susceptible, especially calves and pregnant cows. In the U.S.A. the infection causes a heavy yearly loss of cattle due to jaundice and haemoglobinuria of calves and abortion in cows and pigs. The organism has been isolated in many parts of the world from human and animal sources. Certain species of field-mice may also act as carrier hosts.

Grippotyphosa has been described as the cause of 'swamp fever' of Europe and certain parts of Asia, Africa, Israel and U.S.A. It usually attacks agricultural workers and usually produces a relatively mild illness with a low mortality rate resembling canicola fever. Various species of voles carry the organism. In the U.S.S.R. and Israel, cattle have been seriously affected.

Pyrogenes produces a febrile illness with or without jaundice and varying in its severity. It occurs among field workers in Indonesia and other parts of the Far East. Certain species of rats appear to act as reservoirs of infection.

Zanoni, a serotype within the Pyrogenes serogroup and serotype *australis* are causal agents of 'Cane fever' in North Queensland. Sugarcane workers are mainly affected, but *zanoni* may also infect urban dwellers. The illness is comparatively mild but convalescence is protracted. Lymphadenitis is a common feature. Certain species of rat are the carriers of the organism.

Bataviae. This organism causes leptospirosis of rice-field workers in Italy, where the field-mouse (*Micromys minutus sorcinus*) is the reservoir host. The disease in that part of the world is comparatively mild and jaundice is rare. In S.E. Asia, however, where the chief carrier host is the brown rat (*R. norvegicus*) cases are much more severe, jaundice is common and death may occur.

Sejroe was first observed in human infection in the island of Sejroe (Denmark). It has also been recorded in other parts of Europe. The disease is relatively mild. Certain species of rodents are carriers of the organism, and related strains have been isolated from rodents in Great Britain.

REFERENCES AND FURTHER READING

BROOM, J. C. & COGHLAN, J. D. (1958) Leptospira ballum in small rodents in Scotland. *Lancet*, **ii**, 1041.

BROOM, J. C. & COGHLAN, J. D. (1960) Leptospira bratislava isolated from a hedgehog in Scotland. *Lancet*, **i**, 1326.

CHANG, R. S. & McCOMB, D. E. (1954) Erythrocyte sensitizing substances from five strains of Leptospirae. *American Journal of Tropical Medicine and Hygiene*, **3**, 481.

COGHLAN, J. D., NORVAL, J. & SEILER, H. E. (1957) Canicola fever in man through contact with infected pigs. *British Medical Journal*, **i**, 257.

COX, C. D. (1966) Studies on the isolation and growth of Leptospira from surface waters. *Annales de la Société belge de médecine tropicale*, **46**, 193.

COX, C. D. & LARSON, A. D. (1957) Colonial growth of leptospirae. *Journal of Bacteriology*, **73**, 4, 587.

ELLINGHAUSEN, H. C. & McCULLOCH, W. G. (1965) Nutrition of *Leptospira pomona* and growth of 13 other serotypes. Fractionation of oleic albumin complex and a medium of bovine albumin and polysorbate 80. *American Journal of Veterinary Research*, **26**, 45.

FAINE, S. (1965) Silver staining of spirochaetes in single tissue sections. *Journal of Clinical Pathology*, **18**, 381.

GALTON, M. M., POWERS, D. K., HALL, A. D. & CORNELL, R. G. (1958) A rapid macroscopic-slide screening test for serodiagnosis of leptospirosis. *American Journal of Veterinary Research*, **19**, 71, 505.

KIRSCHNER, L. & GRAHAM, L. (1959) Growth purification and maintenance of Leptospira on solid media. *British Journal of Experimental Research*, **40**, 57.

SHARP, C. F. (1958) Laboratory diagnosis of leptospirosis with the sensitized-erythrocyte lysis test. *Journal of Pathology and Bacteriology*, **76**, 349.

STURDZA, N. & ELIAN, M. (1961) Comparative study on different strains of *L. biflexa* as antigen for the complement fixation test in leptospirosis. *Archives roumaines de pathologie expérimentale et de microbiologie*, **20**, 33.

TURNER, L. H. (1967) Leptospirosis I. *Transactions of the Royal Society of Tropical Medicine and Hygiene*, **61**, No. 6, 842.

TURNER, L. H. (1967) Leptospirosis II. *Transactions of the Royal Society of Tropical Medicine and Hygiene*, **62**, No. 6, 881.

WOLFF, J. W. (1954) *The Laboratory Diagnosis of Leptospirosis.* Springfield: Thomas.

WORLD HEALTH ORGANIZATION (1959) Joint WHO/FAO. Export committee on zoonoses. 2nd report. *World Health Organization Technical Report Series*, No. 180.

WORLD HEALTH ORGANIZATION (1967) Current problems in leptospirosis research. *World Health Organization Technical Report Series*, No. 380.

41. Chlamydia

The chlamydiae are a group of small intracellular parasites. They contain both DNA and RNA; stain poorly with Gram's stain but can be seen after staining by Machiavello, Castenada or Giemsa's method as either elementary bodies (300 nm) or initial bodies (800–1200 nm) in the cytoplasm of infected cells. These microorganisms are sensitive to broad spectrum antibiotics and in laboratory systems to penicillin. They cause a variety of clinical conditions including trachoma, inclusion conjunctivitis, lymphogranuloma venereum and psittacosis (see Vol. 1, Chapter 50).

Laboratory Diagnosis

Specimens

Smears from TRIC infections (i.e. eye, cervix or urethral smears) on clean slides; scrapes or swabs from eye or genital infections in 2SP (sucrose phosphate medium) (Gordon *et al.,* 1969) containing 3 per cent foetal calf serum; sputum from cases of psittacosis, or paired sera. These organisms should *not* be put in viral transport medium, as the organisms are sensitive to penicillin, but in the sucrose phosphate medium, kept as cold as possible and sent to the laboratory without delay (Thygeson and Hanna, 1969).

Laboratory Treatment of Specimens

Smears

After the smears have been fixed with methanol, they may be stained by Giemsa's method and examined for the presence of initial bodies in the cytoplasm of the epithelial cells or for elementary bodies in the cytoplasm or free (see colour plate 13, Vol. 1). Should the smear prove positive, a second smear may be stained with Lugol's iodine and examined for the presence of glycogen matrices; subgroup A chlamydiae have such matrices; subgroup B do not. The type of result is illustrated in the colour plates 13–15 of Vol. 1.

Preparation of Specimens for Isolation

Specimens for isolation collected in 2SP plus 3 per cent foetal calf serum should be disintegrated by glass beads in a Whirlmix for 1 min followed by indirect sonication for 7 min (Gordon *et al.,* 1969). Sputum should be homogenized with glass beads, treated with streptomycin and lightly centrifuged to remove cellular debris.

Culture of the Treated Specimens in Experimental Systems

Seven to eight day old embryos

1. Introduce 0.2 ml by the yolk sac route and incubate at 35°C (Chap. 10).
2. Candle the eggs daily; discard any embryos which die within 24 h post-inoculation.
3. Harvest the yolk sac from any embryos which die subsequently or are sacrificed 12 days post-inoculation.
4. Make yolk sac impression smears from the stalk.
5. Fix and stain by Machiavello, Castenada or Giminez (1964) methods.
6. Examine for initial and elementary bodies.
7. If the smears from the harvested embryos are negative, the yolk sac should be ground up in a Ten Broek tube and the suspension passed to a further batch of embryos; attention is drawn to the hazards of cross-contamination between batches of embryos in this blind passage procedure.

Mice

1. 0.5 ml may be introduced intraperitoneally into mice.
2. At necropsy make impression smears of the spleen.
3. Fix and stain by Giemsa's method.
4. Examine for the presence of initial and elementary bodies.

Tissue Culture in Irradiated McCoy Cells (Darouger, Kinnison and Jones, 1971) or BHK cells (Taverne and Blyth, 1971)

Preparation of McCoy cell cultures.

1. Inoculate a Falcon flask with McCoy cells in Eagle's medium (Chap. 9) containing 5 per cent foetal calf serum, no penicillin but 100 μg/ml vancomycin and 25 units/ml of nystatin in addition to the usual streptomycin.

2. When the monolayer is complete, irradiate the flask with 4500–6000 rad from an X-ray source.

3. Reincubate the culture for five to seven days.

4. Trypsinize, count and resuspend the cells at a concentration of 10^5/ml (Chap. 9) in modified Eagle's medium as above.

5. Dispense the cells in 1 ml amounts in flat-bottomed polystyrene bijou bottles (Sterilin) containing a sterile 13 mm No. 3 Chance glass coverslip.

6. Reincubate for two days to allow the cells to attach to the coverslip.

Inoculation of the tissue culture.

1. Make the specimen up to 2 ml with modified Eagle's medium.

2. Add 0.5 ml specimen to each of two tubes.

3. Centrifuge for 1 h at 2700 g in an MSE 'Super minor' centrifuge.

4. Incubate 2 h at 35°C.

5. Discard the medium containing the inoculum.

6. Add 1 ml fresh growth medium.

7. Incubate for about 60 h at 35°C.

8. Wash the cells several times with phosphate buffer (pH 6.8).

9. Fix in methanol 10 min.

10. Stain by Giemsa's method.

11. Examine by dark field microscopy; Giemsa-stained inclusions appear yellow.

12. If the first coverslip is positive, the second may either be stored at −70°C to act as the inoculum for further studies or stained with iodine to assign the chlamydiae to subgroup A or B. If the first coverslip is negative, incubation of the second one should be continued for a total time of 72 h before being stained by Giemsa's method.

Identification of the Isolated Chlamydiae

The chlamydiae may be provisionally identified by the appearance of the Giemsa and iodine stained smears and confirmed by immunofluorescence using a group antiserum. Subgroup A may now be subdivided for epidemiological purposes by the micro-immunofluorescence test using type-specific antisera (Dwyer et al., 1972).

Examination of Sera

Serological examination of paired sera from patients may be carried out by the complement fixation test using the group antigen (Chap. 11). If avian sera are being examined, the indirect complement fixation test must be employed (Meyer, Eddie and Schachter, 1969).

2SP (Sucrose Phosphate Medium) (Gordon et al., 1969)

0.2M sucrose in 0.02M phosphate buffer pH 7.2. Vancomycin 100 μg/ml, streptomycin 50 μg/ml should be added to this solution which can be stored for short periods at 4°C.

REFERENCES

DAROUGER, S., KINNISON, J. R. & JONES, B. R. (1971) Simplified irradiated McCoy cell culture for the isolation of Chlamydiae. In *Trachoma and Related Disorders Caused by Chlamydial Agents*, p. 63, edited by R. L. Nichols. Amsterdam: Excerpta Medica.

DWYER, R. ST. C., TREHARNE, J. D., JONES, B. R. & HERRING, J. (1972) Results of micro-immunofluorescence tests for the detection of type-specific antibody in certain chlamydial infections. *British Journal of Venereal Diseases*, **48**, 452.

GIMINEZ, D. F. (1964) Staining rickettsiae in yolk sac cultures. *Stain Technology*, **39**, 135.

GORDON, F. B., HARPER, I. A., QUAN, A. L., TREHARNE, J. D., DWYER, R. ST. C. & GARLAND, J. A. (1969). Detection of Chlamydia (Bedsonia) in certain infections of man. 1. Laboratory procedures: Comparison of yolk sac and cell culture for detection and isolation. *Journal of Infectious Diseases*, **120**, 451.

MEYER, K. F., EDDIE, B. & SCHACHTER, J. (1969) Psittacosis—Lymphogranuloma venereum agents. In *Diagnostic procedures for Viral and Rickettsial Infections*, edited by E. H. Lennette and N. J. Schmidt. New York: American Public Health Association Incorporated.

TAVERNE, J. & BLYTH, W. A. (1971) Interactions between trachoma organisms and macrophages. In *Trachoma and Related Disorders Caused by Chlamydial Agents*, p. 88, edited by R. L. Nichols. Amsterdam: Excerpta Medica.

THYGESON, P. & HANNA, L. (1969). TRIC agents. In *Diagnostic Procedures for Viral and Rickettsial Infections*, 4th edn., edited by E. H. Lennette and N. J. Schmidt, New York. American Public Health Association Incorporated.

42. Rickettsiae

Rickettsiae are small coccobacillary or filamentous prokaryotes, about a third of the size of bacteria, that grow in the cytoplasm or nuclei of mammalian and other cells and, with the exception of *Rickettsia quintana*, are unable to grow in cell-free media. They are found in arthropods such as lice, fleas and ticks and also can infect a wide range of vertebrate hosts, including man. Human rickettsial infections include epidemic typhus (*R. prowazekii*); endemic typhus (*R. mooseri*); the spotted fever group (*R. rickettsi, R. conori, R. akari*, etc.); scrub typhus (*R. tsutsugamushi*); trench fever (*R. quintana*) and Q fever (*Coxiella burnetii*). The cell biology of the organisms, their ecology, the clinical aspects of human infection and an outline of laboratory diagnosis is described in Volume 1, Chapter 51.

LABORATORY METHODS FOR DIAGNOSIS OF RICKETTSIAL INFECTIONS

The present chapter describes a limited number of laboratory diagnostic methods; necessarily so because the isolation of rickettsiae in laboratory hosts such as guinea pigs, mice, cotton rats or hamsters, and, in particular, their propagation in the chick embryo (CE) yolk sac is a hazardous operation that should not be attempted in general microbiological or clinical pathology laboratories. Even in specialist laboratories there has been a substantial number of infections with typhus and Q fever rickettsiae. Some of these outbreaks have followed the adaptation of rickettsiae to the CE yolk sac where they grow profusely. The processing of the lungs and spleens of experimentally infected animals, or of naturally infected ruminant placentas or infected arthropods may also be hazardous. *Consequently cultivation of the organisms in animals, eggs or cell cultures should be restricted to laboratory staffed by vaccinated workers and equipped with safety cabinets, centrifuges with windshields, sealed blenders operated in safety cabinets and other 'high risk' facilities* (see Chap. 16). *There should also be segregated animal accommodation.*

Methods for the diagnosis of rickettsial infections within the competence of the general laboratory include serological tests for complement fixing (CF) or other antibodies to typhus or spotted fever rickettsiae or *C. burnetii*, together with the Weil–Felix agglutination reaction with suspensions of non-motile Proteus strains. In addition, guinea pigs may be inoculated with material suspected to contain *C. burnetii* and subsequently tested for development of antibody, but preferably should not be autopsied and their tissues examined for rickettsiae or used for 'blind passage' to fresh animals.

COMPLEMENT FIXATION TESTS FOR TYPHUS AND Q FEVER: SOURCES AND STANDARDISATION OF ANTIGENS

Phase 1 and Phase 2 CF antigens from *C. burnetii* are available from a number of commercial and non-commercial sources, but the availability of typhus and spotted fever CF antigens is now very restricted. For the initial diagnosis of the typhus or spotted fever groups the distinct, specific, soluble CF antigens characteristic of each group, prepared by ether extraction of a saline suspension of infected yolk sacs, are satisfactory. Because of the supply difficulty it may be mentioned that typhus group, spotted fever group and Q fever antigen and antisera are retailed by Beckman Instruments, Diagnostic Operations, 2500 Harbor Blvd., Fullerton, Calif. 92634; soluble typhus and Q fever antigens are also marketed by the Commonwealth Serum Laboratories, Parkville, Melbourne, Australia. Lederles, at one time a prime source of supply for antigens, is no longer producing them and stocks have been transferred to the Communicable Disease Center, Atlanta, Ga., who may be able to assist. A Q fever antigen suitable for the capillary agglutination test is produced by Veterinaria AG, Gruben Str. 40, Zurich 1, Switzerland.

Finally the Standards Laboratory, Central Public Health Laboratory, Public Health Laboratory Service, produce Q fever Phase 1 and 2 CF antigens for restricted distribution. (This list makes no claim to be complete nor does it constitute sponsorship of any particular preparation.)

CF antigens from scrub typhus rickettsiae are more strain specific although group reactions may be obtained by immunofluorescence; the serological diagnosis of these infections is a specialized matter outside the scope of the general laboratory.

The CF test described in Chapter 11 can be used with typhus, spotted fever and Q fever antigens; viz., with the microtitre plates, a unit volume of 0·025 ml, 2 MHD of complement and overnight incubation at 4°C. Antigens should first be titrated in 'chessboard' fashion against a known positive serum from the species to be tested; it is known, for example, that the fixation area and the optimal antigen concentration of *C. burnetii* CF antigen may differ markedly with antisera from human and sheep. The optimal antigen dilution (i.e. that giving the highest serum titre), or 4 to 8 units of antigen if there is no clear optimal concentration, is also tested against 2, 1·5, 1·0 MHD of complement and should show no anticomplementary effect at 1·0 MHD. Antigens may also be checked against Wassermann-positive sera for non-specific reactivity and ideally control antigens from non-infected yolk sac should also be available. Antigens should be stored unfrozen at 4°C.

PREPARATION OF SERA FOR TESTING. Human and guinea pig sera rarely react non-specifically with rickettsial antigens, but sera from other animal species, e.g. sheep, may do so, particularly after storage for long periods. All sera are heat inactivated at 56°C for 30 min. Sera that react non-specifically after this treatment may be treated by the CO_2 method of Imam and Alfy (1966). In this the serum is diluted 1 part in 10 with sterile distilled water and a small piece of dry ice added. After the gas has bubbled off, any precipitate is removed by centrifugation. The tonicity of the supernatant fluid is restored with 8·5 per cent saline solution and the mixture is heat-inactivated before use in the CF test.

A range of serum dilutions from 10 to 1280 will usually bracket the end point. Alternatively, convalescent phase serum specimens may be 'screened' at dilutions of 10 and 40 and positive reactors retitrated over the range of dilutions along with the acute phase serum sample. Test antigens for a patient with suspected Q fever, typhus or Brill's disease in the United Kingdom (UK) would normally include the group soluble CF antigen for epidemic and murine typhus and the Phase 2 CF antigen of *C. burnetii*. Rickettsial pox has not been identified in the UK or Western Europe although present in the USSR; a history of a recent visit to an endemic area of other rickettsioses (e.g. boutonneuse fever in the Mediterranean, see Vol. 1, Table 51.1) might lead to the inclusion of *R. akari* CF antigen to detect infection with the spotted fever group.

INTERPRETATION OF CF RESULTS. CF antibody generally appears in the second week of typhus and Q fever and, given negative results with control antigen, the demonstration of a four-fold or greater rise in antibody level is definitive. The observation of an antibody titre of 160 or more in a single serum specimen may be a pointer to recent or current infection, particularly if surveys of healthy persons in the same geographical area have not revealed antibody at such a level. However, the evidence is still less certain than with a change in antibody level. The antibody response to infection may be delayed by antibiotic treatment; therefore clinically suspect, but seronegative patients should be resampled at 4 and 6 weeks from the onset of illness and the sera titrated in 'chessboard' fashion against antigen so as to detect a feeble antibody response.

Reactions against the group soluble CF antigen of epidemic and murine typhus, or against that of the spotted fever group, do not define the species of rickettsia causing the infection. This may be determined by examination of the sera with washed rickettsial suspensions either in the CF reaction or by agglutination; higher titres are obtained against the infecting organism. However, because of the scarcity of the antigens these procedures are available only in a few reference laboratories (see Elisberg and Bozeman, 1969, for further details). Sera reacting with *C.*

burnetii, Phase 2 CF antigen should be titrated with Phase 1 antigen if there is a clinical suspicion of endocarditis or chronic infection (see Vol. 1, page 528).

WEIL–FELIX REACTION

This reaction depends on the fortuitous similarity of antigenic determinants between various rickettsiae on the one hand, and certain non-motile strains of *Proteus vulgaris* and *Proteus mirabilis* on the other. Agglutinins to the *Proteus* strains (probably in the IgM fraction of the globulins) often appear quickly and this is useful diagnostically. They are heat labile so that sera should not be heat inactivated and the mixtures of Proteus agglutinating suspension and patients' serum should be incubated at 37° or 52°C – temperatures lower than those sometimes employed for the Widal reaction to detect Salmonella agglutinins.

The test can be performed in Dreyer's tubes, as with the Widal reaction. A 'master' set of serum dilutions from 5 to 640 is prepared in normal saline either in Wassermann tubes or Bijou bottles. With an automatic pipette, 0·1 ml amounts of each serum dilution are transferred to Dreyer's tubes in each of 3 rows, starting from the most dilute. Similar volumes (0·1 ml) of each of the three Proteus suspensions, OX_{19}, OX_2, OXK, previously diluted to the optical densities recommended by the manufacturers, are then added, respectively, to a row of serum dilutions and well mixed. Controls should include a tube of each bacterial suspension, mixed with a volume of saline instead of serum, to detect autoagglutinability of the bacterial suspension; ideally, a known positive control serum should be titrated against each of the suspensions to determine if they are of standard agglutinability. The racks of Dreyer's tubes are incubated for 4 h in a 37°C water bath with the bottom third of the tubes in the water, to facilitate mixing by convection. They are placed overnight at 4°C and read the next morning with a × 8 hand lens, in a light box with a dark background. Agglutination is of the granular 'O' type; the walls of the Dreyer's tubes with scratched or eroded glass may be clarified for reading by dipping the tubes in a wide-mouthed bottle containing xylol.

INTERPRETATION OF WEIL–FELIX REACTION. Weil–Felix agglutinins appear around the fifth day after onset and reach peak titres, often in the thousands, in early convalescence. As with the CF reaction a rising antibody level between acute and convalescent samples of serum offers the soundest evidence of infection. Sera from patients with various rickettsioses agglutinate the different Proteus suspensions to different titres (see Vol. 1, Table 51.2); these patterns, together with the CF results, may indicate broadly the infecting species of rickettsia. Note that patients with Q fever, trench fever and rickettsialpox do not develop Weil–Felix agglutinins and that those with the recrudescent form of epidemic typhus (Brill–Zinsser disease) are frequently negative. Consequently a negative result does not finally exclude a rickettsial infection. False positive results, usually lower, unchanging, levels of antibody, may be found in patients with urinary tract infection with *Proteus sp.*, in leptospirosis, liver disease and a variety of other conditions; out-of-date suspensions may give spurious results. Thus confirmation of a positive Weil–Felix reaction by CF or agglutination tests with specific rickettsial antigens is essential.

Other serological tests—macroscopic and microscopic agglutination reactions, immuno-fluorescence, radio-immunoprecipitation, and the agglutination of erythrocytes sensitized with antigenic fractions from typhus and spotted fever rickettsiae—have special applications and references to some of these are given by Elisberg and Bozeman (1969). The CF test is an insensitive way of measuring antibody; thus surveys of populations for evidence of exposure to *C. burnetii* by radioimmunoassay reveal a much wider distribution of reactors than is indicated by CF testing.

DEMONSTRATION OF C. BURNETII IN SPECIMENS FROM HUMAN DISEASE OR ANIMAL HOSTS

The presence of *C. burnetii* in such specimens as heparinized blood from a Q fever patient, vegetations from suspected Q fever endocarditis obtained at operation or at autopsy, or specimens of milk from infected cattle, can be demonstrated by inoculation of guinea pigs or hamsters. The number of organisms in an acute phase blood sample from a Q fever patient, or in an infected milk sample is usually small and the likelihood of the excretion of the organism in the urine of the inoculated guinea pig is also small; as judged by absence of cross-infection of guinea pigs held in the same animal house area or evidence of infection in animal attendants. This may not apply to inoculated mice which may excrete the rickettsia more readily. When larger doses of rickettsiae, for example in an ovine placenta or a cardiac valve vegetation are inoculated, urinary excretion by guinea pigs and cross-infection is more likely. For this reason it is prudent if the processing of such specimens and the handling of inoculated animals is undertaken by persons who either have antibody to *C. burnetii*, or who give a delayed hypersensitivity reaction to intradermal inoculation with *C. burnetii* vaccine. The evidence suggests that Q fever vaccines, which must be given to persons without dermal hypersensitivity, are highly effective in stimulating protection (Report, 1967).

Mature guinea pigs (around 500 g) are anaesthetized and 5 ml of blood taken by cardiac puncture. The serum is separated and tested for antibody against *C. burnetii*, phase 2 CF antigen, and held at $-20°C$. Two sero-negative animals are inoculated intraperitoneally with 3 to 5 ml of the sample (milk, heparinized blood or blood clot, etc.) without antibiotic. Note that streptomycin inhibits rickettsiae and that penicillin in large doses is toxic to guinea pigs. One or more uninoculated animals are placed in cages nearby to monitor possible cross-infection. When the patient has already formed antibody, for example in the mid-stages of an acute rickettsial infection or in Q fever endocarditis, it is probably advantageous to separate the serum from the blood clot and grind the latter in sucrose-glutamate solution with sodium rather than potassium phosphate, or in serum broth, skim milk or other protective medium. Rectal temperatures may be taken to detect a febrile response (over $40°C$ or $104°F$) in the guinea pigs. One month after inoculation all animals are again bled by cardiac puncture and the pre- and post-inoculation samples retested against *C. burnetii* CF antigen and with the typhus soluble CF antigens if indicated. A conversion to sero-positive, with negative results in the control uninoculated animals acting as sentinels for cross-infection, is good evidence of the presence of *C. burnetii* in the inoculum and no further passages nor visualization of the organism in spleen smears or by subculture in the CF yolk sac are required. Negative guinea pigs, or those with equivocal serological responses may be left for another 2 to 3 weeks and retested before disposal; inocula containing small numbers of organisms may not stimulate a rise in CF antibody until 6 or so weeks after inoculation. Although typhus and other rickettsiae are quite sensitive to heat and disinfectants, *C. burnetii* differs markedly and material containing this organism should if possible be autoclaved. If this is not possible formalin or gluteraldehyde should be used; phenolic disinfectants may not be effective unless they are allowed to act for several hours and preferably overnight.

MISCELLANEOUS TECHNIQUES

Microscopy and Staining

Rickettsiae in tissues, impression smears of organs, valve vegetations and the like may be stained by the overnight Giemsa technique (p. 49) or by the Machiavello or Giminez methods (p. 54, 516). Examination of thin sections of valve vegetations from suspected Q fever endocarditis in the electron microscope may be helpful in revealing the shape and internal structure of *C. burnetii* and distinguishing them from cell granules, e.g. of mast cells. Rickettsiae in smears or tissues may be stained by direct or indirect immunofluorescence (Elisberg and Bozeman, 1969) and this technique has, for example, been used in detection of *C. burnetii* in cardiac vegetations.

REFERENCES

IMAM, I. Z. E. & ALFY, L. (1966) The elimination of the anticomplementary reactions of the sera by CO_2. *Journal of the Egyptian Public Health Association*, **41**, 33–36.

ELISBERG, B. L. & BOZEMAN, F. M. (1969) Rickettsiae. In *Diagnostic Procedures for Viral and Rickettsial Infections*. Edited by Lennette, E. H. & Schmidt, N. J., 4th edition, p. 826–868. American Public Health Assoc. Inc.

REPORT (1967). *First International Conference on Vaccines against Viral and Rickettsial Diseases of Man*. PAHO Scientific Publication No. 147, May 1967, p. 517–536.

43. Mycoplasmas: Technical Methods

Mycoplasmas and Acholeplasmas, previously known as pleuropneumonia-like organisms (PPLO), are small prokaryotic cells (200–250 nm diameter). They resemble larger prokaryotic cells (e.g. bacteria) in their ability to grow in cell-free media and in the structure of their nucleus and ribosomes, but have no rigid cell wall. They have a cytoplasmic membrane, but unlike that of bacteria, it contains cholesterol or carotenol in addition to the usual neutral and phospholipids. The mycoplasmas cannot synthesize their own cholesterol and require it as a growth factor in the culture medium. The acholeplasmas synthesize carotenol as a substitute for cholesterol, but will incorporate cholesterol if it is provided. The absence of a rigid cell wall is reflected in branched and other unusual morphological forms of the mycoplasma cell. Cells of some species have a coccobacillary morphology, others are filamentous. Mycoplasmas are not inhibited by penicillin, bacitracin, polymyxin B or sulphonamides; in general they are sensitive *in vivo* to tetracycline, kanamycin, chloramphenicol, streptomycin, tylosin and to arsenical compounds and sodium aurothiomalate. Except for T-strain mycoplasmas they are more resistant to the inhibitory action of thallium salts than bacteria, a difference exploited to isolate the organisms from material contaminated with the latter. Despite some colonial similarities, mycoplasmas are distinct from L-phase variants of bacteria and do not revert to bacteria when cultured in media free of inhibitors of bacterial cell wall synthesis or other L-phase inducers (see Vol. I, Chap. 52).

Mycoplasma cells stain poorly by Gram's method but are negative. Consequently various special staining techniques are used—overnight Giemsa, Dienes' stain, cresyl-fast violet, or orcein—depending on circumstance. The cells from fluid culture may also be visualized by dark ground or phase-contrast methods in the light microscope, or in the electronmicroscope by negative contrast staining or in thin sections; some species have surface projections which resemble those of myxoviruses. The irregular shape in negative contrast preparations may present difficulties in confident identification (Wolanski and Maramorosch, 1970). Examination of thin sections offers more certainty by the recognition within the cell of the nuclear area, ribosome arrays and the trilaminar cytoplasmic membrane.

Mycoplasmas are grown in soft agar medium with a high (10–20 per cent v/v) concentration of serum or other protein such as ascitic fluid. The function of the serum or other protein is to provide a source of cholesterol, fatty acids (or urea for T-strains) and to regulate their availability to the organisms. Yeast extract, nucleic acid mixtures, tissue extracts, coenzymes and other supplements may be required according to species. Many mycoplasma species are aerobes or facultative anaerobes, others grow better in hydrogen or nitrogen with 10 per cent v/v CO_2. The mycoplasma cells multiply initially within the agar to form a ball-shaped colony that grows up to the surface of the agar and spreads along it giving a halo of delicate growth. When viewed from above such a colony presents a 'fried egg' appearance (Vol. I, Plate 52.2) with an agar-embedded centre. Colony size varies from 200–500 μm for the 'large colony' mycoplasmas to 20–50 μm for T (for tiny colony) strain mycoplasmas. Mycoplasmas also grow in broth, or in semisolid agar or diphasic broth-agar culture, with serum and other supplements. Many species grow readily in cell culture where they adhere to the cell surface and are also free in the medium. Isolation of mycoplasmas in laboratory animals does not play an important part in laboratory diagnosis although *M. pneumoniae* was first cultivated in hamsters and cotton rats and in chick embryos.

The established human mycoplasma flora comprises *M. hominis, M. pneumoniae, M. salivarium, M. orale* serotypes 1, 2 and 3, *M. fermentans,* and numerous serotypes of T-strain mycoplasmas. Other occasional isolates from human sources include *M. lipophilum* (Del

Guidice and Carski, 1968), *M. primatum,* primarily a simian mycoplasma but originally designated the 'Navel' strain, and the saprophyte, *A. laidlawii.* Jansson (1971) claims to have isolated mycoplasmas with a colony size between 3 and 30 μm, even smaller than T-strains. They require egg-yolk-containing media and a special microscopic technique for recognition; their nature as biological entities requires confirmation.

The clinical associations of the human mycoplasma flora are:

(1) *M. pneumoniae* with febrile bronchitis or pneumonia, accompanied in a proportion of patients by formation of cold haemagglutinins, *Streptococcus MG* agglutinins, biological false-positive WR, and antitissue antibodies. Also with some cases of Stevens-Johnson syndrome, erythema nodosum, meningoencephalitis, Guillain-Barré syndrome, myringitis and haemolytic anaemia.

(2) *M. hominis, M. fermentans* and T-strains with some cases of salpingitis, tubo-ovarian abscess, pelvic abscess, septic abortion and puerperal infection and fever. There is an emerging association of T-mycoplasmas with infertility, abortion and still-birth, and with prematurity and low birth weights. Colonization of the lower urinary and genital tracts by mycoplasmas is common in both sexes and is broadly related to sexual activity. Although in most studies T-mycoplasmas have been isolated more often from non-gonococcal urethritis, vaginitis and cervicitis than from controls, their etiological role in these conditions is not established (see Vol. I, Chap. 52 and reviews: Lancet, 1973 and McCormack *et al.,* 1973, also Gnarpe and Friberg, 1973).

General information on the cell biology of mycoplasmas may be found in the review by Maniloff and Morowitz (1972) and in Hayflick (1969). General accounts of clinical aspects of infection with mycoplasmas may be found in Hayflick (1969); Marmion (1967); Hodges, Fass and Saslaws (1972); Smith and Sangster (1972); Csonka and Spitzer (1969); Csonka and Corse (1970) and Fleming *et al.* (1967). Recent references to immunopathological and heterogenetic serological reactions and their effects are Clyde (1971); Costea, Yakulis, and Heller (1972); Biberfeld (1970, 1971);

Marmion, Plackett and Lemcke (1967) and Plackett *et al.* (1969).

GENERAL METHODS FOR THE HANDLING OF MYCOPLASMA CULTURES

Media. The formulae and methods of preparation of solid, semisolid and liquid media for 'large colony' and T-strain mycoplasmas are described in detail in Chapter 5, pp. 133–4.

Attention to the following points is important. There is sometimes a difference in growth-promoting properties between sera from different horses and it is advisable to test bleed a series of animals and obtain a large volume of serum from those that are satisfactory and to store it at $-20°C$ or below. Alternatively, tested serum may be available from commercial sources. Serum is used without heat inactivation. Pooled human serum is sometimes used instead of horse serum but may contain antibody to mycoplasmas. Some human mycoplasmas will grow on swine serum but the growth of *M. pneumoniae* is significantly less than on horse serum. The growth-promoting properties of serum from various animal species is related to their cholesterol content. Thus, when it is desired to grow strains of mycoplasma for immunization of rabbits, avoiding the use of a heterologous serum in the medium, it is necessary to add cholesterol to the rabbit serum in the medium (Taylor-Robinson *et al.,* 1963). The source and method of preparation of yeast extracts is important, not all commercially prepared extracts will support the growth of *M. pneumoniae.* The method described in Chapter 5 involves low temperature extraction. It is important that the pH of the extract and of the final medium should be adjusted to pH 7·0 to 8·0. Mycoplasmas are inhibited by some metal ions so it is important to use Analar grade chemicals and double distilled or ion-exchanged water in media preparation. Variation in batches of agar may make it necessary to vary concentration by trial and error; for optimal growth mycoplasmas must have a soft agar. The standard solid medium described in Chapter 5 should grow all members of the human flora, except T-strains, but may not be satisfactory for some avian or animal mycoplasmas. Formulae and supplements for some of these species are described by Lemcke (1965) and in Hayflick (1969).

Much effort has been expended in the search for growth-promoting or inhibitor-neutralizing factors, e.g. nucleic acids, coenzymes, extracts of boiled erythrocytes, bovine lung or staphylococci. These substances may be of use in attempts to isolate fastidious mycoplasmas and are described by Klieneberger-Nobel (1962), Lemcke (1965) and Stewart, Rylance and Marmion (1974). Minimal or partly defined media without serum or meat digests have been developed for some mycoplasmas (see Marmion, 1967). Complex tissue culture media (Jensen *et al.,* 1965; Eagle's basal medium; Quinlan, Liss and Maniloff, 1972) with yeast extract and lipid may be valuable as substitutes for serum-containing medium in antigen preparation or for increasing uptake of isotope labelled precursors from the medium. The semisolid and diphasic versions of the standard medium are valuable in providing a soft yet supporting framework for mycoplasma growth. Growth of glycolytic species, such as *M. pneumoniae,* in broth may be enhanced by addition of glucose and by shaking or rolling the container (Marmion, 1967). Diphasic medium may be made selective for *M. pneumoniae* by incorporation of 0·001 per cent methylene blue. This inhibits other members of the human flora; if glucose and a pH indicator are also added the medium may be monitored for the growth of *M. pneumoniae* by the change of pH to acid. Subculture onto solid medium must then be done to verify the presence of the mycoplasma.

Solid and fluid media for T-strain mycoplasmas described in Chapter 5 are based on media developed by Shepard and alternative formulae are given in Shepard (1969). The media contain serum (a source of urea), yeast extract and added urea. Growth in both solid and liquid medium is rapid and is conveniently monitored by the change of colour of the indicator to alkaline as the result of formation of ammonia from the urea. The alkaline shift is accompanied by a loss of viability and media with HEPES buffer may be used to counteract this and improve growth and colony size (Manchee and Taylor-Robinson, 1969).

Mycoplasma Culture and Identification of Isolates

Culture. Mycoplasma medium is expensive and it is economical to hold it in small plastic disposable Petri dishes, 50 mm × 13 mm (e.g. Sterilin, Falcon, Esco, etc.). A vent may be cut in the edge of the dish with a hot wire to allow gaseous exchange. These dishes have good optical properties and the colonies at the surface of the medium should be visualized without opening the dish by placing it, lid down, on the stage of a microscope without stage clamps and equipped with x 10 and x 4 objectives and x 10 oculars. This combination of lenses is optimal for the range (20–500 μm) of mycoplasma colonies. The larger ones may, of course, be visualized with a plate microscope. Examination without opening the plate is important because incubation has frequently to continue for 2–3 weeks and contamination, particularly with moulds, may be a problem.

Plates may be labelled with white adhesive tape and an indelible pen (e.g. laundry marker). The small size of the plates and the moist atmosphere in which they are held makes labelling with ordinary ball-point or felt-tip pens or grease pencils unsatisfactory. While the plates are being examined it is advisable to hold them upon a tray lined with filter paper soaked in 70 per cent v/v ethanol or methylated spirit and also to wipe the microscope stage with the spirit from time to time to reduce the load of contaminants on the outside of the plates. Moulds may grow over the edge of the lid, into the water of condensation on the inside of the lid and finally onto the medium itself.

Plates are incubated aerobically in plastic lunch boxes or in glass jars with sealed lids (fruit preserving jars) with a roll of cotton wool soaked in water to maintain humidity. It is important to clean, disinfect or autoclave these containers regularly so as to prevent a build-up of fungal contaminants. Anaerobic incubation is effected in a McIntosh and Fildes jar with 90 per cent hydrogen and 10 per cent CO_2 or microaerophilic incubation by flushing the jar with 90 per cent nitrogen and 10 per cent CO_2 mixture.

The technique of subculturing strains of mycoplasmas differs from the standard 'picking' method with bacteria because of the embedded nature of the colony. Small blocks of agar medium, bearing one or more colonies, are cut from the medium and placed colony-side down on fresh medium. A small stainless steel spatula, or scalpel with detachable blades, may be used for this purpose and is held in boiling water and burned off with spirit between transfers. The block is moved an inch or so across the plate so that mycoplasma cells will rub off onto the new medium. When mycoplasmas are first established on solid media of, for example, a different composition to that on which they have been carried, it may be found that growth occurs mainly under the block. Periodic movement of the block around the surface of the medium during the course of incubation may lead to satisfactory establishment of growth.

The colonial morphology of various species of mycoplasmas is often not distinctive and cross-contamination of strains and colonies made up of sectors of different mycoplasmas is a real hazard. For this reason it is important to clone stock strains and isolates by serial subculture from one colony. The culture is grown in broth, filtered, 220 nm APD, and two or three ten-fold serial dilutions prepared from it and plated on solid media to give a plate with well dispersed colonies. A small block with one colony is then removed with a spatula or by aspirating it with a wide bore Pasteur pipette. The colony-bearing block is expelled into semisolid agar, incubated and then subcultured onto solid media. This procedure may be repeated several times to ensure that the strain is pure.

Lyophilized cultures may be recovered by inoculating the material from the ampoule in 'stab' fashion into the centre of a bijou bottle of semisolid medium and later subculturing onto solid media. The initial incubation in semisolid 'agar may help to establish small numbers of organisms in a medium to which they are unaccustomed. Stock strains or isolates may be preserved by lyophilization, or by placing small amounts of a heavy culture in semisolid agar medium at $-70°C$. Strains may be transmitted by mail on sealed plates or, more conveniently, as an agar block with colonies in semisolid agar in a bijou bottle.

Identification of isolates. Mycoplasma colonies are differentiated from small bacterial colonies and pseudocolonies by staining methods. They are further identified by biochemical reactions, by certain biological reactions such as haemolysin production and haemadsorption and, above all, with the large colony mycoplasmas, by serological differentiation into species. Mycoplasmas are differentiated from unstable L-phase organisms by cultivation on the standard medium without penicillin and thallium acetate to allow the latter to revert to bacteria. Various workers have used electrophoretic analysis of mycoplasma and L-phase extracts on polyacrylamide gels; this gives excellent species differentiation and facilitates identification of L-phase organisms with bacterial parents (Theodore, Tully and Cole, 1971). Others have used gas chromatography to differentiate mycoplasma species (Meyer and Blazevic, 1971).

In the general bacteriological laboratory colony size provides a primary differentiation between 'large colony' and T-strain mycoplasmas. The former are identified by biochemical, biological and serological means (Table 43.1). The latter are identified by their ability to split urea, their inhibition by erythromycin and their resistance to lincomycin. They are also inhibited by 5'-Iodo-2'-deoxyuridine and hydroxyurea (Shepard, 1969). Serological identification of T-strains is possible but as there are numerous antigenic subtypes (Lin, Kendrick and Kass, 1972), simple typing by growth inhibition, of such value with the classical mycoplasmas, is not readily applicable, for variables and stringent requirements; see Black (1973). Selected test methods are now given.

Stains for Mycoplasmas

The most generally used stain is that of Dienes (Dienes, 1939; Madoff, 1959).

1. DIENES' STAIN

Formula

Azure II	0·25 g
Methylene blue	0·5 g
Maltose	2·0 g
Na_2CO_3	0·05 g
Benzoic acid . . .	0·04 g
Distilled water	20 ml

Table 43.1 Biological and biochemical reactions of members of the human mycoplasma flora

| Species | Requirement for yeast extract | Inhibition of growth by | | | | Haemolysis | Haemadsorption | Acid from glucose | Ammonia from | | Aerobic reduction of tetrazolium |
		Thallium-acetate (0.01% w/v)	Methylene blue (0.001% w/v)	Erythromycin (100 µg/ml)	Lincomycin (200 µg/ml)				arginine	urea	
M. pneumoniae	+	–	–	+	–	β	+	+	–	–	+
M. fermentans	–	–	+	±	+	–	–	+	+	–	–
M. hominis	–	–	+	–	+	– or α	–	–	+	–	–
M. orale 1	+	–	+	–	+	–	+*	–	+	–	–
M. orale 2	–	–	+	–	–	–	–	–	+	–	–
M. orale 3	+	–	+	–	–	–	+*	–	+	–	–
M. salivarium	–	–	+	–	–	–	–	–	+	–	–
T-mycoplasmas	+	+	–	+	–	β	–	–	–	+	–

*With chicken erythrocytes, not guinea pig or human; variable, but see Purcell and Chanock (1969).

526

Method
(a) Flood the plate, or a portion of the plate containing suspected mycoplasma colonies, with 1/10 Dienes' stain in distilled water. Examine the plate microscopically using a low power objective (x 4 or x 10).
(b) Smear clean coverslips with the 'neat' stain and allow to dry. Cut out a block of agar (5–10 mm square x 1–2 mm thick) from the plate and place colony-side down on the dry stain. Attach a brass ring (15–20 mm diameter x 3–4 mm thick) to a microscope slide by warming the ring in a Bunsen flame, dipping in vaseline and pressing the ring onto a slide. Place the coverslip, agar block side down, on the ring and view the stained preparation microscopically using a low power objective (x 4 or x 10). Colonies of mycoplasma retain the stain for at least two days while those of nearly all bacterial colonies lose the colour in half an hour. Large-colony mycoplasmas stain an intense royal blue, T-mycoplasmas stain reddish or greenish-blue. Colonies which have been transferred to slides by the hot water transfer method may be stained by overnight exposure to Dienes' stain or a mixture of Dienes' and Giemsa in equal proportions. By this method the stained preparation may be viewed microscopically with the oil immersion objective.

2. Cresyl-fast Violet
  Cresyl-fast violet (Shepard, 1967) is also valuable, particularly with T-strain mycoplasmas.

Formula: stock solution
  Adjust distilled water to pH 3·7 with glacial acetic acid (1–5 drops/100 ml). Dissolve 1 g cresyl-fast violet in 100 ml distilled water, pH 3·7. Allow solution to ripen for 48 h.

Working solution (prepared daily)
  Stock solution   .   .   .   . 20 ml
  NaCl   .   .   .   .   . 0·05 g
  Agitate 1 min, filter and add
    maltose   .   .   .   . 7·0 g
  Colonies of mycoplasma, both large and T-strains, stain red-purple.

Method
  The stain may be applied by any of the methods mentioned above although difficulty may be experienced in coating coverslips. If this is so, the block should be stained before applying a coverslip.

3. Giemsa Stain
  Blocks of agar with colonies should be inverted onto microscope slides and immersed in Bouin's fixative overnight. The block is then removed and the slide rinsed in tap water for 1 h. The slide is placed colony-side down on two supports in a Petri dish to which is added 1/20 Giemsa stain in distilled water. Staining is allowed to take place overnight, before rinsing and microscopic examination.

4. Intensified Giemsa
  This method involving pretreatment with potassium permanganate is used for staining smears of exudates, impression smears from organs etc., and is described in detail by Marmion (1967).

Distinction of Mycoplasma Colonies and Artefacts (pseudocolonies)
Although well developed mycoplasma colonies are distinctive enough there may be difficulties in differentiating young or poorly growing colonies from the artefacts known as pseudocolonies (Brown, Swift and Watson, 1940) or from the nuclei of tissue cells from cell cultures or clinical specimens. Pseudocolonies are precipitates arising from the high concentration of serum in mycoplasma media. Although they are not biological entities, they may appear to subculture when a block containing them is pushed over the surface of uninoculated medium as fresh collections of 'colonies' appear in the inoculated area apparently as a result of stress charges in the medium surface or the provision of foci on which precipitates can increase. The agar embedded centre of a mycoplasma colony is slightly granular and extends through several focal planes whereas a pseudocolony may have a central knob but is a superficial structure found in the focal plane of the medium surface. Mycoplasma colonies and pseudocolonies differ in their staining reactions with Dienes' stain, cresyl-fast violet or Giemsa, which reveal the collections of mycoplasma cells making up the colony. In addition pseudocolonies are not, of course,

inhibited by broad spectrum antibiotics, anti-sera, UV or X irradiation, and do not incorporate thymidine or uridine into their structure.

Biochemical and Biological Tests

Fermentation of carbohydrates. A 1 per cent w/v concentration of the carbohydrate under test is incorporated into an agar slope, or in semisolid or fluid preparation of the standard medium together with phenol red (0·002 per cent w/v). The range of sugars fermented is limited and is not of great differential importance. For most purposes it is sufficient to test for acid production from glucose. If other sugars are used it is important to remember that a maltase and a diastase in unheated horse serum may lead to false positive reactions. Fermentation may be weak and small changes of pH may be more accurately detected with a microelectrode than by colour change of the indicator; if semisolid or fluid media are used, growth should be confirmed in negative tubes by subculture. Lemcke (1965) and Freundt (1958) may be consulted for details of other biochemical tests.

Arginine deaminase. The standard liquid medium is supplemented with 1 per cent w/v L-arginine HCl and 0·002 per cent phenol red and adjusted to pH 7·0. Production of ammonia is indicated by a change to a deep red colour. Note that the horse serum in the medium contains urea and that an organism with urease may also produce ammonia.

Urease (Shepard and Lunceford, 1970; Shepard, 1973). Urease activity may be determined in a liquid medium (Shepard's U9 medium) or by plate tests.

(a) Urease colour test liquid medium

Basal broth:

Tryptic digest broth powder
(BBL or Difco)   .   .   . 0·75 g
(not all batches are satisfactory and tests with known T-myco-plasmas are advisable)
Sodium chloride (NaCl)   .   . 0·5 g
Potassium dihydrogen phosphate
(KH_2PO_4)   .   .   . 0·02 g
Deionized water   .   .   . 100 ml

The ingredients are dissolved, pH adjusted to 5·5 with 2N HCl and the basal broth sterilized in the autoclave at 121°C for 15 min.

Complete medium:

Sterile basal broth   .   .   . 95 ml
Unheated normal horse serum   . 4·0 ml
10 per cent w/v urea, stock solution   .   .   .   . 0·5 ml
0·2 per cent w/v phenol red, stock solution   .   .   .   . 1·0 ml
Penicillin G 100,000 units/ml   . 1·0 ml
Adjust to pH 6·0

A high grade (Analar) urea is used and sterilized by filtration.

The complete medium is dispensed in 1·5–2·0 ml volumes in 7 ml screw capped bottles. Preparations should not be kept longer than one week. The medium may also be used for isolation of T-strains from clinical specimens and for this purpose may be supplemented by 2·5 μg/ml of amphotericin B to suppress yeasts and filamentous fungi that give a positive urease test.

(b) Plate spot tests for urease and differential media

A solution containing 1 per cent w/v Analar grade urea and 0·8 per cent w/v manganous chloride is applied to suspected T-strain colonies which must be less than 48 h old. The liberation of ammonia from the urea reacts with the divalent cation indicator—manganous chloride—to give a golden brown precipitate around the colony. Alternatively, 0·03 per cent w/v manganous sulphate may be incorporated in the T-strain solid medium thus giving a differential medium on which T-strains have a golden precipitate around them while 'large colony' mycoplasmas do not change the medium.

Tetrazolium reduction (Kraybill and Crawford, 1965). Plates of standard mycoplasma agar are prepared with the addition of 2·0 ml of 1 per cent w/v stock solution of 2-3-5 triphenyltetrazolium chloride per 100 ml of medium. The stock solution is sterilized in the autoclave. A block of agar containing numerous colonies is placed, colony-side down, on the tetrazolium plate and the plate reincubated *aerobically*. In 3–6 days the colony-containing block becomes pink in colour if *M. pneumoniae* is present. It should be noted that under *anaerobic* conditions many mycoplasmas give a positive tetrazolium reaction and that members of the non-human mycoplasma flora e.g., *M. gallisepticum, A.*

laidlawii—give positive aerobic reduction of tetrazolium. An overlay method has also been described for *M. pneumoniae* (Woods and Smith, 1972).

Haemolysis and Haemadsorption

Isolates of mycoplasmas are inoculated onto standard medium to give well dispersed colonies and incubated until colonies are well grown (5–8 days). The plate is then overlayed with a thin layer of saline-agar containing 1 per cent v/v sheep or guinea pig erythrocytes and reincubated aerobically overnight.

M. pneumoniae produces a maximum clearing resembling β-haemolysis. T-strains also produce β-haemolysis of guinea pig erythrocytes but test conditions are critical. Other mycoplasmas may produce a greenish clearing of the overlay. Haemolysis depends on production of hydrogen peroxide; a simple test for this is described by Lind (1970).

Haemadsorption may be tested by flooding the culture plate, or a block excised from it, with a 1 per cent v/v suspension of sheep erythrocytes in saline and leaving them in contact for 30 min. The erythrocyte suspension is then aspirated and the colonies gently washed with saline and then inspected under the microscope. Positive colonies are seen to be plastered with erythrocytes. Spermatozoa and tissue culture cells may also adsorb to colonies (Taylor-Robinson and Manchee 1967 a and b); the spectrum of activity is not precisely the same as that of haemadsorption but in each instance pretreatment of the colonies with antiserum to the mycoplasma inhibits the reaction.

Serological Identification of Mycoplasmas

Serological methods are the most important means of identifying and classifying mycoplasmas. Almost all the known serological techniques—e.g., agglutination, complement-fixation, gel diffusion, inhibition of haemadsorption, indirect haemagglutination, immunofluorescence, metabolic inhibition, complement-mediated mycoplasmacidal antibody, radioimmunoassay, etc.—have been used either to classify strains or to measure antibody in sera from convalescent patients or hyperimmunized animals (see Purcell, Chanock and Taylor-Robinson, 1969). Some of these techniques recognize intratypic differences and are more relevant for a reference, than a general laboratory. Details are given of two simple methods—growth inhibition on agar and immunofluorescence on colonies transferred to glass slides—that will allow identification of most isolates in a general laboratory.

Growth inhibition on agar. The method follows those developed by Huijsmans-Evers and Ruys (1956) and Clyde (1964). After cloning the isolate, inoculate a mycoplasma broth with a small (5–10 mm²) block containing colonies and incubate for 3–7 days depending on the strain. Dry plates of standard mycoplasma medium at 37°C, then flood seed the plates with the broth culture and dry them again at 37°C. Place filter paper disks containing mycoplasma antisera on the seeded plates. The antisera are prepared by hyperimmunization of animals with representative strains of each of the human mycoplasma species. Up to 4 disks may be placed on each plate; one disk should contain no serum. The disks may be prepared by soaking sterile filter paper disks, 5 mm diameter and either holding them frozen at −20° or by drying them and storing at 4°C. Alternatively a single multiarmed set of disks may be used, with a different serum on each arm (Stanbridge and Hayflick, 1967). Suitable antisera may be prepared in the laboratory by immunization of rabbits or obtained from Microbiological Associates of 2680 Ober-Eschback, Amttang 10, Frankfurt, Germany. The plates are incubated, aerobically or anaerobically, depending on the nature of the isolate and inspected macroscopically and microscopically for a zone of inhibition of growth around the disks (illustrated in Vol. I, Plate 52). The method is highly specific and shows little of the cross-reactions between species revealed by more sensitive methods such as complement fixation. It may be necessary to seed a smaller dose of organisms if there is evidence of partial inhibition around the disks with 'breakthrough' of colonies.

Identification of mycoplasmas by immunofluorescence on slides. Colonies are transferred to microscope slides by placing a 5–10 mm² block with well dispersed colonies face down on an area marked out by glass diamond. The slides should have been chemically cleaned (e.g. chromic acid) and held in ethanol before use. The slide and agar block is lowered into a beaker of water at 85°C. It helps to have a simple platform and handle in light metal to support the slide during this operation. Once in the water the block turns opaque and finally melts over the surface of the slide. At this point a quick swirling motion will dislodge the agar and leave the mycoplasma colonies heat-fixed to the slide. The slide is then removed from the beaker, rinsed briefly in another beaker of water at 85°C to free the preparation of the last traces of agar, then dried and inspected under the low power of the microscope to confirm that colonies have, in fact, been transferred.

The mycoplasma antisera, usually made in rabbit, goat or horse, and the appropriate fluorescein conjugated antiglobulin, are absorbed with a mixture of packed, washed yeast cells and horse liver powder. This is done to cut down possible heterologous reactions between the antisera, the conjugate and residual traces of medium components (yeast extract or horse serum) on the slide. Sera and absorbents are mixed in ratio of approximately 0·5 g to 2 ml of serum and held for 1 hour at room temperature with periodic shaking, then centrifuged and the supernatant fluid passed through a syringe membrane filter to remove fine particles.

The conjugate and mycoplasma antisera have first to be titrated on known strains to determine the dilution for use in the test with unknown colonies. Mycoplasma antisera may be used at a concentration of 8–16 antibody units. A conjugate will usually have a titration end point of 20 to 40 on antibody coated colonies and may be used at a dilution of 5 to 10. Concentrations stronger than 5 are liable to give non-specific staining.

In the first stage of staining the unknown colonies, a drop of diluted, absorbed, antiserum is spread over the colony-bearing area of the slide with a toothpick or bacteriological loop so as to ensure even dispersion. The slide is placed in a closed, humid chamber for 30 minutes at 37°C. Next the slide is washed by placing it in a container of phosphate-buffered saline with a magnetic stirrer for 30 min at room temperature. The excess buffer is then drained from the slide and it is carefully mopped dry with a cellulose wipe without touching the area with colonies. A drop of conjugate is then spread over the colony area and the slide returned to the moist chamber for 30 min at 37°C. The slide is then washed again with fresh buffer and quickly rinsed with distilled water, mopped dry, and the colony area covered with mounting fluid (e.g. buffer pH 7·6 1 part, Analar glycerol 9 parts, or one of the permanent fluorescence-free mountants) and a coverslip; its edges may be sealed with colourless nail varnish. The preparation is viewed in the fluorescence microscope with a dark ground condenser. Colonies with attached antibody show a bright green speckled fluorescence; negative colonies autofluoresce blue or silver-grey depending on the wavelength of the exciting light (Vol. I, Plate 7). Controls should include preparations with buffer as the 'middle layer' rather than antiserum, and also some with buffer instead of conjugate. There should also be a control preparation of a known strain of mycoplasma and its homologous antiserum to check that the diluted, adsorbed, conjugate is still active.

In general this method gives clear-cut differentiation between mycoplasma species when care is taken to use the antisera at a standard unitage. It is also possible to detect mixtures of mycoplasmas by looking for stained and unstained colonies or parts of colonies within the same preparation.

Antibody in human (or animal) convalescent-phase sera may be titrated on colonies but both this method and growth inhibition are of low sensitivity compared with antibody measurement by metabolic inhibition, indirect haemagglutination, or radioimmunoassay. Del Guidice, Robillard and Carski (1967) have developed a method for fluorstaining of colonies directly on agar and detection with the incident illuminator of the microscope.

ISOLATION OF MYCOPLASMAS FROM CLINICAL SPECIMENS

M. pneumoniae infection of the respiratory tract. Patients with bronchiolitis or pneumonia may harbour *M. pneumoniae* in the naso-pharynx or respiratory secretions for substantial periods of time, even after antibiotic therapy and clinical recovery. Nevertheless there are marked variations in the ease with which the organism is grown by different laboratories and frequently laboratory diagnosis depends more on tests of acute and convalescent phase sera than on culture of the mycoplasma.

Throat and nose swabs are taken and the heads broken off into 2 ml of a transport medium in a bijou bottle; the standard myco-plasma fluid medium will do for this purpose or a mixture of basal broth, bovine serum albumin (1 per cent v/v), gelatin (0·3 per cent w/v) and penicillin (1000 units/ml) may be employed.

On arrival at the laboratory the broken end of the swab stick is grasped with forceps (e.g. obsolete Spencer-Wells forceps) and the fluid expelled from the swab head by pressure against the wall of the bijou bottle. One to 1·5 ml of the contents of the bottle is then inoculated into a bottle of diphasic medium containing glucose and methylene blue and one or two drops plated onto the standard solid mycoplasma medium.

Sputum is mixed with an equal volume of mycoplasma broth and lightly homogenized (e.g. in a Nelson blender) and is then inoculated into diphasic medium and onto solid myco-plasma medium. Particularly viscous specimens may be liquefied by digestion with pancreatic dornase. Isolation rates may be improved by inoculation of 10–15 ml volumes of sputum extract into diphasic medium in small medical 'flats'. Pleural fluid, aspirates from otitis media, cerebrospinal fluid and other miscel-laneous specimens for *M. pneumoniae* are also inoculated into diphasic medium.

Tissue specimens from the lungs of fatal cases of atypical pneumonia, or from animals inoculated experimentally, may require special treatment to offset the mycoplasmacidal effects of tissue enzymes released on grinding the tissue (Kaklamanis *et al.*, 1969). Diphasic media should be inoculated with several ten-fold dilutions of the tissue extract as well as with the concentrated material.

In general, plates and diphasic medium are incubated aerobically (at 35·5–36°C) and the latter is inspected each day for acid production and subcultured onto a plate of solid medium if this occurs. The primary plate inoculated with the swab eluates or sputum is inspected at 3–5 day intervals and all media are held up to 3 weeks before discard. At that stage apparently negative plates may be flooded with a saline suspension of human or sheep erythrocytes to detect inconspicuous colonies by haemadsorp-tion. Suspect colonies on the primary plate, or from the subcultures from diphasic medium, are subcultured and identified by biochemical and serological tests already described.

Infections of the genital tract. Clinical speci-mens for isolation of 'large colony' or T-myco-plasmas from the genital tract may include high vaginal or cervical swabs, urethral swabs or urine after massage of prostrate and para-urethral glands, specimens of purulent aspirate from 'non-bacterial' salpingitis, tissue or swabs from membranes or foetus in cases of abortion or prematurity, or semen collected as part of an investigation of infertility. In addition, blood may be taken for culture in puerperal fever. Swabs may be taken into Stuart's transport medium or into mycoplasma broth *without* inhibitors such as thallium acetate or methylene blue. Ampicillin may be added to control bacterial overgrowth.

Swabs are spread on plates of standard and T-mycoplasma media; eluates from the swabs may also be inoculated into diphasic medium without methylene blue and into liquid T-myco-plasma medium. Urine is centrifuged and the deposit inoculated onto plates and into fluid medium. Tissue and pus may be blended with mycoplasma broth, without inhibitors, and the supernatant fluid from a lightly centrifuged suspension inoculated into standard and T-strain media. Blood for culture should be taken into diphasic medium without glucose or methylene blue in a fashion analogous to the Castenada blood culture bottle; also into T-mycoplasma broth; both types of media are subcultured at intervals onto the appropriate solid media. Semen should be lightly blended with T-strain broth and plated onto solid and into liquid media. As there is evidence that *M. hominis* and T-mycoplasmas absorb to the spermatozoa via neuraminidase sensitive re-ceptors, consideration might be given to eluting the organisms with receptor destroying enzyme (RDE) to improve isolation rates.

Incubation of all plates, both for *M. hominis* and *M. fermentans* and for T-strain mycoplasmas, should be under microaerophilic or anaerobic conditions. Suspect colonies are subcultured and identified as already described.

SEROLOGICAL DIAGNOSIS OF MYCOPLASMA INFECTIONS

Mycoplasma Pneumoniae

As indicated, antibody to *M. pneumoniae* may be measured by a wide range of techniques of widely differing sensitivity. The techniques commonly used in the general bacteriological laboratory are complement-fixation and metabolic inhibition.

In addition, about half the patients infected with *M. pneumoniae* develop cold haemagglutinins to their own or Group 'O' erythrocytes and a smaller proportion, agglutinins to *Streptococcus MG*. These heterogenetic reactions depend on fortuitous similarities between glycolipid haptens in the mycoplasma membrane and carbohydrate determinants in the streptococcal cell (Marmion, Plackett and Lemcke, 1967; Plackett *et al.,* 1969) and in the 'I' antigen of the erythrocyte (Costea, Yakulis and Heller, 1972). As cold haemagglutinins develop rapidly it may be of value to estimate them as well as testing for complement-fixing or other antibody to *M. pneumoniae*; techniques are described in Chapter 11.

Preparation of complement-fixing antigens from Mycoplasma pneumoniae and other mycoplasmas.
Methods for growing *M. pneumoniae* and other mycoplasmas on glass surfaces follow those of Somerson *et al.* (1967) and Purcell *et al.* (1971). Roux bottles, or 2 or 16 oz medical 'flats' (prescription) bottles, are washed to tissue culture standards. Standard or modified (see below) PPLO broth, to an amount between 1/4 and 1/10 of the volume of the bottle, is added and inoculated with about 10^7 colony forming units of mycoplasma in the log phase of growth. The bottles are then tightly closed and incubated flat at 36–37°C for 3–5 days. *M. pneumoniae* adheres to glass when the fluid phase contains 20 per cent v/v horse serum, but it and other species of mycoplasma adhere better when 5 per cent v/v Difco PPLO

serum fraction (bovine) is used in place of the horse serum. The medium should be supplemented with 1 per cent w/v glucose for *M. pneumoniae* and other glycolytic species, or with 1 per cent w/v L-arginine HCl for arginine-utilizing strains. A sheet of organisms forms on the glass and may be washed with phosphate buffered saline to free it from medium components. The adherent mycoplasmas are then scraped off with a glass rod tipped in rubber. The suspension of *M. pneumoniae* may then be inactivated by heat (60°C for 30 min) and used in this form as a complement-fixing antigen, or the complement-fixing glycolipids may be extracted with chloroform-methanol.

For lipid extraction, organisms from the fluid phase of the culture may be used as well as those from the glass. They are weighed then suspended in phosphate magnesium buffer (0·02 M phosphate + 0·01 M $MgSO_4$: pH 7·0) (1·0 g wet weight in 8·0 ml of buffer) by grinding in a Ten Broeck grinder. Chloroform-methanol (2:1 v/v) is added in the ratio of 19 volumes of solvent for each volume of organisms suspended in magnesium-phosphate buffer, and is allowed to stand at room temperature for 1 h with occasional shaking. The extract is filtered through a small plug of glass wool in a filter funnel to remove cellular debris, 1/5 of the volume of the extract is estimated and this amount of 0·1 M potassium chloride KCl (Analar reagent in deionized water) added to the extract. This mixture is held in a separating funnel and forms two layers; a heavy one of chloroform and a lighter one of methanol and water. The chloroform layer contains the glycolipids and is stored overnight over anhydrous sodium sulphate at 4°C, then filtered through Whatman No. 1 filter paper. The sodium sulphate is washed with fresh chloroform-methanol and the washing added to the chloroform extract. The volume of resulting harvest is reduced in a rotary evaporator at 37°C. When about 1·0 ml of oily liquid remains it is taken up in approximately 5 ml of ethanol at 56°C and this solution is then rapidly squirted with a syringe and 26 gauge needle into approximately 20 ml of complement-fixation test diluent (Oxoid) to give a dispersed suspension. Sodium azide 0·08 per cent w/v is added as a preservative.

The whole cell or suspended lipid antigens are titrated in 'chessboard' fashion in the CF test against human and rabbit antisera to determine the optimum antigen concentration—i.e. that dilution giving the highest serum titre—for routine tests. The heat inactivated whole cell antigen and the lipid antigen both give good results with acute and convalescent sera from atypical pneumonia patients. As the lipid antigen is free from anticomplementary activity it can be used at high unitage to detect the poor CF antibody responses that occur in some patients with *M. pneumoniae* infections. However, the chloroform methanol extraction also makes accessible cardiolipin-like phosphatides so that the antigen will react with WR-positive sera from syphilitics. Paradoxical or conflicting results should therefore be investigated by testing the sera for specific antitreponemal antibody by the TPHA or other techniques (Vol. II, Chap. 39).

Metabolic inhibition test for measurement of antibody to M. pneumoniae. A large volume of mycoplasma broth without glucose is inoculated with a cloned strain of *M. pneumoniae* and grown for 4 days. The degree of growth is checked by phase contrast examination and subculture and the broth centrifuged lightly to deposit organisms growing as large, suspended colonies. The supernatant fluid is ampouled in convenient volumes and snap-frozen in a bath of ethanol and solid CO_2 and stored at $-70°C$. This constitutes the seed organism for the test proper.

Tests are done in plastic disposable trays with 96 cups arranged in 8 rows of 12 (Cooke microtitre trays with U-shaped cups, Flow Labs). An ampoule of seed is removed from $-70°C$, thawed rapidly and titrated in a row of cups in the tray from 10^0 to 10^{-6} in ten-fold steps; the diluent being the standard mycoplasma broth *with* glucose and phenol red. The unit volume for the doubling dilutions is 0·025 ml and an extra volume of 0·025 ml of medium, representing the serum in the test proper, is added to each cup and the total volume made up to 0·2 ml. The tray is then sealed with wide strip sellotape and incubated. The growth of the mycoplasma is indicated by the acid change in the cups—a change from red to yellow—and at a chosen period, say after 4 days' incubation, the dilution of seed just producing an acid change (=one acid-forming unit) may be determined. $10^{1·3}$ acid-forming units are used in the test proper. Sera for test, and a known positive serum, are diluted 1/5 in saline and inactivated at 56°C for 30 min. They are further diluted in mycoplasma broth with glucose and phenol red over a range from 10 to 2560 and to each dilution is added a dilution of seed corresponding to $10^{1·3}$ acid-forming units. Controls should include the starting dilution of each serum without added organisms and a titration of the working dilution of seed organisms, without antisera, to check that the unitage is correct. Plates are sealed with sellotape and incubated for the period originally used in titrating the seed suspension. Plates are then removed from the incubator and the tape over each cup pierced with a hot surgical needle. This releases CO_2 from those cups in which acid change has not occurred and sharpens the contrast with those that have changed. Inhibition of acid formation indicates antibody. It should be noted, however, that sera from patients receiving broad spectrum antibiotics will give an inhibitory effect that may be mistaken for antibody. The method may be used for ammonia-producing mycoplasmas by substituting arginine or urea for the glucose (Taylor-Robinson *et al.,* 1966; Purcell *et al.,* 1969). (For further practical details see Purcell and Chanock, 1969.)

DETECTION OF MYCOPLASMAS IN CELL CULTURE

The frequency with which various species of mycoplasma are found in cell cultures varies from country to country and reflects local practice in handling cells, local commercial arrangements for supply of cells, or private exchange of cultures (Reviews; Hayflick, 1965; MacPherson, 1968; Stanbridge, 1971). Although initially mycoplasmas are perhaps introduced into cell cultures from the nasopharynx of handlers, or from medium components such as bovine or swine serum, trypsin, chick embryo extract and the like, the prevalence of a single, or limited number of species in many different cell lines argues for cross-contamination between cell lines as an important, and too often unrecognised, mode of infection. Species reported include *M. hominis, M. orale* type I, *M. hyorhinis, M. arginini,* and from time to time, *M. fermentans, M. gallisepticum, A. laidlawii, A. granularum* and *M. pulmonis.*

Mycoplasmas in cell cultures may be detected by light or phase contrast microscopy of cell sheets stained by Giemsa (pp. 48–9), orcein (Fogh and Fogh, 1964), or acridine orange (Ebke and Kuwert, 1972). Cell sheets may also be examined by immunofluorescence with single or pooled antisera to the mycoplasma species likely to be found as cell culture contaminants. Mycoplasmas may be visualized in the electron-microscope in thin sections of cell sheets or, less reliably, in negative contrast preparations of cell lysates.

Other methods involve detection of enzymes characteristic of mycoplasmas and not of their host cells—e.g. arginine deaminase (Schimke and Barile, 1963); such methods have the attraction of speed but suffer from the limitations that not all mycoplasmas have the arginine deaminase pathway and that simple culture of the cells for mycoplasma is more sensitive if somewhat slower. Other workers (Horoszewicz and Grace, 1964; Levine, 1972) have taken advantage of the fact that mycoplasma infected cell cultures exhibit abnormal levels of thymidine and uridine phosphorylase; thus estimation of the uracil split from radio-isotope tagged uridine can be used as an index of contamination. Tagged thymidine and uridine is incorporated into, respectively, the DNA and RNA of the mycoplasmas and the labelled organisms can be located by the increase of silver grains over the cytoplasm of cells in auto-radiographs (Studzinski, Gierthy and Cholon, 1973); however, experience again suggests that the method is less sensitive than culture. Todaro, Aaronson and Rands (1971) have developed an ingenious method in which cell cultures are exposed to tagged thymidine or uridine, the fluid phase or cell elutates are concentrated and centrifuged on a sucrose gradient, and the fractions examined for radio-activity at a characteristic buoyant density (1·20 to 1·24 g/cm^3). This method would be advantageous for detection of mycoplasmas that grow poorly in cell-free media; some mycoplasmas become highly adapted to life at the cell surface and have a low plating efficiency in cell-free media.

Probably the method chosen for detection will depend on the interests and resources of the laboratory; i.e. detection by Todaro's method will appeal to those with isotope counters and ultracentrifuges. Two simple methods—immunofluorescence on 'flying' coverslips of cells and culture on standard mycoplasma medium—are described for the general bacteriological laboratory; the former provides a rapid 'screening' method for frequent testing and the latter, although slower, is still of value in terms of sensitivity.

Detection of Mycoplasmas in Cell Cultures by Immunofluorescence

Tissue culture tubes, e.g. $6 \times \frac{5}{8}$ in tubes, with half coverslips (22 × 6 mm), are seeded with 1×10^5 cells of continuous cell lines, such as HEp 2 or with larger numbers of diploid cells. After closure they are incubated at a low angle so that the cells settle onto the coverslips. After 24–48 h, when a semiconfluent sheet is visible, the coverslip is removed and fixed for 10 min in cold Analar-grade acetone, previously held over dehydrated calcium sulphate. The fixed coverslips may be stored in a closed container at −20°C if they are not to be examined at once. The coverslips, cell monolayer upwards, are attached to the edge of a miscroscope slide by taping about 2–3 mm of the end of the coverslip to the slide; up to six coverslips may be attached to one slide like a comb and the identity of the coverslips may be noted on the tape. The edge of the tape is painted with colourless nail varnish to prevent reagents soaking into it during staining and washing. A drop of absorbed specific mycoplasma antiserum, or pool of antisera, is spread over the cells on the coverslip and the slide held at 37°C for 30 min in a humid container. The antiserum is then washed off and the row of coverslips suspended in a bath of phosphate buffered saline, stirred magnetically. After allowing the buffer to drain away a drop of absorbed, diluted fluorescein conjugated antiglobulin is placed on the coverslip and again left at 37°C for 30 min. In turn this is washed away with phosphate buffer, and then quickly rinsed in distilled water. The coverslip is mounted, cells down, in buffered glycerol or permanent fluorescence-free mountant, and the edges sealed with nail varnish in the case of glycerol mountant.

In the ultraviolet microscope the mycoplasmas are seen on the surface of the cells as green staining particles or clumps, particularly on processes joining cells. Filamentous mycoplasmas may appear as tangled skeins. The mycoplasma antisera are titrated on cells infected with the homologous strain and used at a dilution of 8–16 antibody units. Conjugates are absorbed first with a liver powder corresponding to the species of cell to be tested and then with a pack of the cells under test. Controls of antisera without conjugate and conjugate without antisera are included.

Detection of Mycoplasmas in Cells by Culture

Mycoplasmas are cell-associated; so cells are scraped off into a small volume of the fluid phase of the culture and the suspension inoculated onto two plates of the standard medium and into the centre of one bijou bottle of semisolid medium. At the same time it is of value to inoculate a glucose broth without inhibitor to detect low grade infection of the cells with bacteria or yeasts. One plate is incubated aerobically and the other anaerobically or in nitrogen and CO_2. It is particularly important to use anaerobic conditions to detect *M. orale* in cell culture. The semisolid agar is subcultured at 3, 7 and 14 days and the primary plates and the subcultures are examined at the same intervals. Suspected colonies are stained by Dienes' method or with cresyl-fast violet and the isolates identified by immunofluorescence and by subculture and growth inhibition. The presence of L-phase organisms simulating mycoplasmas is investigated by subculture on standard medium without inhibitors.

Treatment of Contaminated Cells

This is a matter of some difficulty as the antibiotic sensitivity of different mycoplasma species varies. Basic policy should include buying in mycoplasma-free cells (and checking them at time of purchase), growing them up and storing clean stocks in liquid nitrogen or at −70°C. Contaminated sublines are rigorously discarded as infection is liable to spread to other cell lines. Separate hoods must be used for contaminated and clean lines along with separate cell culture media, pipette cans, etc. Hoods should be cleaned between handling different cell lines. Cells which cannot be discarded may be treated with tetracycline, kanamycin, tylosin or other broad spectrum antibiotics to which the organism is demonstrably sensitive (see Stanbridge, 1971; Cross, Goodman and Shaw, 1967; Fogh and Fogh, 1969). Sodium aurothiomalate is effective against some species but disappointing with *M. orale*. Other methods advocated but less effective outside the laboratory of origin are heating cultures at 41°C, treatment with antiserum to the mycoplasma concerned (see Stanbridge, 1971), or the use of Tricine buffered cell culture media (Spendlove *et al.*, 1971).

It must be remembered that even if stock cell lines are mycoplasma free, many virus stocks will be contaminated and will serve as a source of further laboratory outbreaks of contamination. Treatment of virus infected cell cultures with antibiotics and gold salts, or gamma irradiation of virus seeds (Polley and Fanok, 1973) may overcome the problem.

REFERENCES

Biberfeld, G. (1970) Antibodies to tissue antigens in cases of *Mycoplasma pneumoniae* infection. *Acta Pathologica et Microbiologica Scandinavica* (B) **78**, 266.

Biberfeld, G. (1971) Antibodies to brain and other tissues in cases of *Mycoplasma pneumoniae* infection. *Clinical Experimental Immunology*, **8**, 319–333.

Black, F. T. (1973) Modification of the growth inhibition test and application to human T-mycoplasmas. *Applied Microbiology*, **25**, 528–33.

Brown, T. M., Swift, H. F. & Watson, R. F. (1940) Pseudocolonies simulating those of pleuropneumonia-like microorganisms. *Journal of Bacteriology*, **40**, 857–864.

Clyde, W. A. (1964) Mycoplasma species identification based on growth inhibition by specific antisera. *Journal of Immunology*, **92**, 958–65.

Clyde, W. A. (1971) Immunopathology of experimental *Mycoplasma pneumoniae* disease. *Infection Immunity*, **4**, 757–763.

Costea, N., Yakulis, V. J. & Heller, P. (1972) Inhibition of cold agglutinins (anti-I) by *Mycoplasma pneumoniae* antigens. *Proceeding of the Society of Experimental Biology*, **139**, 476–479.

Cross, G. F., Goodman, M. R. & Shaw, E. J. (1967)

Detection and treatment of contaminating mycoplasmas in cell culture. *Australian Journal of Experimental Biology and Medical Sciences*, **45**, 201–212.

CSONKA, G. W. & CORSE, J. (1970) Selective inhibition *in vitro* of *Mycoplasma hominis* by lincomycin. *British Journal of Venereal Diseases*, **46**, 203.

CSONKA, G. W. & SPITZER, R. J. (1969) Lincomycin, non-gonococcal urethritis and mycoplasmata. *British Journal of Venereal Diseases*, **45**, 52–54.

DIENES, L. (1939) L organism of Klieneberger and *Streptobacillus moniliformis* and other bacteria. *Journal of Infectious Diseases*, **65**, 24–42.

DEL GUIDICE, R. A., ROBILLARD, N. F. & CARSKI, T. R. (1967) Immunofluorescence identification of *Mycoplasma* on agar by use of incident illumination. *Journal of Bacteriology*, **93**, 1205–1209.

DEL GUIDICE, R. A. & CARSKI, T. R. (1968) Characterization of a new Mycoplasma species of human origin. *Bacteriological Proceedings*, p. 67.

EBKE, J. & KUWERT, E. (1972) Detection of *Mycoplasma orale* type 1 in tissue cultures by means of acridine orange stain. *Zentralblatt für Bakteriologie und Hygiene, I Abt. Orig. A 221*, 87, 93.

FLEMING, P., KRIEGER, E., WATTY, E. I., QUINN, P. A. & BANNATYNE, R. M. (1967) Febrile mucocutaneous syndrome with respiratory involvement associated with isolation of *M. pneumoniae*. *Canadian Medical Association Journal*, **97**, 1458–1459.

FOGH, J. & FOGH, H. (1964) A method for direct demonstration of pleuropneumonia-like organisms in cultured cells. *Proceedings of the Society of Experimental Biology*, **117**, 899–901.

FOGH, J. & FOGH, H. (1969) Procedures for control of mycoplasma contamination of tissue cultures. *Annals of the New York Academy of Sciences*, **172**, 15–30.

FREUNDT, E. A. (1958) *The Mycoplasmataceae*. Copenhagen; Aarhuus Stiftsbogtry Kkerie.

GNARPE, H. & FRIBERG, J. (1973) T-mycoplasmas as a possible cause of reproductive failure. *Nature*, **242**, 120–121.

HAYFLICK, L. (1965) Tissue cultures and Mycoplasmas. *Texas Reports on Biology and Medicine*, **23**, 285–303.

HAYFLICK, L. (Ed.) (1969) *The Mycoplasmatales and L-phase of Bacteria*. Amsterdam: North-Holland.

HODGES, G. R., FASS, R. J. & SASLAWS, S. (1972) Central nervous system disease associated with *M. pneumoniae* infection. *Archives of Internal Medicine*, **130**, 277–282.

HOROSZEWICZ, J. S. & GRACE, J. T. (1964) PPLO. Detection in cell culture by thymidine cleavage. *Bacteriological Proceedings*, p. 131.

HUIJSMANS-EVERS, A. G. & RUYS, A. C. (1956) Microorganisms of the pleuropneumonia group (Family of Mycoplasmataceae) in Man II. Serological identification and discussion of pathogenicity. *Antonie van Leeuwenhoek*, **22**, 377–384.

JANSSON, E. (1971) Isolation of fastidious mycoplasmas from human sources. *Journal of Clinical Pathology*, **24**, 53–56.

JENSEN, K. E., SENTERFIT, L. B., CHANOCK, R. M., SMITH, C. B. & PURCELL, R. H. (1965) An inactivated *Mycoplasma pneumoniae* vaccine. *Journal of American Medical Association*, **194**, 248–252.

KAKLAMANIS, E., THOMAS, L., STAVROPOULOS, K., BORMAN, I. & BOSHWITZ, C. (1969) Mycoplasmacidal activity of normal tissue extracts. *Nature*, **221**, 860–861.

KLIENEBERGER-NOBEL, E. (1962) *Pleuropneumonia-like Organisms (PPLO): Mycoplasmataceae*. New York: Academic Press.

KRAYBILL, W. H. & CRAWFORD, Y. E. (1965) A selective medium and colour test for *Mycoplasma pneumoniae*. *Proceedings of the Society of Experimental Biology, New York*, **118**, 965–970.

LANCET (1973) Mycoplasmas in human infertility. *Lancet*, **i**, 1162–1163.

LEMCKE, R. M. (1965) Media for the *Mycoplasmataceae*. *Laboratory Practice*, **14**, 712–716.

LEVINE, E. M. (1972) Mycoplasma contamination of animal cell cultures: a simple, rapid detection method. *Experimental Cell Research*, **74**, 99–109.

LIN, J. S. L., KENDRICK, M. I. & KASS, E. H. (1972) Serological typing of human genital T-mycoplasmas by a complement dependent mycoplasmacidal test. *Journal of Infectious Diseases*, **126**, 658.

LIND, K. (1970) A simple test for peroxide secretion by mycoplasma. *Acta Pathologica et Microbiologica Scandinavica* (B) **78**, 256.

MACPHERSON, I. (1968) Mycoplasmas in tissue culture. *Journal of Cell Sciences*, **1**, 145–168.

MCCORMACK, W. M., BRAUN, P., YHU-HSIUNG LEE, KLEIN, J. O. & KASS, E. H. (1973) The genital mycoplasmas. *New England Journal of Medicine*, **288**, 78.

MADOFF, S. (1959) Isolation and identification of PPLO. *Annals of the New York Academy of Sciences*, **79**, 383–392.

MANCHEE, R. J. & TAYLOR-ROBINSON, D. (1969) Enhanced growth of T-strain mycoplasmas with N-2-Hydroxyethylpiperazine-N′-2 Ethane sulfonic acid buffer. *Journal of Bacteriology*, **100**, 78–85.

MANILOFF, J. & MOROWITZ, H. J. (1972) Cell biology of Mycoplasmas. *Bacteriological Reviews*, **36**, 263–290.

MARMION, B. P. (1967) The mycoplasmas: new information on their properties and their pathogenicity for man. In *Recent Advances in Medical Microbiology*. Edited by Waterson, A. P. London: Churchill.

MARMION, B. P., PLACKETT, P. & LEMCKE, R. M. (1967) Immunochemical analysis of *Mycoplasma pneumoniae* 1. Methods of extraction and reactions of fractions from *M. pneumoniae* and from *M. mycoides* with homologous antisera and antisera against *Streptococcus MG*. *Australian Journal of Experimental Biology and Medical Science*, **45**, 163–187.

MEYER, D. M. & BLAZEVIC, D. J. (1971) Differentiation of human mycoplasma using gas chromatography. *Canadian Journal of Microbiology*, **17**, 297–300.

PLACKETT, P., MARMION, B. P., SHAW, E. J. & LEMCKE, R. M. (1969) Immunochemical analysis of *Mycoplasma pneumoniae* 3. Separation and identification of serologically active lipids. *Australian Journal of Experimental Biology and Medical Science*, **47**, 171–195.

POLLEY, J. R. & FANOK, A. G. (1973) Inactivation of mycoplasma in seed virus stocks using gamma radiation. *Canadian Journal of Microbiology*, **19**, 709–714.

PURCELL, R. H. & CHANOCK, R. M. (1969 in *Diagnostic Procedures for Viral and Rickettsial Infections*, Ch. 23, pp. 786–825. Edited by E. H. Lennette and N. J. Schmidt, New York: American Public Health Association.

PURCELL, R. H., CHANOCK, R. M. & TAYLOR-ROBINSON, D. (1969) Serology of the mycoplasmas of man. *The Mycoplasmatales and L-phase of Bacteria*. Edited by Hayflick, L., pp. 221–264. Amsterdam: North-Holland.

PURCELL, R. H., VALDESUSO, J. R., CLINE, W. L., JAMES, W. D. & CHANOCK, R. M. (1971) Cultivation of mycoplasmas on glass. *Applied Microbiology*, **23**, 288–294.

QUINLAN, D. C., LISS, A. & MANILOFF, J. (1972) Eagles basal medium for Mycoplasma studies. *Microbios*, **6**, 179–185.

SCHIMKE, R. T. & BARILE, M. F. (1963) Arginine breakdown in mammalian cell cultures contaminated with pleuropneumonia-like organisms (PPLO). *Experimental Cell Research*, **30**, 593–590.

SHEPARD, M. C. (1967) Cultivation and properties of T-strains of mycoplasma associated with nongonococcal urethritis. *Annals of the New York Academy of Science*, **143**, 505–514.

SHEPARD, M. C. (1969) In *The Mycoplasmatales and L-phase of Bacteria*. Edited by Hayflick, L. Amsterdam: North-Holland.

SHEPARD, M. C. (1973) Differential method for identification of T-mycoplasmas based on demonstration of urease. *Journal of Infectious Diseases*, **127**, Supplement, p. 22.

SHEPARD, M. C. & LUNCEFORD, C. D. (1970) Differential agar medium for identification of T-mycoplasmas in primary culture. *Bacteriological Proceedings*, **70**, 83.

SMITH, C. & SANGSTER, G. (1972) Mycoplasma pneumoniae meningoencephalitis. *Scandinavian Journal of Infectious Diseases*, **4**, 69.

SOMERSON, N. L., JAMES, W. D., WALLS, B. E. & CHANOCK, R. M. (1967) Growth of *Mycoplasma pneumoniae* on a glass surface. *Annals of the New York Academy of Science*, **143**, 384–389.

SPENDLOVE, R. S., CROSBIE, R. B., HAYES, S. F. & KEELER, R. F. (1971) Tricine-buffered tissue culture media for control of mycoplasma contaminants. *Proceedings of the Society for Experimental Biology*, **137**, 258–263.

STANBRIDGE, E. & HAYFLICK, L. (1967) Growth inhibition test for identification of *Mycoplasma* species utilizing dried antiserum impregnated paper discs. *Journal of Bacteriology*, **93**, 1392–1396.

STANBRIDGE, E. (1971) Mycoplasmas and cell cultures. *Bacteriological Reviews*, **35**, 206–227.

STEWART, Sheila M., RYLANCE, H. J. & MARMION, B. P. (1974) Some investigations into artificial media used for the isolation of *Mycoplasma pneumoniae*. Submitted for publication.

STUDZINSKI, G. P., GIERTHY, J. F. & CHOLON, J. T. (1973) An autoradiographic screening test for mycoplasmal contamination of mammalian cell cultures. *In vitro*, **8**, 466–472.

TAYLOR-ROBINSON, D., PURCELL, R. H., WONG, D. C. & CHANOCK, R. M. (1966) A colour test for measurement of antibody to certain mycoplasma species based on the inhibition of acid production. *Journal of Hygiene (Cambridge)*, **64**, 91–104.

TAYLOR-ROBINSON, D. & MANCHEE, R. J. (1967a) Sperm-adsorption and spermagglutination by mycoplasma. *Nature*, **215**, 484–487.

TAYLOR-ROBINSON, D. & MANCHEE, R. J. (1967b). Novel approach to studying relationships between mycoplasmas and tissue culture cells. *Nature*, **216**, 1306–1307.

TAYLOR-ROBINSON, D., SOMERSON, N. L., TURNER, H. C. & CHANOCK, R. M. (1963) Serological relationships among human mycoplasmas as shown by complement fixation and gel diffusion. *Journal of Bacteriology*, **85**, 1261–1273.

THEODORE, T., TULLY, J. G. & COLE, R. M. (1971) Polyacrylamide gel identification of bacterial L forms and mycoplasma species of human origin. *Applied Microbiology*, **21**, 272.

TODARO, G. J., AARONSON, S. A. & RANDS, E. (1971) Rapid detection of mycoplasma-infected cell cultures. *Experimental Cell Research*, **65**, 256–257.

WOLANSKI, B. & MARAMOROSCH, K. (1970) Negatively stained mycoplasmas; fact or artefact? *Virology*, **42**, 319–327.

WOODS, L. L. & SMITH, T. F. (1972) Tetrazolium agar overlay in test for *Mycoplasma pneumoniae*. *Applied Microbiology*, **24**, 148–149.

44. Pathogenic Fungi

In the laboratory confirmation of the existence and nature of infections by fungi and yeasts, direct methods are more important than indirect methods; identification of the organisms is much more useful than demonstrating the humoral and cellular responses of the host.

For the identification of isolates, microscopical and colonial morphology are used much more than metabolic activities, antigenic structure and pathogenicity for experimental animals.

The methods are simple and though fungi grow easily, they grow slowly. Care must be taken in collecting the specimens to avoid contamination; the appearances of fungi in culture are so variable that considerable experience is required to recognize unusual forms of common pathogens and to distinguish the less common pathogens from contaminants. Laboratories carrying out only a limited amount of mycological work may therefore make their most valuable contribution to the

Table 44.1   Characters of dermatophyte genera

Character	*Microsporum*	*Trichophyton*	*Epidermophyton*
Genus of perfect stage where known	Nannizzia	Arthroderma	Not yet known
Keratinized tissue attacked	Hair Skin (Not nails)	Skin Hair Nails	Skin Nails (Not hair)
Characters of hair infection	Bright green-yellow fluorescence Ectothrix Spores many and small (2–3 μm)	No fluorescence except in *T. schoenleinii* infections (dull green) Endothrix (*T. schoenleinii*, *T. tonsurans* and *T. violaceum*) and ectothrix (*T. mentagrophytes*, small spores, 2–3 μm and *T. verrucosum*, larger spores, 3–6 μm)	Fluorescence Does not occur
Macroconidia in culture	Numerous, except in *M. audouinii* Spindle shaped 7–20 × 35–125 μm Surface rough Septa 4–15 Walls thick, up to 4 μm	Scanty and may be distorted Cylindrical or club shaped 4–8 × 8–50 μm Surface smooth Septa usually 2–6 Walls thin, less than 2 μm	Numerous Pear shaped 6–10 × 30–40 μm Surface smooth Septa 2–4 Walls thin, less than 1·5 μm
Microconidia in culture	Pear shaped 2·5–3·5 × 4–7 μm	Spherical or pear shaped 2–3 × 4–5 μm	Not produced

patient and medical mycology by concentrating on isolating possibly pathogenic fungi from specimens and then sending on all but the most easily identified to an experienced mycologist or mycological reference laboratory. They will probably also in this way make the best use of their own resources.

As pathogenic fungi tend to lose their identifying features in subculture, cultures should be sent on to a reference laboratory as soon as the isolate appears to present a problem, even though the isolating laboratory may also continue its own study of the isolate. The work of identifying an organism often resembles a taxonomic investigation more than routine diagnosis.

In this chapter few details of individual fungi will be given beyond those to be found in Table 44.1. The sections below will deal primarily with the methods of isolation of pathogenic fungi from man.

COLLECTION AND TRANSPORT OF SPECIMENS

SKIN SCALES. Ordinary social washing of the skin is an important preliminary and this should be followed by local cleansing with cotton wool and 70 per cent alcohol. When dry, the active edge of the lesion should be scraped with a sterile scalpel (the type with a banana-shaped blade used by some chiropodists is very convenient) or with a fresh clean microscope slide. If vesicles are present, the tops should be taken with fine scissors. The material collected may be sent in small tubes or in folded paper, preferably black so that small fragments are not lost. It is often convenient to place the material between two slides and then wrap them in black paper.

HAIRS. Infected and damaged hairs may be recognizable with the naked eye. In those infections where the infected hairs fluoresce, selection in the clinic and in the laboratory may be made easier by examination under ultraviolet radiation.

The stumps of the infected hairs should be plucked with forceps. When populations are being surveyed for ringworm of the head, small sterile brushes (Mackenzie, 1963; Midgley and Clayton, 1972) may be used on the hair, after

which the bristles or tines are pressed directly into a plate of suitable medium. Transport is as for skin scales.

NAILS. After thorough cleaning, superficial damaged nail should be pared or scraped away and discarded. Finer parings or scrapings should then be taken from the underlying recently invaded nail. Ordinary nail cuttings are difficult to work with in the laboratory and because any dermatophyte present is liable to be overgrown with contaminants, such specimens are much less likely to yield the pathogen than carefully taken parings. Transport is as for skin scales.

SPUTUM. Fresh morning should be collected and sent to the laboratory without delay, since contaminant yeasts or fungi will multiply rapidly in sputum at room temperature. Several specimens should be sent on different days as it may be impossible to assess the significance of a fungus isolated from a single specimen of sputum.

OTHER SPECIMENS. Pus, urine, cerebrospinal fluid, blood, tissue and ulcer curettings should be collected under sterile conditions in the same way as for bacteriological examination.

MICROSCOPICAL EXAMINATION

Specimens are normally examined as wet preparations in which any tissue cells or keratinized material is partially digested and rendered transparent ('cleared'). Dilute NaOH or KOH (5–30 per cent) or dimethyl sulphoxide (10–40 per cent) or a mixture of the two may be used. Some workers also add Parker's ink for the selective staining of the agent, particularly if candida, pityrosporum (malassezia) or a dermatophyte is being sought. The concentrations and proportions of the different ingredients are not important but the caustics work rather slowly unless the wet preparation is warmed up to about 70°C (slide bearable on the back of the hand). Skin scrapings, hairs and thin nail parings are immersed directly in the fluid on a slide and a coverglass is applied, but if ordinary nail cuttings are sent, they will need preliminary digestion in 30 per cent KOH in a test-tube for up to 3 or 4 hours at 37°C, followed by gentle crushing between slide and coverglass. Sputum and pus are best mixed with the clearing solution before being placed on the slide.

Heat-fixed, Gram-stained dry smears as used generally in bacteriology are satisfactory only for specimens containing yeasts, yeast-like fungi and the larger yeast forms of dimorphic fungi. For the small yeast forms of *Histoplasma capsulatum* alcohol-fixed Giemsa-stained preparations are necessary.

Specimens that might contain either fungi or actinomycetes (e.g. from mycetoma) should be examined both as wet preparations and as dry smears, stained by the Gram and Ziehl-Neelsen methods.

CULTURE OF THE SPECIMEN

Specimens are collected and transported in the same way as for microscopy. Fresh material is best but drying does not harm dermatophytes. Refrigeration of specimens (0–4°C) may damage some filamentous fungi, but if material is kept moist at room temperature any contaminants present will soon overgrow any pathogens.

If a mixture of normal and infected hair is sent, UV light may assist in selecting the best fragments for culture. Sputum may yield better results if it is digested with pancreatin and concentrated (Sanford *et al.,* 1965).

Cerebrospinal fluid should be concentrated by centrifuging and heavy inocula made, especially if culture is for *Cryptococcus neoformans.* Tissue obtained by biopsy should be chopped up in a dish under sterile conditions to give fragments not more than 2 mm in diameter.

Inoculation should be made with straight or hooked nickel chrome wires (SWG 18) on to solid medium and wherever possible, inocula should be pressed into the surface. It is rarely helpful to inoculate specimens into fluid media as a single contaminant spore may overgrow any pathogen present.

Medium should be in the form of slants in tubes or bottles. Petri dishes may be very satisfactory, and perfectly safe, when dermatophytes are being grown but fungi of which the spores are pathogenic on inhalation (e.g. *Histoplasma, Coccidioides*) should never be cultivated in this way. Because fungi are strictly aerobic, cotton-wool plugs should be used. Metal caps, if used, must be left loose.

The choice of medium depends on the organism being sought and the likelihood of contamination. In any particular laboratory it is best to choose a limited range of media, keep their constituents and methods of preparation rigidly uniform and become acquainted with the appearance of the common fungi on them.

For general use, malt tellurite agar or one of the modifications of Sabouraud's medium containing antimicrobial agents is very satisfactory. For the isolation of dermatophytes, the additional incorporation of actidione is helpful as it restrains the growth of many saprophytic fungi (and also some pathogenic fungi and yeasts). Dermatophyte test medium is most appropriately used to demonstrate the presence of a dermatophyte where mycological knowledge and skill are very limited. For the culture of dimorphic fungi rich media such as brain heart infusion agar and penicillin streptomycin blood agar are best and for the demonstration of their yeast forms it is important to use cysteine glucose blood agar without any antimicrobial agent.

The best temperature for incubation of most pathogenic fungi is 26° to 28°C. At 37°C many of them do not grow well and some do not grow at all: only a few grow better (*Aspergillus fumigatus* and most yeasts of medical importance) and only the yeast forms of dimorphic fungi require the higher temperature.

Examination of Cultures

Colonies may first be visible after 24 h or not for 2–3 weeks. Identification depends partly on colonial appearances which change slowly with time but principally on the morphology of the spores which are most clearly seen soon after they first develop. Cultures should therefore be examined every day for the first week and thereafter every 2–3 days. They may be discarded as negative if there is no visible growth after three weeks. Spores are produced in relatively greater numbers on media of low nutritional value (e.g. corn-meal agar) where the growth of vegetative mycelium is restricted.

If a contaminant appears anywhere on the slant, material from the site of the original inoculation should be transferred to a fresh tube at once and with all care. If two different colonies appear at the site of inoculation, each should forthwith be transferred to a fresh tube.

The main features of a colony used in identification are the rate of growth, the colour, texture and folding of the surface and the production and diffusion of pigment into the medium. These change as the colony grows and are best observed, if it is safe to do so, in 'giant colonies' prepared by making a single inoculation into the centre of a Petri dish of suitable medium. The standard method of microscopical examination for fungi is the needle mount (see Vol. II, Chap. 2) but the development of a fungus colony and its spores may be studied microscopically without disturbance or staining by setting up a subculture by the agar block technique (Riddell, 1950).

AGAR BLOCK CULTURE. From Sabouraud's agar plates, cut 1 cm square blocks with a scalpel and ruler and place one on a sterile slide. Inoculate two or more of the vertical sides of the block with a small portion of culture using a straight wire. Place a sterile coverglass on the block and transfer the whole preparation to a closed chamber containing blotting paper soaked in 20 per cent glycerol. A Petri dish, Coplin jar or a plastic slide-staining bath with a lid are satisfactory; the Petri dish will need a bent glass rod to keep the slide and the moist blotting paper apart.

This preparation can be examined, without disturbing the coverslip or the culture, as frequently and for as long as is desired by transferring the whole preparation to a microscope and viewing the growth on the vertical surface of the block with the low power and high dry objectives.

Identification of Isolates

The clinical features of the patient's complaint will indicate the likely causes; the basic mycological features of the relevant organisms are given in Volume I and some details of the common dermatophytes in Table 44.1. Identification is primarily by morphology but nutritional requirements and metabolic activi-ties are used to some extent. Antigenic analysis and animal pathogenicity are of very limited application.

Because of the relative frequency with which yeasts and dermatophytes are isolated, two diagnostic tests used in the identification of *Candida albicans* and a table of characteristic features of some common dermatophytes are given below.

GERM TUBE TEST. Grow the yeast on a peptone containing medium and inoculate some into a small volume of human or horse serum. Incubate at 37°C. Make wet films at 30 min intervals up to 3 h and look for a curved germ tube developing from one pole of some of the yeast cells. This occurs only with *C. albicans* and *C. stellatoidea*.

CHLAMYDOSPORE PRODUCTION. Touch a yeast colony with a straight wire and streak it across and through a plate of corn-meal agar. Incubate at room temperature for 12–48 h. Examine the line of inoculation with the 16 mm objective for the chlamydospores which are diagnostic of *Candida albicans*. They are usually found at the ends of the pseudo-mycelium growing out from the inoculum into the agar.

GENERA AND SPECIES OF DERMATOPHYTES

The distinguishing characters of the three genera of dermatophyte (ringworm-producing) fungi are given in Table 44.1. Those of some of the commoner species are given below.

Microsporum audouinii

The colonies grow rather slowly and form a thin grey dense mat with a downy surface, later becoming radially folded. The medium beneath the colony becomes pinkish brown. *M. audouinii* does not grow on polished rice and sporing is poor on media without added yeast extract. Microconidia are few. Macroconidia are very scanty and though rough and spindle shaped, are often small and distorted; in some strains, none is produced. This species is the main cause of tinea capitis (scalp ringworm) in children in Britain and U.S.A. but laboratories may not isolate it as frequently as many other dermatophytes, perhaps because the clinical diagnosis is more obvious and specimens are not submitted. *M. audouinii* is anthropophilic and no perfect state is known.

M. canis

The colonies grow faster than those of *M. audouinii*; they are white at first with a coarse woolly surface and later develop a sharp yellow colour, best seen at the silky, radially striated edge of the colony or from the back. Growth and pigment are produced on rice grains and sporing is vigorous. Macroconidia outnumber the microconidia and are very large (up to 150 μm long), rough and pointed with thick walls and many septa. The species normally infects cats (and dogs) but causes scalp and body ringworm in children. No perfect state has been demonstrated.

Trichophyton mentagrophytes

The colony types vary. Strains from animals or from human infections derived from animals, are pinkish buff with a granular surface and large numbers of spores. Microconidia are abundant, spherical and found in clusters along the sides of hyphae. Trichophyton-type macroconidia are produced in moderate numbers within 5–10 days and are up to 50 μm long with 3 or 4 septa. Strains from tinea pedis in man (previously called *T. interdigitale*) give rise to white floccose colonies only partially covered with spores but the microscopical appearances are similar. Both strains differ from *T. rubrum* in producing a urease and being able to penetrate fragments of hair in artificial culture. Granular (animal) strains may infect hair of both scalp and chin, causing a small-spored ectothrix infection; the reaction to the fungus may be very brisk and lead (without any bacterial secondary infection) to polymorphonuclear microabscesses in the hair follicles. This is called kerion and it may be followed by a natural cure. The floccose (human) strains of *T. mentagrophytes* usually attack the feet (athlete's foot) and occasionally nails but rarely hair. They appear to be man-adapted and genetically deficient; they occasionally produce no spores and they have not been grown in the perfect state. The granular strains are found in dogs and horses as well as man and the perfect state *Arthroderma benhamiae* has been demonstrated in artificial media by mating of compatible strains.

T. rubrum

The colony is velvety and white or reddish. From the back the pigment is cherry red and may first appear at a dry margin. Microconidia are elongated. Macroconidia are typical of the genus, long and narrow but may not be produced except on rich media. This species is differentiated from *T. mentagrophytes* var. *interdigitale* colonies which are very similar by not producing urease. It attacks skin especially if moist or rubbed (toes and groins) and also nails. It is anthropophilic and has not been isolated from soil; no perfect state is known.

T. verrucosum

This species grows very slowly and needs added yeast extract or thiamine and inositol. Unlike most dermatophytes, it grows better at 37°C than at 30°C. On inadequate media, there may be no growth, or poor growth and no spores. Typical colonies are firm, raised and irregular with a smooth, waxy or just velvety surface. There is more colony beneath the surface of the medium than above it. Pigmentation varies from grey to bright ochre. Macroconidia are absent or, if present, very scanty and irregular. Microconidia are rare. *T. verrucosum* (previously *T. discoides*) causes ringworm in cattle. In farm workers it often causes beard and body ringworm, to which there is a vigorous local reaction.

Epidermophyton floccosum

The colony appears first as a white tuft and then spreads out as a flat grey downy growth becoming greenish yellow and powdery as macroconidia are produced. Later central folding and radial furrows develop and at any stage white tufts of 'sterile' mycelium may appear on the surface and overgrow the whole colony. Microconidia are never produced.

Macroconidia are typically smooth and pear-shaped 30–40 μm in length and with up to 4 septa. There is only one species in the genus. *Epidermophyton* infects the skin of the groin (dhobie's itch) and the toes and occasionally toe nails but never hair. It is anthropophilic and no perfect state has been demonstrated.

REFERENCES AND FURTHER READING

EMMONS, C. W., BINFORD, C. H. & UTZ, J. P. (1971) *Medical Mycology*, 2nd ed. London: Henry Kimpton.

GEORG, L. K., AJELLO, L. & PAPAGEORGE, C. (1954) Use of cycloheximide in the selective isolation of fungi pathogenic to man. *Journal of Laboratory and Clinical Medicine*, **55**, 116.

MACKENZIE, D. W. R. (1963) 'Hairbrush diagnosis' in the detection and eradication of hair ringworm. *British Medical Journal*, **ii**, 363.

MIDGLEY, G. & CLAYTON, Y. M. (1972) Distribution of dermatophytes and Candida spores in the environment. *British Journal of Dermatology*, **86** (Suppl. 8), 69.

RIDDELL, R. W. (1950) Permanent stained mycological preparations obtained by slide culture. *Mycologia*, **42**, 265–270.

SANFORD, L. V., MASON, K. N. & HATHAWAY, B. N. (1965) The concentration of sputum for fungus culture. *American Journal of Clinical Pathology*, **44**, 172.

TAPLIN, D., ZAIAS, N., REBELL, G. & BLANK, H. (1969) Isolation and recognition of dermatophytes on a new medium. *Archives of Dermatology*, **99**, 203.

45. Protozoa

Protozoa are unicellular animals whose range of functions is, however, similar to that of metazoan animals. Parts of the single cell are morphologically differentiated (organelles) for the performance of various functions and so the variety of form in the group is extensive. For example, locomotion is served by a wide variety of organelles—pseudopodia, cilia, flagella and undulating membranes, etc. Thus, protozoa are morphologically diverse and morphology plays a large part in their recognition. Nevertheless, there are many examples of organisms of identical morphology (as far as light and electron microscopy is concerned) being associated with widely different pathological lesions. These different pathological effects may, possibly, be correlated with causations by organisms of different potentiality; but attempts to differentiate morphologically-identical organisms by serological and other means have so far not given very useful results.

Protozoa are mainly important as the causes of several of the 'grandes endémies' which are potent factors in delaying the development of the warm countries of the world—malaria, leishmaniasis, trypanosomiasis and amoebiasis. Besides these infections of major importance, there are many of lesser but still of considerable significance—toxoplasmosis, giardiasis, trichomoniasis, balantidiasis and so on. Protozoal infections in general are of increasing importance in temperate climates as the proportions of the populations composed by immigrants from tropical countries rise, and as tourist activities extend.

Protozoal infections will be treated in this chapter in the approximate order of their medical importance. However, it is useful to provide a taxonomic table to show the position of the genera occurring in man and their relationships to one another. The table is a simplification of that given by Honigberg et al. (1964). Semi-colloquially the organisms concerned are referred to four main groups (as indicated in the taxonomic table on page 545)—the flagellates, the amoebae, the sporozoa and the ciliates. Strictly speaking Naegleria is a flagellate but it is often, because of the form in which it appears as a human pathogen, discussed with the amoebae.

Some of the protozoal infections described are exclusive to man but many involve other species of animal; they are zoonoses—infections of animals transmissible to man (WHO Report, 1967).

The immunology of protozoal infections is not yet well understood. However, a great deal of interest has been directed to this subject in recent years. For summaries of methods of demonstration of antibodies to protozoa see Lumsden (1973). A considerable impetus has been given to studies on the immunology of protozoal infections in the last decade or so by the development of methods for the standardization and maintenance of reference organismal materials by means of cryopreservation. For details of methods for this, and other purposes, see Lumsden, Herbert and McNeillage (1973).

MALARIA

The order Eucoccida in the Subphylum Sporozoa contains the genus *Plasmodium*, four species of which cause malaria in man. The disease is widely distributed in both the Old and New Worlds, between about 40°N and 30°S latitude. However, malaria is nowadays frequently transmitted by bizarre routes, such as by blood transfusion or by the artifices of drug addicts.

LABORATORY DIAGNOSIS

It cannot be too strongly stressed that in the early stages of a primary attack of malaria, particularly *P. falciparum* infection, the clinical picture may be quite unlike that classically associated with malaria; it may simulate many other febrile diseases. Diagnosis depends on the recognition of malaria organisms within erythrocytes in stained films of peripheral blood. Meticulous care in the preparation and staining

Phylum Protozoa

Subphylum I	SARCOMASTIGOPHORA	
Superclass I	Mastigophora (of 3 Superclasses)	
Class 2	Zoomastigophorea (of 2 Classes)	
	Orders—9; of which:	
	Order 3 Rhizomastigida	(*Naegleria*)
	Order 4 Kinetoplastida	(*Leishmania, Trypanosoma*)
	Order 5 Retortamonadida	(*Retortamonas, Enteromonas, Chilomastix*)
	Order 6 Diplomonadida	(*Giardia*)
	Order 8 Trichomonadida	(*Trichomonas*)

Flagellates

Superclass III	Sarcodina	
Class 1	Rhizopodea (of 2 Classes)	
Subclass 1	Lobosia (of 5 Subclasses)	
	Orders—2; of which:	
	Order 1 Amoebida	(*Entamoeba, Endolimax, Iodamoeba, Dientamoeba, Hartmanella*)

Amoebae

Subphylum II	SPOROZOA	
Class 1	Telosporea	
Subclass 2	Coccidia (of 2 Subclasses)	
	Orders—2; of which:	
	Order 2 Eucoccida	(*Eimeria, Isospora, Toxoplasma, Plasmodium*)
Class 2	Piroplasmea	
	Orders—1 only:	
	Order 1 Piroplasmida	(*Babesia*)
Class 3	Toxoplasmea[1]	
	Orders—1 only:	
	Order 1 Toxoplasmida[1]	(*Sarcocystis*)
Class 4	Haplosporea	
	Orders—1 only:	
	Order 1 Haplosporida	(*Pneumocystis*[2])

Sporozoa

Subphylum IV	CILIOPHORA	
	Classes—1 only:	
Class 1	Ciliatea	
Subclass 1	Holotrichia (of 4 Subclasses)	
	Orders—7; of which:	
	Order 2 Trichostomatida	(*Balantidium*)

Ciliates

Notes

1. These groups were originally named as including *Toxoplasma*, which is now transferred to the Order Eucoccida.

2. Considered a yeast-like fungus, by some authors.

of blood films is important if scanty or delicate organisms are not to be overlooked, with serious consequences to the patient.

Blood Films

Blood films should be made on new slides, 75 × 25 mm, cleaned and freed from grease by washing in 70 per cent alcohol, and polished and dried with a fine linen cloth. Previously used cleaned slides, or uncleaned new slides, may produce artefacts which are difficult to interpret on microscopical examination. Blood is most conveniently obtained by puncture of the side of the tip of the third finger with a lancet (Steriseal, Redditch, Worcester, England).

Blood films are stained with Romanowsky stains (e.g. Giemsa's, Leishman's, Wright's stains (Chap. 2)). Two types of blood film are used:

Thick blood films. A dried film is made, some six erythrocytes thick, and the haemoglobin is leached out before staining. Thick blood films are designed to allow the examination of a large quantity of blood quickly, so as to discover low levels of parasitaemia. They are less suitable for the examination of individual parasites in order to make a *Plasmodium* species-specific diagnosis.

A drop of blood about 3 mm in diameter is deposited in the centre of a slide and is spread, with the head of a pin, or with the corner of another slide, to cover an area about 10 mm in diameter. The density of the film should be such that the hands of a watch can just be seen through it. The film is then thoroughly dried, e.g. at 37°C in an incubator for 30 minutes. The film is *not fixed* (which would retain the haemoglobin in the cells) but is simply stained in diluted Giemsa's stain (Chap. 2), during which process the haemoglobin is leached out of the cells. Alternatively, the haemoglobin is removed first by treating with acid alcohol (ethanol 100 per cent with 10 drops of HCl per 50 ml) or with a solution of 2 per cent glacial acetic acid and 0·4 per cent crystalline tartaric acid in distilled water; the film is then washed in water and stained with Giemsa's stain.

Thin blood films. These are adapted to show the morphological characteristics of the organisms,

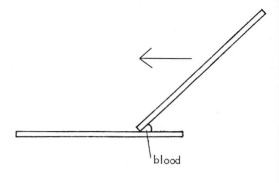

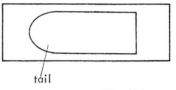

FIG. 45.1
Preparation of blood film.

and of the cells which contain them, most clearly and so aid *Plasmodium* species-specific diagnosis. Ideally, they are one cell thick, i.e. all cells are clearly displayed for examination.

A small drop of blood (about 1·5 mm in diameter) is placed near one end of a slide and, immediately, the end of a second slide is applied to the first slide at an angle of about 45° (Fig. 45.1), the drop of blood being in the re-entrant angle. The end of the second slide is then drawn 'back' to contact the drop, which is then allowed a second or two to spread along the junction of the two slides. The drop is then spread along the first slide by a continuous 'forward' movement of the slide held at 45°. Ideally, the film should cover two-thirds of the centre of the length of the slide, should have a 'tail', and should not extend to the edges of the first slide (Fig. 45.1). The films are allowed to dry, and are then fixed with absolute methanol and stained with Giemsa's stain using a phosphate buffer at pH 7·2.

Thick and thin films are best made on separate slides, so as to avoid the accident of inadvertent fixation of the thick film.

Examination of Films

After the film is stained and dried, immersion oil is spread thinly over its surface with a matchstick and the film is then scanned 'dry' with the ×40 objective; the oil immersion objective is used for a closer examination of possible parasites.

To inexperienced workers, artefacts may sometimes simulate malaria parasites, e.g. a blood platelet overlying a red corpuscle may be mistaken for a *Plasmodium* trophozoite. Essentially, a malaria parasite is recognized by its red-staining nuclear material and blue-staining cytoplasm, and by its occurrence *within* the erythrocyte.

The various species of *Plasmodium* are differentiated not only by their own morphological characteristics but also by the changes which they induce in the cells which they parasitize. These characteristics are summarized in Table 45.1. It must be remembered, however, that the young trophozoites (ring forms) of all four species may be almost indistinguishable from one another, and if only these forms are present in the film, it may be difficult to determine the species.

The most important species diagnosis to be made is that of *P. falciparum*, the parasite of malignant tertian malaria, infections with which may be rapidly lethal in non-immune subjects. The special characteristics of the blood film in infections with this parasite are:

1. The later stages of the asexual reproductive cycle are generally confined to capillaries and deep organs and, therefore, do not appear in the peripheral blood, which contains only early trophozoites (ring forms).

2. Ring forms tend to occur two or more in single cells; *accolé* and *tenué* forms—thin forms applied to the periphery of the erythrocyte or stretched across it—often occur.

3. Gametocytes, if they occur, are crescent-shaped, not round as in the other *Plasmodium* species.

General Comments

Films should, if possible, be taken during the pyrexia and no antimalarial drugs should have been administered beforehand.

It is essential that the film should be well stained; otherwise it is useless searching for parasites. A valuable guide is the staining of the leucocytes in the film; if this is satisfactory any malaria parasites present should be detectable.

It is advisable, in searching thin films for scanty malaria organisms, to examine particularly the edges of the film; parasites may be more numerous there than in the centre. In the diagnosis of clinical malaria, thin blood films are usually sufficient except perhaps in some *P. vivax* and *P. malariae* infections. The absence of parasites during an apyrexial interval, however, by no means excludes malaria and repeated examination of films, including thick films, may be required before the diagnosis can be established.

The diagnosis of malaria by blood examination is exhaustively discussed by Shute and Maryon (1960).

Bone marrow may contain more parasites than occur in peripheral blood and so bone marrow smears, obtained by sternal puncture, may be used for diagnostic purposes.

TRYPANOSOMIASIS

Trypanosoma cruzi and *Tryp. brucei* spp. are the causes of trypanosomiasis in man in, respectively, South and Central America, and Africa. These organisms adopt at different times in their life histories a variety of forms—mainly amastigote, epimastigote and trypomastigote (see Vol. I, Chap. 54). Although the pathological effects of the two diseases differ profoundly, *Tryp. cruzi* exerting its effect mainly through the heart and gut musculature, and *Tryp. brucei* mainly through the CNS, there is a general similarity in the progress of the diseases. A primary lesion may be present at the site of inoculation and multiplication of organisms may take place there locally. This is followed by a stage of general dissemination of the organisms ('early stage') in the body when organisms may be plentiful in the peripheral blood and hence comparatively easily recognized for diagnostic purposes. Later stages of both diseases are slowly progressive and organisms are extremely scarce in peripheral blood and in other fluids which may be

Table 45.1 Differential diagnosis of *Plasmodium* species of man in Romanowsky-stained thin films of peripheral blood

	P. falciparum Malignant tertian	P. vivax Benign tertian	P. malariae Quartan	P. ovale Ovale tertian
			Species and disease	
Trophozoites (a) Ring forms	0·15 to 0·5 of diameter of RBC; RBC normal size Cytoplasm—very fine in young rings; thick irregular in old rings. Marginal (accolé) forms, forms with 2 chromatin dots and multiple infections, common	0·3 to 0·5 of diameter of RBC which is unaltered in size Cytoplasm—circle, thin	0·3 to 0·5 of diameter of RBC which is unaltered in size Cytoplasm—circle, thicker	0·3 of diameter of RBC which is unaltered in size Cytoplasm—circle, thicker
(b) Growing forms	RBC unaltered in size, sometimes stippled, pale Parasite compact; pigment dense brown or black mass *Not usually seen in peripheral blood*	RBC enlarged, stippled Parasite amoeboid, vacuolated; pigment fine and scattered, golden brown	RBC unaltered Parasite compact, rounded or band-shaped; dark brown or black pigments, often concentrates in a line along one edge of band	RBC unaltered in size, or slightly enlarged; stippled; may be oval and fimbriated Parasite compact, rounded; pigment fine brown grains
Mature schizonts	RBC unaltered in size, sometimes stippled, pale Parasite about 0·6 of RBC; nuclei or merozoites 8–24; pigment clumped, black *Not usually seen in peripheral blood*	RBC much enlarged, stippled Parasite large, filling enlarged RBC; nuclei or merozoites 12–24, usually 16; pigment a golden brown central loose mass	RBC unaltered Parasite fills RBC completely; nuclei or merozoites 6–12, usually 8, sometimes forming rosette; pigment, brown black central clump	RBC frequently oval, fimbriated, enlarged, stippled Parasite as for *P. malariae* but does not entirely fill the slightly enlarged RBC; pigment, brown central clump
Gametocytes	RBC distorted Parasite crescentic	RBC enlarged, stippled Parasite large, rounded filling enlarged RBC	RBC unaltered Parasite small, round filling RBC	RBC slightly enlarged, stippled Parasite round
Stippling	Maurer's clefts	Schüffner's dots	None (Ziemann's dots after prolonged Leishman staining)	James's dots

548

sampled. This latter situation provides the main problem in diagnosis.

LABORATORY DIAGNOSIS

Primary Lesion

Aspirates of the lesion should be examined fresh, with phase contrast illumination, searching for active motile organisms (*Tryp. brucei*), or the aspirate should be made into thin films, fixed and stained with Romanowsky stain, and examined in exactly the same manner as blood films for malaria.

Early Stage

During the early (or acute) stage, organisms may often be recognized by simple examinations of the blood or lymphatic fluid, as described below. In cases where these methods are unsuccessful, extend investigations to include the procedures detailed for the late (chronic) stage of the infections.
Blood. Both thin and thick films are prepared and examined as described in examination for malaria parasites. Repeated examinations are desirable, say daily for 7 days.
Lymph. Fluid obtained by aspiration of enlarged lymph nodes is examined fresh, or as thin films stained with Romanowsky stain (*Tryp. brucei*).

Late or Chronic Stage

In general, the concentrations of organisms present in body fluids are very low. Thus direct examinations are usefully reinforced by examination of CSF (*Tryp. brucei*); by concentration of organisms by various techniques, and by multiplicative techniques, i.e. by introducing the sample into an environment, e.g. a culture or a susceptible animal, in which organisms can multiply and thus allow their presence to be detected (see below).
Cerebrospinal fluid. The cell count, the protein content and the occurrence of trypanosomes (*Tryp. brucei*) are of diagnostic importance. First, do the cell count, noting at the same time if trypanosomes are present. If no trypanosomes have been seen, centrifuge the specimen, resuspend the deposit in a small quantity of CSF and examine as a fresh preparation for motile trypanosomes, conveniently also in the counting chamber; or make films of the deposit, fix and stain with Giemsa's stain. Estimate the protein concentration on the supernatant from the centrifugation.

Concentration Methods

Organisms may be concentrated:
1. By centrifuging several millilitres of anticoagulated blood sufficiently to deposit most of the red cells, and then recentrifuging the supernatant to deposit remaining particles. This second deposit is examined, preferably as a fresh film.
2. By centrifugation of heparinized blood in microhaematocrit centrifuge tubes and examining the 'buffy layer' lying over the erythrocytes, either through the wall of the tube or by cutting the tube and expelling the buffy layer on to a slide. Beware of aerosols from tubes fracturing under centrifugation, and the risk of self-inoculation.
3. By passing the heparinized blood through an anion-exchange column with a suitable buffer (Lanham, 1968), and then, after centrifuging the eluate, examining the deposit, either fresh or stained. Because of differences in the surface charge between trypanosomes and blood corpuscles, the corpuscles are preferentially retained on the cellulose while the trypanosomes pass through. Trypanosomes may then be concentrated by centrifugation of the eluate otherwise free of cells. Alternatively the eluate may be filtered ('Millipore') and the filter membrane fixed and stained. This method is very sensitive, and is able to detect trypanosome concentrations as low as 4 per ml. It is, however, easily applicable only to *Tryp. brucei*, not to *Tryp. cruzi*.

Multiplicative Methods

These include introduction of any of the body fluids, already subjected to direct examination, into animals or into culture media, and also xenodiagnosis (allowing known susceptible but uninfected vectors to feed on the suspect host and then examining the gut contents of the vector for organisms, after a period appropriate to allow their multiplication).

Animal inoculation. Inoculate as large volumes as can be accepted by the animal, intraperitoneally, into laboratory animals. For *Tryp. cruzi*, mice are usually susceptible though puppies may sometimes be preferable. For *Tryp. brucei rhodesiense*, mice or rats are usually susceptible. For *Tryp. brucei gambiense*, laboratory rodents are less easily infected and young *Cercopithecus* monkeys or *Cricetomys gambianus* (giant rat) are used. Examine the blood of the inoculated animals, conveniently as fresh films, every 2–3 days till day 30 post-inoculation.

Culture. Inoculate blood, lymph or CSF into blood-agar-slope cultures incubated at 25°–28°C and subsequently examine for developmental forms—epimastigotes and trypomastigotes: useful for *Tryp. cruzi* but not for *Tryp. brucei*, because of general greater difficulty in culturing the latter trypanosomes.

Xenodiagnosis. For *Tryp. cruzi* infections: some 10–20 laboratory-bred triatomid bugs, usually instar 3 or 4 nymphs of *Triatoma infestans* or *Rhodnius prolixus*, are allowed to feed on the suspect host and after at least 14 days the following materials are examined for organisms: faeces expelled by manipulation; dissected gut; or centrifuged suspensions of triturated whole bugs. There is little standardization of techniques as regards the bug instars used, the numbers allowed to feed and the period after which examination takes place. The method is not applicable for diagnosis of *Tryp. brucei* because the trypanosomes produce only very low infection rates in *Glossina* ssp. Beware of the danger of laboratory infection from bug faeces.

Serological Methods

Tryp. cruzi. CF, HA and IF tests are in use, but only CF (Guerreiro-Machado reaction) has been widely used. Procedures vary and antigens are in the process of study for standardization.

Tryp. brucei. IF, agglutination and other tests recently introduced are in process of evaluation. Generally, specific tests may not recognize individuals that can be infected by protozoological means. In this situation much attention has been directed to the estimation of serum and CSF IgM as a diagnostic test.

Mattern *et al.* (1967) cite serum IgM values up to 16 times normal in serum of *Tryp. brucei*-infected patients; this, and more particularly similarly high values in the CSF, are of high diagnostic significance. Serum or CSF IgM concentrations are readily estimated by radial immunodiffusion in agar gel containing anti-IgM serum (Mancini system) or by titration in double-diffusion system (Ouchterlony).

LEISHMANIASIS

Leishmania is closely related to *Trypanosoma*. *Leishmania* spp. infect man, canids, rodents and reptiles. All species, as far as is known, are transmitted by *Phlebotomus* and *Lutzomyia* spp. (Diptera, Nematocera—sandflies). In the mammal host *Leishmania* exist as amastigotes within cells of the mononuclear phagocytic system (MPS) (van Furth *et al.*, 1972).

When the insect ingests infected blood or tissue, the organisms become transformed to promastigotes in the gut where they multiply, ultimately migrating to the buccal cavity from which they are inoculated when the insect bites another host.

Leishmanial infections are classified mainly on the basis of their clinical characteristics: whether they are 'visceral' affecting chiefly the spleen, or 'cutaneous' affecting chiefly the skin. The latter category of infection sometimes also involves the mucous membranes of the nose and pharynx (mucocutaneous leishmaniasis). Although specific names—*L. donovani*, *L. tropica*, *L. mexicana*, *L. brasiliensis*, etc.—are conferred on these organisms, these names are representative of clinical manifestation and geographical distribution, rather than of differences in morphology or biological behaviour in the laboratory.

Leishmania spp. occur intracellularly in the amastigote form in MPS cells of the host, mainly in those of the spleen, liver, bone marrow or lymph nodes in the visceral disease (kala-azar), mainly in the skin and/or mucous membranes in the cutaneous disease (tropical sore, chiclero's ulcer, uta, espundia, etc.). One cell may contain 10 or more organisms.

In films stained with Romanowsky stains, *Leishmania* spp. appear as intracellular round or oval organisms 2–5 μm in their longest diameters. Sometimes in films made from blood, spleen or bone marrow, torpedo-shaped forms occur. Such organisms show two organelles—one large, rounded and palely staining (nucleus); one smaller, rod-shaped, more deeply staining (kinetoplast). Often, since the staining will not differentiate the cytoplasm of an organism from that of the cell in which it occurs, the margins of the organisms will not be distinguishable and organisms will appear simply as pairings of larger paler-staining structures with smaller densely-staining structures. The cytoplasm of the organism may be vacuolated and the organisms may occur in vacuoles in the cytoplasm of the host cell or simply in the continuity of the cytoplasm.

Leishmania spp. are readily cultured in blood agar media (*NNN*, or *4N*; 20 per cent blood agar), incubated at 20°–28°C. In culture the organisms increase in size, elongate and develop a flagellum from the kinetoplast situated near one end, i.e. they develop and reproduce as promastigotes.

Monkeys and dogs may be infected experimentally but *Cricetulus barbarensis griseus* (Chinese hamster) and *Mesocricetus auratus* golden hamster) are extremely susceptible and are the animals of choice for use for diagnostic purposes. All these animals should be inoculated intraperitoneally.

Laboratory Diagnosis

Visceral Leishmaniasis (Kala-azar)—L. donovani

Direct and Multiplicative Methods

L. donovani occurs typically in cells of the spleen, liver, bone marrow and lymph nodes. Material for examination may be obtained by:
1. *Spleen puncture.* This is the most sensitive method of diagnosis. Splenic tissue is obtained by means of a dry hypodermic needle and syringe. The procedure is not without risk and liver puncture, which is nearly as sensitive a method of diagnosis, may be preferred.
2. *Sternal puncture.* This is safer than either spleen or liver puncture.
3. *Lymph node puncture.* The inguinal nodes are those mostly used; but lymph node puncture, though without risk to the patient, is a less sensitive diagnostic method than is spleen or liver puncture.

Blood film

Organisms may occur in blood films, but the method is not sensitive enough for routine diagnosis. Leucopenia is invariable in uncomplicated kala-azar and there is a relative lymphocytosis.

With materials obtained by these methods:
1. Prepare films, stain with Giemsa's stain and examine for amastigotes occurring intracellularly in MPS cells.
2. Inoculate blood-agar cultures incubated at 20°–28°C (*NNN* or *4N*) and examine for promastigotes every few days up to 28 days.
3. Inoculate hamsters intraperitoneally; kill the animals after 5 months and examine spleen smears for amastigotes.

Serological Methods

Formol-gel (aldehyde) reaction (Napier, 1921). This test is mediated by the changes in immunoglobulin quantities and ratios which are characteristic of kala-azar. Immunoglobulins are increased, and the increase is mainly in the IgG fraction. The test is performed as follows:

About 5 ml of blood are withdrawn and allowed to clot. The serum is separated and to 1 ml of it are added two drops of commercial formalin (40 per cent formaldehyde in water). A positive reaction is indicated by an immediate opacity, followed within 20 minutes by the development of a firm white gelatinous coagulum (like hard-boiled egg albumin); mere jellification without opacity is not accepted as a positive result. This method is commonly used in India, but it has been found unreliable in the diagnosis of kala-azar in other countries. It is, of course, not specific, as the globulin changes concerned may occur also in other diseases.

Complement fixation test. This is of definite value; antigens may be prepared from spleens of infected laboratory animals or from *L. donovani* in culture; but antigens prepared from acid-fast bacilli—*Mycobacterium tuberculosis* or *M. phlei*—are equally effective (Monsur, 1956).

Fluorescent antibody test. Promastigotes from cultures are used as slide antigen.

Delayed hypersensitivity skin test (*Leishmanin or Montenegro test*). This test involves the intradermal inoculation of 0·2 ml of a suspension of washed promastigotes (antilog 8 organisms/ml) of *Leishmania* spp. in 0·5 per cent phenol in saline. The test is read at 48 or 72 hours. A positive result is an indurated lesion more than 5 mm in diameter. In kala-azar the test becomes positive only 6–8 weeks after recovery from the disease.

Cutaneous and/or Mucocutaneous Leishmaniasis (Tropical Ulcer, Uta, Chiclero's Ulcer, Pian Bois, Espundia, etc.)—L. tropica, L. mexicana, L. brasiliensis

There is an extremely wide range of pathological lesions in cutaneous/mucocutaneous *Leishmania* infections. In the mildest infections (*L. tropica*), single ulcers on exposed surfaces of the body heal spontaneously in a few years and lead to a condition of permanent immunity, though the scars left by the lesions may be disfiguring. In the most severe infections (*L. brasiliensis*) there is chronic ulceration of skin surfaces and, much more seriously, secondary and extremely disfiguring involvement of the mucosae of the mouth and upper respiratory tract. These severe conditions are intractable to treatment and usually lead to early death by bacterial infection secondary to the gross destruction in the upper respiratory tract. There are immunologically recognizable differences between these *Leishmania* species.

Direct and Multiplicative Methods

The organisms are to be found mainly in the peripheral parts of cutaneous ulcers or in intact mucosa peripheral to mucosal lesions.

Skin ulcers. Films may be made from scrapings of the margin of the ulcer after cleansing of surface discharge which is usually bacterially infected. It is preferable to aspirate the margin of the lesion with a fine needle attached to a 10 ml syringe, just outside the ulcer (with the needle angled so as to penetrate just below the edge of the ulcer), and make films of the aspirate. Films are fixed in absolute methanol and stained with Giemsa's stain, as for thin blood films. Organisms may also be found in films of aspirates of the regional lymph nodes draining the ulcer.

Mucocutaneous lesions. Mucosal lesions are secondary to cutaneous lesions and organisms can usually be found in films prepared from scrapings of the intact mucosae immediately peripheral to the lesion; or in films of nasal secretion.

Sensitivity of diagnosis may be enhanced by inoculation of the materials described above into blood agar culture or into susceptible animals. Cultures, incubated at 25°–28°C, should be maintained for 30 days before discarding but in inoculated hamsters or mice amastigotes should be recognizable in films made from lesions, within 14 days.

Serological Methods

Delayed hypersensitivity skin test (*Leishmanin or Montenegro test*). See above, visceral leishmaniasis. In the less pathogenic infections (*L. tropica* and *L. mexicana*) the reaction becomes positive early in the infection, in the more pathogenic (*L. brasiliensis*), later in the active phase.

AMOEBIASIS

Of the seven species of amoebae occurring in the human intestinal tract, only *Entamoeba histolytica* is pathogenic.

LABORATORY DIAGNOSIS

Faeces

Collection of specimens. Examine the freshly passed faeces in a bedpan and select for examination a portion that looks suspicious, such as bloodstained mucus, which is characteristic of the acute stage of the infection. Alternatively the specimen, unmixed with urine, may be collected in a faeces specimen tube provided with a cork carrying a metal spoon or scoop which fits into the tube.

Microscopic examination. For the recognition of trophozoites the faeces should be examined as soon as possible after being passed and while still warm. The material is emulsified in warmed (solution kept in 37°C incubator) 0·5 per cent eosin saline on a clean microscope slide and covered with a coverslip. Ideally, examination is best carried out on a warm stage; however, as a substitute for this, a small coin previously heated in a bunsen flame can be placed at the end of the prepared slide. The slide is examined using a × 40 objective; trophozoites and cysts are readily identified as they do not stain with eosin.

For the recognition of cysts, place one drop of 2 per cent iodine in 4 per cent potassium iodide solution in water ('double-strength Lugol's iodine') and add to it a small piece of faeces by means of a wire loop or swab stick; mix the faeces in the iodine solution to an even suspension, reject large and coarse particles and cover with a 22 × 22 mm cover slip, so that it adheres firmly (for subsequent examination under oil immersion objective). The finished preparation should not be so thick that single cells and faecal constituents cannot be seen separated from one another ('ground glass' consistency). The preparation is examined with the × 40 objective. When cysts are found, species diagnoses are made using the × 100 oil-immersion objective.

Care and experience in the making and examination of the films are very important.

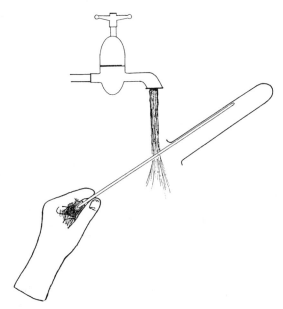

FIG. 45.2
Method of removing debris from inside of centrifuge tube.

The rate of cyst production is not uniform, so that in the case of repeated examinations of faeces it is better to examine three successive specimens at weekly rather than daily intervals.

Preparations stained with iron haematoxylin are useful in the identification of intestinal amoeba. Films from the stool are made on coverslips and are fixed 'wet' by floating the coverslips (film downwards) on a fixing solution consisting of 2 parts saturated mercuric chloride in saline with 1 part absolute ethanol.

Ulcers

Swabs of ulcers, or fragments of tissue from the edge of ulcers, obtained at sigmoidoscopy, examined by the same methods as described for faeces, offer the best chance of finding *E. histolytica* in chronic cases. Alternatively, sections of the tissue obtained may be cut and stained with haemotoxylin and eosin.

Concentration of Cysts (and Helminth Ova) in Faeces

This method (Ridley and Hawgood, 1956) is effective for the concentration of all protozoal cysts and helminth ova, without distortion. It takes only about 5 minutes to perform.

Emulsify with pestle and mortar about 10 g of faeces in approximately 30 ml of 4 per cent formaldehyde in saline (volume of formol saline depends on consistency of faeces). Pass the suspension through a wire sieve (of 250 μm diameter apertures). Pour 15 ml of the sieved suspension into a 25 ml centrifuge tube and add 3 ml of diethyl ether. Shake vigorously, at least 50 times. Centrifuge, at about 650 g for 2 minutes. Using a glass rod, loosen the fatty debris which collects at the liquid interface; keeping the glass rod in position invert the tube boldly to an angle of 45° with the horizontal, pouring away the supernate and the debris. Some of the debris remains attached to the inside of the tube; clear this off with the glass rod by holding the rod under the jet of a running tap allowing the jet to play on the rod and run back inside the tube (Fig. 45.2). Remove samples of the deposit by means of a pasteur pipette, and examine them on a glass slide with a superimposed cover-slip. The factor of concentration is 30–40 times. As the preparations are 'fixed' (by the presence of formalin) cysts will be killed and so eosin staining is valueless; however, iodine or Sargeaunt's stain are useful.

Culture of Intestinal Amoebae
The method of Robinson (1968) (p. 139) is used.

Cultivation

About 50 mg of fresh untreated faeces are added by wire loop to a culture bottle, which receives at the time of inoculation 4 drops (0·12 ml) of 0·5 per cent erythromycin and 10 mg of starch (judged by eye on a knife blade). Basal amoebic medium is added to fill two-thirds of the bottle. After incubating at 37°C for 24 hours, the supernatant is pipetted off and replaced by an equal volume mixture of basal medium and phthalate solution (p. 140) to the same level. Two drops (0·06 ml) of 20 per cent bactopeptone, two drops (0·06 ml) of 0·5 per cent erythromycin and more starch are added. The culture is again incubated at 37°C.

After 24 hours, drops of the culture sediment are examined microscopically in double-strength Lugol's iodine. (The culture should be re-examined after a further 48 hours' incubation.) The presence of *Entamoeba histolytica* is suggested in the first place by the abundance and rapidity of its growth. It is distinguished from *Endolimax nana* and *Entamoeba hartmanni* by being larger; with these smaller species a change from the ×20 to the ×40 objective is necessary to observe detail. *E. coli* is distinguished from *E. histolytica* by being less often bunched, being larger, more rounded and more 'glassy' and staining deep red with iodine. The distinctive nuclear pattern of *Dientamoeba fragilis* is shown by iron haematoxylin staining.

It is recommended that an eye-piece scale is used when reading these cultures.

Morphology of E. histolytica

Trophozoite. Trophozoites measure from 9–30 μm and may be round, elongated or irregular in shape. The cytoplasm consists of a clear hyaline ectoplasm, and a granular, often vacuolated endoplasm, but this differentiation is not always readily observed. In their most

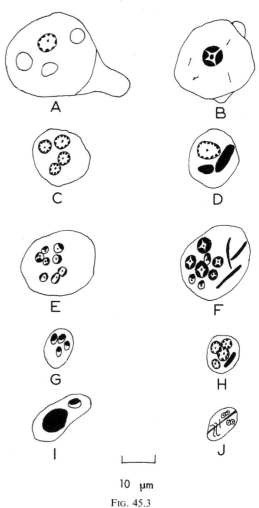

10 μm

FIG. 45.3
Entamoebae in different stages of development.
A = *E. histolytica* trophozoite showing pseudopodium and three included erythrocytes.
B = *E. coli* trophozoite showing pseudopodia and included bacteria.
C = *E. histolytica* cyst with 4 nuclei.
D = *E. histolytica* cyst with one nucleus and chromatoids.
E = *E. coli* cyst.
F = *E. coli* cyst with 8 nuclei, some of which show 'quadrant form' of nuclear chromatin. There are chromatoids present.
G = *Endolimax nana* cyst.
H = *E. hartmanni* cyst with 4 nuclei and a chromatoid.
I = *Iodamoeba buetschlii* cyst showing large discrete 'iodine' vacuole.
J = *Giardia intestinalis* cyst.

active condition the amoebae show flowing movements of their protoplasm and rapidly protrude and retract broad pseudopodia (lobopodia), which may be composed at first mostly of ectoplasm. These movements lead to changes in shape and also to active translatory progression. The nucleus is round or oval, and in the unstained condition is not easily distinguished. It is situated in the endoplasm, usually eccentric in position. It is poor in chromatin, and the nuclear membrane is thin. The chromatin granules are small, and are collected in a ring just inside the nuclear membrane; the nucleus shows a small central karyosome. The amoebae ingest red blood corpuscles, which are observed in the endoplasm, but ingested bacteria are less frequently found. The ingested erythrocytes appear smaller than normal. Ingestion of erythrocytes by amoebae in faecal specimens is pathognomonic of *E. histolytica*. Vegetative forms, after leaving the body, soon become rounded and immobile, die and disintegrate. *Cyst.* Cysts are spherical, with a thin, hyaline, refractile wall, which gives them a distinct double contour. The contents are finely granular, and the average diameter is 12·5 μm. Cysts may contain from one to four nuclei, a diffuse glycogen mass and chromatoid bodies (Fig. 45.3).

Wet preparations stained with iodine are used to show up the nuclei and the glycogen mass. Newly-formed cysts have only one nucleus, and more mature ones, two or four. The glycogen mass is best seen in the newly-formed cyst. The chromatoid bodies remain unstained with iodine, appearing as refractile bodies; however, they stain with Sargeaunt's stain (p. 52) (used after the Ridley and Hawgood concentration method).

Differentiation of E. histolytica from Other Human Intestinal Amoebae and Flagellates

Short descriptions are given which concentrate on useful points for differentiation from *E. histolytica*.

Amoebae

Entamoeba hartmanni. Not often seen in the trophozoite stage in faeces, but frequently as a cyst. The cysts resemble those of *E. histolytica* except that they measure less than 10 μm in diameter (average 8·5 μm) and are frequently immature containing only one nucleus, chromatoid bodies, and diffuse iodine-staining vacuoles.

Entamoeba coli. The trophozoites resemble those of *E. histolytica*, but the cytoplasm is not so distinctly differentiated into endo- and ectoplasm. The pseudopodia are small and blunt and not so refractile as those of *E. histolytica*; translatory movement is negligible. The nucleus is usually central in position, easily distinguishable, rich in chromatin (which is sometimes arranged in 'quadrant form'; Fig. 45.3) and has a thick, refractile, nuclear membrane. The karyosome is larger than in *E. histolytica*. Erythrocytes are not ingested (when this parasite occurs in cases of dysentery) although *E. coli* ingests red cells *in vitro* as readily as does *E. histolytica*. Bacteria are ingested, often in large numbers. The cysts are larger (15–30 μm) than those of *E. histolytica*, the wall is thick, and the mature cyst contains eight nuclei. Chromatoid bodies, when present (usually only seen rarely in immature cysts) are thin, sharp, pointed structures. A diffuse glycogen vacuole may also be present.

Endolimax nana. A frequent intestinal amoeba. The trophozoite is 9 μm in diameter or less. In unstained preparations the single nucleus is not distinct, but haematoxylin staining shows it to have a large, irregular eccentric karyosome. The cysts are usually oval, about 8 μm in diameter. When mature they contain four small nuclei easily seen in wet preparations stained with iodine or with Sargeaunt's stain, similar to the single nucleus seen in the trophozoite, but no chromatoid bodies.

Iodamoeba buetschlii. The trophozoite is very rarely seen in faeces. Cysts measure 9–12 μm in diameter, not usually spherical, and may assume bizarre shapes. They are easily distinguished in iodine preparations by their discrete, deeply-staining, glycogen vacuole. They have a single nucleus.

Dientamoeba fragilis. Rarely seen, since the trophozoites rapidly disintegrate on being passed in the faeces. They are sluggishly motile and have a single massive nucleus. No cyst is known to be formed by this amoeba.

The foregoing comprise the amoebae which may occur in the faeces. There remains:

Entamoeba gingivalis. This organism may occur in considerable numbers in pathological conditions of the mouth, e.g. pyorrhoea, gingivitis, dental caries, but has no definite aetiological relationship to these conditions. The trophozoites are about 10–20 μm in diameter and resemble *E. histolytica* in many respects, showing active amoeboid movement and differentiation of the cytoplasm into ecto- and endo-plasm: the nucleus is indistinct in unstained preparations. The organisms ingest free cells, e.g. leucocytes. They do not form cysts.

Flagellates

Giardia intestinalis. Trophozoites, flattened, pear-shaped; bilaterally symmetrical; 10–18 μm in long diameter; a large sucking disk, on one surface; two nuclei with karyosomes; eight flagella in pairs which arise from the anterior half of the organism (the broad end is called 'anterior'). *Giardia* trophozoites live usually in the duodenum and so only appear in the faeces in diarrhoea. The cysts are characteristic: oval in shape, about 10 μm long, with two or four nuclei (the cyst containing two organisms formed by subdivision); the parallel axostyles are observable, lying diagonally across the length of the cyst.

Giardia infection (giardiasis) is sometimes the cause of dyspepsia, diarrhoea, maladsorption and steatorrhoea, but is often symptomless.

Retortamonas intestinalis. Non-pathogenic. The trophozoite is oval and measures approximately 4·0 × 8·0 μm; it has three flagella. The cyst has four nuclei and measures approximately 4·0 × 7·0 μm.

Chilomastix mesnili. Non-pathogenic. The trophozoite is a pyriform organism having three anterior flagella plus one recurrent and measures 6–20 × 4–10 μm. The cyst is pear-shaped with a single vesicular nucleus and measures approximately 7·0 μm in the long axis.

Enteromonas hominis. Non-pathogenic. Trophozoite oval, 4–10 μm long with three anteriorly directed and one posteriorly directed flagellum. Cysts 6–8 μm long; most binucleate, quadrinucleate when mature.

Serological Diagnosis

Complement fixation tests (Robinson, 1972) and fluorescent antibody tests (Jeanes, 1969) are available. High antibody titres are indicative of extraintestinal involvement such as liver abscess. Jeanes (1969) records titres of up to 32 in symptomless carriers of *E. histolytica* but considers 64 and upwards as indicative of recent active extraintestinal infection. See also Lumsden (1973).

TRICHOMONIASIS

Of the three species of *Trichomonas* infecting man only *Trichomonas vaginalis* is importantly pathogenic, as a cause of vaginitis.

Laboratory Diagnosis

Direct examination. Materials to be examined are:

1. Vaginal exudate. Samples are obtained by swab or pipette or, best, by centrifugation, in 'Hemmings' filter assemblies, of pieces of polyester sponge (Robertson *et al.*, 1969).

2. Centrifugate of urine.

3. For males, urethral secretion or scrapings, with or without prostatic massage.

Specimens are best examined as wet films suspended in isotonic saline by means of phase-contrast illumination, though dried films stained with Giemsa's stain may also be used. Wet films are preferable as the jerky movements of the organism are conspicuous.

Trichomonas vaginalis is a pear-shaped organism 9–15 μm long. Three to five flagella arise from the anterior (broad) end. One flagellum is reflexed posteriorly and forms the border of the undulating membrane. There is a skeletal 'axostyle'.

Culture. The sensitivity of diagnosis may be increased by culturing samples (Robertson *et al.*, 1969). The modification by Lumsden *et al.* (1973) of Feinberg and Whittington's isotonic trichomonas medium is a simple effective culture medium; anaerobiosis of the culture is important.

Two other species of *Trichomonas* infect man, *Trichomonas tenax* in the mouth and *Trichomonas hominis* in the caecum. Neither is pathogenic.

BALANTIDIASIS

Balantidium coli is the only organism in the Ciliophora pathogenic to man; it is found in the faeces and causes ulceration of the large intestine similar to that produced by *Entamoeba histolytica*.

Laboratory Diagnosis

Direct films of faeces and the concentration method described previously for amoebiasis are used. The trophozoite is oval, measuring up to some 140 μm in its long axis. The whole of the body is covered with short cilia which propel the organism in rapid, rolling, directional movements. A large, easily seen, macronucleus is present, situated centrally and just below the funnel-shaped cytostome (mouth). Cysts are formed, which are similar in appearance to the trophozoite, except that they are spherical in shape, thick-walled and lack a cytostome, and are non-motile.

MISCELLANEOUS HUMAN PROTOZOAL INFECTIONS

Toxoplasma

Diagnosis. Dried, methanol-fixed films of body fluids or exudate should be stained with Giemsa's stain and examined for the crescent-shaped zoites which measure 6–7 μm × 2–4 μm and have blue-staining cytoplasm and a red-staining nucleus. The organisms may be inoculated into mice intraperitoneally and their peritoneal fluid examined for zoites in the same way after 7 days.

Serological diagnosis. Several methods are available for the detection of antibodies to *Toxoplasma*: indirect fluorescence, haemagglutination, cytoplasm-modifying, latex agglutination and complement fixation. Of these several tests, those recommended are the Jacobs, Cook and Wilder (1954) modification of the Sabin-Feldman cytoplasm-modifying antibody reaction and the indirect fluorescent antibody technique (Fletcher, 1965).

The Sabin-Feldman test presents difficulties because of the reagents involved and hence is available only at specialized laboratories. However, it is very sensitive, capable of demonstrating significant antibody titres within

two weeks of primary infection. Considerable titres occur among the general population, increasing with age from negative in the newborn (positives in neonates indicate maternal antibody) to 256 in adults: this titre is accepted as the normal limit. The indirect fluorescent antibody test is more easily performed than is the Sabin-Feldman. Results are parallel to those found with the Sabin-Feldman test. With both tests, only rising titres are indicative of current infection, so that two samples of serum should be tested, one original and the other taken two or more weeks later.

Sarcocystis lindemanni

Diagnosis. Biopsy material is sectioned and stained with haematoxylin and eosin. Sarcocysts are fusiform bodies, up to 2 mm in length, lying between the muscle layers. They contain hundreds of round or crescentic zoites which measure some 12 μm in length. They are, therefore, larger than *Toxoplasma* zoites from which they must be differentiated. The sarcocyst is divided up internally by trabeculae.

Pneumocystis carinii

Diagnosis. Lung material, smear or section is stained with haematoxylin and eosin and examination is made for the 10–12 μm diameter cyst-like bodies, containing up to 8 'spores'. Related to interstitial pneumonia in subjects of reduced immunological competence.

Naegleria

Diagnosis. Cerebrospinal fluid from meningitis cases, suspected of containing this amoeba because of the absence of bacteria, is examined direct without centrifugation (Carter, 1972) for this species of amoeba, which has only a single nucleus with a large karyosome, and no other inclusions. Sluggishly motile, short, with irregularly shaped pseudopodia, these organisms can be seen with the transmitted light microscope but are best demonstrated by phase contrast. The organisms are best cultured on non-nutrient agar, previously inoculated with *Aerobacter aerogenes*.

Babesia

These organisms produce disease in animals but are exceedingly rarely found in man, and then usually in subjects who have lost their spleens. They invade red blood cells. Demonstration of the parasite is by blood films prepared and stained as described for the diagnosis of malaria. The parasites are intraerythrocytic pyriform structures measuring 2–4 μm in length with a well-defined nucleus.

REFERENCES

CARTER, R. C. (1972) Primary amoebic meningo-encephalitis. *Transactions of the Royal Society of Tropical Medicine and Hygiene*, **66**, 193.

FLETCHER, S. (1965) Indirect fluorescent antibody technique in the serology of *Toxoplasma gondii*. *Journal of Clinical Pathology*, **18**, 193–199.

GUERREIRO, C. & MACHADO, A. (1913) Da reaccao de Brodet e Gengou na molestia de Carlos Chagas como elemente diagnostico. *Brasil-Medico*, **27**, 225.

HOARE, C. A. (1972) *The Trypanosomes of Mammals.* Oxford: Blackwell Scientific Publications.

HONIGBERG, B. M., BALAMUTH, W., BOVEE, E. C., CORLISS, J. O., GOJDICS, M., HALL, R. P., KUDO, R. R., LEVINE, N. D., LOEBLICH, A. R., WEISER, J. & WENRICH, D. H. (1964) A revised classification of the phylum Protozoa. *Journal of Protozoology*, **11**, 7.

JACOBS, L., COOK, M. K. & WILDER, H. C. (1954) Serologic data on adults with histologically diagnosed toxoplasmic chorioretinitis. *Transactions of the American Academy of Ophthalmics*, **58**, 193.

JEANES, A. L. (1969) Evaluation in clinical practice of the fluorescent amoebic antibody test. *Journal of Clinical Pathology*, **22**, 427.

LANHAM, S. M. (1968) The separation of trypanosomes from blood cells and their behaviour on TEAE- and DEAE-cellulose and on DEAE-Sephadex. *Transactions of the Royal Society of Tropical Medicine and Hygiene*, **62**, 129.

LUMSDEN, W. H. R. (1973) Demonstration of antibodies to Protozoa. In: Weir, D. M. (3rd edn.) *Immunological Methods*. Oxford: Blackwell Scientific Publications.

LUMSDEN, W. H. R., HERBERT, W. J. & McNEILLAGE, G. J. C. (1973) Techniques with trypanosomes. Edinburgh, U.K.: Churchill Livingstone.

MANCINI, G., CARBONARA, A. O. & HEREMANS, J. F. (1965) Immunochemical quantitation of antigens by single radial immunodiffusion. *Immunochemistry*, **2**, 235.

MATTERN, P., KLEIN, F., RADEMA, H. & FURTH, R. VAN (1967) Les γ-macroglobulines reactionnelles et paraproteiniques dans le serum et dans le liquide cephalorachidien humain. *Annales de l'Institut Pasteur*, **113**, 857.

MONSUR, K. A. (1956) Alcoholic extracts of Kedrowsky's bacillus as antigen for complement-fixation tests in kala-azar. *Transactions of the Royal Society of Tropical Medicine and Hygiene*, **50**, 91.

NAPIER, L. E. (1921) A new serum test for kala-azar. *Indian Medical Gazette*, **56**, 238.

RIDLEY, D. S. & HAWGOOD, B. C. (1956) The value of formol-ether concentration. *Journal of Clinical Pathology*, **9**, 74.

ROBERTSON, D. H. H., LUMSDEN, W. H. R., FRASER, K. F., HOSIE, D. M. & MOORE, D. M. (1969) Simultaneous isolation of *Trichomonas vaginalis* and collection of vaginal exudate. *British Journal of Venereal Diseases*, **45**, 42.

ROBINSON, G. L. (1968) The laboratory diagnosis of human parasitic amoebae. *Transactions of the Royal Society of Tropical Medicine and Hygiene*, **62**, 285.

ROBINSON, G. L. (1972) The preparation of amoebic extracts and their testing by complement fixation against clinically proved sera. *Transactions of the Royal Society of Tropical Medicine and Hygiene*, **66**, 435.

SHUTE, P. G. & MARYON, M. (1960) *Laboratory Techniques for the Study of Malaria*. London: J. and A. Churchill.

VAN FURTH, R., COHN, Z. A., HIRSCH, J. G., HUMPHREY, J. H., SPECTOR, W. G. & LANGEWOORT, H. L. (1972) The mononuclear phagocyte system: a new classification of macrophages, monocytes, and their precursor cells. *Bulletin of the World Health Organization*, **46**, 845.

W.H.O. REPORT (1967) *Joint FAO/WHO Expert Committee on Zoonoses. Third Report.* Technical Report Series No. 378. Geneva: World Health Organization.

46. Deoxyriboviruses

In this and the following chapter the properties of the DNA and RNA viruses are briefly listed. The full description of each of the main groups of viruses will be found in Volume I, Chapters 40–49, together with the more important aspects of their epidemiology. The details of the techniques of cultivation and identification of viruses are set out in Chapters 10 and 11, Volume II.

The deoxyviruses include the following groups which now have the approved names of:

1. Poxvirus
2. Herpesvirus
3. Adenovirus
4. Papillomavirus ⎫
5. Polyomavirus ⎬ Papovaviridiae
　　　　　　　　 ⎭
6. Parvovirus
7. Bacterial viruses (e.g. T-even phages)
8. Plant viruses (e.g. Iridovirus group that infects turnips).

Because they are the important pathogens of man the first six are described. The reader interested in groups 6–7 should see Chapter 13, Volume I and for group 8 is referred to Chapter 2 and to Wildy (1971) and Andrewes and Pereira (1972). The polyomaviruses (5) are referred to in Chapter 49.

Poxviruses

The type species is the vaccinia virus and although much dispute continues about its origin it may well derive from the patients that Edward Jenner cared for in the late eighteenth century.

The vaccinia virus contains 5 to 7·5 per cent of double-stranded DNA. Its virions are brick-shaped or ovoid (170–250 × 300–325 nm). The particle is covered by several layers with characteristic surface patterns; as a result a strikingly characteristic appearance is offered under the electron microscope.

All poxviruses share a common nucleo-protein antigen and most contain polymerases, e.g. RNA polymerase; all poxviruses have the capacity for non-genetic reactivation.

Five subgroups of poxviruses have multiple antigens which can combine genetically; subgroups A and B are of special interest in human medicine.

Subgenus A: Smallpox　Alastrim　(variola minor)
　　　　　　 Smallpox
　　　　　　 Cowpox
　　　　　　 Vaccinia
　　　　　　 Infectious ectromelia of mice
　　　　　　 Monkey pox
　　　　　　 Rabbit pox

Subgenus B: Orf
　　　　　　 Milker's nodes
　　　　　　 Bovine papular dermatitis
　　　　　　 Chamois contagious ecthyma

Subgenus C: Goat pox
　　　　　　 Lumpyskin disease
　　　　　　 Sheeppox

Subgenus D: Avianpox diseases
　　　　　　 Canary pox
　　　　　　 Fowl pox
　　　　　　 Pigeon pox
　　　　　　 Turkey pox
　　　　　　 Sparrow pox
　　　　　　 Starling pox
　　　　　　 Junco pox

Subgenus E: Myxomavirus (California) ⎫
　　　　　　 Hare fibroma　　　　　　 ⎪
　　　　　　 Rabbit fibroma　　　　　 ⎪
　　　　　　 Squirrel fibroma　　　　 ⎬ Poxviruses
　　　　　　 Buffalo　　　　　　　　 ⎪
　　　　　　 Camel　　　　　　　　　 ⎪
　　　　　　 Horse　　　　　　　　　 ⎭
　　　　　　 Molluscum　　　　　　　 ⎫
　　　　　　 　contagiosum　　　　　 ⎪
　　　　　　 Swine pox　　　　　　　 ⎬ Viruses
　　　　　　 Tana pox　　　　　　　　⎪
　　　　　　 Yaba monkey　　　　　　 ⎪
　　　　　　 　tumour　　　　　　　　⎭
　　　　　　 Rhinoceros pox

Herpesviruses

The type species is the *Herpesvirus hominis* virus of which there are two distinct serotypes,

1 and 2 (Volume I, Chapter 41). These viruses are relatively large ether-sensitive particles and are covered with a membrane and a protein capsid composed of 162 capsomeres. The nucleic acid core is composed of double-stranded DNA. Characteristically, the herpesviruses replicate within the host cell nucleus where their special quality is that they produce eosinophilic inclusion bodies.

Herpesvirus subgroups are not easy to separate because, in many instances, the virions are intimately united with the component structures of their host cells.

The subgroups include:

(a) Varicella virus
Pseudorabies virus (Aukeszky's disease)
Equine rhinotracheitis viruses
Malignant catarrh virus of cattle
Bovine, canine and feline herpesviruses
Virus III of rabbits.

(b) Herpesvirus simiae (Virus B)
Herpesviruses of monkeys and rabbits
Pulmonary adenomatosis (Jagziegte) of sheep

(c) Epstein-Barr virus (infectious mononucleosis and Burkitt lymphoma)

(d) Herpesviruses of Marek's disease together with many other avian, porcine, frog and reptilian viruses.

Adenoviruses

The type species is Adenovirus type I.

The virus contains in its core double-stranded DNA of a molecular weight of 20 to 25 million daltons. This is covered by a capsid of protein composed of 252 capsomeres disposed in icosahedral symmetry (Volume I, Chapter 12). A common complement-fixing antigen is shared by all mammalian strains. These viruses are ether-resistant and some haemagglutinate the cells of various species.

Human adenoviruses are separated into at least 31 serotypes, which can be placed in three groups according to their patterns of haemagglutination or failure to haemagglutinate. Some human serotypes multiply more readily in monkey cell cultures when there is a concomitant infection with the helper virus of monkeys, SV46. There is a considerable tendency for the adenoviruses to share part of their genomes with the SV (Simian viruses).

Many hybrids of unknown pathogenic qualities may be produced.

Adenoviruses are disseminated universally throughout the animal kingdom. They play an important role in the spread of infection by airborne routes; they also have an affinity for lymph nodes where, after an interval, they may cause local enlargement and swelling that can cause obstruction to major channels in the bronchial tree, in the greater blood vessels, and in the bowels due to mesenteric adenitis. Many are excreted in the faeces.

Other adenoviruses include:

Avian adenoviruses, bovine adenoviruses, canine adenoviruses (e.g. canine infectious hepatitis virus), murine adenoviruses, simian adenoviruses (e.g., SA7), mammalian adenoviruses (e.g. those of sheep, horses, opossum and pigs).

Papovaviridiae

These viruses are recognised as having the status of a family. The type species is the papillomavirus that causes proliferative lesions of skin epithelium but the lesions are almost always innocent. The first papillomavirus described by Shope in 1933 in rabbits still bears his name in general parlance. (Another papilloma of rabbits due to the oral papilloma was described a few years later.) In 1967 came one of the first descriptions of the infectious wart virus in man (*Verruca vulgaris, Myremecia*).

These viruses contain a core of double-stranded DNA within an icosahedral capsid which is probably composed of 72 capsomeres in a skew arrangement. The virions are 52–54 nm in diameter and are stable in the presence of ether, acid and mild heat. All attempts to cultivate human papillomaviruses have completely failed. Serological techniques, however, with viral extracts from human warts as antigens, yield useful information about the immune status of the patient (Cubie, 1972).

Another genus in this family is the polyomavirus which is able to produce in mice and other rodents inoculated experimentally, a multiplicity of tumours in many of their tissues (e.g. the parotid gland). This virus has such interesting biological properties, especially its ability to agglutinate erythrocytes, that it has become a most useful model for the study of the evolution of malignant disease (Andrewes and Pereira, 1972).

Parvoviruses

This group is so-called because its members are all very small with diameters of 18–22 nm. Their shell is a capsid of probably 32 capsomeres. About 34 per cent of the wright of the virion is made up of single-stranded DNA. At one time they were known as *picodna* viruses, but this name has now been abandoned. Parvoviruses are usually propagated in growing cells, e,g. kidney cells, of their own particular host species.

There are two main subgroups of parvoviruses:

Subgroup A: Latent rat virus (type species)
Minute mouse virus
Porcine virus

Subgroup B: Adeno-associated virus types 1, 2–3 and 4 (see Volume I, Chapter 42).

None of the foregoing possesses pathogenicity for man. Some parvoviruses that possibly belong to these groups are feline panleukaemia viruses and the avian and bovine parvoviruses.

REFERENCES

ANDREWES, C. H. & PEREIRA, H. G. (1972). *Viruses of Vertebrates*. London. Ballière Tindall.

CUBIE, H. A. (1972). Serological studies in a student population prone to infection with human pipilloma virus. *Journal of Hygiene (Cambridge)*, **70,** 677.

WILDY, P. (1971). Classification and nomenclature of viruses. *Monographs in Virology*, Vol. 5. Basel, München, Paris and London: S. Karger.

47. Riboviruses

Of the RNA viruses the myxoviruses are ubiquitous and receive their name from their great affinity for mucus. They are divided into two groups—the orthomyxoviruses and para-myxoviruses. Their general properties are described in Volume I, Chapter 44, and the methods used for their propagation and cultivation in Chapters 9 and 10 of this volume.

Orthomyxoviruses

This group is especially associated with epidemic and endemic influenza. The remarkable plasticity and characteristic genetic variability of orthomyxoviruses distinguish them from all the other viruses; thereby they possess great epidemic potentiality.

They contain about 1·0 per cent of single-stranded RNA in probably six pieces, which gives them a helical symmetry. The virion itself is enveloped by a host-cell-derived membrane and the virion is 90–120 nm in diameter. The nucleocapsid within the membrane is composed of a coiled filament of RNA to which *wedge-shaped protein-subunits (five to six) are attached at each turn.* The diameter of this coiled filament is about 18 nm.

Orthomyxoviruses contain lipid and carbohydrate, are ether-sensitive, heat-labile, acid-labile and sensitive to actinomycin-D. Stability is maximal at pH 7·0–8·0. Antigenic variation is frequent. There are three separate and distinct antigenic types A, B and C, distinguishable by *specific* ribonucleoproteins that do not cross-react with each other's antisera.

All the orthomyxoviruses are able to cause haemagglutination of the erythrocytes of various species (see Volume I, Chapter 12).

The various orthomyxoviruses are:

Type A—human influenza viruses, e.g. A0/PR8 34, A1/CAM 46, A2/Singapore 57; porcine influenza virus, e.g. A/Swine/1976/30; equine influenza viruses, e.g. A/Equi–2/Miami/1–63; avian influenza viruses, e.g. fowl plague viruses

Type B—e.g. B/Les/40

Type C—e.g. C/Taylor/47.

Paramyxoviruses

This group has many of the essential qualities of orthomyxoviruses. Individual species vary greatly in their shape and size. Diameters of the enveloped virions are between 100 and 200 nm and they are easily deformed into bizarre forms, some of which may be as long as 600 nm and form sausage-like particles. They contain about 1 per cent RNA. The type species is the Newcastle disease virus, one of the viruses that causes epizootic fowl plague. The virions are about 150 nm in diameter and are enveloped. The capsid is helical and is about 18 nm in diameter and about 1·0 nm thick. These viruses agglutinate and lyse chicken, guinea-pig and human red blood cells and are ether-sensitive; most develop in the cytoplasm and are resistant to actinomycin D. They are antigenically *stable*; genetic recombination does not occur.

The other paramyxoviruses are:

Mumps virus

Parainfluenza virus 1 (Human HA, Sendai, Murine)

Parainfluenza virus 2 (Human CA, SV5, Avian)

Parainfluenza virus 3 (Human HA1, Bovine SF4)

Parainfluenza virus 4

Other possible paramyxoviruses—

Measles virus ⎱
Canine distemper virus ⎰ This triad share antigens in varying proportions
Rinderpest virus ⎰

Pneumonia virus of mice

Respiratory syncytial virus

Rhabdoviruses

These viruses are bullet-shaped and are 130–220 nm long and 60–80 nm wide. They contain about 2 per cent single-stranded RNA and are enclosed by an envelope studded with 10 nm spikes. The symmetry is helical. The virions are sensitive to ether and to acid. Some members haemagglutinate and some of them multiply in arthropods though vertebrates form the principal reservoirs of infection.

The type species is the vesicular stomatitis virus which can *simulate* foot and mouth disease in cattle, horses or sheep.

Subtypes exist—(1) Cocal (Argentinian)
(2) A Brazilian isolate
(3) Indiana C strain.

The important human pathogen of this group is the rabies virus (Volume I, Chapter 48). In addition to it some indigenous viruses carried by bats belong to the group as do many from different plant hosts and some from trout. The monkey (Marburg) virus may also belong to the group.

Togaviridiae

This is a family name for two genera:
Alphavirus (Arbovirus group A)
Flavivirus (Arbovirus group B)
All these viruses are transmitted by arthropods and on account of antigenic sharing are now separated into these two major groups:

1. *Alphaviruses* belong to group A of the arboviruses because they were separated into this group by immunological tests. The virions contain 4–6 per cent single-stranded RNA and are spherical enveloped particles. They contain lipid and are ether-sensitive, but resist the action of trypsin. They haemagglutinate erythrocytes of various species (goose red cells are very sensitive). They multiply in the cytoplasm of their host cells and mature by a process of budding. All the members of the alphaviruses are able to multiply in their arthropod vectors: it is noteworthy that all show serological cross-reactions in haemagglutination inhibition reactions.

The type species is the Sindbis virus (see Chapter 47).

Other members of this genus include:
Chikunguna virus, Middlesburgh virus, O'Nyong-nyong virus, Semlike Forest virus, Venezuelan equine encephalitis virus, Eastern equine encephalomyelitis virus, Western equine encephalomyelitis virus.

Note that there is a considerable number of viruses from various geographical situations which on antigenic grounds belong in this genus.

2. *Flavoviruses* (Arboviruses group B). These viruses have all the general properties of the alphaviruses. They are, however, related to each other by shared antigenic qualities.

The more important viruses of this genus are:
(a) The four serotypes of the dengue viruses
(b) The louping ill virus
The Kyasamur Forest virus
Omsk haemorrhagic fever virus
(c) Japanese encephalitis virus
(d) Powassan virus
(e) St Louis encephalitis virus
(f) West Nile virus.

There are a great many other viruses in this group, each of which is specially related to a particular geographical locality (Andrewes and Pereira, 1972).

Arenaviruses

These are RNA viruses about 100 nm in diameter. Their name comes from a number of electron-dense granules which gives a sandy appearance. They are sensitive to lipid solvents. The viruses grow in the host cell cytoplasm by budding through the cell membrane. All the arenaviruses cross-react antigenically.

The type species is the lymphocytic choriomeningitis virus, which causes an acute benign meningitis in man. It is carried as a commensal in strains of wild and laboratory mice.

The virion seems to contain RNA and to be about 85–95 nm in diameter. It is ether-sensitive, grows in the host cell cytoplasm and matures by a process of budding from the cell membrane. All the strains share a group-specific antigen which can be demonstrated by immunofluorescence. Other members of the arenaviruses include a series of viruses among which are the Tacaribe virus and many others, probably insect-borne natives of South America.

Reoviruses

The interest of groups of viruses lies more in their physical characters than in their pathogenicity.

They have an isometric capsid with icosahedral symmetry. Usually they are naked. They contain 10–20 per cent of double-stranded RNA in several pieces. The diameter of the capsid, which is double-layered, is 75–80 nm and resists lipid solvents. Virus maturation occurs in the host cell cytoplasm with the formation of crystalline arrays of virions symmetrically arranged to form characteristic inclusions.

Reoviruses have the ability to cause minor intestinal or occasionally respiratory illness but they lack the power to originate any epidemiological episodes.

Picornaviridiae

These small riboviruses are the cause of much illness, major or trivial, in man and in animals. They are ubiquitous and their incidence varies from time to time, in many countries and in many climates. The polioviruses (Volume I, Chapter 45) are the most important of them all, but since the use of live poliovaccines their epidemiological patterns and power to cause paralysis have been controlled in many countries. The separation of wild from vaccine strains has become a difficult task suitable only for the specialized virus laboratory (see Chapter 45). The *enteroviruses* are the type species and form a group that contains the 3 polioviruses, the 24 Coxsackie viruses and the 34 echoviruses (see Chapter 45). Other members of the group which infect animals (but not man) include porcine, bovine and a variety of avian species (Wildy, 1971).

The picornaviridiae contain in the cores of their virions about 20–30 per cent of single-stranded RNA which has a molecular weight of about 2·5 million daltons. They have an icosahedral symmetry and measure 20–30 nm in diameter. They are naked, acid-stable and ether-resistant. Primarily these viruses inhabit the intestine. Some strains of the echo- and coxsackie viruses have the ability to haemagglutinate and are potential pathogens of the respiratory tract.

Calciviruses belong to the picornaviridiae. They are the cause of vesicular exanthema of pigs and epidemic respiratory disease of catteries. They do not appear to have human pathogenicity.

Rhinoviruses

These viruses are the most common cause of the human common cold. There are some 90 human strains and a smaller number of equine and bovine strains. The rhinoviruses contain 30 per cent of RNA with a molecular weight of 2·4–2·8 million daltons. They have naked particles, probably with icosahedral symmetry and measure 20–30 nm in diameter. They are acid-labile, and are ether-stable. They have a low ceiling temperature of growth and multiply within the host cell cytoplasm. Of course, their primary habitat is the human respiratory tract.

Included taxonomically in rhinoviruses are the O, A, C, SAT, 23 and Asia serotypes of the foot and mouth disease viruses.

Leukoviruses

These are RNA viruses that belong to four groups, many are oncogenic:
  (1) The avian leucosis-sarcoma complex
  (2) The avian reticulosis-endotheliosis viruses
  (3) The viruses causing leukosis and those of some sarcomata of felines
  (4) The viruses of the mammary tumours of mice.

The type species is the Rous sarcoma virus (RSV). These viruses contain single-stranded RNA of a molecular weight of about 10–12 million daltons. They are heat-labile, ether-sensitive and sensitive to actinomycin D. There is sharing of antigens in groups 1 and 2.

Coronaviruses

These viruses owe their name to the petal-like protrusions some 20 nm long that form a characteristic fringe on the surface of the roughly spherical virions and confer the appearance of a crown from which the generic name is obtained.

Coronaviruses contain RNA but their *strandedness* and their molecular weight is not yet certainly determined. These viruses grow in the cytoplasm of their host cells and they mature by budding into cytoplasmic vesicles. Antigenically, they are heterogeneous, but there is a relationship between some of the human and murine strains. They are *labile* below pH 3.

Coronaviruses have pathogenic qualities for four (perhaps more) mammalian species:

1. Human coronaviruses of a considerable number of serotypes cause common colds and acute respiratory illness.

2. Murine coronaviruses by themselves are harmless to mice, but in the presence of *Eperythrazoon coccoides* (which is also harmless) they cause hepatitis.

3. Porcine coronaviruses cause a highly fatal transmissible disease of young pigs which takes the form of gastroenteritis.

4. A number of other coronaviruses have been described in association with feline infectious peritonitis; other possible members of the group are avian pneumotropic viruses and one virus isolate from horses.

REFERENCES

ANDREWES, C. H. & PEREIRA, H. G. (1972). Viruses of Vertebraes. London: Ballière Tindall.

WILDY, P. (1971). Classification and nomenclature of viruses. *Monographs in Virology*, Vol. 5. Basel, München, Paris and London: S. Karger.

Index

Index

Filmset by Typesetting Services Ltd., Glasgow
Printed by T. and A. Constable Ltd., Edinburgh